**Clinical Atlas of Small Animal Cytology
and Hematology**

Clinical Atlas of Small Animal Cytology and Hematology

Second Edition

Andrew G. Burton, BVSc, DACVP
Clinical Pathologist
IDEXX Laboratories, Inc.
North Grafton, Massachusetts, USA

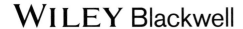

Published by John Wiley & Sons, Inc., Hoboken, New Jersey.
Published simultaneously in Canada.

For general information on our other products and services or for technical support, please contact our Customer Care Department within the United States at (800) 762-2974, outside the United States at (317) 572-3993 or fax (317) 572-4002.

Wiley also publishes its books in a variety of electronic formats. Some content that appears in print may not be available in electronic formats. For more information about Wiley products, visit our web site at www.wiley.com.

Library of Congress Cataloging-in-Publication Data

Names: Burton, Andrew G., author.
Title: Clinical atlas of small animal cytology and hematology / Andrew G.
   Burton.
Description: Second edition. | Hoboken: Wiley, 2024. | Includes
   bibliographical references and index.
Identifiers: LCCN 2023043778 (print) | LCCN 2023043779 (ebook) | ISBN
   9781119985624 (hardback) | ISBN 9781119985631 (adobe pdf) | ISBN
   9781119985648 (epub)
Classification: LCC QH582 (print) | LCC QH582 (ebook) | DDC
   571.6–dc23/eng/20231027
LC record available at https://lccn.loc.gov/2023043778
LC ebook record available at https://lccn.loc.gov/2023043779

Cover Design: Wiley
Cover Images: Courtesy of Andrew G. Burton

Set in 9.5/12.5pt STIXTwoText by Straive, Pondicherry, India

SMI10065013_011824

Dedication

To the veterinarians, technicians, and veterinary professionals who dedicate so much of themselves to the care, health, and well-being of animals. Your passion and sacrifices are seen, and so deeply appreciated.

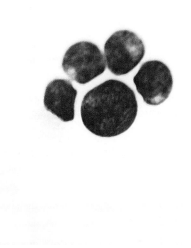

Contents

Preface *xi*
Acknowledgments *xiii*

1 Cytology Sampling and Preparation *1*
1.1 Cytology *1*
1.2 Sample Collection and Preparation *1*
1.3 Sample Staining *7*
1.4 Sample Handling and Storage *8*
References *9*

2 Cytologic Analysis of Cells *11*
2.1 Approach to Cytology Samples *11*
2.2 Sample Quality and Background *11*
2.3 Cell Types *15*
2.4 Cell Shape, Distribution, and Features *29*
2.5 Benign Versus Malignant *30*
References *43*

3 Infectious Agents *45*
3.1 Fungi *45*
3.2 Oomycetes *56*
3.3 Algae *56*
3.4 Mesomycetozoea *58*
3.5 Protozoa *58*
3.6 Helminths *65*
3.7 Bacteria *69*
3.8 Ectoparasites *75*
References *78*

4 Integument *85*
4.1 Cutaneous and Subcutaneous Lesions *85*
References *133*

5 Hemolymphatic *139*
5.1 Lymph Nodes *139*
5.2 Spleen *153*
5.3 Thymus *167*
5.4 Bone Marrow *170*
References *188*

6   Body Cavity Fluids   *193*
6.1   General Classification   *193*
6.2   Specific Effusions   *197*
         References   *208*

7   Musculoskeletal   *211*
7.1   Bone   *211*
7.2   Joints   *219*
7.3   Muscle   *226*
         References   *230*

8   Hepatobiliary   *235*
8.1   Liver   *235*
8.2   Biliary Tract   *250*
         References   *252*

9   Digestive System   *255*
9.1   Salivary Glands   *255*
9.2   Stomach/Intestines   *258*
9.3   Feces   *267*
9.4   Pancreas   *272*
         References   *279*

10   Urinary   *285*
10.1   Kidney   *285*
10.2   Bladder   *291*
10.3   Urine   *294*
10.4   Urinary Crystals   *298*
10.5   Urinary Casts   *303*
         References   *307*

11   Respiratory   *311*
11.1   Nasal Cavity   *311*
11.2   Lung   *317*
11.3   Bronchoalveolar Lavage/Transtracheal Wash   *320*
         References   *328*

12   Endocrine   *331*
12.1   Thyroid   *331*
12.2   Parathyroid   *335*
12.3   Chemoreceptor Tumors   *336*
12.4   Adrenal Gland   *338*
12.5   Pituitary Gland   *340*
         References   *342*

13   Reproductive   *345*
         Male   *345*
13.1   Testes   *345*
13.2   Semen Analysis   *350*
13.3   Prostate   *350*
13.4   Penis   *358*

Female *358*
13.5   Ovary   *358*
13.6   Mammary Glands   *361*
13.7   Vaginal Cytology   *366*
        References   *375*

14   **Neurologic**   *379*
14.1   Brain   *379*
14.2   Cerebrospinal Fluid   *386*
14.3   Spinal Cord   *400*
        References   *402*

15   **Ocular and Special Senses**   *405*
15.1   Eyes: Cornea   *405*
15.2   Eyes: Conjunctiva   *409*
15.3   Ears   *412*
        References   *417*

16   **Blood Smear Preparation and Evaluation**   *421*
16.1   The Importance of Blood Smear Evaluation   *421*
16.2   Making a Blood Smear   *421*
16.3   Blood Smear Staining and Handling   *425*
16.4   Blood Smear Evaluation   *427*
16.5   Hematology Procedures and Techniques   *430*
        References   *432*

17   **Erythrocytes**   *433*
17.1   Approach to Evaluating Red Blood Cells   *433*
17.2   Red Blood Cell Distribution   *433*
17.3   Red Blood Cell Morphology   *438*
17.4   Red Blood Cell Inclusions   *456*
17.5   Red Blood Cell Neoplasia   *461*
17.6   Red Blood Cell Infectious Agents   *462*
        References   *468*

18   **Leukocytes**   *475*
18.1   Approach to Evaluating Leukocytes   *475*
18.2   Neutrophils   *476*
18.3   Neutrophil Inclusions   *484*
18.4   Eosinophils   *488*
18.5   Basophils   *489*
18.6   Mast Cells   *491*
18.7   Monocytes   *492*
18.8   Lymphocytes   *495*
18.9   Leukocyte Neoplasia   *498*
18.10   Leukocyte Infectious Agents   *504*
        References   *509*

19   **Platelets**   *515*
19.1   Approach to Evaluating Platelets   *515*
19.2   Platelet Distribution   *515*

19.3   Platelet Morphology   *518*
19.4   Platelet Neoplasia   *522*
19.5   Platelet Infectious Agents   *524*
        References   *525*

20   Background Features and Miscellaneous Cells   *527*
20.1   Approach to Blood Smear Background Features   *527*
20.2   Acellular Elements   *527*
20.3   Miscellaneous Cells   *528*
20.4   Infectious Agents   *533*
        References   *536*

        Index   *537*

Preface

The *Clinical Atlas of Small Animal Cytology and Hematology* returns, with brand new hematology chapters and fully updated cytology sections. More comprehensive than ever, the mission of this textbook remains unchanged: to empower veterinary medical professionals with increased knowledge and confidence in cytology and hematology through exceptional images, a guided approach to interpretation, and succinct yet thorough supporting text.

Images form the keystone of this atlas, and this extensive collection is unparalleled for the size, clarity, completeness, and representative nature of the photomicrographs. The images have been carefully curated to mimic the experience of microscopy and highlight the important diagnostic features that lead to the confident interpretation of samples. The power of these uniquely large images is perhaps best highlighted in the new hematology chapters, where they readily showcase the frequently small cells, infectious agents, and inclusions present in the blood.

Multiple examples of common conditions are provided to highlight the exciting (though often challenging) variations that may be encountered in practice. Additionally, images of different cells that may be confused with each other have been thoughtfully arranged for easy side-by-side comparison. Photomicrographs are accompanied by detailed descriptions, figure legends and annotated with arrows when needed to guide readers through the diagnostic process and ensure all important elements of samples are appreciated. Chapter 2 provides a guided approach to the interpretation of cytology samples, including cell types, criteria of malignancy, and common artifacts. This atlas contains only images of conditions where the diagnosis was confirmed by histopathology, special stains, infectious disease testing, pathognomonic cytologic features, or other confirmatory tests. All samples are stained with Romanowsky stains unless otherwise specified.

An in-depth hematology section is an exciting new addition to this textbook. Chapter 16 provides detailed instructions to prepare and stain high-quality blood smears, and a step-by-step guide that can be used at the microscope for a complete evaluation of the smear. Common hematology procedures are also described, with easy-to-follow instructions. Subsequent chapters in the hematology section provide a comprehensive catalog of cells, inclusions, infectious agents, and other components seen in blood, both common and rare, accompanied by interpretive guides, helpful hints, and fully referenced text.

The cytology chapters have been fully revised, and all contain new conditions and images. A new chapter detailing sample acquisition, preparation, and staining opens the textbook to help ensure the creation of the highest quality samples – important for viewing in-house, with point-of-care analyzers, or submission to the laboratory. Our knowledge of the complex world of pathology is constantly changing, and this edition has been critically referenced with the most current, relevant, and scientifically robust studies to aide in optimal, evidence-based decision-making. This edition retains the popular easy-to-read bullet point format, which increases efficiency without compromising the completeness or scientific rigor of the information.

From practitioners to pathologists, trainees to technicians, and every professional that makes veterinary medicine great, may the *Clinical Atlas of Small Animal Cytology and Hematology* be a powerful resource to help in our collective endeavor for the best possible patient care.

Acknowledgments

My sincerest gratitude to Wiley Publishers and the incredible team that continues to believe in the vision and impact of this book.

Thank you to the veterinary community for your support. You inspire this textbook and my work as a pathologist.

I would like to acknowledge the unwavering and generous support of my colleagues – most notably Cathy Greene, Dr. Maria Vandis, Dr. Raquel Walton, Dr. Karl Jandrey, and Dr. Bill Vernau.

And with all my heart, thank you to my family, especially Dr. Eric Franson – your love is the fuel for it all.

1

Cytology Sampling and Preparation

1.1 Cytology

Cytology is a useful, rapid, noninvasive, and safe diagnostic procedure with often strong correlation to histopathology, including high specificity for the diagnosis of neoplasia in cutaneous and subcutaneous masses [1, 2], lymph nodes [3], and oral tumors [4] in dogs and cats as well as bacterial infection in fluid samples [5]. Importantly, the quality of the sample, especially cellularity, has a significant effect on the interpretation and accuracy of results [6, 7].

Quality of cytology samples depends on four major factors:

1) Sample collection.
2) Slide preparation.
3) Staining.
4) Sample handling.

The ideal sample is adequately cellular, distributed in a monolayer, free of artifacts or contaminants, and is well stained. Point-of-care options for cytology have increased dramatically in recent years, further necessitating the need for clinics to be confident and proficient in the preparation and staining of high-quality cytology samples. This chapter provides a detailed description of how to collect, prepare, stain, and handle cytology samples. Following these steps will increase the chance of creating excellent quality cytology samples that maximize accurate interpretation, which is described in Chapter 2.

1.2 Sample Collection and Preparation

1.2.1 Selecting Lesions for Cytology

Not all masses or lesions are amenable to cytologic evaluation, and thoughtful selection of suitable lesions for cytology is an important component of obtaining diagnostic samples. Highly vascular lesions may yield only blood, while some mesenchymal lesions exfoliate cells poorly for cytology. It is also important to be mindful of the limitations of cytology. Only a small portion of the lesion or organ of interest is sampled, and the limited number of cells available may not represent the underlying pathologic process. Additionally, cytology cannot evaluate tissue architecture such as tissue or vessel invasion, sometimes limiting the evaluation of biologic behavior, which does not always correlate with cytomorphology. Specificity is usually higher than sensitivity when comparing cytologic and histopathologic interpretations, which is often directly related to the aforementioned limitations of reviewing only a small number of cells from a focal area of a lesion or an organ [2]. Agreement between cytology and histopathology can also be low due to limitations of focal sampling and lack of tissue architecture; particularly relevant when evaluating lymph nodes for metastatic disease [3, 8].

1.2.2 Preparing the Site

Special preparation of the site (e.g., clipping of surrounding fur or sterile preparation of the skin) is not required for most lesions. If excessive surface debris, dirt, or gel (from topical medications or ultrasound procedures) is present, this may be cleaned with sterile saline or alcohol; however, ensure that the area is completely dry prior to sampling. For sampling of internal organs, the skin should be clipped and surgically prepared prior to the procedure.

1.2.3 Sampling Techniques and Slide Preparation

Cytology samples may be obtained by numerous techniques including needle collection, swabs, scrapes, impressions, and brushes, which can be tailored to the nature and accessibility of the lesion, organ, or region of interest. Needle and impression sampling are best performed in areas free of ulceration or tissue necrosis, and it may be helpful to sample from multiple areas, including the center

Clinical Atlas of Small Animal Cytology and Hematology, Second Edition. Andrew G. Burton.
© 2024 John Wiley & Sons, Inc. Published 2024 by John Wiley & Sons, Inc.

and edges of the lesions as well as deep and superficial regions to increase the probability of a diagnostic sample. If possible, multiple slides should be made to increase cell yield and the likelihood of diagnostic samples, and using different techniques to make multiple slides may be helpful. The following sections will describe common sampling techniques in more detail.

1.2.3.1 Needle Collection

Needle collection (with or without syringe aspiration) is the most common and usually the most effective technique to obtain diagnostic cytology samples, as it can collect cells from different areas and depths of the lesion. It is commonly used to sample cells from skin masses, lymph nodes, and internal organs.

Supplies Slides must be made immediately after sample collection to avoid clotting or drying of the aspirated material, so it is important to have all supplies ready prior to sampling. Supplies needed include the following:

- Latex or nitrile gloves.
- Glass microscope slides with a frosted edge.
- A pencil.
- Sterile needles (20, 22, or 25 gauge).
- Syringes (3, 6, or 12 ml).

Procedure

1) Select appropriate needle.

    Starting with a 22-gauge needle is recommended. In one study, there was no difference in cellularity when using 22- and 25-gauge needles; however, 25-gauge needles were associated with greater cellular trauma, while 22-gauge needles had greater blood contamination [9]. Importantly, there was no difference between the needle gauges in the ability to make a diagnosis. A 20-gauge needle may sometimes be appropriate (e.g., for some mesenchymal lesions, and bone lesions); however, blood contamination may be an issue.

2) Start with a non-aspiration technique.

    For most masses and lymph nodes, it is recommended to start by using just the needle. Stabilize the mass or lymph node as appropriate/possible with one hand and hold the hub of the needle in the dominant hand (Figure 1.1). Direct the needle into the mass and collect material using short, sharp movements, redirecting within the mass in multiple different planes without leaving the skin. Typically, 3–5 redirections are sufficient to collect adequate material. *Note*: Material may not be visible within the needle, even if an adequate sample has been collected. If blood is seen in the needle, stop the procedure immediately and make slides

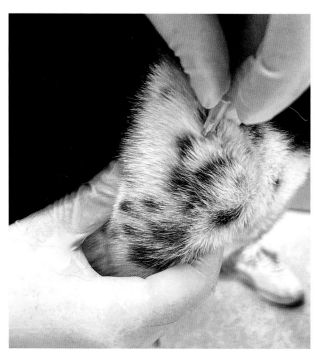

Figure 1.1 Non-aspiration needle collection technique. Note that the mass is stabilized in one hand, while the other hand directs the needle into the mass in short, sharp movements through different planes without leaving the skin. Courtesy of Dr. Eric Franson.

with that sample. Resampling with a smaller needle gauge or less redirection of the needle should be attempted to obtain samples with no or minimal blood contamination.

3) Add aspiration if needed.

    If no material is retrieved, or cellularity is very low, applying negative pressure using a syringe attached to the needle during collection may increase cellular yield (Figure 1.2). This technique can increase blood contamination and may result in cell damage or rupture, especially if using large syringes or if excessive pressure is applied. In one study investigating lymph node aspiration, there was no difference in sample quality (including cellularity, blood contamination, and cell preservation) between aspiration and non-aspiration techniques [10]. *Note*: It is important that no aspiration or negative pressure is applied when removing the needle and syringe from the lesion, as this can disperse the sampled material irretrievably throughout the syringe.

Internal organs are sampled using needle collection and is ideally performed with ultrasound guidance. Longer spinal needles are usually required to reach the organ of interest. For highly vascular organs, including the spleen and liver, the needle-only technique may be helpful.

Fluid-filled lesions are also best sampled with a needle aspiration technique. The aspirated fluid can be used to make slides, and any additional fluid can be stored in EDTA tubes to make additional slides at a later time, or in plain tubes for microbial culture and susceptibility testing if desired. When fluid is drained from some lesions, a solid component of the mass may become apparent, and sampling of this region can be fruitful to further evaluate the mass or underlying process that may be causing the fluid accumulation.

Slide Preparation It is important that slides be made immediately after collection of material, as any delay risks clotting or coagulation of the sample or desiccation of cells.

1) Lay multiple, clean slides on a solid, flat surface and label those by writing patient details on the frosted edge of the slide with a pencil.
2) Attach an air-filled syringe (typically 6 or 12 ml) to the needle hub (this can be the same syringe if the aspiration technique was used).
3) Touch the needle to the glass slide near the frosted edge with the bevel facing downward (Figure 1.3). Touching the glass surface will help prevent material spraying over a large distance and trauma to the cells.
4) Depress the syringe with gentle force, using air pressure to expel a small amount of the contents from the needle hub. *Note*: Greater pressure can always be used to expel more material if needed, so start with gentle force. Repeat this step on multiple slides if enough material is present in the needle hub.

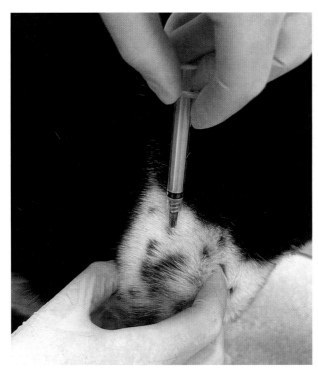

Figure 1.2 Aspiration needle collection technique. A syringe can be attached to the needle and used to apply negative pressure to help increase cellular yield in poorly exfoliating lesions. Courtesy of Dr. Eric Franson.

Conversely, for intra-abdominal lymph nodes, the aspiration technique has been shown to provide higher cellularity and was more likely to be diagnostic than non-aspiration techniques [11].

Figure 1.3 Transferring the sample to glass slides. Note that the bevel of the needle is facing downward and is touching the glass slide to ensure the sample remains in a focal area for optimal spreading.

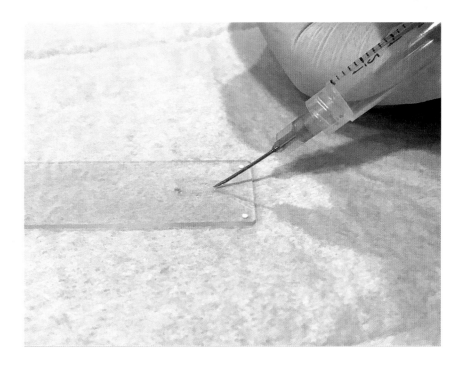

5) Rest a clean glass slide on top of the slide with the material (Figure 1.4). Using only the weight of the top slide, with no or minimal downward pressure, pull this along the lower slide to spread the material in a monolayer (Figure 1.5). *Note*: Do not use the needle to disperse the material on the slide. This often results in trauma to the cells and thick linear aggregates of material that are difficult to evaluate (Figure 1.6).

6) Air-dry the slides by blowing on them or using the cool setting on a hair dryer [12].

Slides should be left for an additional 1–2 minutes prior to staining to ensure they are completely dry. *Note*: Slides should *never* be heat fixed. Heat fixing does not improve cellular yield, including for bacteria and infectious agents, and may cause heat damage to cells [13, 14].

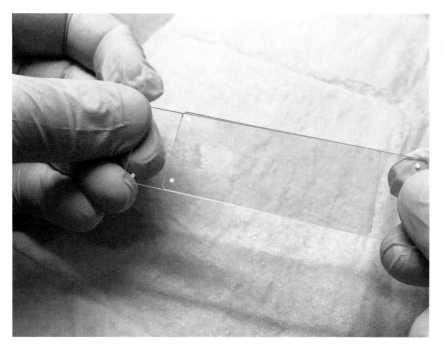

Figure 1.4 Spreading the sample. Rest a clean glass slide on top of the slide with the sample and allow the sample to spread.

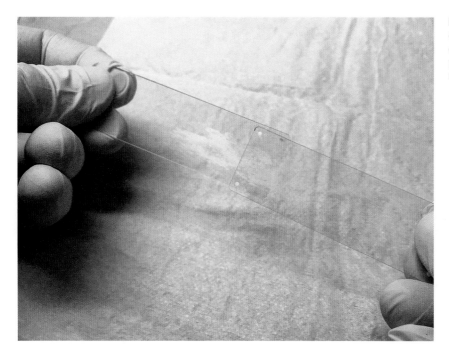

Figure 1.5 Spreading the sample. Use only the weight of the top slide, with no or minimal additional downward pressure to spread the sample in a monolayer across the slide.

Figure 1.6 An ideal cytology slide is present on the right, with a monolayer of cells. A needle was used to disperse the material on the slide on the left, which can rupture cells, and create linear areas that are too thick for cell evaluation.

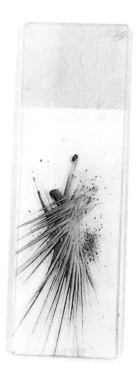
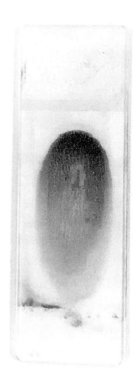

For fluid samples, a direct smear should always be made at the time of sampling, either using the technique described earlier or using a blood smear technique (see Chapter 16). This is essential to appreciate the cellularity and distribution of cells. Concentrated samples may also be created by spinning down the fluid in a centrifuge, removing two-thirds of the supernatant, and reconstituting the concentrated cell pellet within the remaining fluid and then making the slide as described. Squash preparations of any chunks of tissue or material may also be helpful to increase cellularity, especially for bronchoalveolar lavage (BAL) or transtracheal wash (TTW) samples.

1.2.3.2 Swab Sampling

Swabs are most commonly used for sampling from ears, vaginal cytology, and exuding lesions including fistulous tracts or nasal discharge.

Supplies Similar to needle aspirates, slides must be made immediately after sample collection to avoid drying of the aspirated material, so it is important to have all supplies ready prior to sampling. Supplies needed include the following:

- Latex or nitrile gloves.
- Glass microscope slides with a frosted edge.
- A pencil.
- Sterile cotton swab.
- ± Sterile water.

Procedure Introduce the cotton swab into the area of interest, being careful to avoid contamination with surrounding tissue (e.g., the outer pinna for ear canal swabs or the vestibule for vaginal cytology samples) (Figure 1.7). If the area is dry or crusted, the tip of the cotton swab may be moistened with sterile saline to aid in collection, cell yield, and sample preparation. The swab may be spun or gently pressed against the lesion or tissues to collect material.

Slide Preparation For swabs, roll the samples with gentle pressure to create a thin, linear row of material along the slide (Figure 1.8). Do not wipe or use excessive downward pressure, as this may rupture or damage cells.

1.2.3.3 Scrapes

Scrapes are most commonly used to evaluate for ectoparasites, but may also be useful for dry, flat, or crusted skin lesions, including those associated with other infectious agents including dermatophytes [15]. They may also be used to collect cells from masses removed for histopathology prior to placing these in formalin.

Supplies

- Latex or nitrile gloves.
- Glass microscope slides with a frosted edge.
- A pencil.
- Scalpel blade.
- Immersion oil.

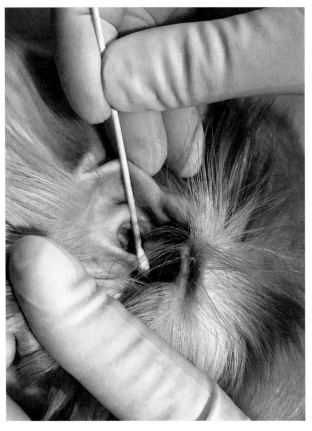

Figure 1.7 Swab collection method for external ear cytology.

Procedure Stabilize the skin or lesion with one hand and hold the scalpel in the dominant hand at a slight angle. Scrape the surface of the lesion with short, moderately firm strokes toward the angle of the tilted scalpel. For deep skin scrapings, continue to scrape until a small amount of serosanguinous material is noted, and collect this material with a scooping action using the scalpel blade.

Slide Preparation For superficial hair scrapings, place a small drop of immersion oil on the slide for the collected hair to remain in place. For deeper scrapings, use the scalpel blade to gently spread the material over the slide. If abundant material was collected and remains thick, use another glass slide to spread the material in a manner similar to that described in Section 1.2.3.1.

1.2.3.4 Impression Smears

These are often used to evaluate biopsy samples prior to being placed in formalin. They may be less useful for exuding lesions on the skin, as often only surface material is obtained, which may not be representative of deeper portions.

Supplies
- Latex or nitrile gloves.
- Glass microscope slides with a frosted edge.
- A pencil.
- ± Gauze swabs.

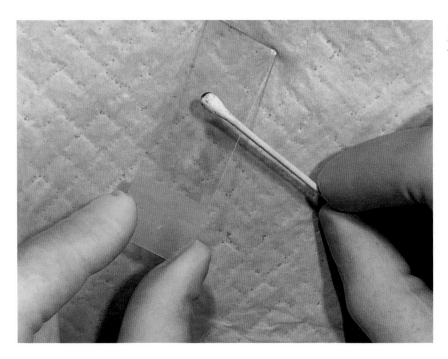

Figure 1.8 The swab is gently rolled along the slide to transfer material in a thin monolayer for review. Courtesy of Dr. Eric Franson.

Procedure and Slide Preparation For skin lesions, the slide is directly applied to the area, with care to avoid contamination from surrounding skin. Cleaning the lesions of any topical medications or excessive debris is recommended if possible. For biopsy samples, it is ideal to use a cut surface for access to cells deep within the tissue. Excess blood should be removed by blotting the cut surface on gauze prior to gently pressing on multiple areas of the glass slide.

1.2.3.5 Brushings

Cytology brushes are commercially available and can be useful for collecting cells from many surface locations, including ocular samples (cornea and conjunctiva) [16, 17] and the airways [18].

Supplies
- Latex or nitrile gloves.
- Glass microscope slides with a frosted edge.
- A pencil.
- Cytology brush.

Procedure The brush is gently moved and rotated over the surface of interest. Focusing on visibly abnormal areas free of excessive surface material (e.g., mucus or hemorrhage in the airways) will help maximize cellular yield.

Slide Preparation The material collected from the brushing procedure should be immediately transferred to the glass slides by gently rolling the brush in a thin linear row, similar to that described for swab samples in Section 1.2.3.2.

1.3 Sample Staining

Cytology samples are typically stained with Romanowsky-type stains for routine assessment. Examples of Romanowsky stains include Wright stain, Giemsa stain, May-Grünwald Giemsa, and Leishman stain. These stains contain eosin, which binds to basic components of the cells and stains them pink (e.g., hemoglobin in erythrocytes), and methylene blue, which binds to the acidic components of cells and stains them blue (e.g., nuclei).

1.3.1 Rapid Romanowsky-type Stains

Rapid Romanowsky-type stains are the most common stains used in clinic, for example, Diff-Quik (Siemens, Munich, Germany) and Hema 3® (Fisher Scientific, Pittsburgh, PA) (Figure 1.9). Methanol is used as fixative; however, these stains are aqueous-based.

1.3.1.1 Rapid Stain Procedure

The following steps detail how to maximize the stain quality of cytology samples using rapid Romanowsky-type stains:

1) Ensure slides are completely dry prior to staining.
2) Gloves should be worn when staining slides, and forceps or a wooden peg can be used to hold the slide during staining.
3) Fix slides for 1–2 minutes. Slides cannot be over-fixed; however, under-fixation of slides greatly affects stain quality and may lead to cellular lysis or poor stain uptake.

Figure 1.9 Rapid Romanowsky-type stains (Diff Quik).

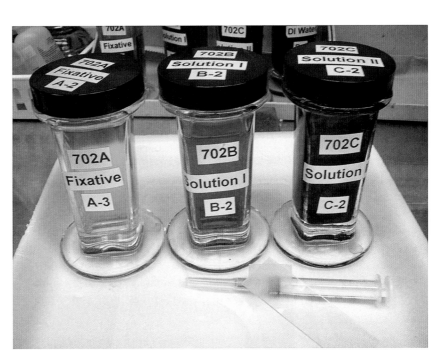

Increasing fixation time greatly increases stain quality of the sample. Slides should be dipped in the fixative until evenly and completely covered and then allowed to sit in the fixative for 1–2 minutes. After this time, remove them and allow excess fixative to drain by standing the lower edge of the slide onto an absorbent pad.

4) Dip the slide into solution 1 (eosin) to completely and evenly cover it and then dip the slide a further 4–6 times for approximately 1 second per dip.

5) Allow excess stain to drain before repeating this step for solution 2 (methylene blue).
Note: The number of dips and time spent in the eosin and methylene blue stains can and should be tailored to the needs of the sample and preference of the observer to increase or decrease stain intensity. For example, thicker preparations will likely require more time in each stain.

6) Rinse the slide thoroughly with water (ideally deionized water) and stand it vertically to dry.
Note: Even if slides are being sent to a laboratory for evaluation, it is advisable to stain the slides one at a time and review them (until a diagnostic slide is confirmed) to ensure that intact cells are present and that the slide quality is adequate for interpretation, especially as non-diagnostic samples (often due to low or acellular samples) are frequently encountered in a diagnostic laboratory setting [19].

1.3.1.2 Advantages and Disadvantages

When using stains for cytology and hematology, it is important to appreciate their strengths and weaknesses, which can have an important impact on interpretation. The following lists summarize some of the important advantages and disadvantages of rapid Romanowsky-type stains [20].

Advantages
- Readily available and cost effective.
- Ease of use and fast turnaround time for staining samples.
- Good cytoplasmic detail.
- Excellent staining of background material and extracellular matrix.
- Typically stain infectious agents well (especially bacteria and Distemper viral inclusions) [21, 22].

Disadvantages
- Reduced nuclear detail (though nucleoli stain prominently).
- Diff-Quik may stain mast cell, basophil, and granular lymphocyte granules poorly, or not at all [21]. This is

especially important when evaluating metastatic mast cell disease in lymph nodes [23].

1.3.2 Stain Care and Quality Assurance

Careful maintenance of stains dramatically affects stain quality. Ensure that fresh, clean stains are used to prevent excessive stain precipitation or contamination artifacts. Excessive stain precipitation (see Figure 2.9) may be seen on stained cytology slides with prolonged stain time, insufficient washing of slide, or use of old or unfiltered stains, and replacing or filtering stains on a regular basis is recommended.

Sometimes, changes in the color or intensity of the stain of blood smears may be appreciated: [24]

- Too pink: Low stain pH, inadequate time in methylene blue stain, degraded stain.
- Too blue: High stain pH, prolonged time in methylene blue stain, insufficient washing, exposure to formalin fumes.

1.4 Sample Handling and Storage

The following tips will help maintain slide quality during storage and transport:

- It is ideal to store and transport slides in plastic slide containers to prevent slide breakage or damage.
- If oil was used on the slides, resting the slides face down on microscope cleaning wipes for 1–2 hours will absorb much of the oil, allowing for cleaner storage.
- If slides are being kept for long-term use, store them in a dark, dry place. Dry, stained slides can be effectively and efficiently stored in empty microscope slide boxes with a reference list of the slides on a piece of paper that can be stored folded in the lid of the box.
- Never place slides in the refrigerator, especially if unfixed/unstained. Also avoid exposure to extreme temperatures, including leaving slides outside for transport pick up in winter or summer.
- It is imperative that unstained slides are not exposed to formalin fumes, which fix the cells and prevent appropriate uptake of cytologic stains, causing pale staining and preventing evaluation of nuclear and cytoplasmic detail (see Figure 2.19). Unstained cytology slides should therefore never be stored with histopathology samples in formalin and are ideally stored and transported in their own airtight bags.

References

1 Ghisleni, G., Roccabianca, P., Ceruti, R., *et al.* (2006) Correlation between fine-needle aspiration cytology and histopathology in the evaluation of cutaneous and subcutaneous masses from dogs and cats. *Vet. Clin. Pathol.*, **35** (1), 24–30.

2 Cohen, M., Bohling, M.W., Wright, J.C., *et al.* (2003) Evaluation of sensitivity and specificity of cytologic examination: 269 cases (1999-2000). *J. Am. Vet. Med. Assoc.*, **222** (7), 964–967.

3 Ku, C.-K., Kass, P.H., Christopher, M.M. (2017) Cytologic-histologic concordance in the diagnosis of neoplasia in canine and feline lymph nodes: a retrospective study of 367 cases. *Vet. Comp. Oncol.*, **15** (4), 1206–1217.

4 Bonfanti, U., Bertazzolo, W., Gracis, M., *et al.* (2015) Diagnostic value of cytological analysis of tumours and tumour-like lesions of the oral cavity in dogs and cats: a prospective study on 114 cases. *Vet. J.*, **205** (2), 322–327.

5 Allen, B.A., Evans, S.J.M. (2022) Diagnostic accuracy of cytology for the detection of bacterial infection in fluid samples from veterinary patients. *Vet. Clin. Pathol.*, **51** (2), 252–257.

6 Berzina, I., Sharkey, L.C., Matise, I., *et al.* (2008) Correlation between cytologic and histopathologic diagnoses of bone lesions in dogs: a study of the diagnostic accuracy of bone cytology. *Vet. Clin. Pathol.*, **37** (3), 332–338.

7 Sontas, B.H., Yüzbaşıoğlu Öztürk, G., Toydemir, T.F., *et al.* (2012) Fine-needle aspiration biopsy of canine mammary gland tumours: a comparison between cytology and histopathology. *Reprod. Domest. Anim.*, **47** (1), 125–130.

8 Grimes, J.A., Matz, B.M., Christopherson, P.W., *et al.* (2017) Agreement between cytology and histopathology for regional lymph node metastasis in dogs with melanocytic neoplasms. *Vet. Pathol.*, **54** (4), 579–587.

9 Arai, S., Rist, P., Clancey, N., *et al.* (2019) Fine-needle aspiration of cutaneous, subcutaneous, and intracavitary masses in dogs and cats using 22- vs 25-gauge needles. *Vet. Clin. Pathol.*, **48** (2), 287–292.

10 Karakitsou, V., Christopher, M.M., Meletis, E., *et al.* (2022) A comparison in cytologic quality in fine-needle specimens obtained with and without aspiration from superficial lymph nodes in the dog. *J. Small Anim. Pract.*, **63** (1), 16–21.

11 Whitlock, J., Taeymans, O., Monti, P. (2021) A comparison of cytological quality between fine-needle aspiration and non-aspiration techniques for obtaining ultrasound-guided samples from canine and feline lymph nodes. *Vet. Rec.*, **188** (6): e25. doi: 10.1002/vetr.25. Last accesses October 15, 2023.

12 De Witte, F.G., Hebrard, A., Grimes, C.N., *et al.* (2020) Effects of different drying methods on smears of canine blood and effusion fluid. *Peer. J.*, **8**, e10092. doi: 10.7717/peerj.10092. Last accesses October 15, 2023.

13 Griffin, J.S., Scott, D.W., Erb, H.N. (2007) Malassezia otitis externa in the dog: the effect of heat-fixing otic exudate for cytologic analysis. *J. Vet. Med. A Physiol. Pathol. Clin. Med.*, **54** (8), 424–427.

14 Toma, S., Comagliani, L., Persico, P., *et al.* (2006) Comparison of 4 fixation and staining methods for the cytologic evaluation of ear canals with clinical evidence of ceruminous otitis externa. *Vet. Clin. Pathol.*, **35** (2), 194–198.

15 Caruso, K.J., Cowell, R.L., Cowell, A.K., *et al.* (2002) Skin scraping from a cat. *Vet. Clin. Pathol.*, **31** (1), 13–15.

16 Ripolles-Garcia, A., Sanz, A., Pastor, J., *et al.* (2021) Comparison of the use of a standard cytology brush versus a mini cytology brush to obtain conjunctival samples for cytologic examination in healthy dogs. *J. Am. Vet. Med. Assoc.*, **259** (3), 288–293.

17 Perazzi, A., Bonsemiante, F., Gelain, M.E., *et al.* (2017) Cytology of the healthy canine and feline ocular surface: comparison between cytobrush and impression technique. *Vet. Clin. Pathol.*, **46** (1), 164–171.

18 Zhu, B.Y., Johnson, L.R., Vernau, W. (2015) Tracheobronchial brush cytology and bronchoalveolar lavage in dogs and cats with chronic cough: 45 cases (2012-2014). *J. Vet. Intern. Med.*, **29** (2), 526–532.

19 Skeldon, N., Dewhurst, E. (2009) The perceived and actual diagnostic utility of veterinary cytological samples. *J. Small Anim. Pract.*, **50** (4), 180–185.

20 Krafts, K.P., Pambuccian, S.E. (2011) Romanowsky staining in cytopathology: history, advantages and limitations. *Biotech. Histochem.*, **86** (2), 82–93.

21 Allison, R.W., Velguth, K.E. (2010) Appearance of granulated cells in blood films stained with automated aqueous versus methanolic Romanowsky methods. *Vet. Clin. Pathol.*, **39** (1), 99–104.

22 Harvey, J.W. (1982) Hematology tip – stains for distemper inclusions. *Vet. Clin. Pathol.*, **11** (1), 12.

23 Sabattini, S., Renzi, A., Marconato, L., *et al.* (2018) Comparison between May-Grünwald-Giemsa and rapid cytological stains in fine-needle aspirates of canine mast cell tumour: diagnostic and prognostic implications. *Vet. Comp. Oncol.*, **16** (4), 511–517.

24 Houwen, B. (2002) Blood film preparation and staining procedures. *Clin. Lab. Med.*, **22** (1), 1–14.

2

Cytologic Analysis of Cells

2.1 Approach to Cytology Samples

Adopting a routine approach to evaluating cytology samples makes cytopathology easier to approach, more efficient, and increases the chance of making a diagnosis. Four major components of every sample should be evaluated:

1) Sample quality and background.
2) Cell types.
3) Cell shape, distribution, and features.
4) Benign versus malignant.

2.2 Sample Quality and Background

The background of the sample is the first component to be evaluated, as it can provide important clues about underlying pathology. Some common background changes include:

- *Cystic material*: Cystic lesions often have a thick blue, purple, or pink background that may be scalloped. Cholesterol crystals are a hallmark of cell degeneration that occurs commonly in cystic lesions. These appear cytologically as rectangular, flat, non-staining crystals, often with a notched corner (Figure 2.1).
- *Necrosis*: Necrotic debris is seen as amorphous, globular, blue/purple/gray material (Figure 2.2). This material may predominate and obscure cellular detail.
- *Hemorrhage*: Blood often is present in the background of samples as a consequence of sampling, which may be supported if platelets are present. Prior hemorrhage within the lesion is confirmed when macrophages are erythrophagocytic and/or contain heme breakdown pigment such as hemosiderin or hematoidin (Figure 2.3).

Figure 2.1 Cholesterol crystals, 20× objective. Note the common notched corners.

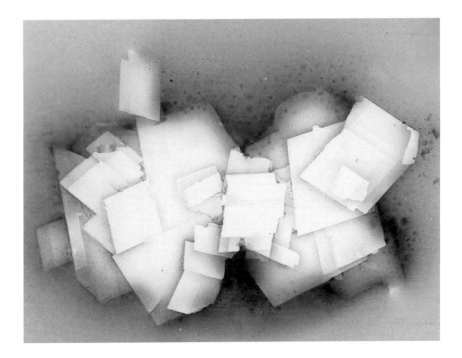

Clinical Atlas of Small Animal Cytology and Hematology, Second Edition. Andrew G. Burton.
© 2024 John Wiley & Sons, Inc. Published 2024 by John Wiley & Sons, Inc.

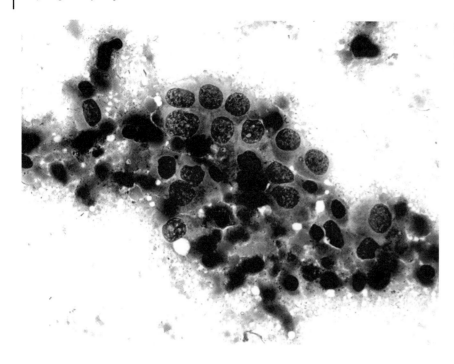

Figure 2.2 Necrotic material, 50× objective. Intact prostatic carcinoma cells are surrounded by globular, blue/purple necrotic material.

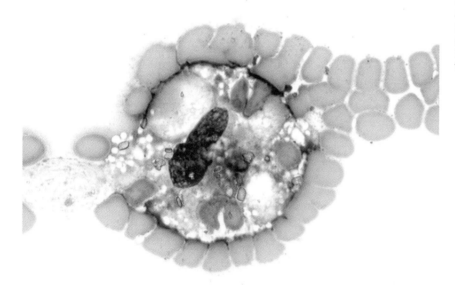

Figure 2.3 Hemorrhage, 100× objective. A macrophage is seen with a central purple nucleus. Red blood cells, blue/green hemosiderin, and golden hematoidin crystals are present within the cytoplasm.

- *Extracellular matrix*: Extracellular matrix is mostly bright pink and may be smooth, fibrillar, or stippled (Figure 2.4). It is most common with mesenchymal proliferation, but the basement membrane of epithelium can appear similarly. Collagen may also be seen, often as pale pink serpiginous ribbons (Figure 2.5).
- *Cytoplasmic fragments*: Fragments of cytoplasm (Figure 2.6) may be seen with any cell type; however,

they are most commonly associated with lymphocytes (and have previously been called 'lymphoglandular bodies') [1].
- *Mineralization*: Mineralized debris is seen as clear, irregular/gritty, refractile aggregates, and often is seen outside the plane of focus of cells in the sample (Figure 2.7). It may be seen in chronic, cystic, or necrotic lesions.

Figure 2.4 Extracellular matrix, 50×
objective. Note the bright pink, smooth,
streaming matrix material intimately
associated with spindle cells (synovial
cell sarcoma).

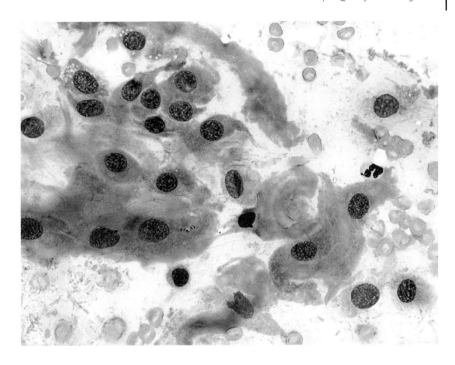

Figure 2.5 Collagen, 50× objective.
Delicate tendrils of pink collagen swirl
around well-differentiated mesenchymal
cells (fibroma).

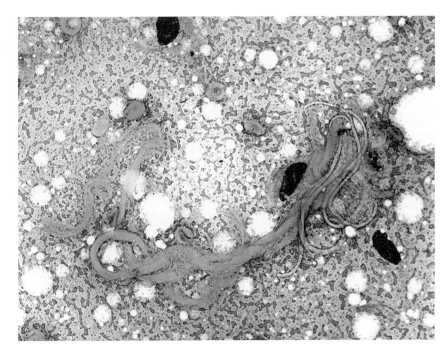

2.2.1 Artifacts and Incidental Findings

It is also important to recognize artifacts or incidental
findings in samples. Glove powder starch crystals are
round with a characteristic cross in the middle (Figure 2.8)
and should be distinguished from mineralized debris.
Precipitation of stain appears as variably coarse, granular
pink/purple material (Figure 2.9). It may be seen in the

background, but can cover cells, and care should be taken
to distinguish it from cytoplasmic granules, intracellular
bacteria, and lubricant/ultrasound gel which also appears
granular/globular and stains bright purple/magenta
(Figure 2.10). Crystals may form incidentally in the background of thick samples, making geometric patterns
(Figure 2.11). Hemoglobin crystals may also form if

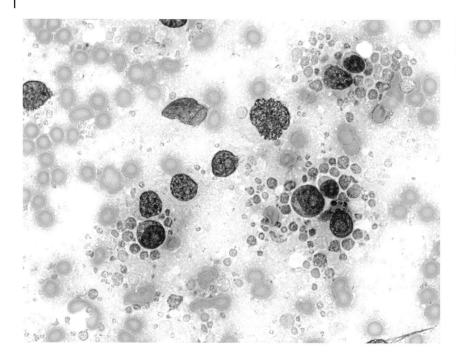

Figure 2.6 Cytoplasmic fragments, 50× objective. Note the small round fragments of pale-blue cytoplasm surrounding lymphocytes in a case of canine lymphoma.

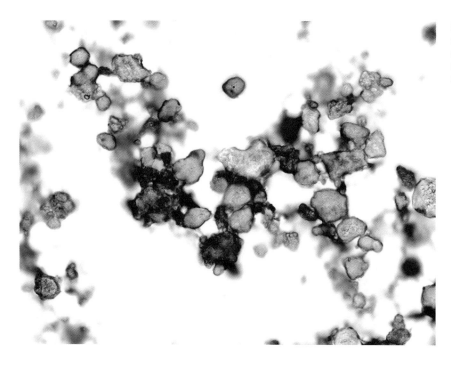

Figure 2.7 Mineralized debris, 50× objective. The material is seen in different planes of focus highlighting the three-dimensional nature of the mineralized debris.

hemodiluted samples are exposed to humidity or extreme temperatures (Figures 2.12 and 2.13), and clotted blood may produce striking colorful patterns (Figure 2.14). Other common artifacts/incidental findings include nuclear material and bare nuclei from lysed cells (Figures 2.15 and 2.16), apoptotic cells (Figure 2.17), and environmental contaminants including pollen grains (Figure 2.18). Formalin artifact results in a pale, homogeneous blue appearance to cells, and cellular detail is obscured (Figure 2.19). Cytologic samples should be transported separately from samples in formalin or should be in separate, airtight containers.

Figure 2.8 Glove powder starch crystals, 50× objective. Note the characteristic cross in the center of the crystals.

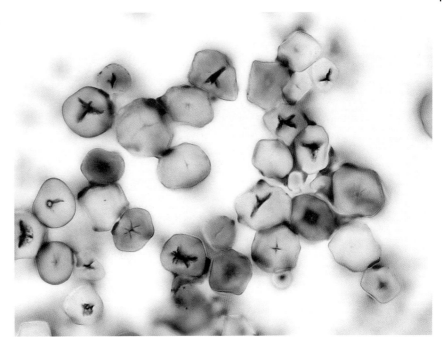

Figure 2.9 Stain precipitate, 50× objective. Stain precipitate is granular and may be pink, purple, or deeply basophilic and varies from fine (center/right) to coarse (lower left).

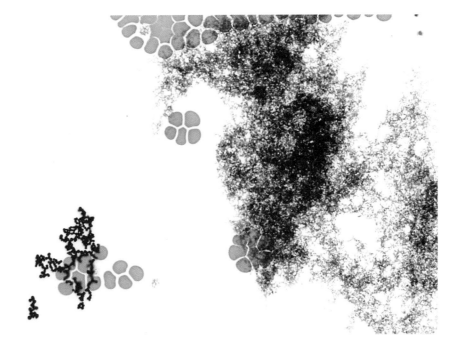

Some normal tissue components are commonly seen as incidental findings in fine-needle aspirate samples, including capillaries (Figures 2.20 and 2.21), adipose and lipid (Figures 2.22 and 2.23), skin surface keratin debris (Figure 2.24), skeletal muscle (Figure 2.25), and normal mesothelium (Figure 2.26).

2.3 Cell Types

If nucleated cells are seen, it is important to determine if the cell types present are of inflammatory or tissue origin, or if both are present.

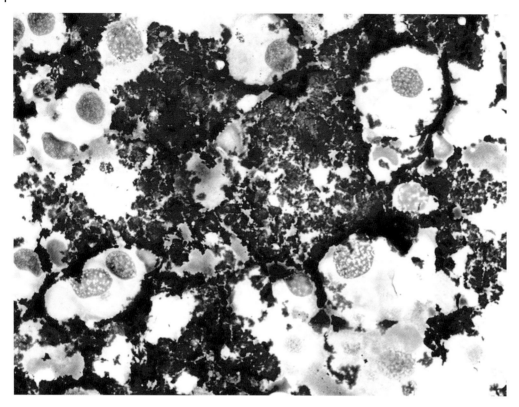

Figure 2.10 Ultrasound/lubricant gel, 50× objective. Bright purple granular material (ultrasound gel) surrounds transitional epithelial cells in a catheter urine sample from a dog.

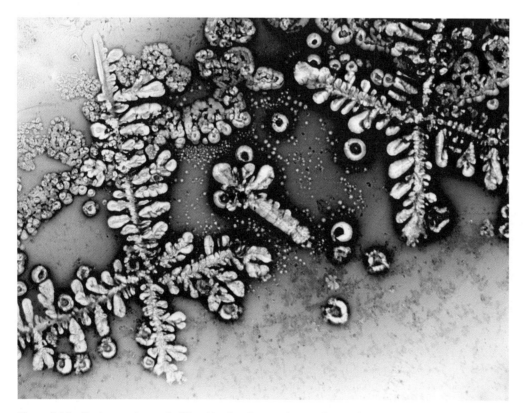

Figure 2.11 Background crystals, 20× objective. Geometric crystals may form incidentally in the background of thick samples.

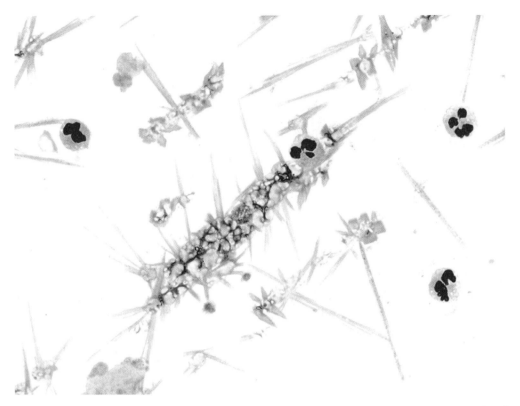

Figure 2.12   Hemoglobin crystals, 50× objective. These crystals are needle-shaped and have the color of red blood cells. Note the blood-associated neutrophils.

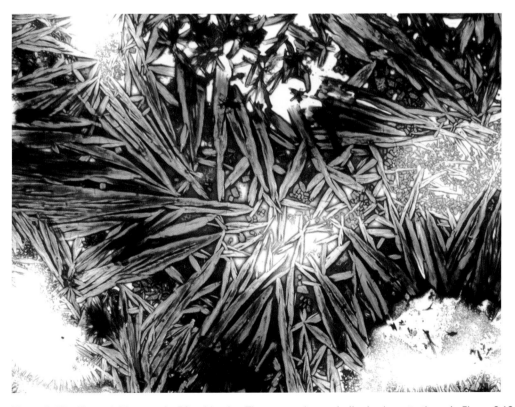

Figure 2.13   Hemoglobin crystals, 50× objective. These crystals are similar in shape to those in Figure 2.12, but are variably sized and pink/orange due to the increased amount of blood.

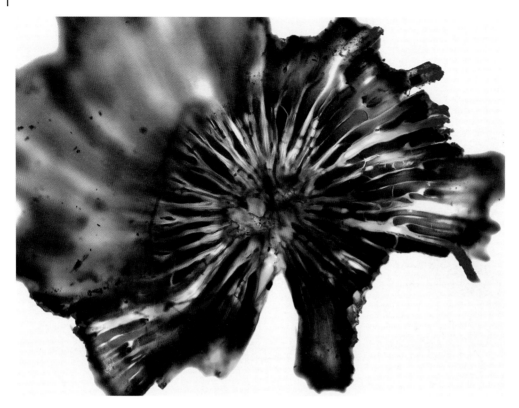

Figure 2.14   Blood clot, 50× objective. Clotted blood may form colorful patterns.

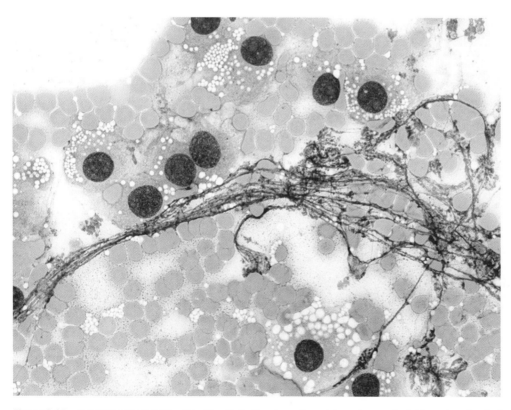

Figure 2.15   Nuclear material, 50× objective. Note the streaming pink nuclear material from lysed cells in an ovarian granulosa cell tumor.

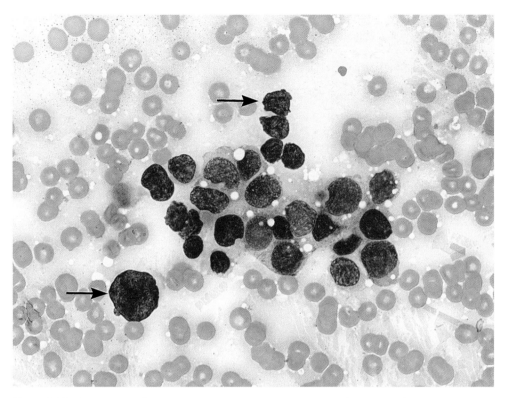

Figure 2.16 Bare nuclei, 50× objective. Nuclei from lysed cells (arrows) appear puffy and lack surrounding cytoplasm. The origin of these cells cannot be accurately determined.

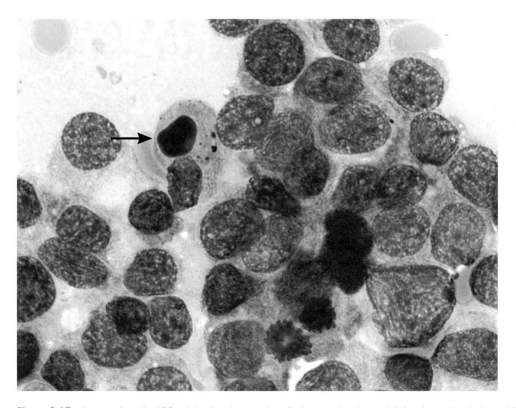

Figure 2.17 Apoptotic cells, 100× objective. Apoptotic cells have pyknotic nuclei that have deeply basophilic, dense chromatin (arrow). Pyknotic nuclei may break apart into variably sized, dense nuclear fragments.

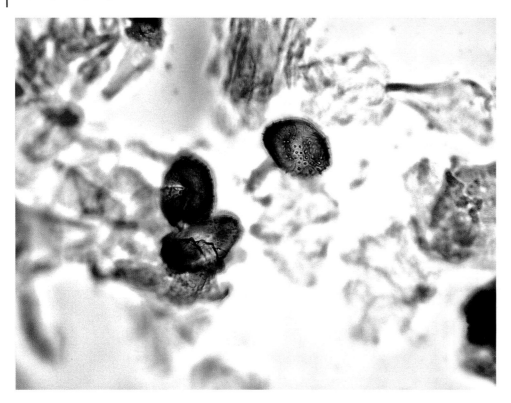

Figure 2.18 Pollen grains, 50× objective. Skin impression smear from a dog. Note the prominent spikes protruding from the surface. Pollen grains are highly variable in shape, color, and texture depending on species.

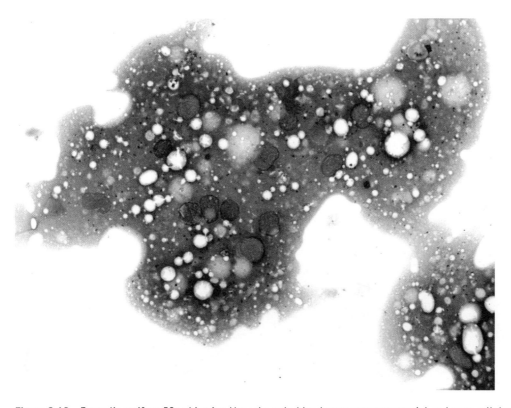

Figure 2.19 Formalin artifact, 50× objective. Note the pale-blue homogeneous material and poor cellular detail precluding evaluation of cellular morphology.

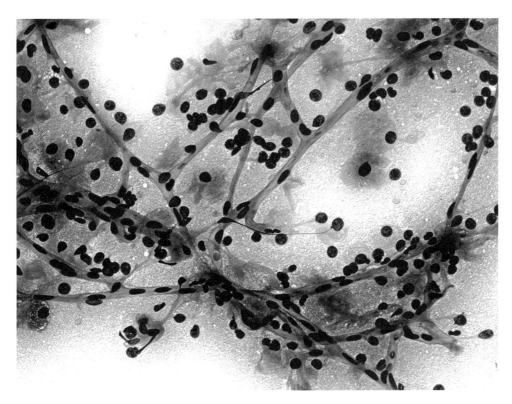

Figure 2.20 Capillaries, 20× objective. Linear pink capillaries course between hepatocytes (well-differentiated hepatocellular carcinoma).

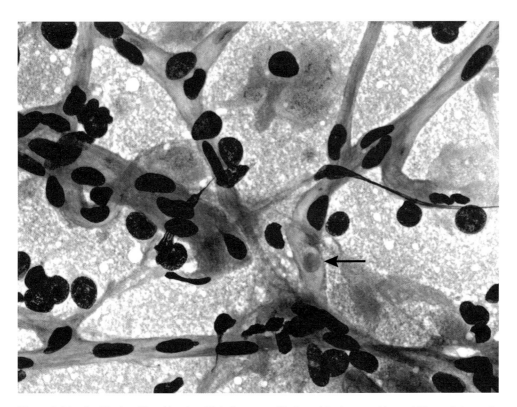

Figure 2.21 Capillaries, 50× objective. Pink, linear capillaries with elongated basophilic nuclei seen in rows. Note the red blood cell traveling within the capillary (arrow).

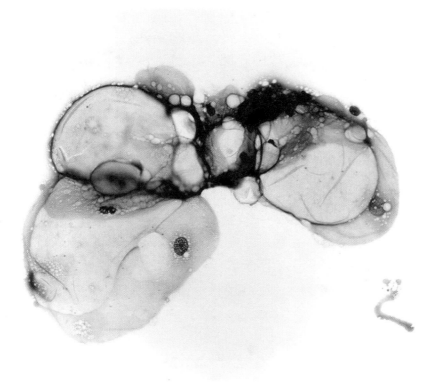

Figure 2.22   Mature, fat-laden adipocytes, 50× objective.

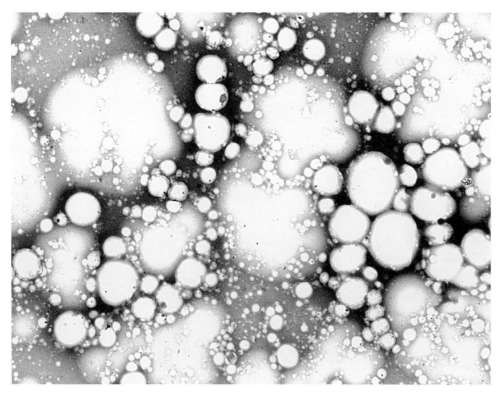

Figure 2.23   Lipid vacuoles, 50× objective.

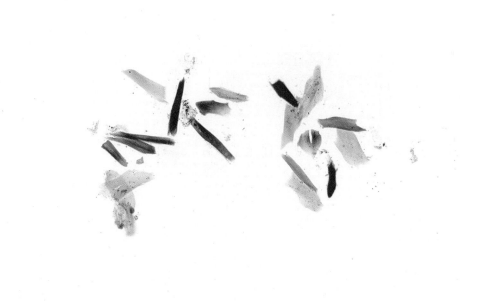

Figure 2.24 Keratin debris from the skin surface, 20× objective.

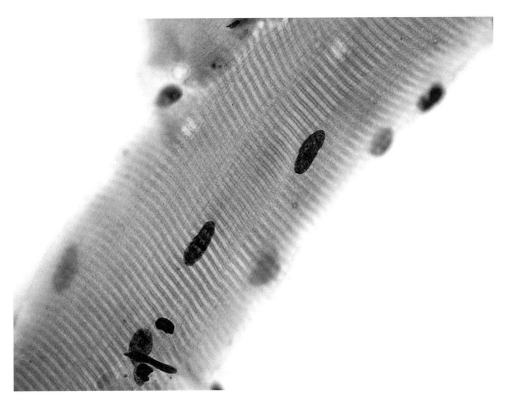

Figure 2.25 Skeletal muscle, 100× objective. Skeletal muscle has medium-blue cytoplasm with subtle parallel striations often easier to see on higher objectives.

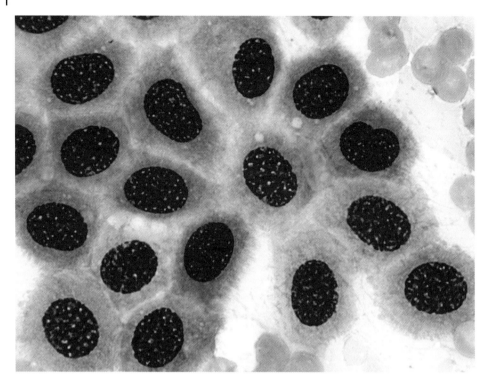

Figure 2.26 Normal mesothelium, 100× objective. Note the pink fringe border.

2.3.1 Inflammatory Cells

Inflammatory cells in tissues often appear similar to their counterparts in blood (Figures 2.27A–F). The types of inflammatory cells present may give clues as to the underlying cause:

- Neutrophils = Bacteria, immune-mediated disease, and tissue injury.
- Eosinophils = Fungal agents, protozoa, parasites, allergy/hypersensitivity, and some neoplasms (e.g., mast cell tumors and T-cell lymphoma) [2].
- Macrophages = Fungi, *Mycobacteria*, tissue injury/necrosis, and cystic lesions.
- Lymphocytes = Chronic disease and immune-mediated disease.
- Plasma cells = Chronic disease and immune-mediated disease. Plasma cells are terminally differentiated B lymphocytes and may accumulate immunoglobulins in their cytoplasm seen as blue (or rarely pink) smooth globular inclusions (Mott cells) [3] or bright-pink peripheral cytoplasmic coloration (flame cells).

The morphology of inflammatory cells is also important. Neutrophils are more likely to be degenerative with an infectious etiology. Degenerative changes include swelling of the nuclei, loss of lobulation, and karyorrhexis/karyolysis (Figure 2.28). Degenerative changes are not to be confused with toxic changes. Degenerative changes affect the *nuclei*, occur in tissues, and may help raise suspicion for an infectious etiology. Toxic changes mostly affect the *cytoplasm* of neutrophils (Döhle bodies, increased basophilia, vacuolation; Figure 2.29) and are only assessed on peripheral blood smears (see Chapter 18) [4, 5]. Neutrophils are more likely to be apoptotic or pyknotic (Figure 2.30) in sterile inflammatory lesions.

2.3.2 Tissue Cells

If the cells present are not recognizably inflammatory, they likely represent the aspiration of tissue cells. These cells are further investigated based on their shape, distribution/interactions with each other, and criteria of malignancy.

(A)

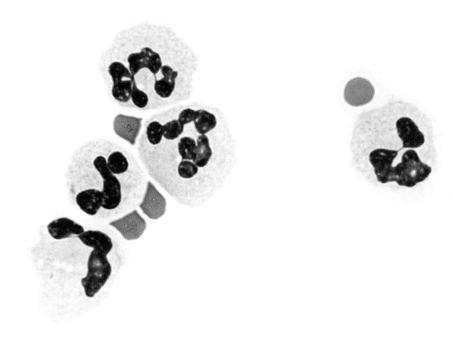

(B)

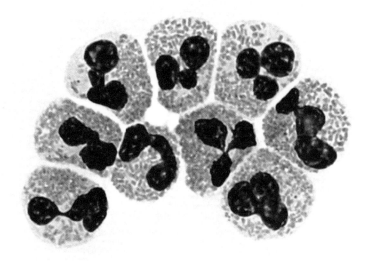

Figure 2.27 Inflammatory cells, all 100× objective. (A) Neutrophils. (B) Eosinophils.

(C)

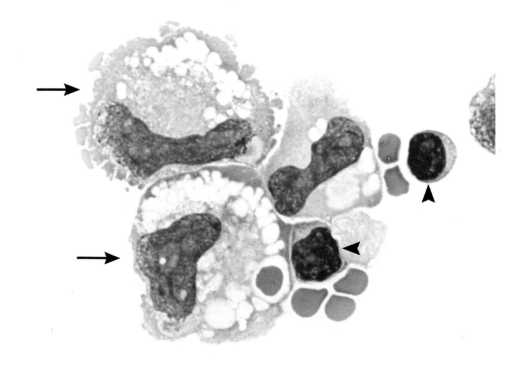

(D)

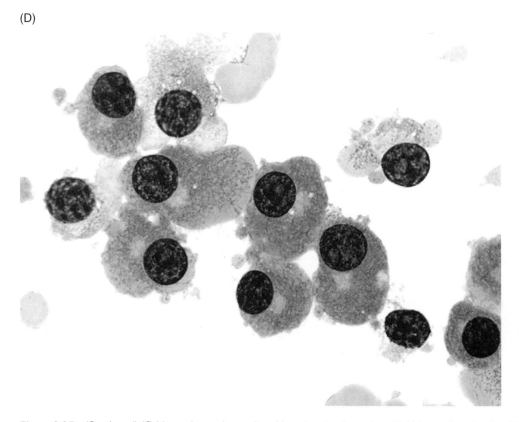

Figure 2.27 (Continued) (C) Macrophages (arrows) and lymphocytes (arrowheads). Note erythrophagia within one of the macrophages (lower left). (D) Plasma cells. Note the prominent perinuclear clearing (Golgi zone).

(E)

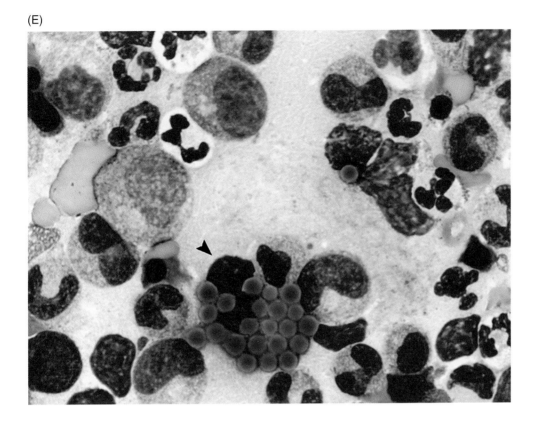

(F)

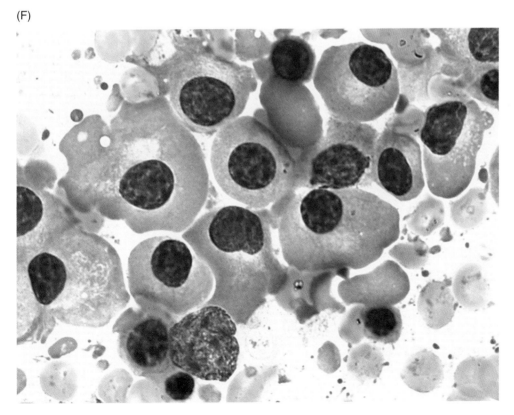

Figure 2.27 (Continued) (E) Mott cells. A Mott cell (arrowhead) contains numerous bright-blue aggregates of immunoglobulin. (F) Flame cells.

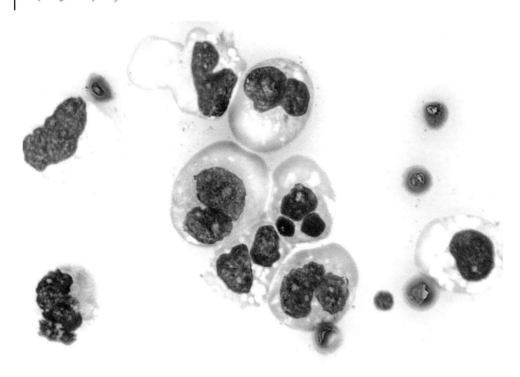

Figure 2.28 Degenerative neutrophils, 100× objective. Note the swollen nuclei, loss of lobulation, and karyorrhexis (compare to non-degenerative neutrophils in Figure 2.27A).

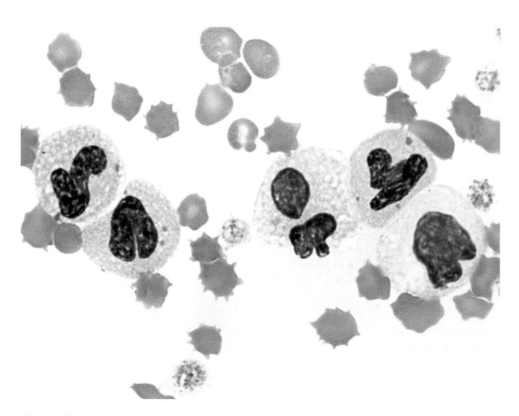

Figure 2.29 Toxic neutrophils, blood, cat, 100× objective. Note the cytoplasmic changes including small blue inclusions (Döhle bodies), cytoplasmic basophilia, and vacuolation.

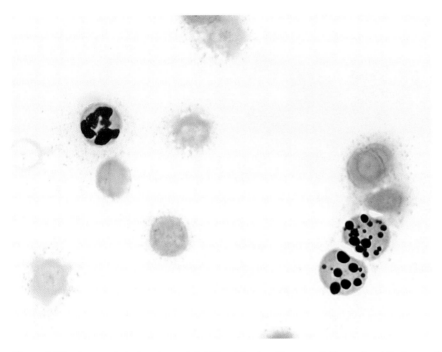

Figure 2.30 Apoptotic/pyknotic nuclei, 100× objective. Two apoptotic neutrophils (lower right) with multiple variably sized, deeply basophilic, pyknotic nuclear fragments.

2.4 Cell Shape, Distribution, and Features

The shape of cells and the way they interact with each other can give valuable information regarding the origin of the cells. In cytopathology, cells often are grouped into one of three clinically useful categories: round cells, epithelial cells, and mesenchymal cells [6].

2.4.1 Epithelial Cells

Cells of epithelial origin often exfoliate in large numbers and are seen mostly in cohesive sheets whereby cells share prominent intercellular borders with each other, like bricks and mortar (Figure 2.31).

2.4.2 Mesenchymal Cells

Mesenchymal cells exfoliate variably well. They generally are fusiform or spindloid with tapering ends (Figure 2.32). Some cells of mesenchymal origin are round (e.g., osteosarcoma; see Figure 2.33 and Chapter 7). Mesenchymal tumors also are most likely to be associated with extracellular matrix production (see Figure 2.4).

2.4.3 Round Cells

Round cell tumors technically are mesenchymal in origin (derived embryologically from mesoderm) [7]. However, it is clinically useful to consider common round cell neoplasms separately, including mast cell tumors, lymphoma, plasma cell tumors, histiocytic neoplasia, and transmissible venereal tumors (see Chapter 5 for details). Cells from these neoplasms often exfoliate in large numbers and mostly are individualized or discrete (Figure 2.34).

It is important to note that cytology is not always able to accurately assign cells into one of these categories. While such generalizations are useful, they do not replace histopathologic assessment of tissue architecture for accurate assessment of cell type and origin. Some common exceptions to the rules described earlier include the following:

- Round cell tumors may be so cellular that cells are pushed together and appear cohesive (Figure 2.35).
- Anaplastic carcinomas often lose the ability to form cell junctions and may appear as individualized or round cells (Figure 2.36).
- Melanoma cells may be round or spindloid, seen individually, in aggregates or sheets, and may be

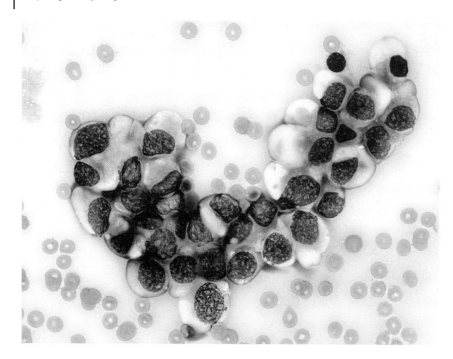

Figure 2.31 Epithelial cells, prostatic carcinoma, dog, 50× objective. Cells are cohesive and 'sticky' with prominent intercellular borders.

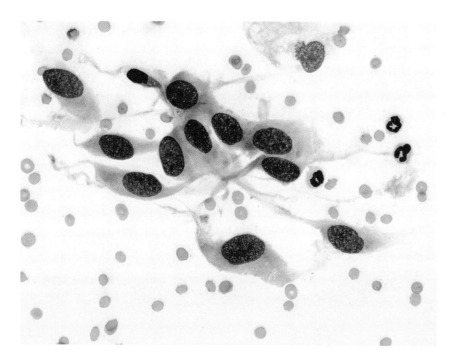

Figure 2.32 Mesenchymal cells, leiomyosarcoma, cat, 50× objective.

associated with extracellular matrix (Figure 2.37; see Chapter 4 for details).

- Cells of some mesenchymal tumors are round (e.g., osteosarcoma, chondrosarcoma, and rhabdomyosarcoma) (Figure 2.33; see Chapter 7 for details).

2.5 Benign Versus Malignant

Benign lesions typically are composed of well-differentiated, uniform populations of cells (Figures 2.38 and 2.39). Variation in cellular features between cells is more

Figure 2.33 Mesenchymal cells, osteosarcoma, dog, 50× objective. The neoplastic mesenchymal cells are discrete and round.

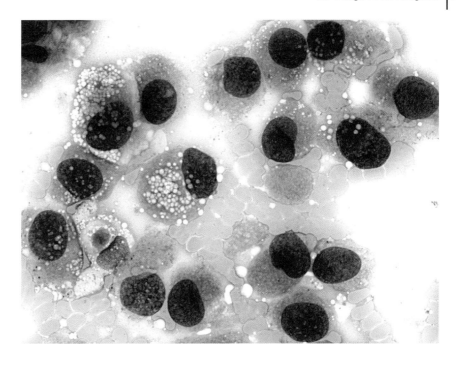

Figure 2.34 Round cell tumor, mast cell tumor, dog, 50× objective.

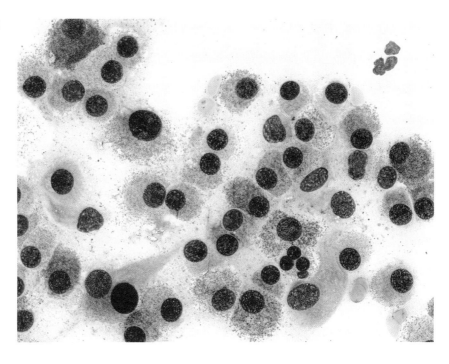

suggestive of malignancy. Criteria of malignancy are listed below, according to the cell features affected:

- *Cellular*: **Anisocytosis** (variation in cell size) (Figure 2.40); cell piling (Figure 2.41); **cell cannibalism** [8, 9]

(Figure 2.42); poor cohesion in epithelial tumors; and poor differentiation.

- *Cytoplasmic*: **High nuclear to cytoplasmic (N/C) ratios** (decreased volume of cytoplasm) (Figure 2.43); increased cytoplasmic basophilia.

- *Nuclear*: **Anisokaryosis** (variation in nuclear size) (Figure 2.44); **mitotic figures**; **multinucleation** (Figure 2.45); **satellite nuclei** (Figure 2.46); **nuclear fragmentation** (Figure 2.47); **hyperchromasia** (Figure 2.48); and nuclear crowding/molding.

- *Nucleolar*: **Prominent nucleoli** (Figure 2.49); **multiple nucleoli** (Figure 2.50); anisonucleosis (variation in nucleolar size); and abnormal nucleolar shape.

Criteria of malignancy that are most common and/or reliable are shown in bold type. Most of these affect the

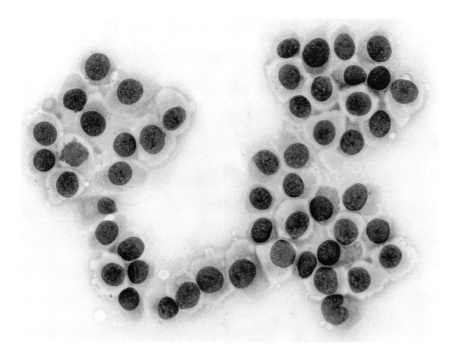

Figure 2.35 Round cell tumor, histiocytoma, dog, 50× objective. The cells are pushed into sheets, which can mimic epithelial cells, but still appear discrete, without prominent intercellular borders.

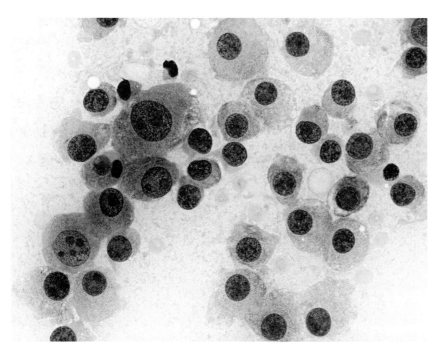

Figure 2.36 Poorly cohesive carcinoma (hepatocellular carcinoma), dog, 50× objective.

Figure 2.37 Malignant melanoma, dog, 50× objective. The cells are vaguely cohesive, round to spindloid and associated with pink extracellular matrix. Note the green/black pigment in the cytoplasm of some cells (arrowheads) and the mitotic figure (arrow).

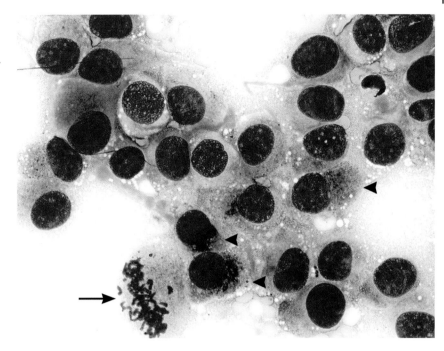

Figure 2.38 Benign mesenchymal neoplasia, fibroma, dog, 50× objective. Note the minimal variation between cells.

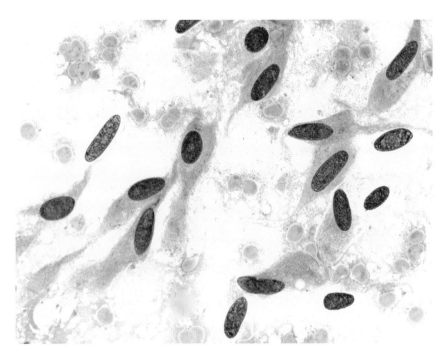

nucleus, and careful examination of nuclei in suspected neoplastic lesions is recommended.

2.5.1 Mitotic Figures

Increased numbers of mitotic figures indicate increased proliferation in tissues. Stages of normal mitosis include prophase, metaphase, anaphase, and telophase (Figure 2.51A–E) [10].

- Prophase: Chromatin condenses into coarse, ropey clumps of similar size, giving the chromatin pattern a marbled appearance. This is a subtle change that can be easily overlooked.
- Metaphase: Metaphase may appear different depending on the orientation of the cell. A ring of uniform chromosomes may be seen when viewed end-on, or the chromosomes may be seen in a linear arrangement in the center of the cell.

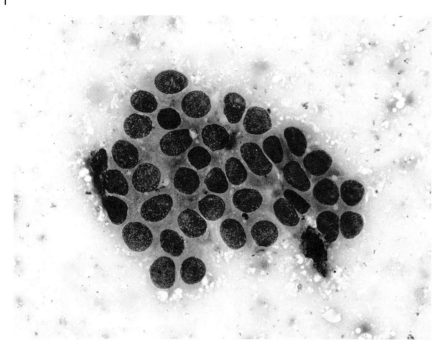

Figure 2.39 Benign epithelial neoplasia, mammary adenoma, dog, 50× objective. Note the minimal variation between cells.

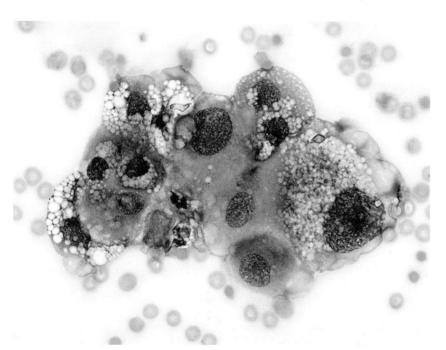

Figure 2.40 Anisocytosis, mesothelioma, dog, 50× objective. Note the variation in size between cells.

- Anaphase: In anaphase, two uniform clusters of chromosomes are separated from each other within a single cytoplasmic border.
- Telophase: Telophase is characterized by a nuclear envelope forming around two uniform clusters of chromosomes prior to the separation of the cells (cytokinesis).

These may be seen in normal tissues with high turnover rates of cells, such as bone marrow, gastrointestinal tract, and even in hyperplastic lymph nodes. Mitoses frequently are seen in increased numbers in neoplastic lesions and are an important criterion of malignancy.

Deviations in the appearance of these mitotic figures described earlier are often called *bizarre mitotic figures*

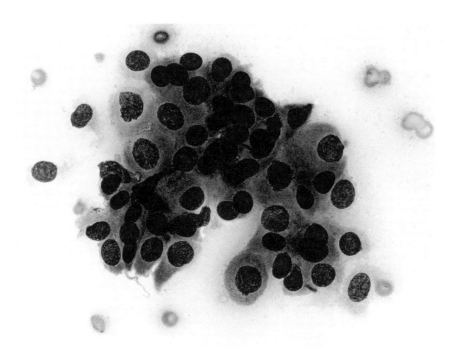

Figure 2.41 Cell piling, perianal gland carcinoma, dog, 50× objective. The cells are overlapping, crowded, and disorganized.

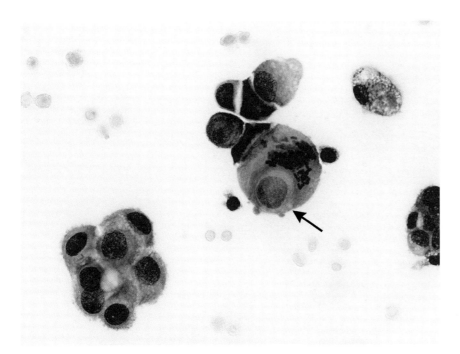

Figure 2.42 Cell cannibalism, mesothelioma, dog, 50× objective. A mitotic neoplastic cell has phagocytosed another neoplastic cell (arrow).

and may be characterized based on spindle symmetry (including spindle multipolarity) and abnormal sister chromatid segregation (including chromosome bridges, chromatid bridges, and chromosome lagging) (Figure 2.52) [10]. Combinations of these abnormalities may result in complex bizarre mitotic figures (Figure 2.53). Bizarre mitoses, even in low numbers, are highly suggestive of malignancy.

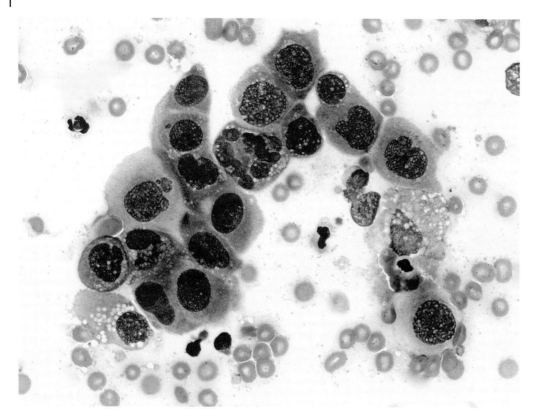

Figure 2.43   High N/C ratios, mammary carcinoma, dog, 50× objective.

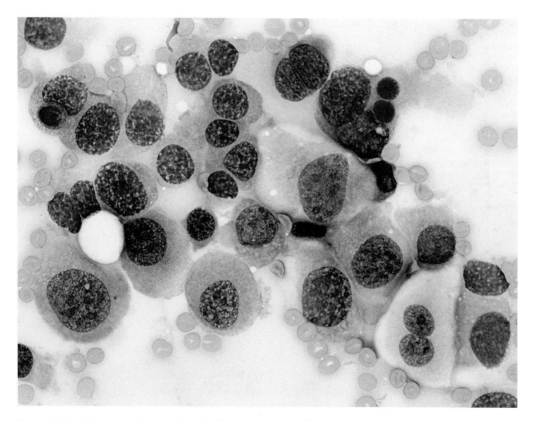

Figure 2.44   Anisokaryosis, transitional cell carcinoma, dog, 50× objective. Some nuclei are 3–4× the size of others.

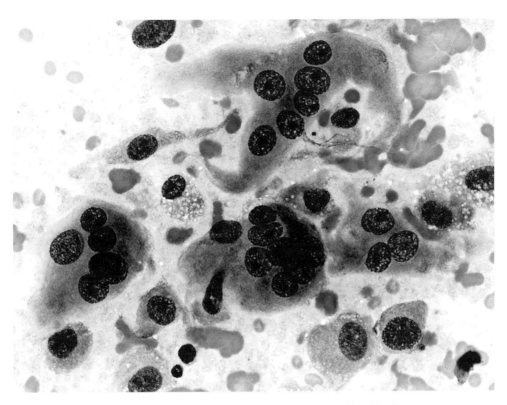

Figure 2.45 Multinucleation, anaplastic sarcoma with giant cells, cat, 50× objective.

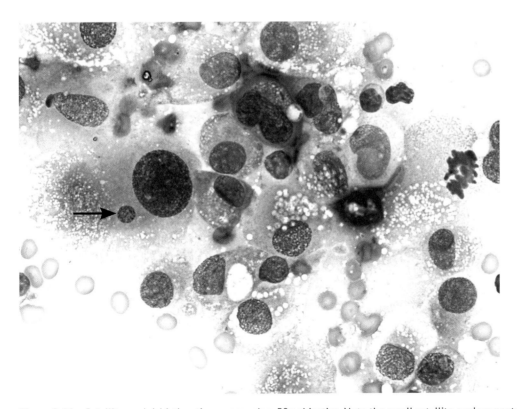

Figure 2.46 Satellite nuclei, histiocytic sarcoma, dog, 50× objective. Note the small satellite nucleus next to the larger nucleus (arrow).

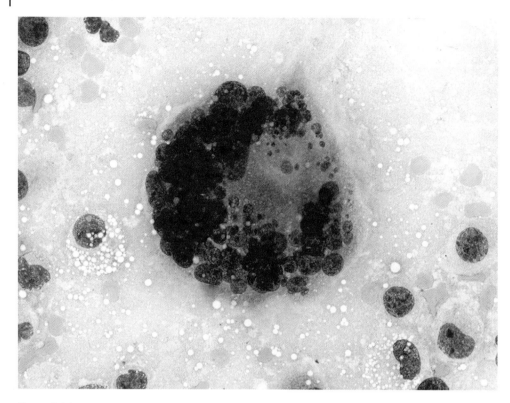

Figure 2.47   Nuclear fragmentation, histiocytic sarcoma, dog, 50× objective.

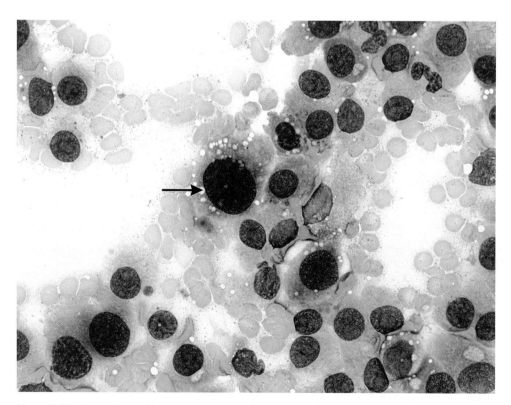

Figure 2.48   Hyperchromasia, osteosarcoma, dog, 50× objective. Note how dark the chromatin is (arrow) relative to other cells.

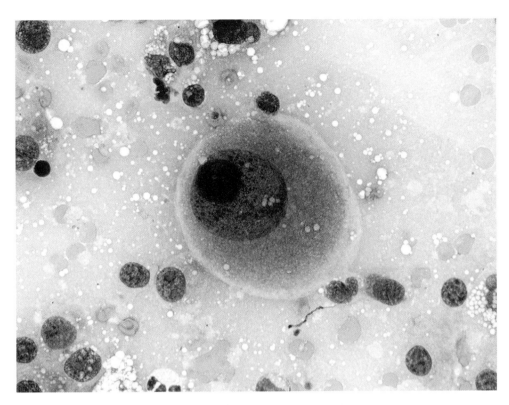

Figure 2.49 Prominent nucleoli, histiocytic sarcoma, dog, 50× objective.

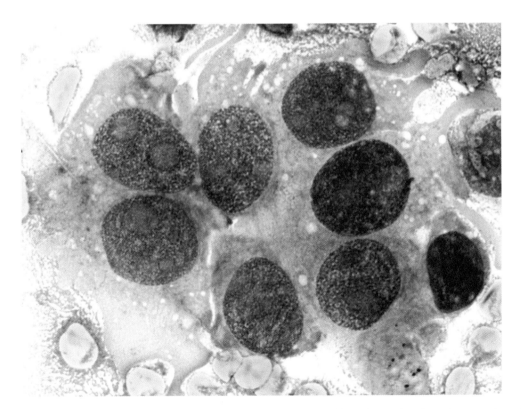

Figure 2.50 Multiple nucleoli, osteosarcoma, dog, 100× objective. Note the varying sizes, shapes, and number of nucleoli in each nucleus.

(A)

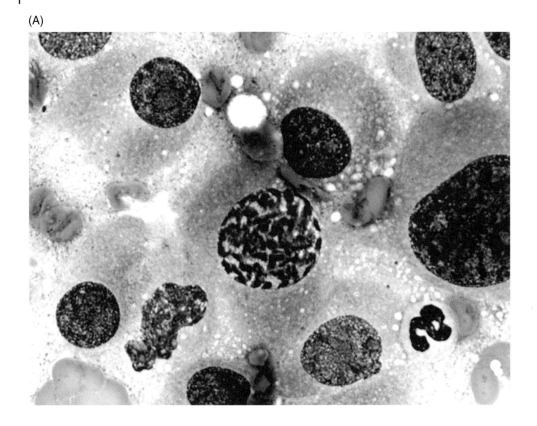

(B)

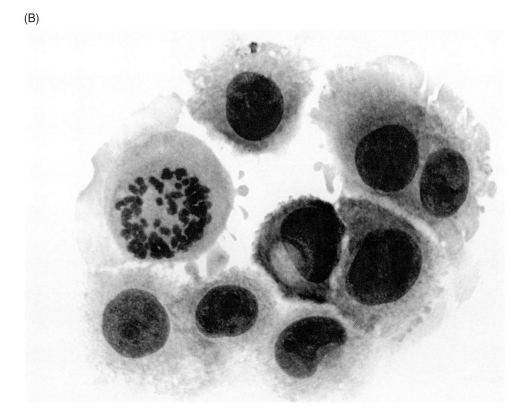

Figure 2.51   Stages of normal mitosis. (A) Prophase. (B) Metaphase (end on).

(C)

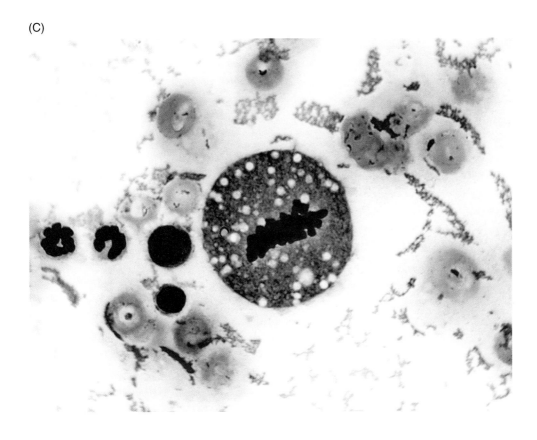

(D)

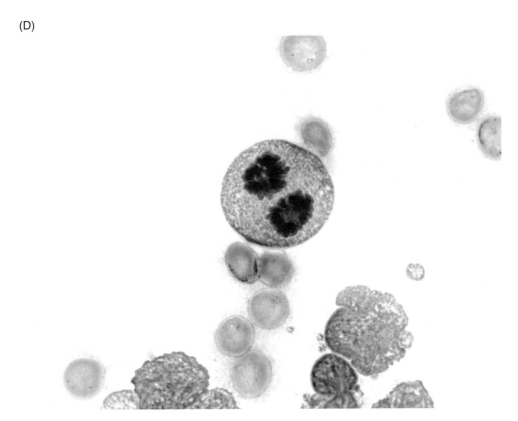

Figure 2.51 (Continued) (C) Metaphase (side on). (D) Anaphase.

(E)

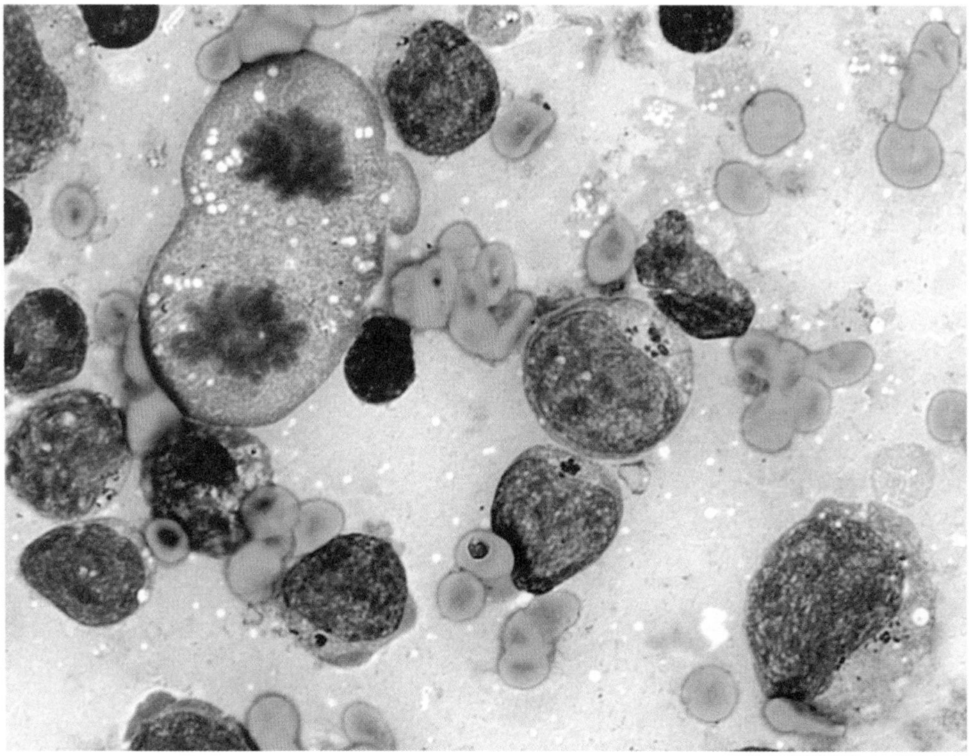

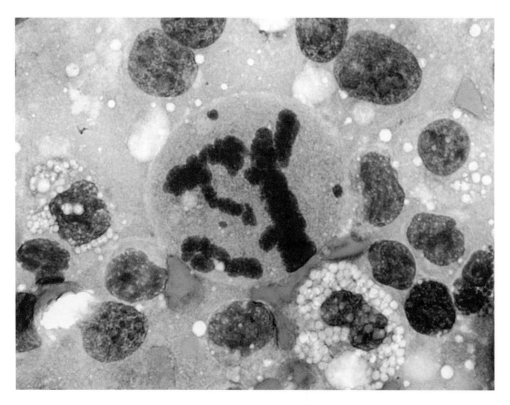

Figure 2.51 (Continued) (E) Telophase.

Figure 2.52 Bizarre mitotic figure, histiocytic sarcoma, dog, 100× objective. Note the multipolar mitosis with lagging chromosomes.

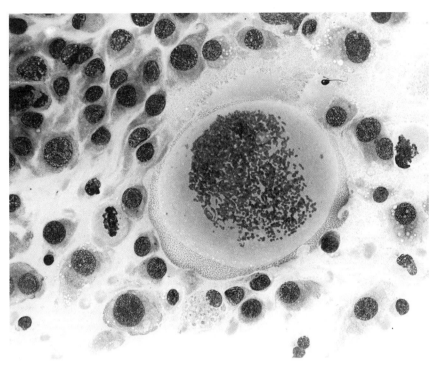

Figure 2.53 Giant and complex mitosis, soft tissue sarcoma, dog, 50× objective. A smaller mitotic cell in metaphase is seen to the left of the giant bizarre mitotic cell.

References

1 Francis, I.M., Das, D.K., al-Rubah, N.A., *et al.* (1994) Lymphoglandular bodies in lymphoid lesions and nonlymphoid round cell tumours: a quantitative assessment. *Diagn. Cytopathol.*, **11** (1), 23–27.

2 Bray, K.Y., Muñana, K.R., Meichner, K., *et al.* (2016) Eosinophilic meningomyelitis associated with T-cell lymphoma in a cat. *Vet. Clin. Pathol.*, **45** (4), 698–702.

3 Cazzini, P., Watson, V.E., Brown, H.M. (2013) The many faces of Mott cells. *Vet. Clin. Pathol.*, **42** (2), 125–126.

4 Aroch, I., Klement, E., Segev, G. (2005) Clinical, biochemical, and hematological characteristics, disease prevalence, and prognosis of dogs presenting with neutrophil cytoplasmic toxicity. *J. Vet. Intern. Med.*, **19** (1), 64–73.

5 Segev, G., Klement, E., Aroch, I. (2006) Toxic neutrophils in cats: clinical and clinicopathologic features, and disease prevalence and outcome – a retrospective case control study. *J. Vet. Intern. Med.*, **20** (1), 20–31.

6 Meinkoth, J.H., Cowell, R.L. (2002) Recognition of basic cell types and criteria of malignancy. *Vet. Clin. North Am. Small Anim. Pract.*, **32** (6), 1209–1235.

7 Andrew, A., Rawdon, B.B. (1987) The embryonic origin of connective tissue mast cells. *J. Anat.*, **150**, 219–227.

8 Meléndez-Lazo, A., Cazzini, P., Camus, M., *et al.* (2015) Cell cannibalism by malignant neoplastic cells: three cases in dogs and a literature review. *Vet. Clin. Pathol.*, **44** (2), 287–294.

9 Yang, C., McAloney, C.A., Jennings, R.N., *et al.* (2019) What is your diagnosis? Thoracic mass in a dog. *Vet. Clin. Pathol.*, **48** (4), 774–776.

10 Tvedten, H. (2009) Atypical mitoses: morphology and classification. *Vet. Clin. Pathol.*, **38** (4), 418–420.

3

Infectious Agents

3.1 Fungi

3.1.1 *Cryptococcus*

3.1.1.1 Cytologic Features
Small and large forms exist. Organisms are round, ranging from ~5 to 20 μm in diameter. They have basophilic cytoplasm with a thick capsule and a prominent nonstaining encircling halo (Figure 3.1). The organisms divide via narrow-based budding, which is a helpful distinguishing feature from *Blastomyces*, which divide via broad-based budding. Variation in size is common with cryptococcal organisms compared to uniform *Histoplasma*. Infection is often associated with granulomatous inflammation (Figures 3.2 and 3.3).

3.1.1.2 Clinical Considerations
- Cats > dogs.
- *Cryptococcus neoformans* and *Cryptococcus gattii* most common species [1].
- Most common in nasal cavity or skin, but also lungs, lymph nodes, central nervous system (CNS), eyes, and may be disseminated [1–3].

3.1.1.3 Prognosis
Cats = generally good with appropriate therapy, though relapse can occur, even after long periods of remission [4]. CNS involvement carries a poor prognosis [5, 6].
Dogs = guarded to poor [4, 6, 7].

3.1.2 *Histoplasma capsulatum*

3.1.2.1 Cytologic Features
Small, uniform, round yeast organisms ~2–5 μm in diameter, with deep purple cytoplasm that frequently forms an eccentric purple crescent. A small, clear halo encircles the cells (Figure 3.4). Narrow-based budding rarely is seen. The organisms usually are seen within macrophages.

3.1.2.2 Clinical Considerations
- Dogs and cats [8, 9].
- Mostly affects the respiratory tract but may disseminate to many organs, especially the gastrointestinal tract, liver, spleen, bone marrow, and lymph nodes [8–10].

3.1.2.3 Prognosis
Guarded prognosis for cats, and prolonged therapy often required [9]. Dogs with respiratory histoplasmosis have a good prognosis with appropriate therapy [11]. Negative prognostic factors in dogs may include dyspnea, need for oxygen supplementation, palpable abdominal organomegaly, anemia, and thrombocytopenia [8]. Disseminated disease in cats and dogs carries a guarded to poor prognosis [11].

3.1.3 *Sporothrix* spp.

3.1.3.1 Cytologic Appearance
Mostly ovoid to cigar-shaped (Figure 3.5), ~4–10 μm in length, and 1–3 μm wide. The elongated shape helps distinguish *Sporothrix* spp. from perfectly round *H. capsulatum*. The organisms have pale-blue cytoplasm, with prominent pink to purple nuclei that often are eccentrically placed. They have a thin clear capsule. Organisms divide via narrow-based budding. Mostly accompanied by pyogranulomatous inflammation.

3.1.3.2 Clinical Considerations
- Cats > dogs.
- *Sporothrix schenckii* most common species in dogs and cats. *Sporothrix humicola* and *Sporothrix brasiliensis* also reported in cats, with the latter an important emerging pathogen [12].
- Cutaneous lesions around the face most common. Pulmonary and generalized disease possible [13].
- Zoonotic potential.

Clinical Atlas of Small Animal Cytology and Hematology, Second Edition. Andrew G. Burton.
© 2024 John Wiley & Sons, Inc. Published 2024 by John Wiley & Sons, Inc.

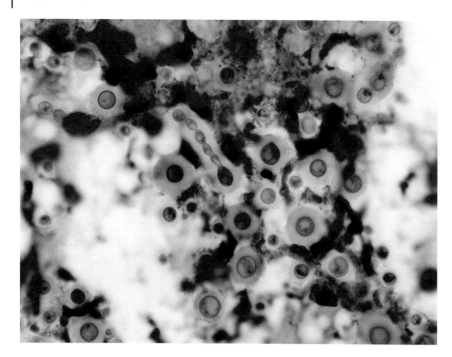

Figure 3.1 *Cryptococcus neoformans*, cat, 50× objective. Note the narrow based budding forming a chain of organisms.

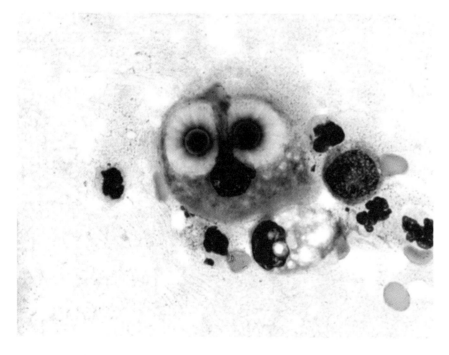

Figure 3.2 *Cryptococcus neoformans*, cat, 50× objective. Two organisms are phagocytosed by a macrophage.

3.1.3.3 Prognosis

Cure rates are good in cats with prolonged therapy, but relapse can occur [14]. Cats with respiratory signs have a poorer prognosis [15]. Spontaneous regression may occur in a small number of dogs [16].

3.1.4 Dermatophytes

3.1.4.1 Cytologic Appearance

Fungal arthrospores often are associated with hair shafts and are ovoid, 2–4 μm in diameter, and stain deeply basophilic, with a thin clear capsule (Figure 3.6) [17]. They may be

Figure 3.3 *Cryptococcus neoformans*, cat, 50× objective. Multiple organisms with prominent encircling clear halos are phagocytosed by macrophages and seen in the background.

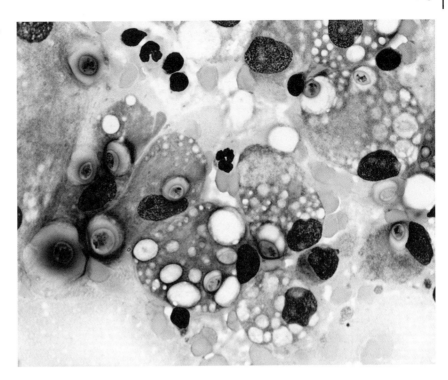

Figure 3.4 *Histoplasma capsulatum*, cat, 100× objective. Abundant organisms seen within a macrophage and in the background.

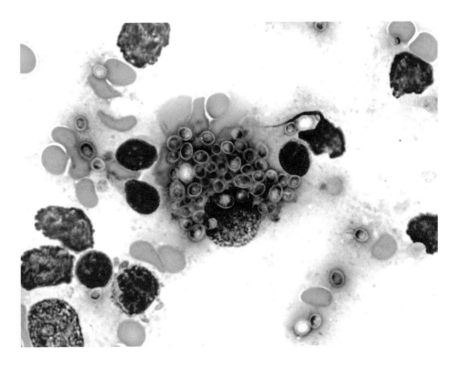

associated with an inflammatory response in kerions, characterized by macrophages, neutrophils, and eosinophils.

3.1.4.2 Clinical Considerations

- Cats > dogs.
- Caused by *Microsporum* and *Trichophyton* spp. [18]
- Mainly seen in young or immunocompromised patients [18].
- Classically present as circular regions of alopecia, often around the face and limbs. Raised nodules (kerions) may also be seen [19, 20].
- Zoonotic potential [21].

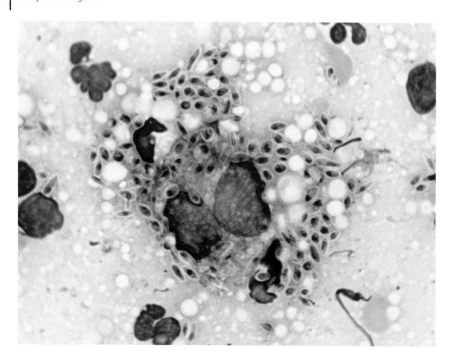

Figure 3.5 *Sporothrix schenkii*, cat, 100× objective. Organisms seen within and around a macrophage. Note their elongated, slender shape.

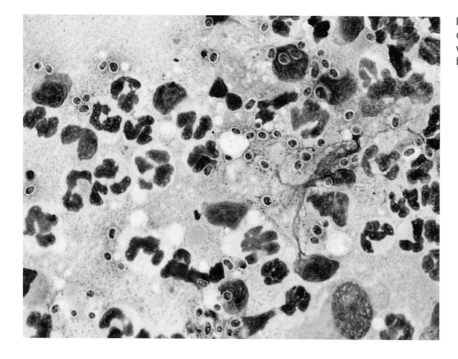

Figure 3.6 Dermatophytes, dog, 100× objective. Small basophilic organisms with a clear halo are noted in the background.

3.1.4.3 Prognosis

Good. Healthy animals usually clear infection within 3 months [19]. Prognosis may be worse in persistently immunocompromised patients.

3.1.5 *Blastomyces dermatitidis*

3.1.5.1 Cytologic Appearance

Organisms exfoliate variably well, ranging from single organisms, to abundant. They are ~10–20 μm in diameter, and round with a thick, refractile, deep-blue cell wall, but lack a capsule (compared to *Cryptococcus*) and divide via broad-based budding (Figure 3.7). Typically, they are associated with a mixed inflammatory response, with extracellular organisms (rarely phagocytosed by macrophages).

3.1.5.2 Clinical Considerations

- Dogs (typically large breed) >> cats.
- Pulmonary disease most prevalent [22]. Common extrapulmonary sites include skin, bone, lymph nodes, liver, and CNS [22, 23].

Figure 3.7 *Blastomyces dermatitidis*, dog, 100× objective.

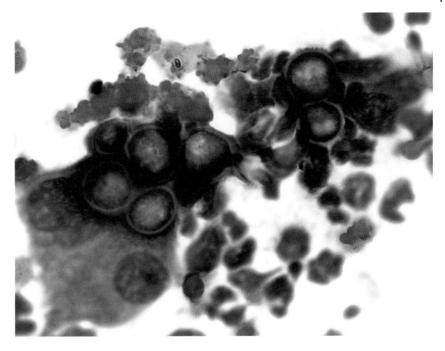

Figure 3.8 *Coccidioides immitis* spherule, dog, 50× objective. Note the large size relative to red blood cells and the folded capsule.

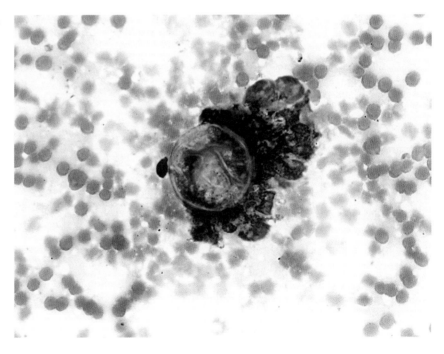

- Urine antigen testing has a high sensitivity for the diagnosis of active disease [24].

3.1.5.3 Prognosis
Variable. Cure rates range from 50% to 75%, and recurrence may occur [25, 26]. CNS involvement, severe pulmonary pathology, and disseminated disease confer a poor prognosis [25, 27].

3.1.6 Coccidioides

3.1.6.1 Cytologic Appearance
Coccidioides spherules generally are very large but range from 10 to 200 μm in diameter. The spherules have a thick, double-contoured wall that may fold on itself (Figure 3.8). Some spherules contain numerous small, spherical endospores (2–5 μm) (Figure 3.9). The size and presence of endospores make distinguishing *Coccidioides* spp. from

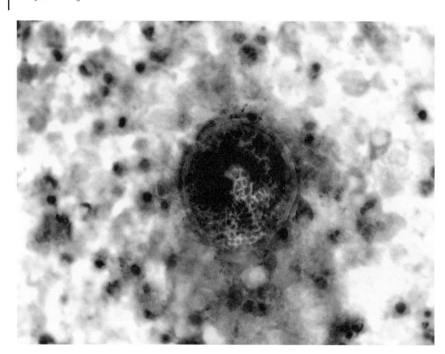

Figure 3.9 *Coccidioides immitis*, dog, 50× objective. Note the spherule containing numerous small endospores.

other fungal agents generally straightforward. They often are seen in low numbers, and incite a marked pyogranulomatous response.

3.1.6.2 Clinical Considerations
- Dogs > cats [28].
- Causative agent of Valley Fever.
- *Coccidioides immitis* and *Coccidioides posadasii* spp. [28]
- Primarily pulmonary disease ± bone, skin, ocular, or disseminated disease [28–30].

3.1.6.3 Prognosis
Response to therapy is variable based on location and extent of disease but is generally good with prompt therapy, especially for localized disease [28, 29]. Cats often have a good prognosis with prolonged therapy, though recurrence is common [28]. Dogs with intracranial coccidioidomycosis have a fair to good prognosis with appropriate therapy, and dogs with osteomyelitis may have a good prognosis with prolonged treatment [30, 31].

3.1.7 *Candida*

3.1.7.1 Cytologic Appearance
Candida spp. are budding yeast that can form long pseudohyphae (chains of yeast organisms), germ tubes, or true non-constricted hyphae, giving them a highly variable appearance (Figure 3.10). Neutrophils play a key role in defense against *Candida* spp. and usually predominate [32].

3.1.7.2 Clinical Considerations
- Dogs and cats.
- Common commensal in the gastrointestinal tract, urogenital tract, and skin.
- Disease may be localized or generalized and often is associated with predisposing disease or antimicrobial therapy [33, 34].

3.1.7.3 Prognosis
Generally good for localized infection, and with control of any underlying predisposing factors. Guarded prognosis for disseminated disease.

3.1.8 *Pneumocystis*

3.1.8.1 Cytologic Appearance
Cysts and trophozoites may be present in pulmonary secretions. Cysts are round, ~5 µm in diameter, and have clear cytoplasm with 1–2 µm round, purple inclusions, often arranged in a ring formation (Figures 3.11 and 3.12). Trophozoites are more variable in shape and range from 2 to 5 µm, often seen extracellularly. Often accompanied by granulomatous or eosinophilic inflammation.

3.1.8.2 Clinical Considerations
- Clinical disease in dogs. Subclinical disease reported rarely in cats.
- Dachshunds and Cavalier King Charles Spaniels overrepresented [35–37].

Figure 3.10 *Candida albicans*, dog, 100× objective, urine. Note the elongated germ tubes and chains of organisms forming pseudohyphae.

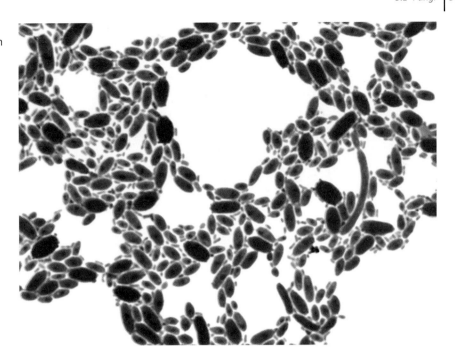

Figure 3.11 *Pneumocystis* spp., dog, 100× objective. Note the small size relative to the red blood cell and the small purple inclusions.

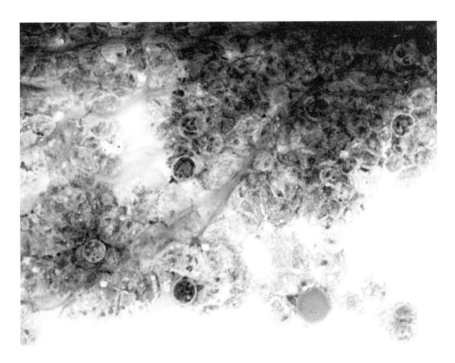

- Mostly seen in young or immunocompromised patients [35, 37].
- Clinical signs = exercise intolerance, cough, dyspnea, severe weight loss, and fever [35].

3.1.8.3 Prognosis

Guarded. Mortality rates are moderate to high, but survival possible with appropriate therapy, especially early in the disease [35]. Disseminated disease reported rarely and carries a poor prognosis [38].

3.1.9 *Malassezia*

3.1.9.1 Cytologic Appearance

Malassezia yeast stain intensely basophilic and are ovoid but divide via broad-based budding, frequently giving them a bilobed 'peanut' or 'snowman' appearance (Figure 3.13).

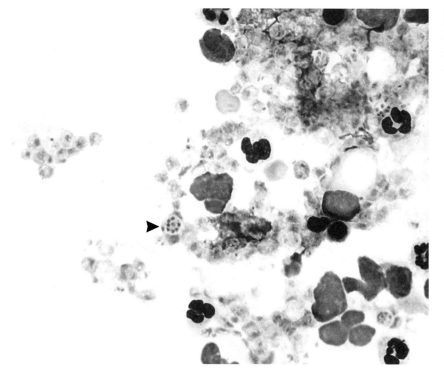

Figure 3.12 *Pneumocystis* spp., dog, 100× objective. The characteristic ring of purple inclusions is present in some organisms (arrowhead). Note also the neutrophilic inflammation.

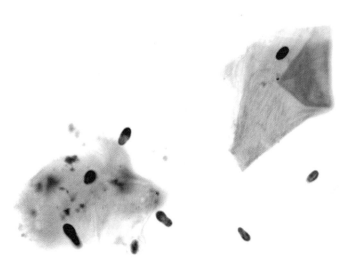

Figure 3.13 *Malassezia*, dog, 100× objective.

3.1.9.2 Clinical Considerations

- Dogs > cats.
- Commensal organisms of skin found in low numbers in healthy animals [39].
- Disease manifests mostly on the skin (periocular, perioral, inguinal region, and interdigital) and in the ears (otitis externa; see Chapter 15).
- Predisposing conditions include skin folds, hypersensitivity disorders, and endocrinopathies [39].

3.1.9.3 Prognosis

Good with appropriate therapy and treatment of any predisposing disorders.

3.1.10 *Cyniclomyces*

3.1.10.1 Cytologic Appearance
Cyniclomyces guttulatus are large (10–20 μm long and 5 μm wide), cylindrical yeast found individually or in forking chains (Figure 3.14). They have a clear cell wall and a centrally placed basophilic band.

3.1.10.2 Clinical Considerations
- Mostly an incidental finding in feces, resulting from coprophagia [40].
- Rarely found in urine, nasal cavity, bile, and bronchoalveolar lavage from a dog with aspiration pneumonia [40–42].
- Rare cases of chronic diarrhea linked to overgrowth of *Cyniclomyces*, though the organisms likely are opportunists rather than primary agents [43].

3.1.10.3 Prognosis
Excellent.

3.1.11 *Penicillium* spp.

3.1.11.1 Cytologic Appearance
Penicillium spp. are characterized by septate hyphae approximately 2–5 μm wide, which give rise to branched or unbranched conidiophores with secondary branching giving them a brush-like appearance (Figure 3.15). They may be associated with pyogranulomatous inflammation.

3.1.11.2 Clinical Considerations
- Saprophytic fungi, ubiquitous in the environment [44].
- Dogs > cats. German Shepherds predisposed [44, 45].
- Typically opportunistic infections in immunocompromised patients [44, 46].
- Disease may be localized (often in the nasal cavity, lungs, lymph nodes, and bone) or disseminated [44–48].

3.1.11.3 Prognosis
Guarded for localized disease depending on the area affected. Disseminated disease associated with a poor prognosis [44, 45, 48].

3.1.12 *Aspergillus*

3.1.12.1 Cytologic Appearance
Hyphae from *Aspergillus* spp. have parallel sides, are septate and branching, with branches mostly emanating at 45° angles (Figure 3.16). Fungal hyphae appear similar to other fungal diseases, and culture is required for definitive diagnosis.

3.1.12.2 Clinical Considerations
- Dogs and cats. German Shepherds predisposed [49, 50].
- Most common in the nasal cavity, but may affect any organ system (e.g., keratitis, otitis, or disseminated) [50].
- Nasal aspergillosis most common in dolichocephalic dog breeds.

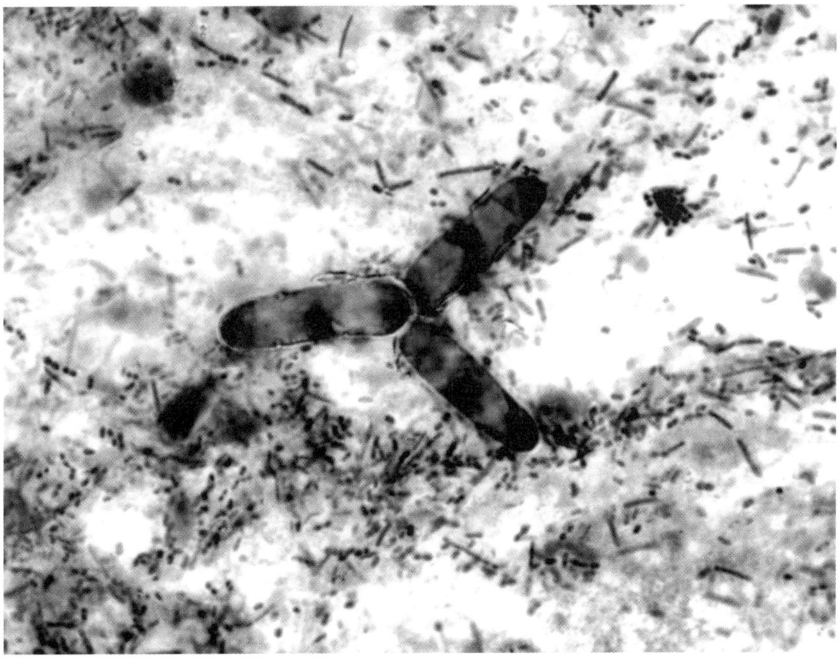

Figure 3.14 *Cyniclomyces guttulatus*, dog, 50× objective. Three organisms in a characteristic forking arrangement. Note the large size relative to bacteria in the background.

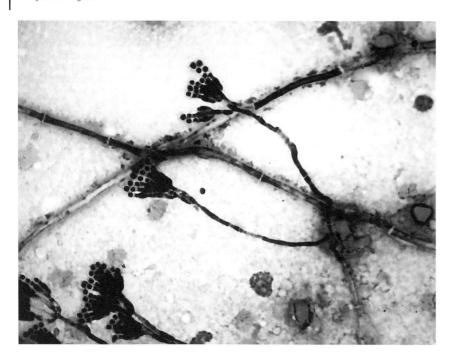

Figure 3.15 *Penicillium* spp., dog, 50× objective. Note the brush-like appearance of the branching conidiophores. Photo courtesy of Dr. Laura V. Lane.

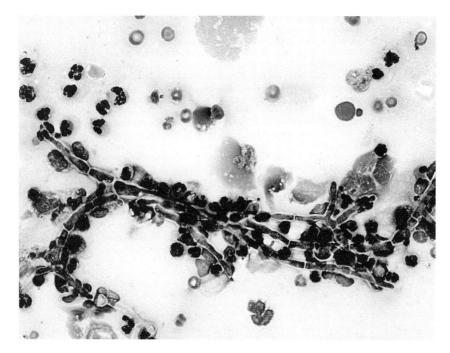

Figure 3.16 *Aspergillus* spp. hyphae, dog, 20× objective. Note the characteristic 45° angle branching of fungal hyphae.

3.1.12.3 Prognosis

Highly variable based on location and extent of disease, but often guarded with failure of treatment and relapse common [49]. Prognosis for disseminated disease is poor [50, 51].

3.1.13 Phaeohyphomycosis

3.1.13.1 Cytologic Appearance

Fungi that cause phaeohyphomycosis have variably pigmented cell walls, which can vary from blue/green to green/

brown; however, pigment may be absent. They are also recognized as ovoid to ellipsoid yeast or irregularly septate hyphae with nonparallel walls and irregular branching that may be seen singly or in chains. They often form prominent constrictions at septa, giving them a characteristic beaded (toruloid) appearance (Figure 3.17). They are often accompanied by pyogranulomatous inflammation. Fontana–Masson stains may be helpful to confirm melanin in lightly pigmented organisms, especially to differentiate these from cytologically similar fungi in the group hyalohyphomycosis

Figure 3.17 Phaeohyphomycosis, dog, 50× objective. The hyphae have a characteristic beaded (toruloid) appearance.

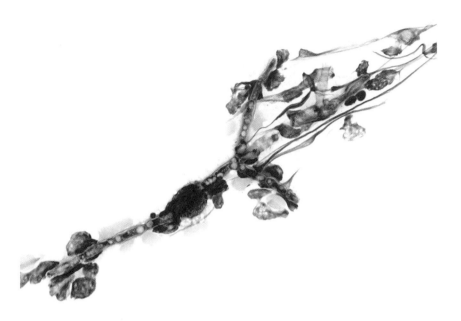

Figure 3.18 Phaeohyphomycosis, dog, 50× objective (same case as Figure 3.17). GMS stain highlighting the fungal hyphae.

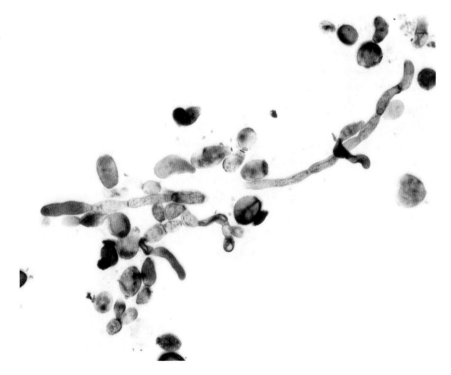

which lack pigment [52]. Grocott methenamine silver (GMS) stain can also be helpful in highlighting fungal organisms in cytologic samples (Figure 3.18).

3.1.13.2 Clinical Considerations

- Caused by a group of pigmented (dematiaceous) fungi that contain melanin in their cell walls [53].

- Fungal genera within this category include *Alternaria*, *Bipolaris*, *Cladophialophora*, *Curvularia*, *Fonsecaea*, and *Phialophora* among many others [52].
- Cats are usually immunocompetent, while dogs are usually immunocompromised [52, 54].
- Disease may be localized or disseminated. Localized lesions usually cutaneous, and commonly affect the

digits, pinnae, and nasal planum [53]. Disseminated disease more common in immunocompromised patients and may involve lymph nodes, CNS, liver, and kidneys [53, 55, 56].

3.1.13.3 Prognosis
Typically good for focal lesions with surgery and medical therapy [52]. Disseminated disease has a guarded prognosis [56], but immunocompetent patients may have a good prognosis with appropriate therapy [57].

3.2 Oomycetes

3.2.1 *Pythium insidiosum*

3.2.1.1 Cytologic Appearance
Hyphae are broad (~5 μm wide) with parallel walls, and stain poorly with routine stains (compared to *Aspergillus* spp.). They are branching and infrequently septate with rounded tapering ends (Figure 3.19). Infection frequently is associated with a marked pyogranulomatous inflammatory response that may include eosinophils.

3.2.1.2 Clinical Considerations
- Dogs >> cats [58].
- Gastrointestinal and cutaneous forms [58].
- Gastrointestinal pythiosis = focal or multifocal segmental thickening or granulomatous masses, most common at gastric outflow region or ileocecocolic junction [59].

- DDx = Lagenidiosis and Zygomycosis. Culture is required for a definitive diagnosis.

3.2.1.3 Prognosis
Guarded based on location and stage of disease. Surgical excision of lesions with wide margins may be curative. Non-resectable lesions carry a poor prognosis [60], but may respond to medical therapy [61]. Colonic pythiosis may respond well to medical therapy [59].

3.3 Algae

3.3.1 *Prototheca*

3.3.1.1 Cytologic Appearance
Prototheca are round to ovoid (width and length vary from 5 to 15 μm) with thick, clear cell walls and granular basophilic cytoplasm. Organisms may undergo endosporulation, forming multiple endospores within the cell wall (Figure 3.20). A granulomatous or mixed inflammatory response frequently is present.

3.3.1.2 Clinical Considerations
- Dogs > cats.
- *Prototheca zopfii* and *Prototheca wickerhamii* major pathogenic species in dogs [62, 63].
- Often associated with immunosuppression [62].
- Disease manifests in the skin (dogs and cats) or systemically (dogs), primarily affecting the gastrointestinal tract, CNS, and eyes [62, 64].

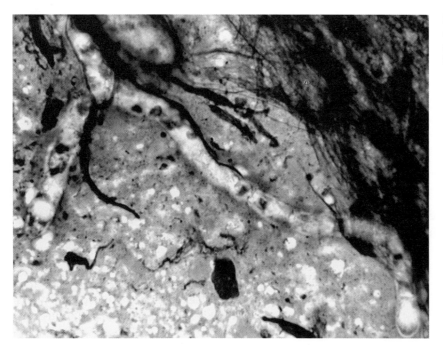

Figure 3.19 *Pythium insidiosum* hyphae, dog, 100× objective. Note the characteristic rounded tapering ends of the poorly staining hyphae.

Figure 3.20 *Prototheca*, dog, 100× objective. Slide courtesy of Dr. Ty McSherry.

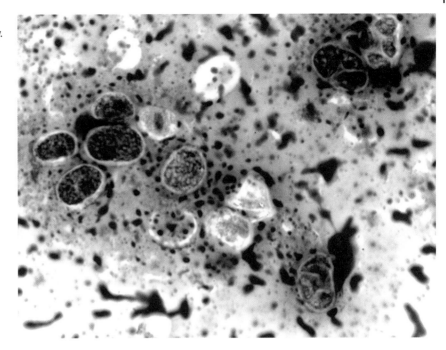

Figure 3.21 Diatoms, dog, 50× objective, bronchoalveolar lavage. The organisms are elongated with prominent capsular striations and internal organelles.

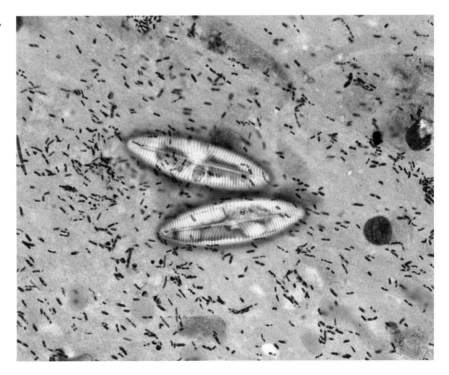

3.3.1.3 Prognosis

Surgical excision of cutaneous disease can be curative. Prognosis for disseminated disease in dogs is poor [65, 66].

3.3.2 Diatoms

3.3.2.1 Cytologic Appearance

Diatoms have highly variable morphology which is often geometric, and shapes range from fusiform, elongated, and rectangular to triangular or ovoid. They are clear to pale blue and are characterized by a nonstaining central core with emanating refractile capsular striations (Figure 3.21). Internal organelles (nucleus, mitochondria, and chromatophores) may be visible.

3.3.2.2 Clinical Considerations

- Unicellular algae found in freshwater, saltwater, and terrestrial environments [67, 68].

- Large numbers in pulmonary tissues may be an important marker of drowning or near drowning [69].
- Rare diatoms could represent contamination if tap water used to rinse slides during staining [68].

3.3.2.3 Prognosis
Guarded due to high rates of complication and mortality associated with cases of near drowning, especially in cats [70].

3.4 Mesomycetozoea

3.4.1 *Rhinosporidium seeberi*

3.4.1.1 Cytologic Appearance
Mature endospores are most commonly seen, which are round, 10–15 µm in diameter, with a thick cell wall and an intensely purple cytoplasm (Figure 3.22). Immature endospores are 2–4 µm in diameter, and stain pale pink with purple areas thought to represent nuclear material [71]. Large, round sporangia may be present that contain numerous endospores. Mixed inflammation is common.

3.4.1.2 Clinical Considerations
- Dogs >> cats. Most common in young-to-middle aged and large breed dogs [72].
- Unilateral > bilateral [72].
- Presents as a pale tumor-like mass in the nasal cavity, usually in the rostral third [72–74].
- Difficult to culture.

3.4.1.3 Prognosis
Good with surgical removal of polyps, though repeat surgery may be required [72, 74].

3.5 Protozoa

3.5.1 *Neospora caninum*

3.5.1.1 Cytologic Appearance
Tachyzoites of *N. caninum* are crescent or 'banana' shaped, ~5 µm long, and ~1 µm wide. They have pale purple cytoplasm and round pink/purple nuclei that may be centrally or eccentrically placed (Figure 3.23). They are cytologically indistinguishable from *Toxoplasma gondii*.

3.5.1.2 Clinical Considerations
- Dogs > cats. Dogs are the definitive host and cats may act as an intermediate host [75].
- Most common in young or immunocompromised animals [76].
- Neuromuscular signs most common (ataxia, tetraparesis, head tilt, and muscle atrophy). Cardiac, gastrointestinal, pulmonary, and cutaneous diseases may be seen [76, 77].
- PCR most reliable test to distinguish from *T. gondii*.

3.5.1.3 Prognosis
Variable based on severity and stage of disease. Recovery is less likely in peracute cases with severe clinical signs, and when therapy is delayed [77].

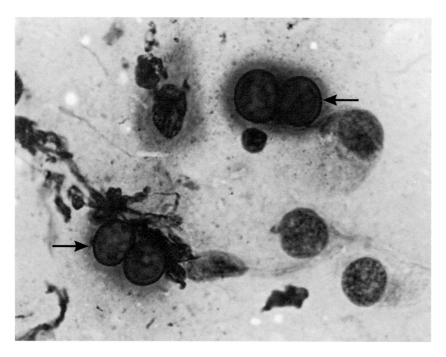

Figure 3.22 *Rhinosporidium seeberi* endospores (arrows), dog, 100× objective, nasal mass.

Figure 3.23 *Neospora caninum*, dog, 100× objective. Multiple crescent-shaped organisms present within neutrophils.

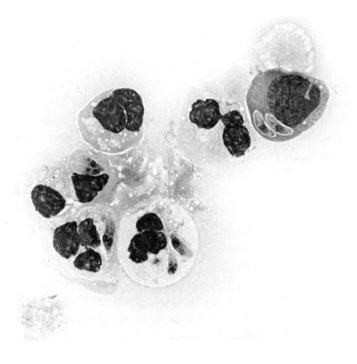

3.5.2 *Toxoplasma gondii*

3.5.2.1 Cytologic Appearance
Tachyzoites are cytologically similar to *Neospora caninum* and cannot be distinguished cytologically (compare Figures 3.24 and 3.23).

3.5.2.2 Clinical Considerations
- Cats > dogs. Cats are definitive host.

- Organ systems commonly affected include CNS, muscles, lungs, and eyes [78].
- Clinical signs = fever, retinitis, seizures, ataxia, and respiratory distress.
- Clinical disease more common in immunosuppressed patients (e.g., FIV+) [77–80].
- Zoonotic potential. *Note*: Cats with antibodies no longer shed oocysts in feces and neither are, nor will become, a zoonotic risk [78].

Figure 3.24 *Toxoplasma gondii*, dog, 100× objective. Three extracellular crescent-shaped organisms are accompanied by mixed inflammatory cells.

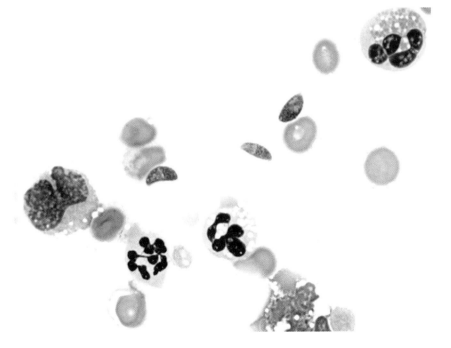

3.5.2.3 Prognosis

Variable, but mostly good. Most disease is subclinical. Appropriate therapy is successful in most patients. CNS involvement, especially in immunocompromised patients, carries a poor prognosis [81].

3.5.3 *Leishmania*

3.5.3.1 Cytologic Appearance

Leishmania amastigotes are small (~2–4 μm long, 1–2 μm wide), ovoid, and have pale cytoplasm with prominent, pink, round nuclei. A characteristic feature is a deep purple kinetoplast (a single large mitochondrion) that forms a right angle with the nucleus, often forming a 'T' shape (Figure 3.25). This is an important feature used to distinguish *Leishmania* spp. from other small infectious organisms. They induce mostly granulomatous inflammation.

3.5.3.2 Clinical Considerations

- Dogs > cats [82].
- Mostly affect skin, spleen, bone marrow, and lymph nodes [83].
- Clinical signs = lymphadenomegaly, splenomegaly, cutaneous lesions, ocular lesions, and onychodystrophy [82].
- Zoonotic potential.

3.5.3.3 Prognosis

Variable. High rates of full or partial remission and long survival times are possible with appropriate therapy [84].

Concurrent kidney disease and advanced stage of disease are poor prognostic markers [85].

3.5.4 *Cytauxzoon felis*

3.5.4.1 Cytologic Appearance

Tissue macrophages are distended by schizonts, which contain numerous small purple granular developing merozoites (Figure 3.26). Macrophages have a characteristic prominent nucleolus. Merozoites will then enter the circulation and infect red blood cells as characteristic ring-formed 'piroplasms.' These are small (~0.5–1 μm in diameter), round to signet-ring-shaped, intracellular organisms (Figure 3.27). They are mostly seen singly but can also be seen in pairs or tetrads. See also Chapter 17 for descriptions of cytauxzoonosis in blood.

3.5.4.2 Clinical Considerations

- Cats only.
- Schizonts most common in liver, spleen, lungs, lymph nodes, and blood [86, 87].
- Clinical signs = fever, jaundice, anemia, thrombocytopenia, and neurologic signs (including seizures) [86].
- PCR is highly sensitive for diagnosis and may be positive several days prior to clinical signs [88].

3.5.4.3 Prognosis

Guarded to poor and mortality rates are high, especially in untreated patients [89]. Some cats may survive with aggressive therapy [90]. Subclinical disease may occur in some cats [91].

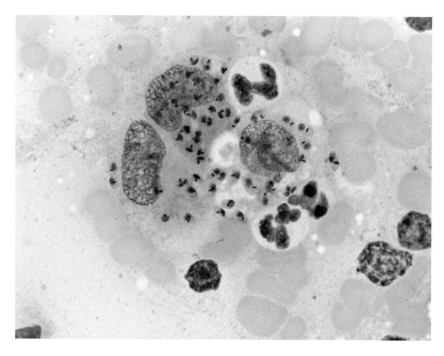

Figure 3.25 *Leishmania* spp., dog, 100× objective. Note the characteristic 'T' shape of the organisms.

Figure 3.26 *Cytauxzoon felis* schizont, cat, 100× objective. A large macrophage contains numerous mature merozoites, and an early schizont is present (lower right). Note the macrophage nuclei with their prominent nucleoli. Slide courtesy of Dr. Maggie McCourt.

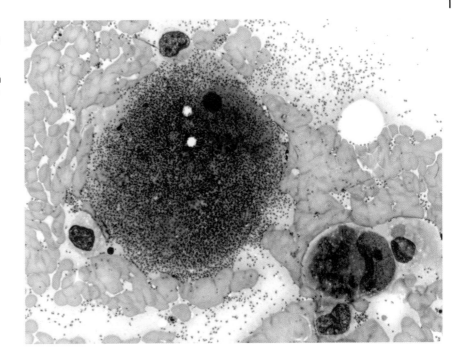

Figure 3.27 *Cytauxzoon felis*, cat, peripheral blood, 100× objective. Note the round piroplasms within the red blood cells (arrowheads).

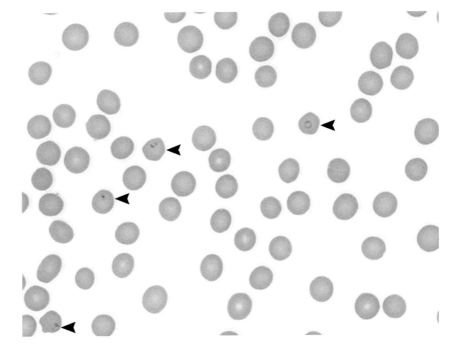

3.5.5 *Giardia*

3.5.5.1 Cytologic Appearance

Giardia spp. may be seen as either trophozoites or cysts in feces. Trophozoites are round to pear-shaped, ~10 μm in length, and have four pairs of flagella, making them highly motile. They have two nuclei, separated by a longitudinal axoneme (Figure 3.28). Cysts are ovoid, ~12 μm long and ~7 μm wide, and often have a folded or concave surface (Figure 3.29). When viewed in fresh fecal samples, *Giardia* spp. have a smooth, deliberate movement across the slide (compared to Trichomonads).

3.5.5.2 Clinical Considerations

- Common parasite in dogs and cats [92].
- Clinical signs = diarrhea (mucoid, pale, soft ± steatorrhea), and weight loss. Some infected patients may be asymptomatic [92].
- Zoonotic potential [92, 93].

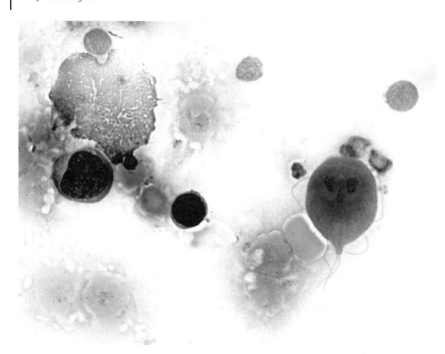

Figure 3.28 *Giardia lamblia* trophozoite, dog, 100× objective. Slide courtesy of Dr. Heather L. Wamsley.

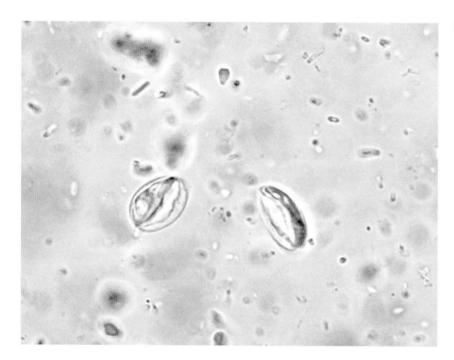

Figure 3.29 *Giardia lamblia* cysts, dog, 50× objective.

3.5.5.3 Prognosis
Good with appropriate therapy.

3.5.6 Trichomoniasis

3.5.6.1 Cytologic Appearance
Trichomonads are fusiform to pear-shaped organisms that have undulating membranes and flagella that make them highly motile (Figure 3.30). When fresh fecal samples are inspected, the movement of Trichomonads is more 'jerking' and random than that of *Giardia* spp., which is smooth and deliberate.

3.5.6.2 Clinical Considerations
- *Tritrichomonas foetus* (cats > dogs) and *Pentatrichomonas hominis* (dogs > cats).
- Many animals are asymptomatic carriers. Disease mostly seen in young animals [94].

Figure 3.30 *Tritrichomonas fetus*, cat, 100× objective, feces. Note the flagella and undulating membrane. Slide courtesy of Dr. Emily Walters.

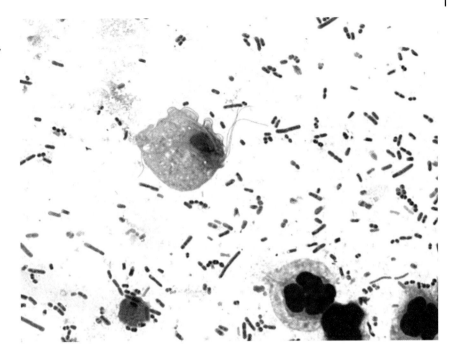

Figure 3.31 *Blastocystis* spp., dog, 50× objective, feces. Note the large central vacuoles and eccentric pink nuclei.

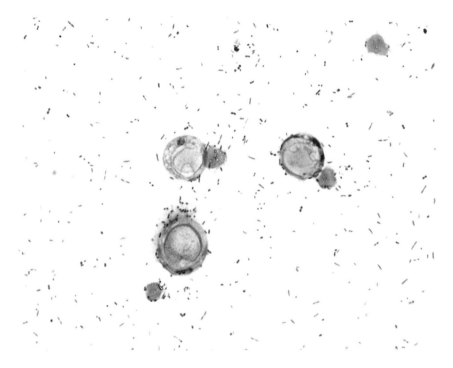

- Clinical signs = chronic diarrhea often with mucus and fresh blood [94, 95].
- PCR used for differentiation [96].

3.5.6.3 Prognosis

Excellent. Spontaneous resolution of disease secondary to *T. foetus* occurs in many cats but may take months [97].

3.5.7 Blastocystis

3.5.7.1 Cytologic Appearance

Blastocystis organisms are round, approximately 10–20 μm in diameter with pale-blue cytoplasm, and usually have a single, small, round, pink nucleus. The vacuolar form is most common, with a single large vacuole that pushes the cytoplasm and nucleus to the edge of the organism (Figure 3.31). Pink granular material may also be present within the vacuole.

3.5.7.2 Clinical Considerations

- Ubiquitous, unicellular protozoan of the gastrointestinal tract, common in dogs and cats [98, 99].
- Pathogenicity is uncertain [99, 100].
- Zoonotic potential [98].

3.5.7.3 Prognosis

Good.

3.5.8 *Cryptosporidium*

3.5.8.1 Cytologic Features

Cryptosporidium oocysts can be difficult to identify in feces, as they are colorless and small (~5 μm in diameter). Stained samples (with Romanowsky stains or Kinyoun acid-fast) highlight oocysts, which often appear 'crinkled' (Figure 3.32).

3.5.8.2 Clinical Considerations

- *Cryptosporidium canis* (dogs) and *Cryptosporidium felis* (cats) [101].
- Mostly subclinical infections. Clinical signs = watery diarrhea.
- Immunocompromised patients (e.g., FeLV+ cats) predisposed [102].
- Zoonotic potential (mainly in immunocompromised people) [101].

3.5.8.3 Prognosis

Mostly excellent. Investigation for underlying disease in clinical patients is recommended.

3.5.9 *Hepatozoon* spp.

3.5.9.1 Cytologic Appearance

Gamonts most frequently are seen in blood, and also rarely in cytologic samples from tissues. These are ovoid, ~8–11 μm long, and ~4 μm wide, mostly seen phagocytosed by leukocytes (Figure 3.33). They stain pale blue or may be negatively staining. Nuclei are variably visible. *Hepatozoon canis* gamonts are slightly larger than those of *Hepatozoon americanum* but cannot be reliably distinguished by cytology [103]. Evaluation of buffy coat smears increases the sensitivity of detection, especially for *H. americanum* where gamonts are usually present in low numbers [104].

3.5.9.2 Clinical Considerations

- Dogs > cats.
- *H. canis* and *H. americanum* (dogs); *Hepatozoon felis*, *Hepatozoon silvestris*, and *H. canis* (cats) [104].
- Affected tissues include skeletal muscle and bone (*H. americanum*); spleen, bone marrow, lymph nodes, liver, kidney, lungs ± bone (*H. canis*); skeletal and cardiac muscle (*H. felis, H. silvestris*). Affected tissues include skeletal muscle and bone (*H. americanum*); spleen, bone marrow, lymph nodes ± bone (*H. canis*) [104, 105].
- Clinical signs: Subclinical infection common with *H. canis* in dogs and *H. felis* in cats [104, 106]. *H. canis* = Lethargy, lymphadenomegaly, splenomegaly. *H. americanum* = Musculoskeletal signs (altered gait, weakness, and muscle atrophy), pyrexia, ocular discharge [104, 105].

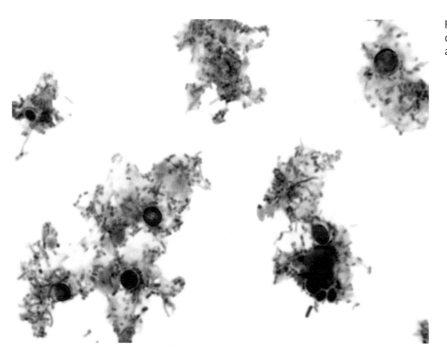

Figure 3.32 *Cryptosporidium canis* oocysts, dog, 100× objective, Kinyoun acid-fast stain.

Figure 3.33 *Hepatozoon americanum*, dog, peripheral blood, 100× objective.

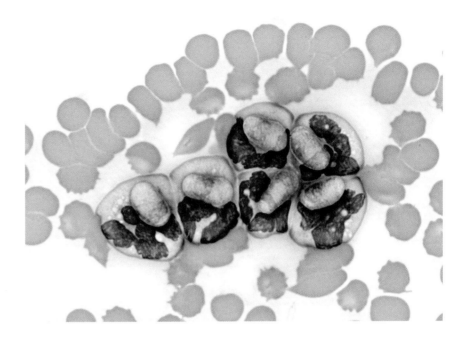

3.5.9.3 Prognosis

Short- and long-term control can be achieved with appropriate therapy [107]. Relapse may occur with *H. americanum*, and persistent infections may carry a more guarded prognosis due to complications from amyloidosis, glomerulopathy, and vasculitis [104, 108].

3.6 Helminths

3.6.1 *Mesocestoides*

3.6.1.1 Cytologic Appearance

Parasites are mostly detected in peritoneal fluid, which has a characteristic flocculent gross appearance with yellow particulate matter (Figure 3.34). Larvae and their fragments are large (200–2000 μm), tubular/verminous with deep blue cytoplasm, and often clear/tan refractile structures (~10 μm) that are calcareous corpuscles (calcium deposits unique to cestodes) (Figure 3.35). Rarely, tetrathyridia – the asexual reproductive form which has round parasitic suckers – may be present.

3.6.1.2 Clinical Considerations
- Dogs > > cats.
- Usually causes peritonitis but can be found in organs (liver and lymph node) [109].
- Clinical signs = ascites, anorexia/weight loss, and vomiting [110, 111].

3.6.1.3 Prognosis

Guarded. Aggressive therapy is required for a positive outcome [110, 111].

3.6.2 *Filaroides hirthi*

3.6.2.1 Cytologic Appearance

Larvae are large (~250–300 μm in length, ~15 μm wide), verminous, and tightly coiled. They stain pale blue, with basophilic internal organs. Concurrent inflammation is usually neutrophilic or eosinophilic (Figure 3.36).

3.6.2.2 Clinical Considerations
- Dogs.
- Immunosuppressed patients at increased risk [112].
- Clinical signs = cough and dyspnea.
- Peripheral eosinophilia inconsistently reported [112].
- DDx = *Oslerus osleri*, which appear similar, but have a kinked distal tail.

3.6.2.3 Prognosis

Generally good to excellent.

3.6.3 *Aelurostrongylus abstrusus*

3.6.3.1 Cytologic Appearance

Larvae are large (~400 μm long, ~20 μm wide), verminous, pale purple to unstained, and often tightly coiled on

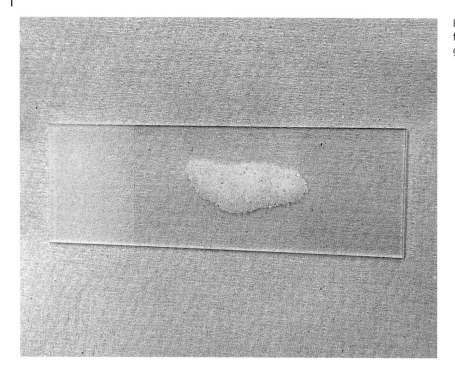

Figure 3.34 *Mesocestoides*, abdominal fluid gross appearance, dog. Note the granular texture of the fluid.

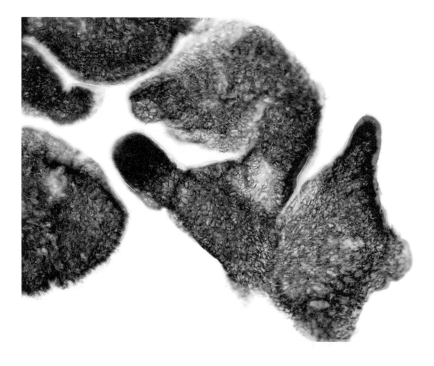

Figure 3.35 *Mesocestoides*, abdominal fluid, dog, 20× objective. Note the refractile, clear-to-tan calcareous corpuscles.

themselves. Characteristic features include a dorsal spine, and a short, kinked tail (Figure 3.37).

3.6.3.2 Clinical Considerations
- Cats.
- Animals may be asymptomatic. Clinical signs = cough, nasal discharge, and dyspnea [113].

- Disease more pronounced in young or immunosuppressed patients [114].

3.6.3.3 Prognosis
Generally good to excellent, with mortality and uncommon outcomes [113].

Figure 3.36 *Filaroides hirthi*, dog, 50× objective.

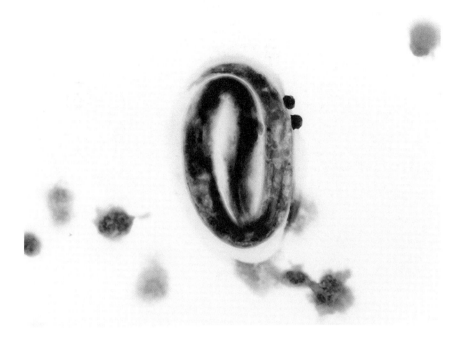

Figure 3.37 *Aelurostrongylus abstrusus*, cat, 50× objective. Note the prominent dorsal spine down the center.

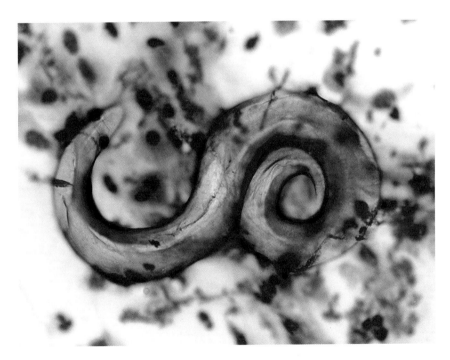

3.6.4 *Dracunculus*

3.6.4.1 Cytologic Appearance
Larvae are ~500 μm in length and ~25 μm wide and have a characteristic whip-like tail (Figure 3.38). Often accompanied by a marked neutrophilic/eosinophilic inflammatory response.

3.6.4.2 Clinical Considerations
- Dogs > cats [115].

- Associated with subcutaneous nodules that may be pruritic and form fistulae [116].
- Lesions most common on distal extremities, and also reported on the head, chest, abdomen, and flank [115].
- Infection most common between late winter and early spring [115].

3.6.4.3 Prognosis
Excellent.

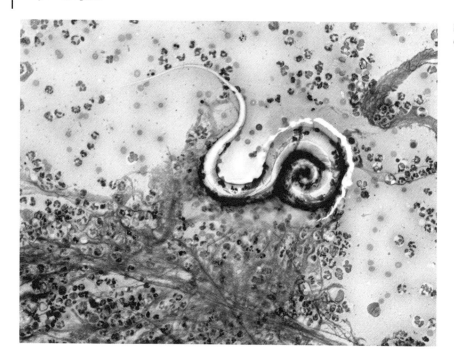

Figure 3.38 *Dracunculus*, dog, 20× objective.

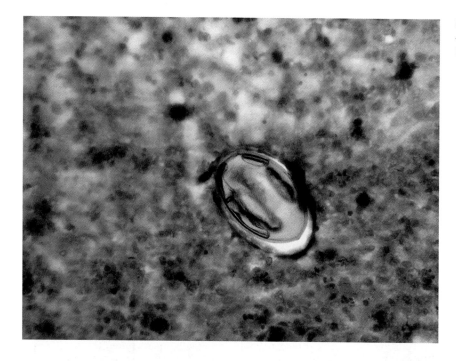

Figure 3.39 *Paragonimus kellicotti*, cat, 40× objective. Photo courtesy of Drs. Michelle Plier and Lon Rich.

3.6.5 *Paragonimus*

3.6.5.1 Cytologic Appearance

Paragonimus ova are most frequently encountered in either lung aspirates or feces. They are ovoid, ~100 μm in length and ~50 μm wide, tan-colored, and often have thick ridges (Figure 3.39). A unipolar operculum may be observed.

3.6.5.2 Clinical Considerations

- Cats > dogs.
- *Paragonimus kellicotti* most common [117].
- Infection may be asymptomatic, but may cause respiratory signs of cough, dyspnea, nasal discharge, or rarely pneumothorax [117–119].

- Ova may be detected in respiratory washes, fecal sedimentation, or less commonly aspiration of lung nodules [120, 121].

3.6.5.3 Prognosis
Good with appropriate therapy [117–119].

3.7 Bacteria

3.7.1 Mycobacteria

3.7.1.1 Cytologic Appearance
Mycobacterium spp. do not stain with routine stains (due to high concentrations of mycolic acid in their cell walls) and appear as clear to refractile, rod-shaped organisms that may be found within macrophages, or scattered across the background of the sample (Figures 3.40 and 3.41) [122]. They induce a mostly granulomatous inflammatory response.

3.7.1.2 Clinical Considerations
- Dogs and cats [122, 123].
- Aerobic, Gram-positive, acid-fast bacilli (Figure 3.42) [123].
- Numerous *Mycobacterium* spp. exist that cause different diseases. Infections may affect skin, lymph nodes, respiratory tract, gastrointestinal tract, bone, or be disseminated [122–124].

- Zoonotic potential for some mycobacterial species [123, 125].

3.7.1.3 Prognosis
Variable based on organ involvement and severity of disease. Disseminated disease is associated with a poor prognosis [123].

3.7.2 *Actinomyces/Nocardia*

3.7.2.1 Cytologic Appearance
Actinomyces and *Nocardia* spp. are cytologically similar, appearing as slender, filamentous bacteria with characteristic branching (Figure 3.43). They are lightly basophilic and have red, beaded areas. They may be seen in macrophages or extracellularly, and occasionally in large bacterial mats. They are mostly accompanied by a granulomatous or pyogranulomatous inflammatory response.

3.7.2.2 Clinical Considerations
- Dogs and cats. Actinomycosis more common than nocardiosis.
- Both Gram-positive. *Nocardia* spp. are variably acid-fast positive [126].
- Subcutaneous masses with draining lesions and pulmonary disease most common [127]. Disseminated disease may occur, especially in immunocompromised patients [126].

Figure 3.40 *Mycobacteria* spp., cat, 100× objective. A macrophage contains numerous clear, rod-shaped bacteria.

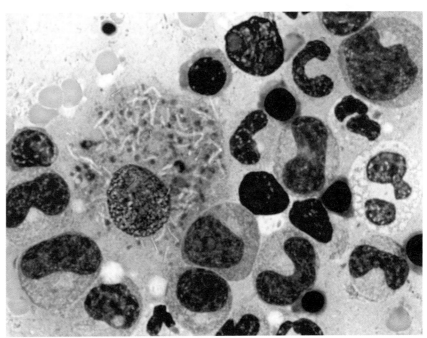

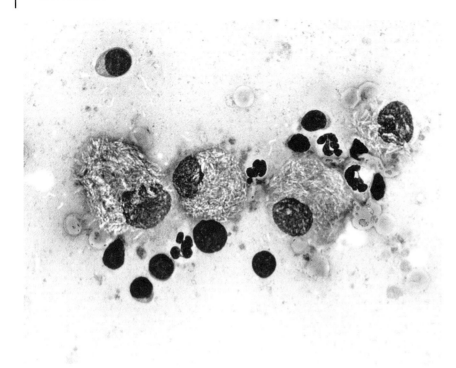

Figure 3.41 *Mycobacteria* spp., dog, 100× objective. Macrophages are distended with slender, negatively staining bacterial rods that are also seen in the background.

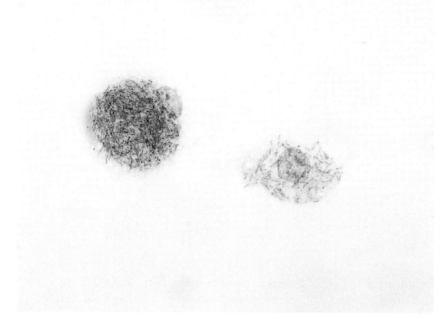

Figure 3.42 *Mycobacteria* spp., dog, 100× objective, acid-fast stain (same case as Figure 3.41). Note the bright-pink positive staining of organisms within macrophages.

3.7.2.3 Prognosis

Actinomycosis has a good prognosis with appropriate therapy [128, 129]. Nocardiosis is more commonly associated with underlying immunosuppression, and overall carries a poorer prognosis [130, 131].

3.7.3 *Bordetella bronchiseptica*

3.7.3.1 Cytologic Appearance

B. bronchiseptica may be seen as coccobacilli adhered to cilia and interciliary spaces of respiratory epithelial

Figure 3.43 *Actinomyces* spp., cat, 100× objective. Note the long, fine, branching filamentous bacteria.

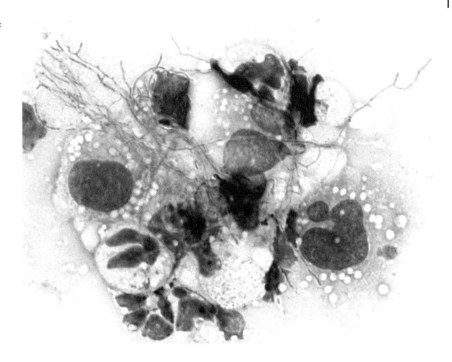

Figure 3.44 *Bordetella bronchiseptica*, dog, 100× objective. Note the basophilic coccobacilli adhered to the cilia of the columnar respiratory epithelial cells.

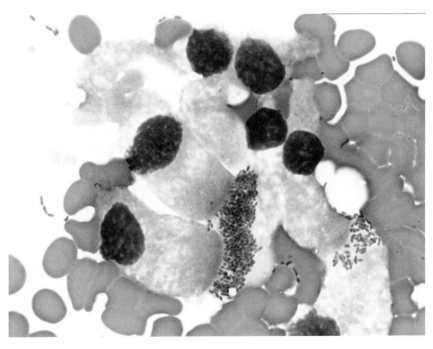

cells (Figure 3.44). They mostly induce a neutrophilic response, but mononuclear inflammation may predominate [132].

3.7.3.2 Clinical Considerations
- Dogs and cats. More prevalent in young and group-housed animals [133].
- Clinical signs = productive hacking cough, lethargy, fever ± serous or seromucous nasal discharge [134].

- Cytologic identification of bacteria more likely to diagnose infection than microbial culture, but quantitative PCR is the best diagnostic test [132].
- Zoonotic potential, but rare [135].

3.7.3.3 Prognosis
Good to excellent with appropriate therapy. Mild/uncomplicated cases may be self-limiting. Severe cases may, however, be fatal [134, 136].

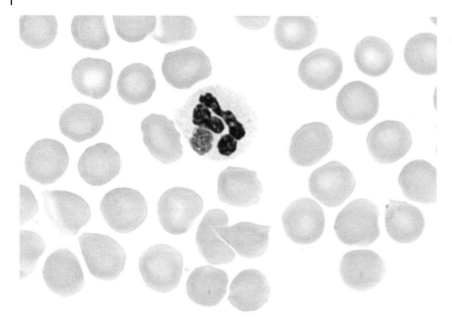

Figure 3.45 *Anaplasma phagocytophilum*, dog, 100× objective. A morula of basophilic staining organisms is seen within a neutrophil.

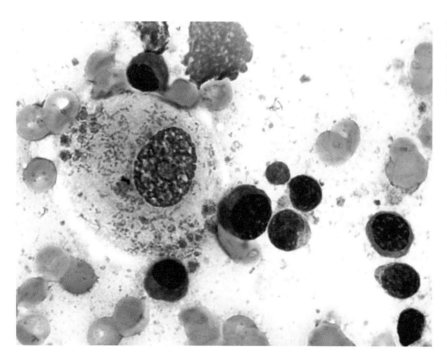

Figure 3.46 *Neorickettsia helminthoeca* (salmon poisoning disease), lymph node, dog, 100× objective. A macrophage contains many small blue/gray curvilinear organisms that are also seen in the background.

3.7.4 Rickettsial Bacteria

3.7.4.1 Cytologic Appearance

Rickettsial bacteria form morulae (round aggregates of bacteria) within phagosomes of leukocytes (Figure 3.45). They most commonly are seen in circulating leukocytes but may also be seen in joint fluid or organs (see Chapter 7). *Ehrlichia canis* infects monocytes and lymphocytes, while *Ehrlichia ewingii* and *Anaplasma phagocytophilum* infect granulocytes [137]. *Neorickettsia helminthoeca* is the causative agent of salmon poisoning disease and is seen in lymph node aspirates of affected dogs (see Figure 3.46 and Chapter 5).

3.7.4.2 Clinical Considerations

- Gram-negative, intracellular bacteria.
- Dogs >> cats. *N. helminthoeca* infects dogs only.
- Clinical signs = lethargy, fever, lymphadenopathy, neurologic signs, and polyarthropathy [137, 138].

- Hematologic changes = thrombocytopenia, neutrophilia (*A. phagocytophilum*, *E. ewingii*), neutropenia (*E. canis*), and anemia [138].

3.7.4.3 Prognosis

Generally good with appropriate therapy. Severe acute cases of *E. canis* and *N. helminthoeca* have a guarded prognosis [138, 139].

3.7.5 *Clostridium* spp.

3.7.5.1 Cytologic Appearance

Clostridium spp. (*Clostridium perfringens* and *Clostridium difficile*) are rod-shaped bacteria that often have a characteristic 'safety pin' appearance due to the presence of endospores (Figure 3.47). The presence of even large numbers of these bacteria in fecal samples does not correlate with disease or toxin production, and while they may raise suspicion of *Clostridium* spp. diarrhea, further testing is recommended [140].

3.7.5.2 Clinical Considerations

- Gram-positive, spore-forming, anaerobic rods.
- Commensal bacteria in the gastrointestinal tract of dogs and cats. Overgrowth and toxin production associated with disease [140].
- Clinical signs = diarrhea, lethargy, and anorexia ± vomiting [141].

3.7.5.3 Prognosis

Generally good, but severe disease can be life threatening [140, 141].

Figure 3.47 *Clostridium perfringens*, dog, 100× objective. Note the characteristic clear spores in the bacteria giving them a 'safety pin' appearance.

3.7.6 *Campylobacter* spp.

3.7.6.1 Cytologic Appearance

Campylobacter spp. are thin, curved to spiral bacteria that often have a characteristic 'gull-wing' shape when seen in fecal samples (Figure 3.48). The presence of such bacteria is suggestive of campylobacteriosis; however, further diagnostics are warranted as non-pathologic spiral bacteria may appear similar.

3.7.6.2 Clinical Considerations

- Dogs and cats, mostly affect young patients.
- Isolated from feces of normal and diseased animals [140, 142].
- Clinical signs = diarrhea, lethargy, and anorexia ± vomiting [140].
- Zoonotic potential [143].

3.7.6.3 Prognosis

Good to excellent with appropriate therapy. Mild/uncomplicated cases generally are self-limiting.

3.7.7 *Helicobacter* spp.

3.7.7.1 Cytologic Appearance

Helicobacter-like organisms are long (5–10 μm), tightly spiral-shaped bacteria that mostly are thicker than other spiral-shaped bacteria, and have a textured basophilic appearance. Infection may be accompanied by inflammatory cells (Figure 3.49).

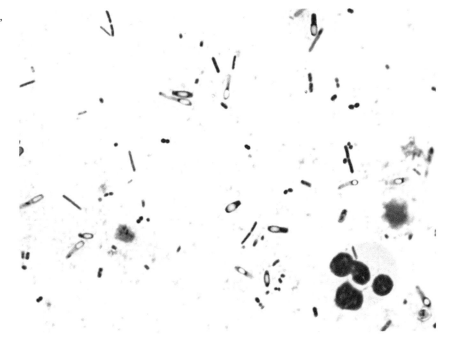

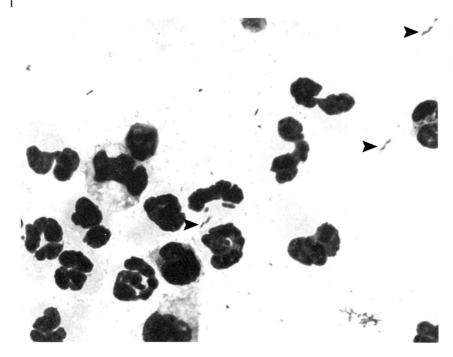

Figure 3.48 *Campylobacter* spp., dog, 100× objective. Note the small, 'gull-wing' or 'M'-shaped bacteria (arrowheads) accompanied by neutrophilic inflammation.

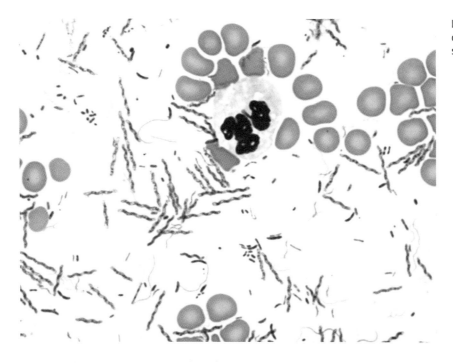

Figure 3.49 *Helicobacter* spp., dog, 100× objective. Note the large size and tight spirals.

3.7.7.2 Clinical Considerations

- Gram-negative, microaerophilic, spiral-shaped bacteria.
- *H. pylori* (an important gastric pathogen in humans) is extremely rare in cats and dogs [144]. Other *Helicobacter* spp. are common in dogs and cats [145].
- Clinical signs = chronic intermittent vomiting, inappetence, pica, and weight loss [146]. *Note*: The majority of dogs and cats with infection are asymptomatic, and strong evidence for *Helicobacter* spp. as a primary pathogen is lacking.
- Associated with gastric lymphofollicular hyperplasia in dogs [147].

3.7.7.3 Prognosis

Good with appropriate therapy, but recurrence of infection can be high [148].

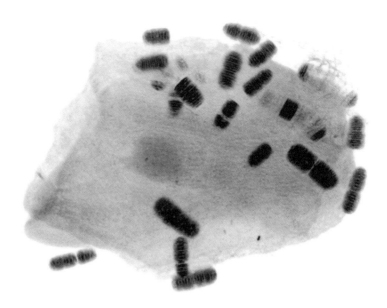

Figure 3.50 *Simonsiella*-like bacteria, dog, 100× objective. Bacteria are present in characteristic linear stacks.

3.7.8 *Simonsiella*-like Bacteria

3.7.8.1 Cytologic Appearance
Simonsiella-like bacteria are large, rod-shaped bacteria that align in rows after division, and have a characteristic, stacked appearance (Figure 3.50).

3.7.8.2 Clinical Considerations
- Rod-shaped, Gram-negative commensals of the oropharynx, gastrointestinal tract, and conjunctiva [149].
- *Simonsiella*-like bacteria belong to three genera of the Neisseriaceae family (*Simonsiella, Conchiformibius,* and *Alysiella*) collectively referred to as multicellular longitudinally dividing (MuLDi) Neisseriaceae [149].
- Incidental finding.
- Their presence is a hallmark of oropharyngeal contamination of airway samples (see Chapter 11).

3.7.8.3 Prognosis
Excellent.

3.8 Ectoparasites

3.8.1 Myiasis

3.8.1.1 Cytologic Appearance
Cases of myiasis associated with *Cuterebra* spp. larvae contain a heterogeneous mixture of cells, cellular debris, and often cylindrical, spiraled tubular, and branching structures representing fragments of larval bronchial tree (Figures 3.51 and 3.52). Variably intact cells may be present that are large (70–120 μm diameter) with ropey chromatin and prominent nucleoli (Figure 3.52) [150]. An inflammatory process is also commonly present, including increased eosinophils, neutrophils, and macrophages. Conical to hook-shaped spines (cuticular spines) may also be seen in cytology samples [151].

3.8.1.2 Clinical Considerations
- Cats and dogs [152].
- Caused by Diptera larvae, most commonly associated with *Cuterebra* spp. [153].
- Infestation most frequent in late summer months [153].
- Cutaneous/subcutaneous form most common, frequently around the head, neck, shoulders, or thorax [152, 153].
- Lesions form a mass or nodule (warble), often with a central hole/pore that may ooze purulent material, and larvae may be seen through this pore.
- Aberrant migration may affect CNS (feline ischemic encephalitis in cats), respiratory tract, and eyes, among other sites [152, 154–156].

3.8.1.3 Prognosis
Good prognosis for localized cutaneous lesions with careful surgical extraction of larvae. Mortality may occur with systemic disease and appears more common in dogs than cats [152], and brain involvement carries a grave prognosis [154].

3.8.2 *Demodex* spp.

3.8.2.1 Cytologic Appearance
Demodex spp. are elongated (cigar-shaped), with four pairs of short legs grouped in the podosoma region (Figure 3.53). Adults typically are 150–250 μm in length, while nymphs

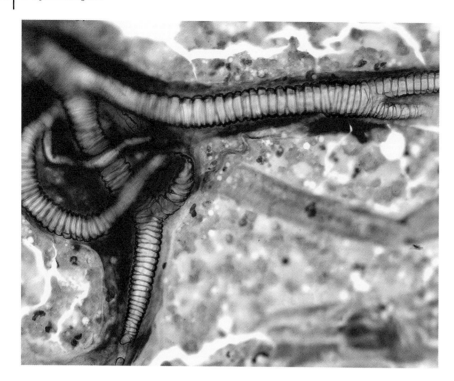

Figure 3.51 *Cuterebra* spp., cat, 20×
objective. Note the branching, annular
structures (parasitic bronchial tree).

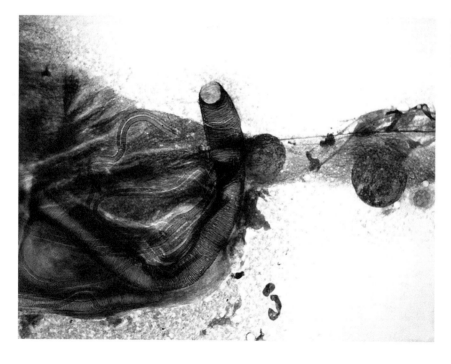

Figure 3.52 *Cuterebra* spp., cat, 20×
objective. Note the cylindrical, circular
bronchial tree fragments, and cells with
large nuclei and ropey chromatin.

are shorter. Deep skin scrapes or hair plucks usually are
required to find mites.

3.8.2.2 Clinical Considerations
- Dogs > cats.
- Local (four or fewer lesions) or generalized disease may
  be seen. Generalized disease in adults is mostly associated with immunosuppression [157, 158].

- Predilection sites = face, ventrum, and limbs [158].
- Skin is crusted, alopecic (often symmetrical), thickened,
  or hyperpigmented.

3.8.2.3 Prognosis
Good to excellent with appropriate therapy. Investigation
for concurrent disease is warranted for generalized disease
in dogs aged >18 months [157].

Figure 3.53 *Demodex canis* nymph, dog, 50× objective.

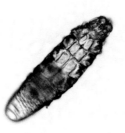

Figure 3.54 *Sarcoptes scabii*, dog, 20× objective.

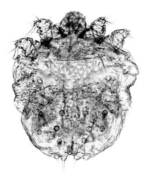

3.8.3 *Sarcoptes scabiei*

3.8.3.1 Cytologic Appearance

These mites are circular (200–600 μm in diameter, with females twice as large as males), and have two pairs of legs at their anterior portion and two pairs at the posterior portion that do not extend beyond the body margin (Figure 3.54).

3.8.3.2 Clinical Considerations

- Dogs > cats.
- Young dogs most susceptible [157].
- Predilection sites = limbs (especially elbow and hock), pinnae, and ventral abdomen.
- Lesions are intensely pruritic and vary from papules to thick crusts with poor hair condition [158].

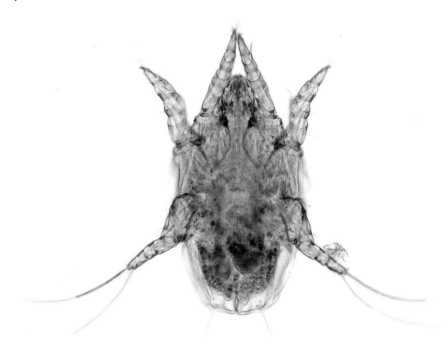

Figure 3.55 *Otodectes cynotis*, dog, 20× objective.

3.8.3.3 Prognosis
Excellent.

3.8.4 *Otodectes cynotis*

3.8.4.1 Cytologic Appearance
Adult mites range from 250 to 450 μm in length (females are larger than males). They have two anterior and two posterior pairs of legs (Figure 3.55). Eggs often are also present that are ovoid and ~200 μm long (see Chapter 15, Figure 15.19).

3.8.4.2 Clinical Considerations
- Common primary cause of otitis externa in cats and dogs [159].
- Clinical signs = head shaking, ear scratching, and ear droop [158].
- May be accompanied by neutrophilic inflammation and ceruminous, black, and granular discharge [158].

3.8.4.3 Prognosis
Excellent.

References

1 Trivedi, S.R., Malik, R., Meyer, W., *et al.* (2011) Feline cryptococcosis: impact of current research on clinical management. *J. Feline. Med. Surg.*, **13** (3), 163–172.

2 Cooley, S., Galustanian, G., Moon, A., *et al.* (2022) CT findings of nasal cryptococcosis in cats and dogs: a case series. *Vet. Radiol. Ultrasound*, **63** (4), 422–429.

3 Myers, A., Meason-Smith, C., Mansell, J., *et al.* (2017) Atypical cutaneous cryptococcosis in four cats in the USA. *Vet. Dermatol.*, **28** (4), 405-e97.

4 O'Brien, C.R., Krockenberger, M.B., Martin, P., *et al.* (2006) Long-term outcome of therapy for 59 cats and 11 dogs with cryptococcosis. *Aust. Vet. J.*, **84** (11), 384–392.

5 Duncan, C., Stephen, C., Campbell, J. (2006) Clinical characteristics and predictors of mortality for *Cryptococcus gattii* infection in dogs and cats of southwestern British Columbia. *Can. Vet. J.*, **47** (10), 993–998.

6 Sykes, J.E., Sturges, B.K., Cannon, M.S., *et al.* (2010) Clinical signs, imaging features, neuropathology, and outcome in cats and dogs with central nervous system cryptococcosis from California. *J. Vet. Intern. Med.*, **24** (6), 1427–1438.

7 McGill, S., Malik, R., Saul, N., *et al.* (2009) Cryptococcosis in domestic animals in Western Australia: a retrospective study from 1995–2006. *Med. Mycol.*, **47** (6), 625–639.

8 Wilson, A.G., KuKanich, K.S., Hanzlicek, A.S., *et al.* (2018) Clinical signs, treatment and prognostic factors for dogs with histoplasmosis. *J. Am. Vet. Med. Assoc.*, **252** (2), 201–209.

9 Aulakh, H.K., Aulakh, K.S., Troy, G.C. (2012) Feline histoplasmosis: a retrospective study of 22 cases (1986-2009). *J. Am. Anim. Hosp. Assoc.*, **48** (3), 182–187.

10 Davies, C., Troy, G.C. (1996) Deep mycotic infections in cats. *J. Am. Anim. Hosp. Assoc.*, **32** (5), 380–391.

11 Brömel, C., Sykes, J.E. (2005) Histoplasmosis in dogs and cats. *Clin. Tech. Small Anim. Pract.*, **20** (4), 227–232.

12 Gremião, I.D.F., Martins da Silva da Rocha, E., *et al.* (2021) Guideline for the management of feline sporotrichosis caused by *Sporothrix brasiliensis* and literature revision. *Braz. J. Microbiol.*, **52** (1), 107–124.

13 Gremião, I.D., Menezes, R.C., Schubach, T.M., *et al.* (2015) Feline sporotrichosis: epidemiological and clinical aspects. *Med. Mycol.*, **53** (1), 15–21.

14 Crothers, S.L., White, S.D., Ihrke, P.J., *et al.* (2009) Sporotrichosis: a retrospective evaluation of 23 cases seen in northern California (1987–2007). *Vet. Dermatol.*, **20** (4), 249–259.

15 Pereira, S.A., Passos, S.R., Silva, J.N., *et al.* (2010) Response to azolic antifungal agents for treating feline sporotrichosis. *Vet. Rec.*, **166** (10), 290–294.

16 Schubach, T.M., Schubach, A., Okamoto, T., *et al.* (2006) Canine sporotrichosis in Rio de Janeiro, Brazil: clinical presentation, laboratory diagnosis and therapeutic response in 44 cases (1998–2003). *Med. Mycol.*, **44** (1), 87–92.

17 Caruso, K.J., Cowell, R.L., Cowell, A.K., *et al.* (2002) What is your diagnosis? Skin scraping from a cat. *Vet. Clin. Pathol.*, **31** (1), 13–15.

18 Long, S., Carveth, H., Chang, Y.M., *et al.* (2020) Isolation of dermatophytes from dogs and cats in the South of England between 1991 and 2017. *Vet. Rec.*, **187** (10), e87. doi: 10.1136/vr.105957. Last accessed October 15, 2023.

19 Frymus, T., Gruffydd-Jones, T., Grazia Pennisi, M., *et al.* (2013) Dermatophytosis in cats: ABCD guidelines on prevention and management. *J. Feline. Med. Surg.*, **15** (7), 598–604.

20 Logan, M.R., Raskin, R.E., Thompson, S. (2006) 'Carry-on' dermal baggage: a nodule from a dog. Pyogranulomatous inflammation with intralesional fungal agents. *Vet. Clin. Pathol.*, **35** (3), 329–331.

21 Moskaluk, A.E., VandeWoude, S. (2022) Current topics in Dermatophyte classification and clinical diagnosis. *Pathogens*, **11** (9), 957. doi: 10.3390/pathogens11090957. Last accessed October 15, 2023.

22 Marin, J.K., Savage, M.Y., Adley, B.D., *et al.* (2019) What is your diagnosis? *J. Am. Vet. Med. Assoc.*, **254** (1), 61–64.

23 Rudmann, D.G., Coolman, B.R., Perez, C.M., *et al.* (1992) Evaluation of risk factors for blastomycosis in dogs: 857 cases (1980–1990). *J. Am. Vet. Med. Assoc.*, **201** (11), 1754–1759.

24 Foy, D.S., Trepanier, L.A., Kirsch, E.J., *et al.* (2014) Serum and urine Blastomyces antigen concentrations as markers of clinical remission in dogs treated for systemic blastomycosis. *J. Vet. Intern. Med.*, **28** (2), 305–310.

25 Legendre, A.M., Rohrbach, B.W., Toal, R.L., *et al.* (1996) Treatment of blastomycosis with itraconazole in 112 dogs. *J. Vet. Intern. Med.*, **10** (6), 365–371.

26 Legendre, A.M., Selcer, B.A., Edwards, D.F., *et al.* (1984) Treatment of canine blastomycosis with amphotericin B and ketoconazole. *J. Am. Vet. Med. Assoc.*, **184** (10), 1249–1254.

27 Demeter, E.A., Canales, G.M., Scrivani, P.V., *et al.* (2019) Pathology in practice. *J. Am. Vet. Med. Assoc.*, **254** (11), 1287–1290.

28 Arbona, N., Butkiewicz, C.D., Keyes, M., *et al.* (2020) Clinical features of cats diagnosed with coccidioidomycosis in Arizona, 2004-2018. *J. Feline. Med. Surg.*, **22** (2), 129–137.

29 Davidson, A.P., Shubitz, L.F., Alcott, C.J., *et al.* (2019) Selected clinical features of Coccidioidomycosis in dogs. *Med. Mycol.*, **57** (Suppl 1), S67–S75.

30 Shaver, S.L., Foy, D.S., Carter, T.D. (2021) Clinical features, treatment, and outcome of dogs with Coccidioides osteomyelitis. *J. Am. Vet. Med. Assoc.*, **260** (1), 63–70.

31 Kelley, A.J., Stainback, L.B., Knowles, K.E., *et al.* (2021) Clinical characteristics, magnetic resonance imaging features, treatment, and outcome for presumed intracranial coccidioidomycosis in 45 dogs (2009–2019). *J. Vet. Intern. Med.*, **35** (5), 2222–2231.

32 Cheng, S.C., Joosten, L.A., Kullberg, B.J., *et al.* (2012) Interplay between *Candida albicans* and the mammalian innate host defense. *Infect. Immun.*, **80** (4), 1304–1313.

33 Pressler, B.M., Vaden, S.L., Lane, I.F., *et al.* (2003) *Candida* spp. urinary tract infections in 13 dogs and seven cats: predisposing factors, treatment, and outcome. *J. Am. Anim. Hosp. Assoc.*, **39** (3), 263–270.

34 Reagan, K.L., Dear, J.D., Kass, P.H., *et al.* (2019) Risk factors for Candida urinary tract infections in dogs and cats. *J. Vet. Intern. Med.*, **33** (2), 648–653.

35 Weissenbacher-Lang, C., Fuchs-Baumgartinger, A., Guija-De-Arespacochaga, A., *et al.* (2018) Pneumocystosis in dogs: meta-analysis of 43 published cases including clinical signs, diagnostic procedures and treatment. *J. Vet. Diagn. Investig.*, **30** (1), 26–35.

36 Lobetti, R.G., Leisewitz, A.L., Spencer, J.A. (1996) *Pneumocystis carinii* in the miniature dachshund: case report and literature review. *J. Small Anim. Pract.*, **37** (6), 280–285.

37 Watson, P.J., Wotton, P., Eastwood, J., *et al.* (2006) Immunoglobulin deficiency in Cavalier King Charles Spaniels with *Pneumocystis* pneumonia. *J. Vet. Intern. Med.*, **20** (3), 523–527.

38 Sakashita, T., Kaneko, Y., Izzati, U.Z., *et al.* (2020) Disseminated Pneumocystosis in a Toy Poodle. *J. Comp. Pathol.*, **175**, 85–89.

39 Guillot, J., Bond, R. (2020) Malassezia yeasts in veterinary dermatology: an updated overview. *Front. Cell. Infect. Microbiol.*, **10**, 79. doi: 10.3389/fcimb.2020.00079. Last accessed October 15, 2023.

40 Winston, J.A., Piperisova, I., Neel, J., *et al.* (2016) *Cyniclomyces guttulatus* infection in dogs: 19 cases (2006–2013). *J. Am. Anim. Hosp. Assoc.*, **52** (1), 42–51.

41 Neel, J.A., Tarigo, J., Grindem, C.B. (2006) What is your diagnosis? Gallbladder aspirate from a dog. *Vet. Clin. Pathol.*, **35** (4), 467–470.

42 Gomez, Y., Gull, T., Merrill, K.M., *et al.* (2019) What is your diagnosis? BAL fluid from a dog. *Vet. Clin. Pathol.*, **49** (2), 356–358.

43 Mandigers, P.J., Duijvestijn, M.B., Ankringa, N., *et al.* (2014) The clinical significance of *Cyniclomyces guttulatus* in dogs with chronic diarrhoea, a survey and a prospective treatment study. *Vet. Microbiol.*, **172** (1–2), 241–247.

44 Acierno, M.M., Ober, C.P., Goupil, B.A., *et al.* (2016) Ureteral obstruction secondary to disseminated penicilliosis in a German shepherd dog. *Can. Vet. J.*, **57** (12), 1242–1246.

45 Zanatta, R., Miniscalco, B., Guarro, J., *et al.* (2006) A case of disseminated mycosis in a German shepherd dog due to *Penicillium purpurogenum*. *Med. Mycol.*, **44** (1), 93–97.

46 Miyakawa, K., Swenson, C.L., Mendoza, L., *et al.* (2011) Pathology in practice: *Penicilliosis*. *J. Am. Vet. Med. Assoc.*, **238** (1), 51–53.

47 Harvey, C.E., O'Brien, J.A., Felsburg, P.J., *et al.* (1981) *Nasal penicilliosis* in six dogs. *J. Am. Vet. Med. Assoc.*, **178** (10), 1084–1087.

48 Rothacker, T., Jaffey, J.A., Rogers, E.R., *et al.* (2020) Novel *Penicillium* species causing disseminated disease in a Labrador Retriever dog. *Med. Mycol.*, **58** (8), 1053–1063.

49 Elad, D. (2019) Disseminated canine mold infections. *Vet. J.*, **243**, 82–90.

50 Schultz, R.M., Johnson, E.G., Wisner, E.R., *et al.* (2008) Clinicopathologic and diagnostic imaging characteristics of systemic aspergillosis in 30 dogs. *J. Vet. Intern. Med.*, **22** (4), 851–859.

51 Cormack, C.A., Donahoe, S.L., Talbot, J.J., *et al.* (2021) Disseminated invasive aspergillosis caused by *Aspergillus felis* in a cat. *J. Vet. Intern. Med.*, **35** (5), 2395–2400.

52 Dehghanpir, S.D. (2023) Cytomorphology of deep mycoses in dogs and cats. *Vet. Clin. North Am. Small Anim. Pract.*, **53** (1), 155–173.

53 Dedeaux, A., Grooters, A., Wakamatsu-Utsuki, N., *et al.* (2018) Opportunistic fungal infections in small animals. *J. Am. Anim. Hosp. Assoc.*, **54** (6), 327–337.

54 McAtee, B.B., Cummings, K.J., Cook, A.K., *et al.* (2017) Opportunistic invasive cutaneous fungal infections associated with administration of cyclosporine to dog with immune-mediated disease. *J. Vet. Intern. Med.*, **31** (6), 1724–1729.

55 Añor, S., Sturges, B.K., Lafranco, L., *et al.* (2001) Systemic phaehyphomycosis (Cladophialophora bantiana) in a dog – clinical diagnosis with stereotactic computed tomographic-guided brain biopsy. *J. Vet. Intern. Med.*, **15** (3), 257–261.

56 Rothenburg, L.S., Snider, T.A., Wilson, A., *et al.* (2017) Disseminated Phaeohyphomycosis in a dog. *Med. Mycol. Case. Rep.*, **15**, 28–32.

57 Crespo-Szabo, S.M., Stafford, J.R. (2021) Diagnosis, treatment and outcome in a dog with systemic Mycoleptodiscus indicus infection. *J. Vet. Intern. Med.*, **35** (4), 1972–1976.

58 Nguyen, D., Vilela, R., Miraglia, B.M., *et al.* (2021) Geographic distribution of *Pythium insidiosum* infections in the United States. *J. Am. Vet. Med. Assoc.*, **260** (5), 530–534.

59 Reagan, K.L., Marks, S.L., Pesavento, P.A., *et al.* (2019) Successful management of 3 dogs with colonic pythiosis using itraconazole, terbinafine, and prednisone. *J. Vet. Intern. Med.*, **33** (3), 1434–1439.

60 Berryessa, N.A., Marks, S.L., Pesavento, P.A., *et al.* (2008) Gastrointestinal pythiosis in 10 dogs from California. *J. Vet. Intern. Med.*, **22** (4), 1065–1069.

61 Cridge, H., Hughes, S.M., Langston, V.C., *et al.* (2020) Mefenoxam, itraconazole and terbinafine combination therapy for management of pythiosis in dogs (six cases). *J. Am. Anim. Hosp. Assoc.*, **56** (6), 307.

62 Whipple, K.M., Wellehan, J.F., Jeon, A.B., *et al.* (2020) Cytologic, histologic, microbiologic and electron microscopic characterization of canine *Prototheca wickerhamii* infection. *Vet. Clin. Pathol.*, **49** (2), 326–332.

63 Migaki, G., Font, R.L., Sauer, R.M., *et al.* (1982) Canine protothecosis: review of the literature and report of an additional case. *J. Am. Vet. Med. Assoc.*, **181** (8), 794–797.

64 Shank, A.M.M., Dubielzig, R.D., Teixeira, L.B.C. (2015) Canine ocular protothecosis: a review of 14 cases. *Vet. Ophthalmol.*, **18** (5), 437–442.

65 Stenner, V.J., Mackay, B., King, T., *et al.* (2007) Prototothecosis in 17 Australian dogs and a review of the canine literature. *Med. Mycol.*, **45** (3), 249–266.

66 Walker, A., MacEwen, I., Fluen, T., *et al.* (2022) Disseminated protothecosis with central nervous system involvement in a dog in New Zealand. *N. Z. Vet. J.*, **70** (4), 238–243.

67 Benson, C.J., Edlund, M.B., Gray, S., *et al.* (2013) The presence of diatom algae in a tracheal wash from a German Wirehaired Pointer with aspiration pneumonia. *Vet. Clin. Pathol.*, **42** (2), 221–226.

68 Martínez-Girón, R., Ribas-Barceló, A., García-Miralles, T., *et al.* (2003) Diatoms and rotifers in cytological smears. *Cytopathology*, **14** (2), 70–72.

69 Piegari, G., De Biase, D., d'Aquino, I., *et al.* (2019) Diagnosis of drowning and the value of the diatom test in veterinary forensic pathology. *Front. Vet. Sci.*, **6**, 404. doi: 10.3389/fvets.2019.00404. Last accessed October 15, 2023.

70 Heffner, G.G., Rozanski, E.A., Beal, M.W., *et al.* (2008) Evaluation of freshwater submersion in small animals: 28 cases (1996–2006). *J. Am. Vet. Med. Assoc.*, **232** (2), 244–248.

71 Meier, W.A., Meinkoth, J.H., Brunker, J., *et al.* (2006) Cytologic identification of immature endospores in a dog with rhinosporidiosis. *Vet. Clin. Pathol.*, **35** (3), 348–352.

72 Cridge, H., Mamaliger, N., Baughman, B., *et al.* (2021) Nasal rhinosporidiosis: clinical presentation, clinical findings, and outcome in dogs. *J. Am. Anim. Hosp. Assoc.*, **57** (3), 114–120.

73 Hill, S.A., Sharkey, L.C., Hardy, R.M., *et al.* (2010) Nasal rhinosporidiosis in two dogs native to the upper Mississippi river valley region. *J. Am. Anim. Hosp. Assoc.*, **46** (2), 127–131.

74 Caniatti, M., Roccabianca, P., Scanziani, E., *et al.* (1998) Nasal rhinosporidiosis in dogs: four cases from Europe and a review of the literature. *Vet. Rec.*, **142** (13), 334–338.

75 Nazari, N., Khodayari, M.T., Hamzavi, Y., *et al.* (2023) Systematic review and meta-analysis of role of felids as intermediate hosts in the life cycle of *Neospora caninum* based on serological data. *Acta Parasitol.*, **68** (1), 266–276.

76 Curtis, B., Harris, A., Ullal, T., *et al.* (2020) Disseminated *Neospora caninum* infection in a dog with severe colitis. *J. Vet. Diagn. Investig.*, **32** (6), 923–927.

77 Barber, J.S., Trees, A.J. (1996) Clinical aspects of 27 cases of neosporosis in dogs. *Vet. Rec.*, **139** (18), 439–443.

78 Hartmann, K., Addie, D., Belák, S., *et al.* (2013) *Toxoplasma gondii* infection in cats: ABCD guidelines on prevention and management. *J. Feline. Med. Surg.*, **15** (7), 631–637.

79 Ludwig, H.C., Schlicksup, M.D., Beale, L.M., *et al.* (2021) *Toxoplasma gondii* infection in feline renal transplant recipients: 24 cases (1998-2018). *J. Am. Vet. Med. Assoc.*, **258** (8), 870–876.

80 Davidson, M.G., Rottman, J.B., English, R.V., *et al.* (1993) Feline immunodeficiency virus predisposes cats to acute generalized toxoplasmosis. *Am. J. Pathol.*, **143** (5), 1486–1497.

81 Singh, M., Foster, D.J., Child, G., *et al.* (2005) Inflammatory cerebrospinal fluid analysis in cats: clinical diagnosis and outcome. *J. Feline Med. Surg.*, **7** (2), 77–93.

82 Baneth, G., Solano-Gallego, L. (2022) Leishmaniasis. *Vet. Clin. North Am. Small Anim. Pract.*, **52** (6), 1359–1375.

83 Paltrinieri, S., Gradoni, L., Roura, X., *et al.* (2016) Laboratory tests for diagnosing and monitoring canine Leishmaniasis. *Vet. Clin. Pathol.*, **45** (4), 552–578.

84 Torres, M., Bardagí, M., Roura, X., *et al.* (2011) Long term follow-up of dogs diagnosed with leishmaniasis (clinical stage II) and treated with meglumine antimoniate and allopurinol. *Vet. J.*, **188** (3), 346–351.

85 Roura, X., Fondati, A., Lubas, G., *et al.* (2013) Prognosis and monitoring of leishmaniasis in dogs: a working group report. *Vet. J.*, **198** (1), 43–47.

86 Cohn, A.L. (2022) Cytauxzoonosis. *Vet. Clin. North Am. Small Anim. Pract.*, **52** (6), 1211–1224.

87 Sleznikow, C.R., Granick, J.L., Cohn, A.L., *et al.* (2022) Evaluation of various sample sources for the cytologic diagnosis of *Cytauxzoon felis*. *J. Vet. Intern. Med.*, **36** (1), 126–132.

88 Kao, Y.F., Peake, B., Madden, R., *et al.* (2021) A probe-based droplet digital polymerase chain reaction assay for early detection of feline acute cytauxzoonosis. *Vet. Parasitol.*, **292**, 109413.

89 Sherrill, M.K., Cohn, A.L. (2015) Cytauxzoonosis: diagnosis and treatment of an emerging disease. *J. Feline. Med. Surg.*, **17** (11), 940–948.

90 Cohn, L.A., Birkenheuer, A.J., Brunker, J.D., *et al.* (2011) Efficacy of atovaquone and azithromycin or imidocarb dipropionate in cats with acute cytauxzoonosis. *J. Vet. Intern. Med.*, **25** (1), 55–60.

91 Wikander, Y.M., Anantatat, T., Kang, Q., *et al.* (2020) Prevalence of *Cytauxzoon felis* infection-carriers in Eastern Kansas domestic cats. *Pathogens*, **9** (10), 854.

92 Bouzid, M., Halai, K., Jeffreys, D., *et al.* (2015) The prevalence of *Giardia* infection in dogs and cats, a systematic review and meta-analysis of prevalence studies from stool samples. *Vet. Parasitol.*, **207** (3–4), 181–202.

93 Murnik, L.C., Daugschies, A., Delling, C. (2023) Gastrointestinal parasites in young dogs and risk factors associated with infection. *Parasitol. Res.*, **122** (2), 585–596.

94 Bastos, B.F., Almeida, F.M., Brener, B. (2019) What is known about *Tritrichomonas foetus* infection in cats? *Rev. Bras. Parasitol. Vet.*, **28** (1), 1–11.

95 Yao, C., Köster, L.S. (2015) *Tritrichomonas foetus* infection, a cause of chronic diarrhea in the domestic cat. *Vet. Res.*, **46** (1), 35.

96 Jones, D., Jones, I.D., Buckeridge, D.M., *et al.* (2022) What is your diagnosis? Pancreatitis in a cat. *Vet. Clin. Pathol.*, **51** (1), 146–148.

97 Foster, D.M., Gookin, J.L., Poore, M.F., *et al.* (2004) Outcome of cats with diarrhea and *Tritrichomonas foetus* infection. *J. Am. Vet. Med. Assoc.*, **225** (6), 888–892.

98 Shams, M., Shamsi, L., Yousefi, A., *et al.* (2022) Current global status, subtype distribution and zoonotic significance of Blastocystis in dogs and cats: a systematic review and meta-analysis. *Parasit. Vectors*, **15** (1), 225. doi: 10.1186/s13071-022-05351-2. Last accessed October 15, 2023.

99 Duda, A., Stenzel, D.J., Boreham, P.F. (1998) Detection of Blastocystis sp. in domestic dogs and cats. *Vet. Parasitol.*, **76** (1–2), 9–17.

100 Chapman, S., Thompson, C., Wilcox, A., *et al.* (2009) What is your diagnosis? Rectal scraping from a dog with diarrhea. *Vet. Clin. Pathol.*, **38** (1), 59–62.

101 Li, J., Ryan, U., Guo, Y., *et al.* (2021) Advances in molecular epidemiology of cryptosporidiosis in dogs and cats. *Int. J. Parasitol.*, **51** (10), 787–795.

102 Monticello, T.M., Levy, M.G., Bunch, S.E., *et al.* (1987) Cryptosporidiosis in a feline leukemia virus-positive cat. *J. Am. Vet. Med. Assoc.*, **191** (6), 705–706.

103 Vincent-Johnson, N.A., Macintire, D.K., Lindsay, D.S., *et al.* (1997) A new Hepatozoon species from dogs: description of the causative agent of canine hepatozoonosis in North America. *J. Parasitol.*, **83** (6), 1165–1172.

104 Baneth, G., Allen, K. (2022) Hepatozoonosis of dogs and cats. *Vet. Clin. North Am. Small Anim. Pract.*, **52** (6), 1341–1358.

105 Marchetti, V., Lubas, G., Baneth, G., *et al.* (2009) Hepatozoonosis in a dog with skeletal involvement and meningoencephalomyelitis. *Vet. Clin. Pathol.*, **38** (1), 121–125.

106 Baneth, G., Aroch, I., Tal, N., *et al.* (1998) Hepatozoon species infection in domestic cats: a retrospective study. *Vet. Parasitol.*, **79** (2), 123–133.

107 Macintire, D.K., Vincent-Johnson, N.A., Kane, C.W., *et al.* (2001) Treatment of dogs infected with *Hepatozoon americanum*: 53 cases (1989–1998). *J. Am. Vet. Med. Assoc.*, **218** (1), 77–82.

108 Macintire, D.K., Vincent-Johnson, N.A., Dillon, A.R., *et al.* (1997) Hepatozoonosis in dogs: 22 cases (1989–1994). *J. Am. Vet. Med. Assoc.*, **210** (7), 916–922.

109 Patten, P.K., Rich, L.J., Zaks, K., *et al.* (2013) Cestode infection in 2 dogs: cytologic findings in liver and a mesenteric lymph node. *Vet. Clin. Pathol.*, **42** (1), 103–108.

110 Boyce, W., Shender, L., Schultz, L., *et al.* (2011) Survival analysis of dogs diagnosed with canine peritoneal larval cestodiasis (*Mesocestoides* spp.). *Vet. Parasitol.*, **180** (3–4), 256–261.

111 Carta, S., Corda, A., Tamponi, C., *et al.* (2021) Clinical forms of peritoneal larval cestodiasis by Mesocestoides spp. in dogs: diagnosis, treatment and long-term follow up. *Parasitol. Res.*, **120** (5), 1727–1735.

112 Genta, R.M., Schad, G.A. (1984) *Filaroides hirthi*: hyperinfective lungworm infection in immunosuppressed dogs. *Vet. Pathol.*, **21** (3), 349–354.

113 Crisi, P.E., Aste, G., Traversa, D., *et al.* (2017) Single and mixed feline lungworm infections: clinical, radiographic and therapeutic features of 26 cases (2013–2015). *J. Feline. Med. Surg.*, **19** (10), 1017–1029.

114 Traversa, D., Di Cesare, A. (2016) Diagnosis and management of lungworm infections in cats: Cornerstones, dilemmas and new avenues. *J. Feline Med. Surg.*, **18** (1), 7–20.

115 Williams, B.M., Cleveland, C.A., Verocai, G.G., *et al.* (2018) Dracunculus infections in domestic dogs and cats in North America; an under-recognized parasite? *Vet. Parasitol. Reg. Stud. Rep.*, **13**, 148–155.

116 Langlais, L. (2003) Dracunculosis in a German shepherd dog. *Can. Vet. J.*, **44** (8), 682.

117 Pechman, R.D., Jr (1980) Pulmonary paragonimiasis in dogs and cats: a review. *J. Small Anim. Pract.*, **21** (2), 87–95.

118 Saini, N., Ranjan, R., Singla, L.D., *et al.* (2012) Successful treatment of pulmonary paragonimiasis in a German shepherd dog with fenbendazole. *J. Parasit. Dis.*, **36** (2), 171–174.

119 Charlebois, P.R., Bersenas, A.M., Yiew, X.T., *et al.* (2023) Local outbreak of spontaneous pneumothorax secondary to paragonimosis in southwestern Ontario dogs. *Can. Vet. J.*, **64** (7), 643–649.

120 Lawson, C.A. (2020) What is your diagnosis? Endotracheal tube wash from a Labrador Retriever. *Vet. Clin. Pathol.*, **49** (1), 156–157.

121 Palić, J., Hostetter, S.J., Riedesel, E., *et al.* (2011) What is your diagnosis? Aspirate of a lung nodule in a dog. *Vet. Clin. Pathol.*, **40** (1), 99–100.

122 Ghielmetti, G., Giger, U. (2020) *Mycobacterium avium*: an emerging pathogen for dog breeds with hereditary immunodeficiencies. *Curr. Clin. Microbiol. Rep.*, **7** (3), 67–80.

123 Lloret, A., Hartmann, K., Pennisi, M.G., *et al.* (2013) Mycobacterioses in cats: ABCD guidelines on prevention and management. *J. Feline. Med. Surg.*, **15** (7), 591–597.

124 Malik, R., Smits, B., Reppas, G., *et al.* (2013) Ulcerated and non-ulcerated nontuberculous cutaneous mycobacterial granulomas in cats and dogs. *Vet. Dermatol.*, **24** (1), 146–153.

125 Barandiaran, S., Martínez Vivot, M., Falzoni, E., *et al.* (2017) Mycobacterioses in dogs and cats from Buenos Aires, Argentina, *J. Vet. Diagn. Investig.*, **29** (5), 729–732.

126 Faccin, M., Wiener, D.J., Rech, R.R., *et al.* (2023) Common superficial and deep cutaneous bacterial infections in domestic animals: a review. *Vet. Pathol.*, **60** (6), 796–811.

127 Siak, M.K., Burrows, A.K. (2013) Cutaneous nocardiosis in two dogs receiving ciclosporin therapy for the management of canine atopic dermatitis. *Vet. Dermatol.*, **24** (4), 453–456.

128 Hardie, E.M., Barsanti, J.A. (1982) Treatment of canine actinomycosis. *J. Am. Vet. Med. Assoc.*, **180** (5), 537–541.

129 Kirpensteijn, J., Fingland, R.B. (1992) Cutaneous actinomycosis and nocardiosis in dogs: 48 cases (1980–1990). *J. Am. Vet. Med. Assoc.*, **201** (6), 917–920.

130 Malik, R., Krockenberger, M.B., O'Brien, C.R., *et al.* (2006) *Nocardia* infections in cats: a retrospective multi-institutional study of 17 cases. *Aust. Vet. J.*, **84** (7), 235–245.

131 Marino, D.J., Jaggy, A. (1993) Nocardiosis. A literature review with selected case reports in two dogs. *J. Vet. Intern. Med.*, **7** (1), 4–11.

132 Canonne, A.M., Billen, F., Tual, C., *et al.* (2016) Quantitative PCR and cytology of bronchoalveolar lavage fluid in dogs with *Bordetella bronchiseptica* infection. *J. Vet. Intern. Med.*, **30** (4), 1204–1209.

133 Binns, S.H., Dawson, S., Speakman, A.J., *et al.* (1999) Prevalence and risk factors for feline *Bordetella bronchiseptica* infection. *Vet. Rec.*, **144** (21), 575–580.

134 Chalker, V.J., Toomey, C., Opperman, S., *et al.* (2003) Respiratory disease in kenneled dogs: serological responses to *Bordetella bronchiseptica* lipopolysaccharide do not correlate with bacterial isolation or clinical respiratory symptoms. *Clin. Diagn. Lab. Immunol.*, **10** (3), 352–356.

135 Egberink, H., Addie, D., Belák, S., *et al.* (2009) *Bordetella bronchiseptica* infection in cats. ABCD guidelines on prevention and management. *J. Feline Med. Surg.*, **11** (7), 610–614.

136 Taha-Abdelaziz, K., Bassel, L.L., Harness, M.L., *et al.* (2016) Cilia-associated bacteria in fatal *Bordetella bronchiseptica* pneumonia of dogs and cats. *J. Vet. Diagn. Investig.*, **28** (4), 369–376.

137 Allison, R.W., Little, S.E. (2013) Diagnosis of rickettsial diseases in dogs and cats. *Vet. Clin. Pathol.*, **42** (2), 127–144.

138 Diniz, P.P.V.P., Moura de Aguiar, D. (2022) Ehrlichiosis and Anaplasmosis: an update. *Vet. Clin. North Am. Small Anim. Pract.*, **52** (6), 1225–1266.

139 Johns, J.L. (2011) Salmon poisoning in dogs: a satisfying diagnosis. *Vet. J.*, **187** (2), 149–150.

140 Marks, S.L., Rankin, S.C., Byrne, B.A., *et al.* (2011) Enteropathogenic bacteria in dogs and cats: diagnosis, epidemiology, treatment, and control. *J. Vet. Intern. Med.*, **25** (6), 1195–1208.

141 Schlegel, B.J., Van Dreumel, T., Slavić, D., *et al.* (2012) *Clostridium perfringens* type A fatal acute hemorrhagic gastroenteritis in a dog. *Can. Vet. J.*, **53** (5), 555–557.

142 Kim, M.W., Sharp, C.R., Boyd, C.J., *et al.* (2021) A survey of enteric organisms detected by real-time PCR assay in faeces of dogs in Western Australia. *Aust. Vet. J.*, **99** (10), 419–422.

143 Iannino, F., Di Donato, G., Salucci, S., *et al.* (2022) Campylobacter and risk factors associated with dog ownership: a retrospective study in household and in shelter dogs. *Vet. Ital.*, **58** (1), 59–66.

144 Handt, L.K., Fox, J.G., Dewhirst, F.E., *et al.* (1994) *Helicobacter pylori* isolated from the domestic cat: public health implications. *Infect. Immun.*, **62** (6), 2367–2374.

145 Van den Bulck, K., Decostere, A., Baele, M., *et al.* (2005) Identification of non-*Helicobacter pylori* spiral organisms in gastric samples from humans, dogs, and cats. *J. Clin. Microbiol.*, **43** (5), 2256–2260.

146 Lecoindre, P., Chevallier, M., Peyrol, S., *et al.* (2000) Gastric helicobacters in cats. *J. Feline Med. Surg.*, **2** (1), 19–27.

147 Biénès, T., Leal, R.O., Domínguez-Ruiz, M., *et al.* (2022) Association of gastric lymphfollicular hyperplasia with Helicobacter-like organisms in dogs. *J. Vet. Intern. Med.*, **36** (2), 515–524.

148 Anacleto, T.P., Lopes, L.R., Andreollo, N.A., *et al.* (2011) Studies of distribution and recurrence of *Helicobacter* spp. gastric mucosa of dogs after triple therapy. *Acta Cir. Bras.*, **26** (2), 82–87.

149 Conrado, F.O., Stacy, N.I., Wellehan, J.F.X. Jr. (2023) Out with the old, in with the new: What's up with Simonsiella spp.? *Vet. Clin. Pathol.*, **52** (2), 208–209.

150 French, T.W., Blue, J.T. (1986) What is your diagnosis? *Vet. Clin. Pathol.*, **15** (4), 18–19.

151 Bau-Gaudreault, L., Overvelde, S., Martin, D. (2018) What is your diagnosis? Subcutaneous temporal mass from a cat. *Vet. Clin. Pathol.*, **47** (2), 324–325.

152 Rutland, B.E., Byl, K.M., Hydeskov, H.B., *et al.* (2017) Systemic manifestations of *Cuterebra* infection in dogs and cats: 42 cases (2000-2014). *J. Am. Vet. Med. Assoc.*, **251** (12), 1432–1438.

153 Pezzi, M., Bonacci, T., Leis, M., et al. (2019) Myiasis in domestic cats: a global review. *Parasit. Vectors*, **12** (1), 372. doi: 10.1186/s13071-019-3618-1. Last accessed October 15, 2023.

154 Rissi, D.R., Howerth, E.W. (2013) Pathology in practice. Ischemic encephalopathy caused by aberrant migration of a Cuterebra larva. *J. Am. Vet. Med. Assoc.*, **243** (4), 493–495.

155 Schlesener, B.N., Peck, E.A., Ledbetter, E.C. (2021) Feline ophthalmomyiasis externa caused by *Cuterebra* larvae: four cases (2005–2020). *J. Feline. Med. Surg.*, **24** (2), 189–197.

156 Glass, E.N., Cornetta, A.M., deLahunta, A., *et al.* (1998) Clinical and clinicopathologic features in 11 cats with *Cuterebra* larva myiasis of the central nervous system. *J. Vet. Intern. Med.*, **12** (5), 365–368.

157 Sood, N.K., Mekkib, B., Singla, L.D., *et al.* (2012) Cytopathology of parasitic dermatitis in dogs. *J. Parasit. Dis.*, **36** (1), 73–77.

158 Thomson, P., Carreño, N., Núñez, A. (2023) Main mites associated with dermatopathies present in dogs and other members of the Canidae family. *Open Vet. J.*, **13** (2), 131–142.

159 Rosser, E.J., Jr (2004) Causes of otitis externa. *Vet. Clin. North Am. Small Anim. Pract.*, **34** (2), 459–468.

4

Integument

4.1 Cutaneous and Subcutaneous Lesions

4.1.1 Mast Cell Tumor: Dog

4.1.1.1 Cytologic Features

Mast cell tumors are characterized by individualized cells that can be pushed into crowded aggregates. They usually have a large volume of cytoplasm that contains abundant purple/metachromatic granules. Nuclei are round, often centrally located, and have stippled chromatin with small basophilic nucleoli. Cytoplasmic granules may obscure nuclear features. Mast cell tumors frequently are accompanied by bright-pink ribbons of collagen (Figure 4.1), fibroplasia (Figure 4.2), and eosinophilic inflammation (Figure 4.3).

Cytology can be used to estimate a high or low tumor grade for canine cutaneous mast cell tumors [1, 2]. Cytologic criteria supportive of a high-grade mast cell tumor include a predominance of poorly granulated/agranular cells, the presence of mitotic figures, binucleated or multinucleated cells, anisokaryosis (twofold variation in nuclear size),

and nuclear pleomorphism (shapes other than round or ovoid) (Figures 4.3–4.6) [2]. Additionally, collagen and fibroblasts are noted to be more abundant in low-grade tumors [3]. *Note*: Grading systems (both for cytology and histopathology) apply only to cutaneous (and not subcutaneous) tumors.

Mast cell granules stain variably well with aqueous Romanowsky stains (e.g., Diff-Quik) (Figure 4.7) which may affect the ability to grade these tumors [4, 5]. Agranular or poorly staining mast cell tumors can be difficult to differentiate from histiocytomas or transmissible venereal tumors (TVT) (compare to Figures 4.12 and 4.27).

4.1.1.2 Clinical Considerations

- Most are solitary, dermal, or subcutaneous and occur commonly on the trunk, limbs, perineum, inguinal, and genital regions [6].
- Primarily seen in older dogs (8–10 years) but can be present in dogs <1 year, including multiple tumors (cutaneous mastocytosis) [7, 8].

Figure 4.1 Mast cell tumor, dog, 40× objective. Note the linear ribbons of bright-pink collagen.

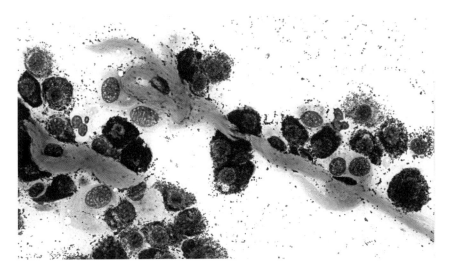

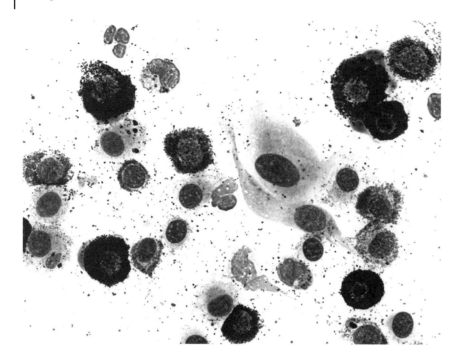

Figure 4.2 Mast cell tumor, dog, 50× objective. Two reactive fibroblasts (center/right) are present.

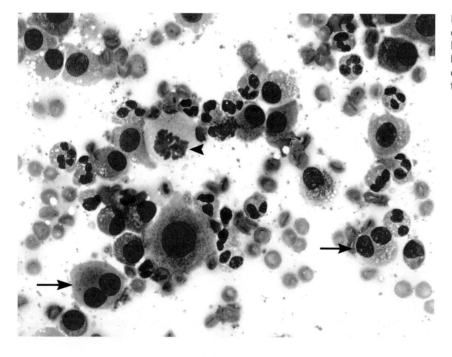

Figure 4.3 Mast cell tumor (histologic grade III, high grade), dog, 50× objective. Note the many eosinophils in the background, poor granulation of mast cells, binucleation (arrows), and mitotic figure (arrowhead).

- Seen in a diverse range of breeds. Some predisposed breeds include dogs of Bulldog descent (including Boxers and Pugs), Golden Retrievers, and Weimaraners [6].
- Metastatic potential increases with tumor grade and occurs most commonly in the regional lymph nodes, skin, spleen, and liver [6].

4.1.1.3 Prognosis

Highly variable based on numerous factors including histologic tumor grade (considered most important), clinical stage, location, and cell proliferation rate [1, 9]. Increased fibroblasts and collagen fibrils in cytology samples have been associated with lower tumor grade and prolonged

Figure 4.4 Mast cell tumor, dog, 50× objective. Note the variable granulation of the cells and occasional binucleation.

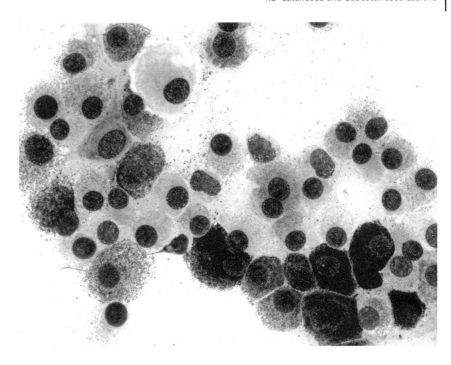

Figure 4.5 Mast cell tumor (histologic grade III, high grade), dog, 50× objective. Numerous features of a high cytologic grade are present including poor granulation, many mitotic figures, and multinucleated cells (including a trinucleated cell, upper center).

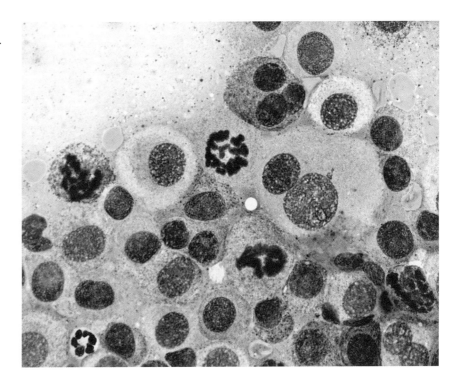

survival [3]. Surgical excision with wide margins can be curative. Subcutaneous mast cell tumors typically have a less aggressive biologic behavior and good long-term prognosis; however, a subset of these tumors (especially those with increased mitotic counts) can have an aggressive disease course [10], and metastatic disease significantly reduces survival time [11].

4.1.2 Mast Cell Tumor: Cat

4.1.2.1 Cytologic Features

Mast cell tumors from cats comprise individualized cells, though they frequently exfoliate in crowded sheets. They are variably granular, often more subtly so than canine mast cell tumors (Figures 4.8 and 4.9). The cells tend to be

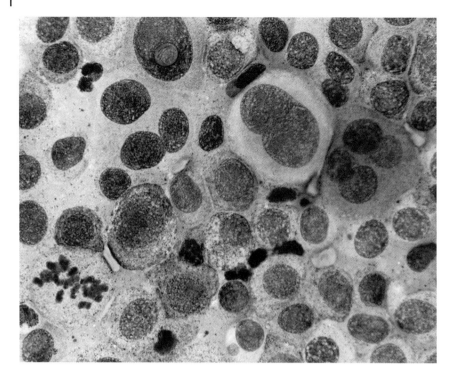

Figure 4.6 Mast cell tumor (histologic grade III, high grade), dog, 50× objective. Note the nuclear pleomorphism in the largest mast cell, accompanied by poor granulation, mitotic figures, and multinucleation

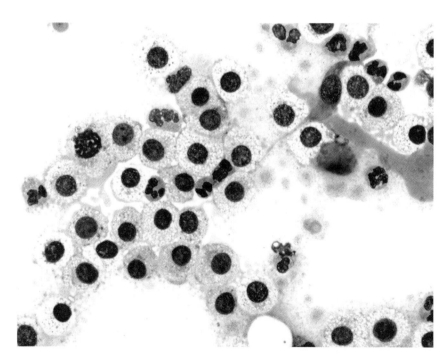

Figure 4.7 Mast cell tumor, dog, 50× objective, Diff Quik stain. Although granules stain poorly, the cells are uniform and minimally pleomorphic (histologic grade I, low grade).

uniform in appearance with abundant cytoplasm and round, centrally located nuclei. Similar to dog mast cell tumors, the granules stain variably well with aqueous Romanowsky stains (e.g., Diff-Quik) (Figure 4.10). Skin tumors may rarely represent part of an aggressive, malignant process, and in such cases typically are poorly granulated and have high N/C ratios, mitotic figures, and increased anisocytosis/anisokaryosis (Figure 4.11).

4.1.2.2 Clinical Considerations

- Mostly single (though may be multiple), raised, hairless dermal nodules, common around the head, neck, limbs, and trunk [12].
- Most common in middle-aged to older cats but can occur in patients <1 year of age [13].
- Solitary tumors typically are benign, though a subset (~20%) may show aggressive behavior with lymph node

Figure 4.8 Mast cell tumor, cat, 50× objective.

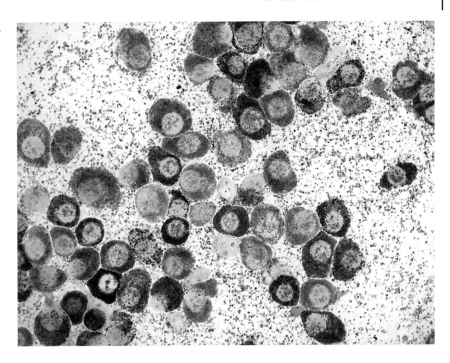

Figure 4.9 Mast cell tumor, cat, 50× objective. Note the more subtle, fine granulation relative to mast cell tumors in dogs.

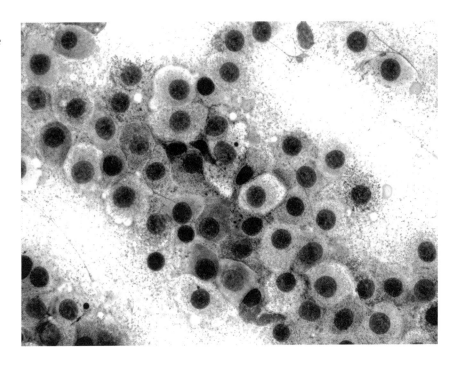

metastases, visceral organ involvement, or cutaneous dissemination [14, 15].

- Cutaneous mast cell tumors in cats not currently graded; however, features associated with more aggressive tumors include increased mitotic count, tumor size >1.5 cm, irregular nuclear shape, and prominent nucleoli [15].
- Metastatic disease to regional lymph nodes may occur even with histologic low-grade tumors [12].

- Multiple nodules may be associated with visceral mast cell disease, and evaluation of the spleen or gastrointestinal tract may be warranted [16].

4.1.2.3 Prognosis
The prognosis for solitary lesions with no evidence of metastasis is excellent, with surgical excision generally curative, and low rates of recurrence and prolonged

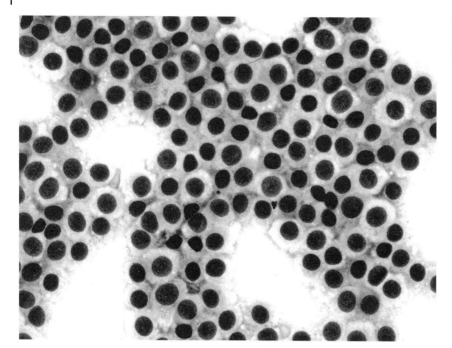

Figure 4.10 Mast cell tumor, cat, 50× objective, Diff Quik stain. Granules stain poorly.

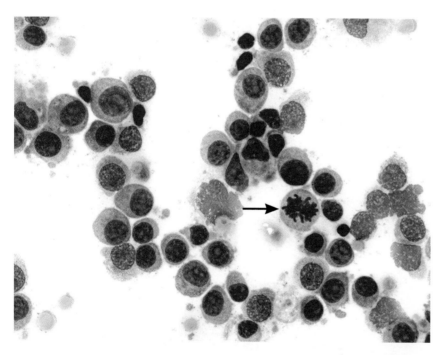

Figure 4.11 Mast cell tumor, cat, 50× objective. This aggressive tumor contained cells that were poorly granular and had high N/C ratios. Note the mitotic figure (arrow).

survival [15, 17]. Histologic tumor grading is not as defined as for canine tumors; however, increased mitotic count, tumors >1.5 cm diameter, and prominent nucleoli are associated with aggressive biologic behavior and reduced survival times [15, 18].

4.1.3 Histiocytoma

4.1.3.1 Cytologic Features

Histiocytomas are characterized by a uniform population of individualized cells that may be pushed together into aggregates. The cells have a moderate to abundant volume of watery-blue cytoplasm. Nuclei are round to reniform and have finely granular chromatin with small nucleoli (Figures 4.12 and 4.13). Small mature lymphocytes are often seen in regressing histiocytomas and may be the predominating cell types (Figure 4.14).

4.1.3.2 Clinical Considerations

- Dogs only.
- Occur at any age, but most dogs are aged <3 years (reported from 2 months to 12 years in one study) [19].

Figure 4.12 Histiocytoma, dog, 50× objective. Note the abundant watery blue cytoplasm.

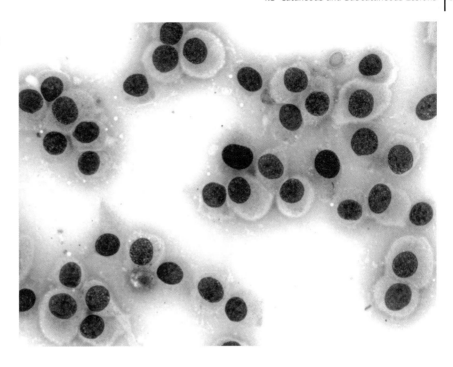

Figure 4.13 Histiocytoma, dog, 50× objective. Note the abundant watery blue cytoplasm and monomorphism of the cell population.

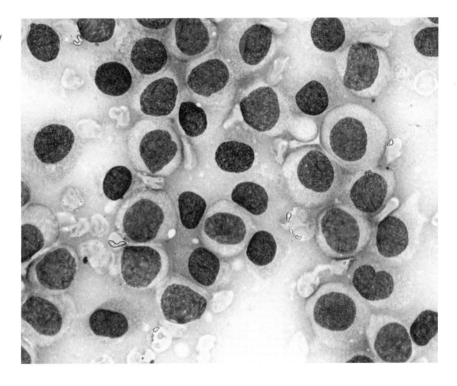

Reported as the most common skin tumor in dogs <1 year of age [20].

- Usually solitary lesions around the head (particularly pinnae) and limbs.
- Most spontaneously regress within 1–2 months. Ulceration is common [21].

- Multiple cutaneous histiocytomas = cutaneous Langerhans cell histiocytosis [22].

4.1.3.3 Prognosis

Excellent for solitary lesions, which typically spontaneously regress. Surgical excision, if required, is generally curative.

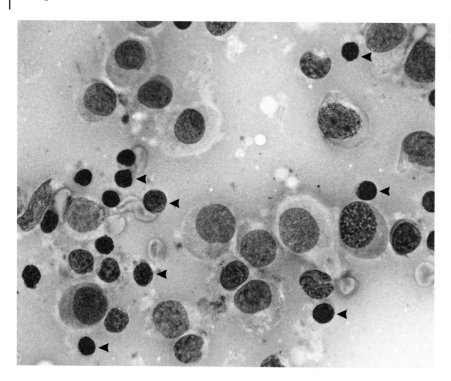

Figure 4.14 Regressing histiocytoma, dog, 50× objective. Note the many small mature lymphocytes (arrowheads).

Cutaneous Langerhans cell histiocytosis carries a guarded to poor prognosis, especially if lymph node involvement is present [23].

4.1.4 Histiocytic Sarcoma

4.1.4.1 Cytologic Features

Histiocytic sarcoma (HS) is characterized by individualized cells that are ovoid with a variable volume of pale-blue cytoplasm that frequently contains clear vacuoles (Figure 4.15). Nuclei are ovoid to ameboid or pleomorphic (Figure 4.16) with finely stippled chromatin and often multiple, prominent basophilic nucleoli of varying size and shape. Marked criteria of malignancy, including multinucleation, nuclear fragmentation, marked anisocytosis/anisokaryosis, karyomegaly, and increased mitotic figures (including bizarre mitoses), are common (Figure 2.52).

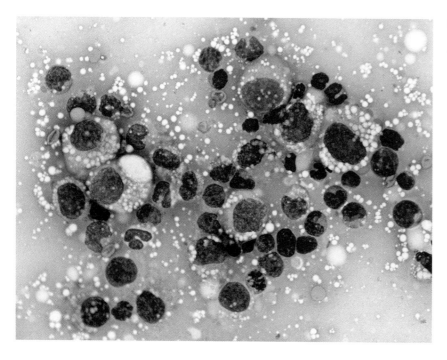

Figure 4.15 Histiocytic sarcoma, dog, 50× objective. Note the prominent cytoplasmic vacuolation.

Figure 4.16 Histiocytic sarcoma, dog, 50× objective. Note the nuclear pleomorphism.

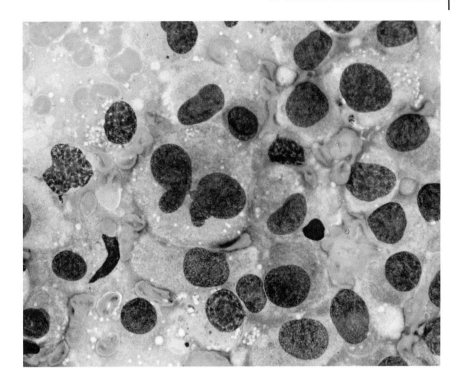

4.1.4.2 Clinical Considerations

- Dogs > > cats.
- Disease may be localized to a single organ or generalized.
- Reported in many dog breeds, but Bernese Mountain Dogs, Rottweilers, Golden Retrievers, Labrador Retrievers, and Flat-Coated Retrievers predisposed [24].
- Organs commonly affected by disseminated HS = spleen, liver, lung, bone marrow, lymph nodes [22].

4.1.4.3 Prognosis

Dependent on whether localized or generalized. Prognosis for disseminated HS is grave, with short survival times even with treatment [25]. Localized HS and periarticular location (see Chapter 7) are associated with a better prognosis [26].

4.1.5 Cutaneous Lymphoma

4.1.5.1 Cytologic Features

Lymphocytes in these cases are monomorphic and may be small or intermediate, but are frequently large, with round nuclei that have finely stippled chromatin and variably prominent nucleoli (Figure 4.17). The cells have a small to moderate volume of medium-blue cytoplasm that may contain a perinuclear packet of pink granules, compared to diffuse granules in mast cells (Figure 4.18). Cutaneous lymphomas frequently are associated with concurrent inflammation, which may predominate and obscure the neoplastic cells (Figure 4.19).

4.1.5.2 Clinical Considerations

- Generally middle-aged to older dogs and cats.
- Epitheliotropic and non-epitheliotropic forms exist and most have a T-cell phenotype.
- May be solitary or generalized. The non-epitheliotropic form usually presents as solitary or multiple nodules, while the epitheliotropic form progresses from alopecia or erythema in the early stages to plaques or masses in the later stages [27].
- Commonly affect haired skin, lips, nasal planum, and paw pads [27].
- Feline cutaneous lymphoma is not associated with FeLV or FIV status [28].

4.1.5.3 Prognosis

Dogs = poor to grave for diffuse cutaneous forms, with ulceration, crusting, and nodule formation associated with reduced survival times [27]. Indolent, T-cell cutaneous lymphomas are rare but carry a better prognosis [29].

Cats = more variable than dogs, with some indolent forms that are slowly progressive [28].

4.1.6 Merkel Cell Carcinoma

4.1.6.1 Cytologic Features

Merkel cell carcinomas are characterized by round cells that are often seen individually, but also in variably sticky aggregates that may form palisading rows (Figure 4.20). They have round nuclei, with coarsely granular chromatin

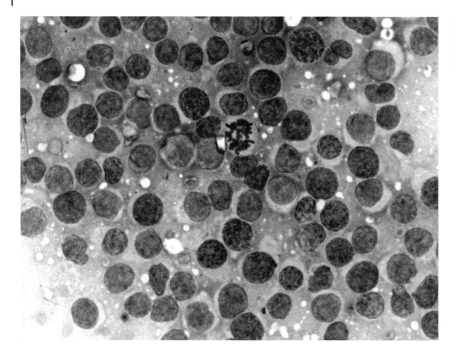

Figure 4.17 Cutaneous lymphoma, dog, 50× objective. Note the high N/C ratios and monomorphism of the population. A mitotic figure is seen (center).

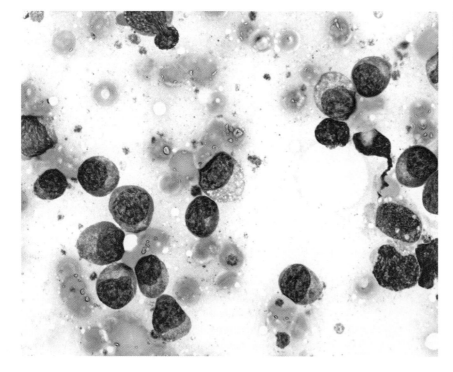

Figure 4.18 Cutaneous lymphoma (granular), dog, 50× objective. Note the perinuclear packet of azurophilic granules in the cytoplasm.

and prominent nucleoli. The cells have a small to moderate volume of pale-blue cytoplasm that may contain punctate clear vacuoles. The frequent individual, discrete appearance of the cells can mimic cutaneous lymphoma (compare to Figure 4.17).

4.1.6.2 Clinical Considerations

- Rare cutaneous tumor of dogs and cats.
- Arise from Merkel cells which are widely disseminated throughout the skin, residing at the bulge of the follicular isthmus [30, 31].

Figure 4.19 Cutaneous lymphoma, dog, 50× objective. Large, neoplastic lymphocytes are accompanied by many neutrophils.

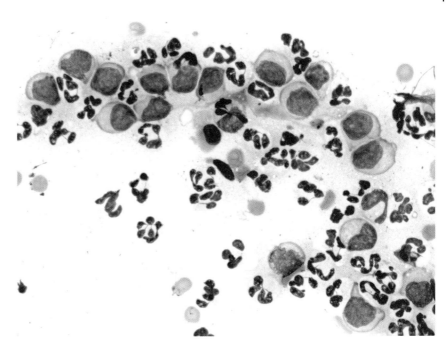

Figure 4.20 Merkel cell carcinoma, dog, 50× objective. The cells are seen both individually and in variably sticky sheets, often in palisading rows.

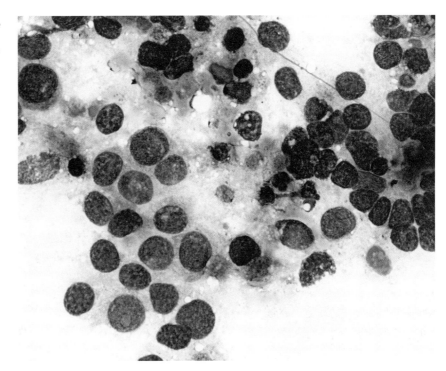

- Often solitary lesions in cats (common around the head and neck); multiple lesions more common in dogs [31–33].

4.1.6.3 Prognosis

Poor prognosis in cats, with short survival times and high rates of recurrence [33]. Disease in dogs is generally more indolent and slowly progressive; however, aggressive variants have been reported [30, 31].

4.1.7 Cutaneous Extramedullary Plasmacytoma

4.1.7.1 Cytologic Features

Plasmacytomas are often vascular lesions and cytology samples may have a moderate to dense background of blood (Figures 4.21 and 4.22). They consist of discrete cells with distinct cell borders, though they may be pushed together into aggregates that can mimic epithelial tumors.

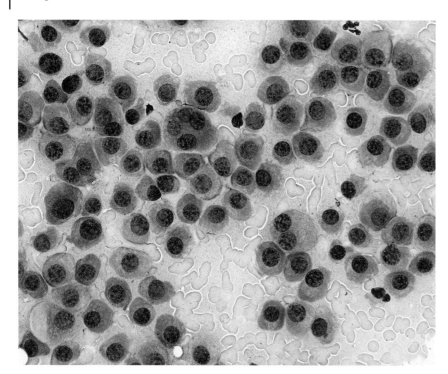

Figure 4.21 Plasmacytoma, dog, 50× objective. Note the moderate background of blood which is common in plasmacytomas.

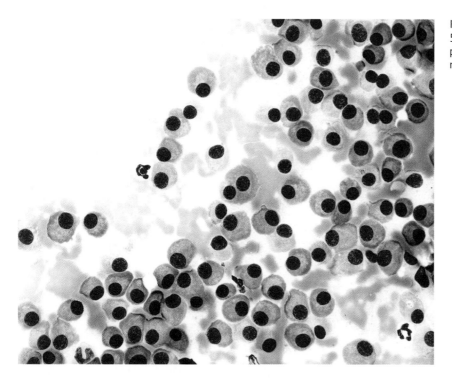

Figure 4.22 Plasmacytoma, dog, 50× objective. Note the prominent perinuclear clearing (golgi zone) in most cells.

The cytologic appearance of plasmacytomas can vary greatly. Cells mostly have a small to moderate volume of mid-blue cytoplasm that frequently has a pale, perinuclear clearing (Golgi zone) (Figures 4.22 and 4.23). The cells may have a bright-pink, peripheralized border due to the production of immunoglobulins (flame cells) (Figure 4.24).

Nuclei are eccentrically placed with regularly clumped chromatin. Binucleation, multinucleation, and mitotic figures are common (Figure 4.25). Anisocytosis and anisokaryosis mostly are mild to moderate, but can be marked, and cellular pleomorphism is not associated with biologic behavior [34].

Figure 4.23 Plasmacytoma, dog, 50× objective.

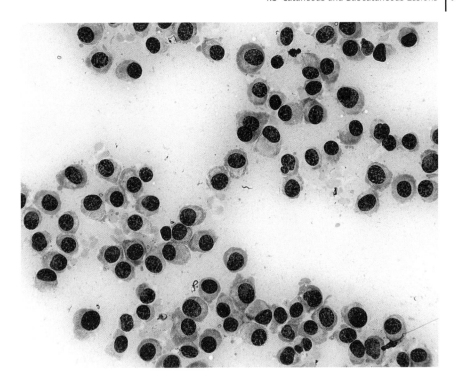

Figure 4.24 Plasmacytoma, dog, 50× objective. Note the peripheralized pink coloration of the cytoplasm.

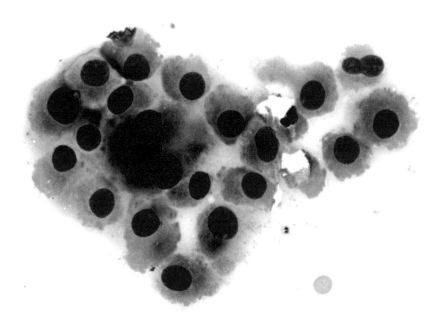

4.1.7.2 Clinical Considerations

- Middle-aged to older dogs. Rare in cats.
- Most are solitary, raised, pink/red, smooth nodules, commonly seen on the limbs (especially digits) and head (especially margins of the lips and ears) [34, 35].
- Multiple tumors may indicate cutaneous plasmacytosis [36].

4.1.7.3 Prognosis

Solitary cutaneous plasmacytomas mostly are benign neoplasms and have an excellent prognosis, with surgical excision generally curative, and low rates of recurrence. Metastatic spread or a manifestation of multiple myeloma is rare [34]. Dogs with cutaneous plasmacytosis have a guarded prognosis [36].

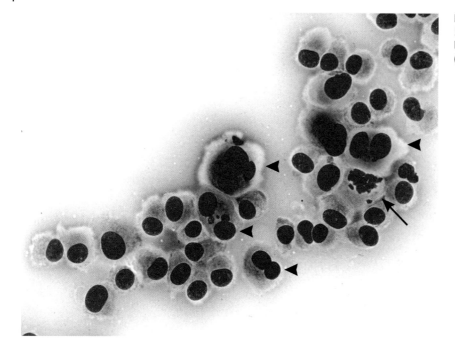

Figure 4.25 Plasmacytoma, dog, 50× objective. Note the frequent binucleation/multinucleation (arrowheads) and mitotic figure (arrow).

4.1.8 Transmissible Venereal Tumor (TVT)

4.1.8.1 Cytologic Features

TVT is characterized by a monomorphic population of large, round cells that have a moderate volume of pale-blue cytoplasm. The cytoplasm of many cells contains characteristic punctate clear vacuoles (Figure 4.26). Nuclei are round, with reticulated/ropey chromatin and prominent, mostly single, basophilic nucleoli. Mitotic figures are common, and increased eosinophils are often present (Figure 4.27).

TVT can appear similar to lymphoma or histiocytomas; however, the cytoplasmic vacuoles, chromatin pattern, and prominent nucleoli of TVT cells are helpful in differentiating these lesions.

4.1.8.2 Clinical Considerations

- Thought to be of histiocytic origin [37].
- Lesions are nodular to multilobulated with an erythemic, ulcerated surface.

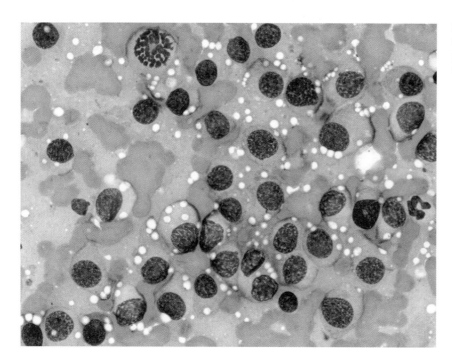

Figure 4.26 Transmissible venereal tumor, dog, 50× objective. Note the prominent clear vacuoles in the cytoplasm and the mitotic figure (top left).

Figure 4.27 Transmissible venereal tumor, dog, 50× objective. The cells have characteristic finely granular chromatin, prominent single nucleoli, and increased mitotic figures. Eosinophilic inflammation is present.

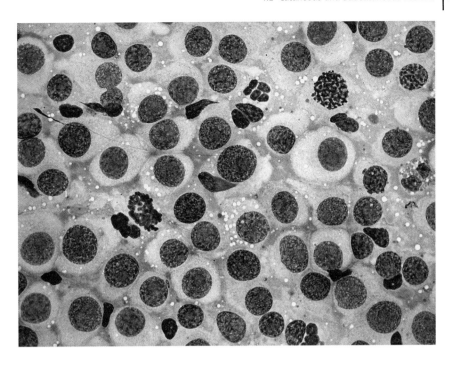

- External genitalia most commonly affected, but lesions may be found around the nose, oral cavity, and eyes [38].
- Usually localized but can spread to local lymph nodes (see Chapter 5), skin, and rarely other locations [39, 40].

4.1.8.3 Prognosis

Good to excellent. TVT may spontaneously regress in some dogs over a period of 3–6 months. Those that require treatment still carry an excellent prognosis [38]. Disseminated disease may confer a poor prognosis [40].

4.1.9 Melanomas

The cytologic appearance and biologic behavior of melanomas are highly variable. The anatomic site, stage, and certain histologic findings may all affect outcome [41]. The following sections describe benign (melanocytomas) and malignant melanomas separately (as defined by the World Health Organization nomenclature) [42] as the two distinct, and usually distinguishable, ends of a continuous spectrum. It is imperative, however, to correlate findings with clinical staging and histopathologic evaluation.

4.1.10 Benign Melanoma (Melanocytoma)

4.1.10.1 Cytologic Features

Melanocytomas often are highly cellular and comprise aggregates of round to spindloid melanocytes. They mostly have a large volume of cytoplasm containing abundant green/black melanin pigment granules (Figure 4.28).

Nuclei, when visible, are ovoid with stippled chromatin and small basophilic nucleoli. Anisocytosis/anisokaryosis are mild and N/C ratios are low.

4.1.10.2 Clinical Considerations

- Benign tumors in older dogs and cats.
- Usually cutaneous, well-circumscribed, pigmented/black, alopecic nodules found in haired skin, commonly affecting the face (especially near the eyelids), neck, trunk, and extremities [43].
- *Note*: tumors of adnexal origin can be pigmented and can be confused with melanocytomas/melanomas (see Figure 4.36).

4.1.10.3 Prognosis

Mostly excellent, with surgical excision often curative. Cutaneous tumors generally have a good prognosis; however, tumors on the lip or digit have a worse prognosis [41]. Highly pigmented tumors carry a favorable prognosis.

4.1.11 Malignant Melanoma

4.1.11.1 Cytologic Features

Malignant melanomas comprise a highly heterogeneous category and can be difficult to diagnose via cytology, and even histopathology, without special stains. Many tumors will contain green/black melanin pigment granules (Figure 4.29), but some may lack melanin pigment (poorly melanotic melanoma; Figure 4.30). Cells may be

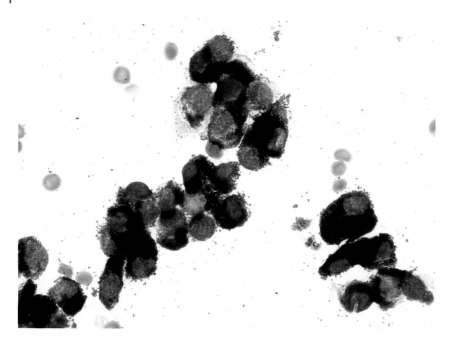

Figure 4.28 Melanocytoma, dog, 50× objective. Note the abundant green/black pigment in cells and in the background.

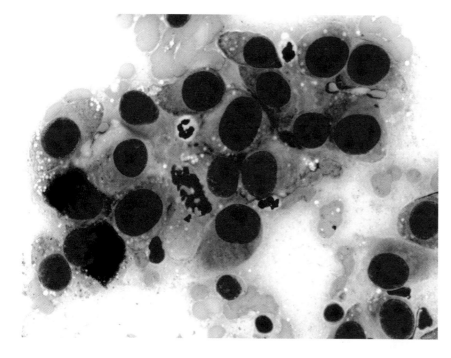

Figure 4.29 Malignant melanoma, dog, 50× objective. Cells mostly lack pigment, with rare heavily pigmented cells (left), and have multiple, prominent basophilic nucleoli. Note the mitotic figure (middle).

round or spindloid, and arranged individually, in sheets or aggregates. In general, malignant melanomas have many criteria for malignancy, including marked anisocytosis/ anisokaryosis, prominent basophilic nucleoli, and mitotic figures.

4.1.11.2 Clinical Considerations
- Dogs > cats. Mostly middle-aged to older patients [43].
- Frequently larger than melanocytomas and variably pigmented.
- Often found in and around the mouth, mucocutaneous junctions, as well as feet (including nail bed) and ventral abdomen [43, 44].
- Evaluation of lymph nodes is strongly recommended, as metastatic disease may be present even in the absence of lymphadenomegaly [45].

4.1.11.3 Prognosis
Malignant melanomas often have a poor to grave prognosis, especially if distant metastatic disease is present [41].

Figure 4.30 Malignant melanoma (poorly melanotic), dog, 50× objective. Note the bizarre mitotic figure on the left.

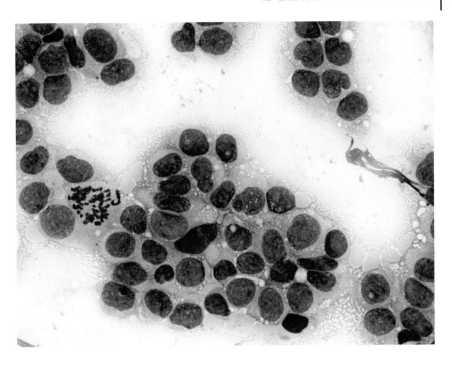

Poorly pigmented tumors also confer a worse prognosis. Many histopathologic parameters (e.g., invasion, Ki67 index) may offer important prognostic information.

4.1.12 Infundibular/Epidermal Cysts

4.1.12.1 Cytologic Features
Samples vary greatly in appearance, but almost all contain many anucleated squamous epithelial cells and aggregates of keratinized debris (Figure 4.31). Cholesterol crystals are

a frequent finding (see Figure 2.1). Other common cytologic features include mineralization (Figure 4.32), hair shaft/bulb fragments (Figure 4.33), and melanin pigment granules. If the cysts rupture and keratin leaks into the dermis, a mixed inflammatory response may ensue (Figure 4.34).

4.1.12.2 Clinical Considerations
- Dogs and cats. Most common in middle-aged to older dogs.
- Grossly = variably firm, well-circumscribed, smooth masses, found mostly on the dorsum and extremities.

Figure 4.31 Infundibular/epidermal cyst, dog, 10× objective. Many anucleated squamous epithelial cells are seen.

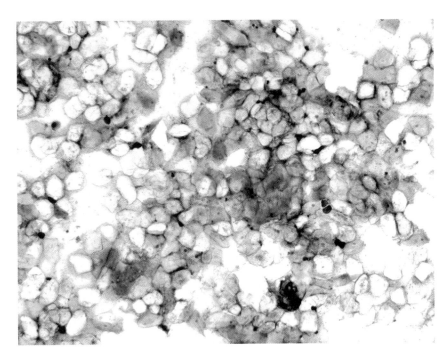

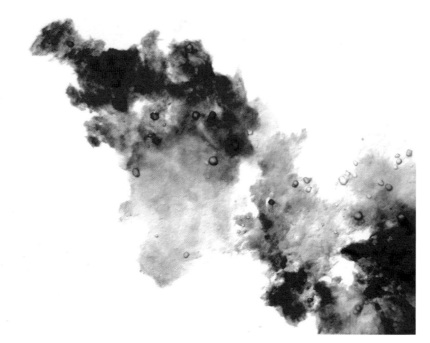

Figure 4.32 Infundibular/epidermal cyst, dog, 20× objective. Keratinized debris is studded with aggregates of refractile, mineralized debris.

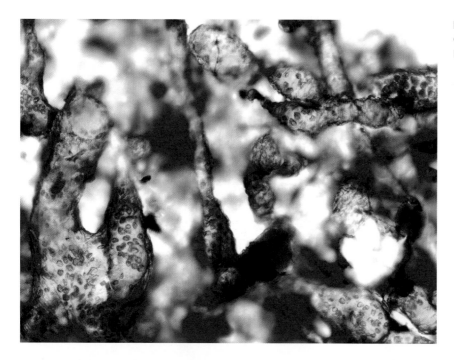

Figure 4.33 Pigmented hair shafts/bulbs, dog, 50× objective. Note the different plane of focus from other material.

- Waxy or gritty, gray/tan material may express from lesions.
- Often solitary, but multiple masses may be present.
- Note: Similar cystic material may exfoliate from tumors of adnexal/hair follicular origin (see Section 4.1.13).

4.1.12.3 Prognosis

Excellent. Surgical excision may be required to treat persistent inflammation from ruptured cysts and generally is curative.

4.1.13 Cutaneous Basilar Epithelial Neoplasia

4.1.13.1 Cytologic Features

Samples contain tight sheets of uniform cuboidal epithelial cells, distributed in papillary arrangements. They may be associated with a bright-pink, smooth extracellular matrix (basement membrane) (Figure 4.35). The cells have a scant volume of pale-blue cytoplasm. Some tumors may contain melanin pigment, often seen as a unipolar cap (Figure 4.36). Granular variants are also reported, where basal epithelial

Figure 4.34 Infundibular/epidermal cyst, dog, 20× objective. Aggregates of anucleated squamous epithelial cells with marked mixed inflammation.

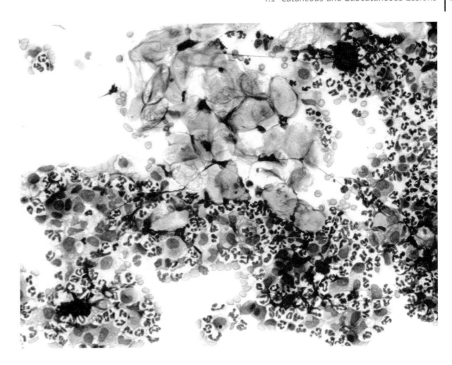

Figure 4.35 Cutaneous basilar epithelial neoplasm (trichoblastoma), dog, 50× objective. Note the bright-pink basement membrane material.

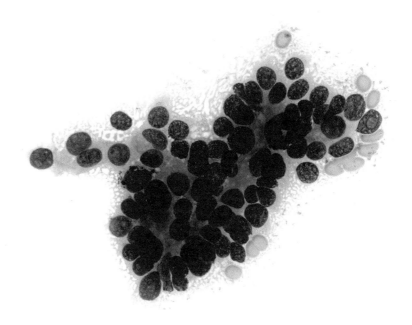

cells are accompanied by granular cells with an abundant cytoplasm containing fine, pink granular material, and care should be taken to differentiate from mast cells (compare Figures 4.37 and 4.4) [46]. Nuclei are round and centrally located with small or inapparent nucleoli. Anisocytosis/anisokaryosis are mild and N/C ratios are high. Cystic material may predominate (see Section 4.1.12).

4.1.13.2 Clinical Considerations

- Large category of tumors arising from basal epithelial cells that differentiate toward epidermal, trichofollicular, or adnexal structures. These include trichoblastomas (most common), trichoepitheliomas, pilomatricomas, and many others. Histopathology is required for differentiation [47].

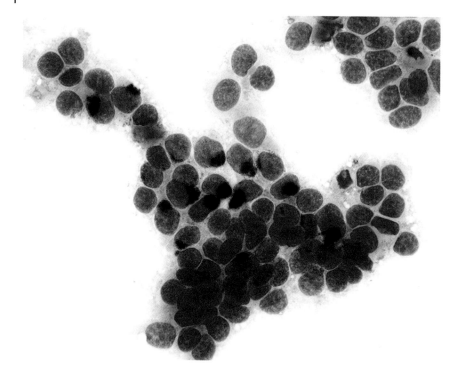

Figure 4.36 Cutaneous basilar epithelial neoplasm (trichoepithelioma), dog, 50× objective. Note the unipolar cap of green/black melanin pigment granules in the cytoplasm of some cells.

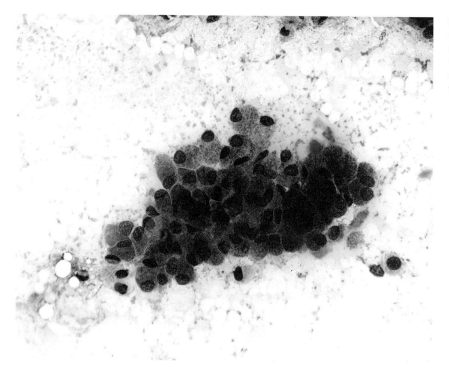

Figure 4.37 Cutaneous basilar epithelial neoplasm (trichoblastoma; granular variant), dog, 50× objective. Cohesive cells often have more abundant cytoplasm than typical basilar cells, with fine purple granules.

- Common around the head and neck in older dogs and cats [47].
- Usually solitary, firm, well-demarcated, hairless, variably pigmented masses.

4.1.13.3 Prognosis
Excellent. Malignant variants are rare.

4.1.14 Basal Cell Carcinoma

4.1.14.1 Cytologic Features
These are similar to those seen in cutaneous basilar epithelial neoplasms, with sheets of cuboidal epithelial cells noted; however, greater criteria of malignancy typically are seen, including cellular piling and crowding, anisokaryosis, and prominent basophilic nucleoli (Figure 4.38).

Figure 4.38 Basal cell carcinoma, cat, 50× objective. Note the cell piling and prominent nucleoli compared to Figure 4.35.

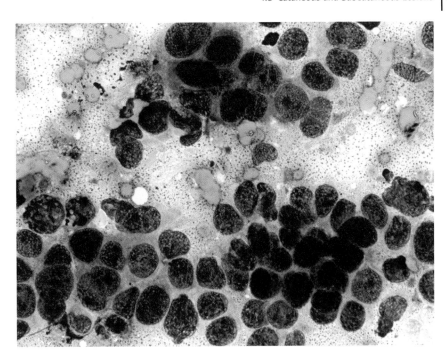

4.1.14.2 Clinical Considerations

- Uncommon tumors in dogs and cats.
- Grossly = variably pigmented and haired, raised plaques or nodules.
- Pleomorphism can be seen in benign cutaneous basilar epithelial neoplasms (usually <30% of cells), and histopathology is required for the evaluation of biologic behavior [47].

4.1.14.3 Prognosis

Good. Basal cell carcinomas are generally considered low-grade malignancies in both dogs and cats. Surgical excision appears to provide good long-term control. Local recurrence and metastatic disease are rare [48].

4.1.15 Sweat Gland Adenomas

4.1.15.1 Cytologic Features

Sweat gland adenomas are characterized by sheets of cuboidal to short columnar epithelial cells with round, eccentrically placed nuclei that have condensed chromatin. Intercellular borders often are poorly defined. Anisocytosis/anisokaryosis are mild (Figure 4.39). These tumors can appear similar to cutaneous basilar epithelial tumors and can become cystic.

4.1.15.2 Clinical Considerations

- Single lesions mostly around the head and limbs [49].
- Adenomas more common than adenocarcinomas [50].
- Multiple histological subtypes.

4.1.15.3 Prognosis

Excellent.

4.1.16 Sweat Gland Adenocarcinomas

4.1.16.1 Cytologic Features

Sweat gland adenocarcinomas are seen as cohesive sheets and nests of cells. Cells are round, with a small to moderate volume of pale-blue cytoplasm, and often eccentrically placed nuclei. Anisocytosis/anisokaryosis are moderate to marked and N/C ratios are moderate to high (Figure 4.40).

4.1.16.2 Clinical Considerations

- Occur mostly on the legs, thorax, and head in dogs and cats [51, 52].
- Well circumscribed. Majority are solitary, but multiple masses may be seen.
- Tumors in dogs may be associated with ultraviolet (UV) radiation exposure [53].
- Multiple histological subtypes.

4.1.16.3 Prognosis

Generally good with surgical excision. May be locally invasive. Distant metastases occur rarely in dogs, and confer a poor prognosis [51].

4.1.17 Sebaceous Adenoma

4.1.17.1 Cytologic Features

Sebaceous adenomas exfoliate variably well as uniform sheets of tightly cohesive cells with abundant clear, foamy cytoplasm (Figure 4.41). Nuclei are centrally located with

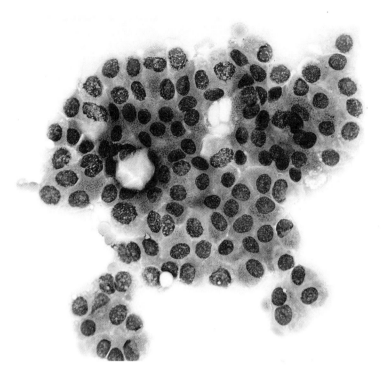

Figure 4.39 Sweat gland adenoma, dog, 50× objective.

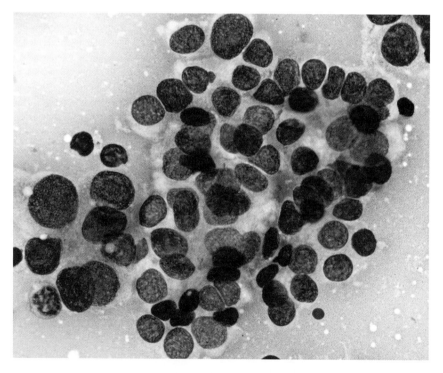

Figure 4.40 Sweat gland adenocarcinoma, dog, 50× objective.

condensed chromatin and small or inapparent nucleoli. Nodular sebaceous hyperplasia appears cytologically similar.

4.1.17.2 Clinical Considerations
- Dogs > cats. Typically older patients.
- Common in many dog breeds, but Miniature Schnauzers, Poodles, and Cocker Spaniels are overrepresented [54].

- Grossly = single, raised, hairless, smooth to wartlike, red lesions.
- Predilection sites = limbs, trunk, eyelids (dogs) and head, back (cats) [54].

4.1.17.3 Prognosis
Excellent. Surgical excision (if required) is curative.

Figure 4.41 Sebaceous adenoma, dog, 50× objective.

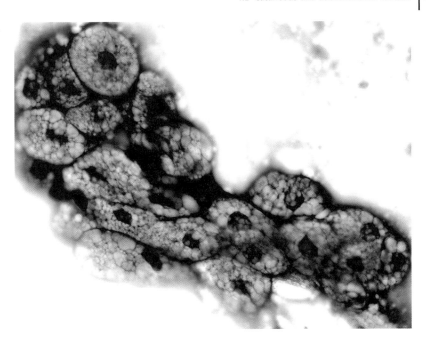

4.1.18 Sebaceous Epithelioma

4.1.18.1 Cytologic Features

Sebaceous epitheliomas comprise well-differentiated basal epithelial cells intimately associated with nests of mature sebaceous epithelial cells (Figure 4.42). Basilar epithelial cells often predominate; however, the ratio of the two populations varies, with no effect on biologic behavior [55].

4.1.18.2 Clinical Considerations

- Common in dogs, uncommon in cats.
- Similar gross appearance to sebaceous adenomas.

4.1.18.3 Prognosis

Generally good with wide surgical excision. Sebaceous epitheliomas may behave as low-grade malignancies, recurring at sites of excision or invading local lymphatics, and rarely are metastatic [56].

4.1.19 Sebaceous Carcinoma

4.1.19.1 Cytologic Features

Often highly cellular, with large cohesive sheets of epithelial cells that have prominent intercellular borders, though individualized cells may predominate [57]. The cells have

Figure 4.42 Sebaceous epithelioma, dog, 50× objective.

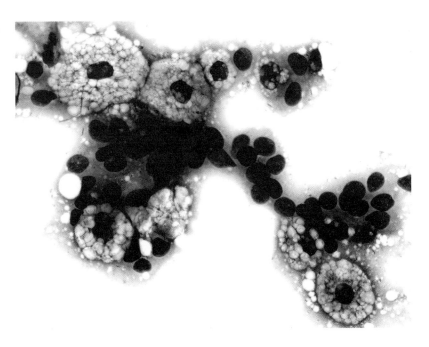

clear to medium-blue cytoplasm with numerous fine clear vacuoles and round, central nuclei with stippled chromatin and prominent nucleoli (Figure 4.43). Anisocytosis/anisokaryosis are moderate to marked and N/C ratios are high.

4.1.19.2 Clinical Considerations
- Uncommon tumors in older dogs and cats [54, 58].
- Grossly = pink, exophytic, wartlike lesions. Ulceration is common.
- Predilection sites = head/neck (dogs) and head, thorax, and perineum (cats).
- Predisposed dog breeds = Cocker Spaniels, West Highland White Terriers, Scottish Terriers, and Siberian Huskies [57].

4.1.19.3 Prognosis
Fair to good. Sebaceous carcinomas are considered low-grade malignancies and are locally invasive. Wide surgical excision can be curative, but recurrence is common. Metastatic disease is rare, usually in local lymph nodes.

4.1.20 Cutaneous Metastatic Carcinoma

4.1.20.1 Cytologic Features
Carcinomas may metastasize to the skin. These mostly appear as cohesive sheets of cells with prominent intercellular borders; however, anaplastic variants may lose cohesion. Criteria of malignancy often are marked, including anisocytosis/anisokaryosis, high N/C ratios, and increased mitotic activity (Figure 4.44).

4.1.20.2 Clinical Considerations
- Many tumor types reported, including mammary, urinary, and pulmonary [59–61].
- Pulmonary carcinomas in cats have a propensity for cutaneous metastasis, often to digits, but also the abdominal wall [61, 62].

4.1.20.3 Prognosis
Poor.

4.1.21 Squamous Papilloma

4.1.21.1 Cytologic Features
Squamous papillomas are characterized by ovoid to polygonal squamous cells that have an abundant cytoplasm containing bright-pink keratohyaline granules. Nuclei are large, round, and pyknotic with condensed chromatin. Squamous papillomas frequently are inflamed (see Figure 4.45).

4.1.21.2 Clinical Considerations
- Often caused by infection with canine papilloma viruses [63].
- Grossly = wartlike or cauliflower-like lesions.
- Common locations = head, eyes, mouth, and feet [63].
- Mostly seen in young, stressed, or immunocompromised patients [20].

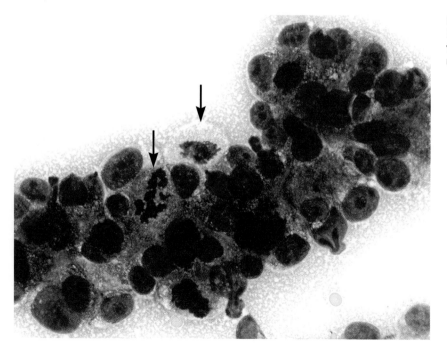

Figure 4.43 Sebaceous carcinoma, dog, 50× objective. Note the fine clear vacuoles, prominent nucleoli, and mitotic figures (arrows).

Figure 4.44 Cutaneous metastatic carcinoma (pulmonary carcinoma), cat, 50× objective.

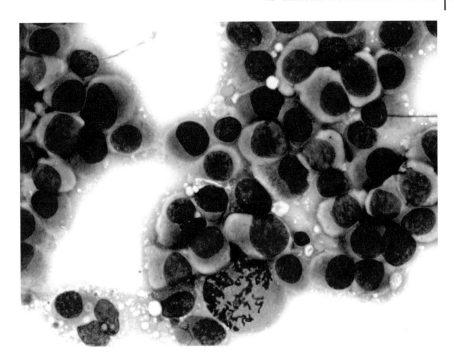

Figure 4.45 Squamous papilloma, dog, 50× objective. Note the characteristic prominent, pink keratohyaline granules in the cytoplasm, and large nuclei.

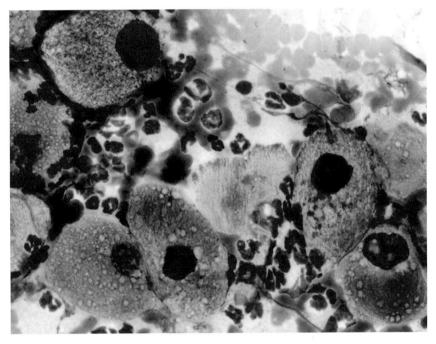

4.1.21.3 Prognosis

Excellent. Most spontaneously regress over a period of 1–6 months, but may persist for up to a year [63, 64]. Surgical excision, if required, is curative.

4.1.22 Squamous Cell Carcinoma (SCC)

4.1.22.1 Cytologic Features

Variably cohesive sheets of cells that range from ovoid to polygonal. They often have prominent criteria of malignancy, with marked anisocytosis and anisokaryosis. The cells frequently have a keratinized cytoplasm, which appears as bright sky-blue and hyalinized (Figure 4.46). Keratinized squamous cells should have small, pyknotic nuclei with dense chromatin. The finding of large, immature nuclei in keratinized cells suggests nuclear to cytoplasmic dissociation and can be seen with both neoplasia and dysplasia. Perinuclear vacuolation is a common finding in SCC. Inflammation (usually neutrophilic) is commonly seen and is not associated with tumor differentiation [65].

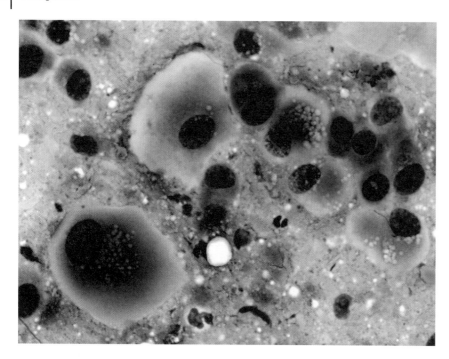

Figure 4.46 Squamous cell carcinoma, cat, 50× objective. Note the sky-blue cytoplasm, immature nuclei, and perinuclear vacuolation.

4.1.22.2 Clinical Considerations

- Cats > dogs [66].
- Common sites = nasal planum, pinnae, eyelids (cats) and flank, abdomen, and nail bed (dogs).
- Metastatic disease to lymph nodes common [66].

4.1.22.3 Prognosis

Variable based on location and presence of metastatic disease. SCC of the digit in dogs has a greater metastatic potential than those elsewhere in the body, with metastasis of cutaneous SCC uncommon [67].

4.1.23 Perianal Gland Adenoma

4.1.23.1 Cytologic Features

Perianal gland adenomas exfoliate as cohesive sheets of ovoid cells with an abundant, medium-blue/purple cytoplasm and round, centrally located nuclei with prominent, single, basophilic nucleoli (Figure 4.47). This appearance gives them a 'hepatoid' look (compare to normal hepatocytes in Figure 8.1). Small, cuboidal cells with higher N/C ratios (basilar reserve cells) may be present and intimately associated with the perianal gland cells, often surrounding

Figure 4.47 Perianal gland adenoma, dog, 50× objective. Smaller reserve cells are seen around the periphery of the epithelial sheets.

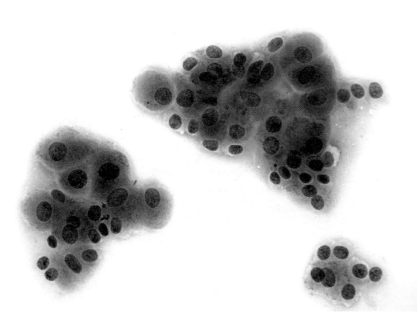

clusters in linear rows. They often are highly vascular tumors, and abundant blood may be present in the background.

4.1.23.2 Clinical Considerations
- Mostly seen in hairless areas around the anus but may be seen in haired skin around the tail base, perineum, posterior pelvic limbs, ventral abdomen, and dorsum [68].
- Multiple masses may be present.
- Older, intact males are at increased risk due to androgen-mediated growth, but tumors are seen in both sexes (neutered or intact) [69].
- Tumors have a tendency to ulcerate.
- Proportion of basal (reserve) cells to perianal gland cells is not associated with malignant potential [70].

4.1.23.3 Prognosis
Excellent. Tumors may regress with castration alone for intact dogs. Surgical excision generally is curative.

4.1.24 Perianal Gland Adenocarcinoma

4.1.24.1 Cytologic Features
Perianal gland adenocarcinomas can look very similar to adenomas, and accurate differentiation requires evaluation of tissue architecture via histopathology. In general, adenocarcinomas have a tendency toward higher N/C ratios and crowding of cells (compare Figures 4.48 and 4.47). Increased numbers of reserve cells are not associated with malignant potential [70].

4.1.24.2 Clinical Considerations
- Less common than adenomas [68, 71].
- No sex predilection.
- Often adherent to underlying tissues and tendency to ulcerate. Usually larger than adenomas [68].
- Some morphologic features that may support carcinoma over adenoma include: lack of distinction between perianal and reserve cells, nodular foci of reserve cells, anisocytosis/anisokaryosis within perianal and reserve cells, perianal gland cells with high N/C ratios, vacuolation of perianal gland cells or sebaceous differentiation, irregular cluster margins, and the presence of lymphoplasmacytic inflammation [68].
- Well-differentiated carcinomas may lack pleomorphism, and histopathology is required for appreciation of tissue architecture for evaluation of biologic behavior [72].

4.1.24.3 Prognosis
Fair to good based on the stage and size of the tumor, with tumors <5 cm carrying a better prognosis [73]. Metastatic spread is typically low and usually occurs late in the course of the disease, but may occur in the regional lymph nodes, lungs, liver, and kidney, and confers a poor prognosis [68, 73].

4.1.25 Anal Sac Apocrine Gland Adenocarcinoma

4.1.25.1 Cytologic Features
These tumors are characterized by sheets of cells that frequently lack defined intercellular borders (compared to

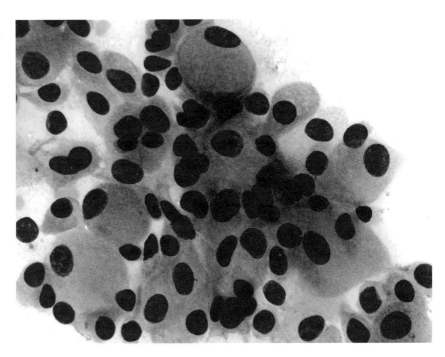

Figure 4.48 Perianal gland adenocarcinoma, dog, 50× objective. Note the higher N/C ratios and cellular crowding relative to perianal gland adenomas.

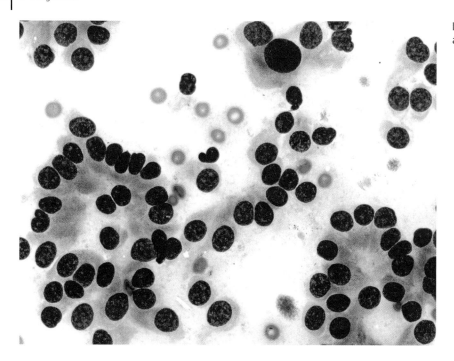

Figure 4.49 Anal sac apocrine gland adenocarcinoma, dog, 50× objective.

perianal gland tumors) and are arranged in palisading rows and acinar formations (Figure 4.49). Nuclei are round with granular chromatin and multiple small nucleoli. Despite an aggressive biologic behavior, anisokaryosis often is mild, and mitotic figures are rare.

4.1.25.2 Clinical Considerations
- Dogs > > cats [74].
- No sex predisposition [75].
- Mostly unilateral, but bilateral tumors reported [76, 77].
- Hypercalcemia seen in ~25% of cases [77, 78].
- High metastatic rate in sublumbar lymph nodes, less commonly to the lungs, liver, and spleen.

4.1.25.3 Prognosis
Fair to poor based on the stage of disease and treatment. Hypercalcemia confers a poor prognosis [78]. Larger tumor size is associated with higher rates of metastatic disease; however small tumors (<2 cm) still have high metastatic rates [77, 79, 80].

4.1.26 Clear Cell Adnexal Carcinoma

4.1.26.1 Cytologic Features
Although of epithelial origin, these tumors contain cells that mostly are individualized and are round to spindloid, which can make differentiating these from a mesenchymal tumor difficult (Figure 4.50). Cells may contain an abundant clear secretory material or cytoplasmic clearing, and pink inclusions may be present. Criteria of malignancy are marked, including anisokaryosis, prominent basophilic nucleoli, and multinucleation. These tumors frequently have a pale gray, 'tigroid' background of streaming cytoplasm from ruptured cells.

4.1.26.2 Clinical Considerations
- Rare tumors, only reported in dogs [81].
- Likely originate from epithelial stem cells, with no definitive apocrine, sebaceous, or follicular differentiation.

4.1.26.3 Prognosis
Mostly good. Complete surgical excision is curative in the majority of cases, with a low recurrence rate, and metastasis is rare [82].

4.1.27 Reactive Fibroplasia

4.1.27.1 Cytologic Features
Reactive fibroplasia is characterized by variable numbers of spindle cells. These cells often have a maturational gradient, ranging from mature cells with a scant volume of cytoplasm and elongated nuclei to plump spindle cells with an abundant deep-blue cytoplasm and ovoid nuclei with stippled chromatin. The reactive response can be florid, and differentiating reactive fibroplasia from spindle cell neoplasms is not always possible with cytology (compare Figures 4.51 and 4.52).

4.1.27.2 Clinical Considerations
- May present as firm nodules or diffuse thickening.
- Commonly associated with trauma or chronic inflammation.
- Often self-limiting but may take many months to resolve.

Figure 4.50 Clear cell adnexal carcinoma, dog, 50× objective. Note the prominent tigroid background and pink cytoplasmic material in some cells.

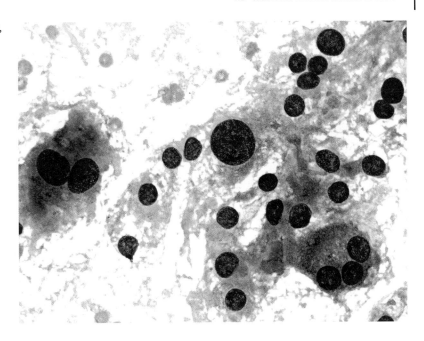

Figure 4.51 Reactive fibroplasia, dog, 50× objective. Note the accompanying inflammation.

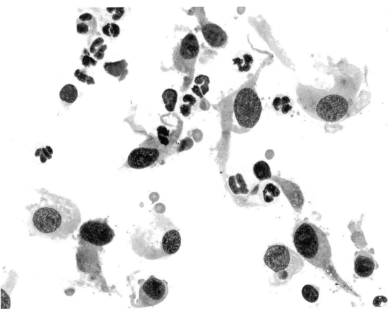

- Cytologic features reported to be more common in reactive versus neoplastic populations include low cellularity, individualized spindle cells, and an increased inflammatory-to-spindle cell ratio [83].

4.1.27.3 Prognosis
Excellent.

4.1.28 Fibroma

4.1.28.1 Cytologic Features
Fibromas often exfoliate poorly. When present, cells are spindloid and seen individually or in small aggregates, which may be accompanied by a pink extracellular matrix. The cells have a scant volume of pale cytoplasm that forms delicate bipolar tendrils and wisps. Nuclei are elongated, with granular chromatin and small basophilic nucleoli. Anisocytosis/anisokaryosis are mild and N/C ratios are high. These often are cytologically indistinguishable from reactive fibroplasia (compare Figures 4.52 and 4.51).

4.1.28.2 Clinical Considerations
- Uncommon tumors in older dogs and cats [84, 85].
- Grossly = firm, well-circumscribed, solitary lesions, most commonly found on the extremities (especially in cats), flank, or head [84].

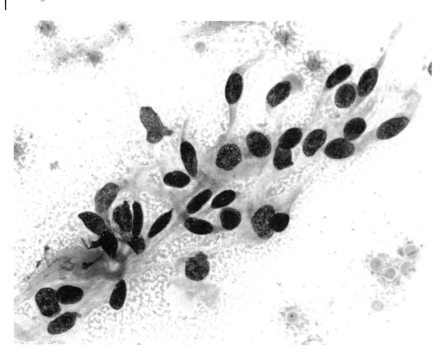

Figure 4.52 Fibroma, dog, 50× objective.

4.1.28.3 Prognosis

Excellent with surgical removal. Recurrence is rare but may occur if excision is incomplete.

4.1.29 Fibrosarcoma

4.1.29.1 Cytologic Features

Fibrosarcomas exfoliate variably well, either individually or in aggregates. The background often contains bright-pink extracellular matrix (Figure 4.53). The cells have a variable volume of cytoplasm forming tapering ends or tendrils and wisps and may contain fine pink granules or clear vacuoles. Nuclei are ovoid to elongated, with finely granular chromatin and prominent nucleoli. Anisocytosis/anisokaryosis often are marked, and multinucleation and mitotic figures may be present.

4.1.29.2 Clinical Considerations

- Generally firm and adherent to surrounding tissue.
- Locally aggressive/invasive.

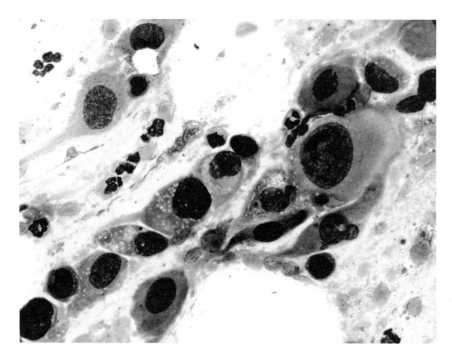

Figure 4.53 Fibrosarcoma, dog, 50× objective.

4.1.29.3 Prognosis

Good with wide surgical excision, which can result in prolonged survival times. Metastatic rates generally are low to moderate, ranging from 8% to 17%, but recurrence of tumors is high [86, 87]. Histologic tumor grade is an important prognostic determinant for metastatic potential (up to 44% of grade III tumors metastasize) [88].

4.1.30 Keloidal Fibroma/Fibrosarcoma

4.1.30.1 Cytologic Features

Keloidal fibromas and fibrosarcomas contain aggregates of spindle cells often centered around characteristic, polygonal to rounded or blunt-ended aggregates of bright-pink, smooth collagen (Figure 4.54). Differentiating keloidal fibromas from keloidal fibrosarcomas cytologically is difficult; however, anisokaryosis often is greater in fibrosarcomas [89].

4.1.30.2 Clinical Considerations

- Dogs only.
- Males (neutered and intact) predisposed [90].
- Fibromas are more common but may undergo malignant transformation to fibrosarcomas [90].

4.1.30.3 Prognosis

Excellent for keloidal fibromas, with surgical excision generally curative [90]. Wide excision is warranted due to the potential for malignant transformation.

4.1.31 Soft-tissue Sarcoma

4.1.31.1 Cytologic Features

Frequently highly exfoliative with aggregates of spindle cells often centered around capillaries (Figure 4.55). Cells have a pale-blue cytoplasm forming delicate wisps and tendrils, which may contain fine, clear vacuoles. Nuclei are ovoid with granular chromatin and small nucleoli (Figure 4.56). Anisocytosis/anisokaryosis are mild and N/C ratios are moderate to high. Multinucleated cells with peripheralized nuclei forming a ring ('crown cells') may be seen and are suggestive of perivascular wall tumors (Figure 4.57) [91]. High-grade soft-tissue sarcomas can have marked criteria of malignancy (Figure 4.58).

4.1.31.2 Clinical Considerations

- A diverse category of tumors that appear similar cytologically and may even be difficult to differentiate with histopathology [92]. Notably, this category includes peripheral nerve sheath tumors and perivascular wall tumors (e.g., hemangiopericytomas). Other soft-tissue sarcomas (e.g., fibrosarcomas, liposarcomas, hemangiosarcomas) are described separately in this text due to often having distinct morphologic features and clinical considerations.
- Common in middle-aged to older dogs > cats.
- Mostly solitary, haired, soft to firm tumors, common on extremities and thorax [93].

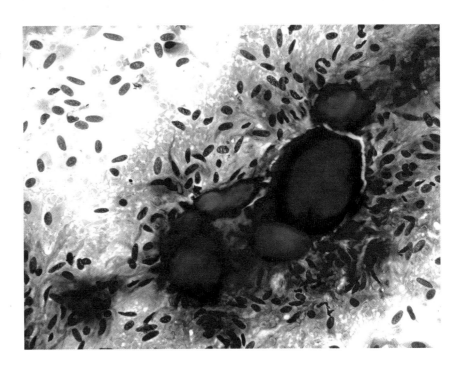

Figure 4.54 Keloidal fibroma, dog, 20× objective. Note the characteristic large, smooth, bright-pink aggregates of collagen.

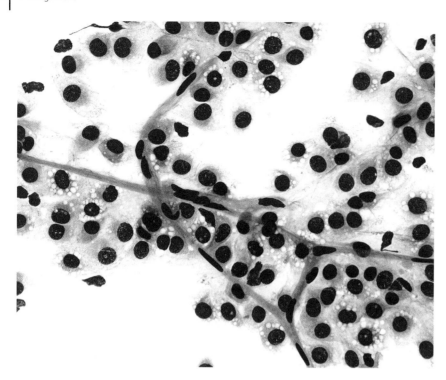

Figure 4.55 Soft tissue sarcoma (perivascular wall tumor), dog, 20× objective. Note the cells emanating from linear, streaming capillaries.

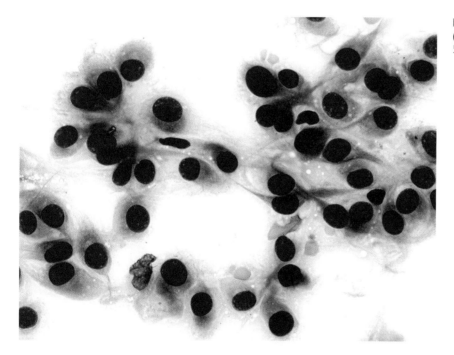

Figure 4.56 Soft tissue sarcoma (perivascular wall tumor), dog, 50× objective.

4.1.31.3 Prognosis

Complete, wide excision generally is curative, especially for low- to intermediate-grade tumors, but recurrence is common with conservative surgical excision as well as for tumors that are ulcerated and located on distal extremities [93]. The propensity for recurrence increases with histologic tumor grade, necrosis, mitotic count, and infiltrated margins, which are also associated with shorter survival times [92, 94]. Metastatic potential generally is low, but also increases with histologic tumor grade.

4.1.32 Hemangioma

4.1.32.1 Cytologic Features

Hemangiomas frequently have a densely bloody background and may only yield a small number of cells.

Figure 4.57 Soft tissue sarcoma (perivascular wall tumor), dog, 50× objective. Note the characteristic 'crown cell' (arrow).

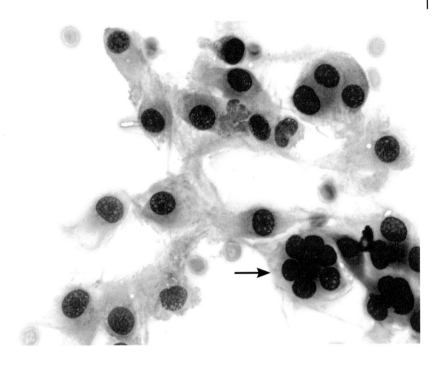

Figure 4.58 Grade III soft tissue sarcoma, dog, 50× objective. Note the multinucleation and increased mitotic figures.

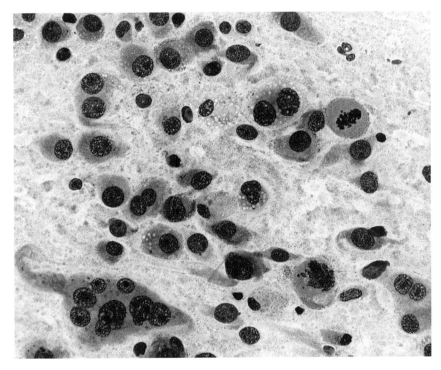

When cells are present, they mostly are individualized spindle cells, with a scant volume of pale-blue cytoplasm that forms delicate bipolar tendrils and wisps (Figure 4.59). Nuclei are ovoid to elongated, with finely granular chromatin and small, single basophilic nucleoli. Anisocytosis/ anisokaryosis are mild, while N/C ratios are high. Low numbers of well-granulated mast cells may be present. Macrophages may be present, with evidence of chronic hemorrhage (erythrophagia or hemosiderin pigment) (see Figure 2.3).

4.1.32.2 Clinical Considerations
- Grossly = hairless, smooth, red/purple dermal nodules.
- Solitary or multiple, often found on the head, limbs, trunk, and ventral abdomen.
- Most are <5 cm in diameter [95].

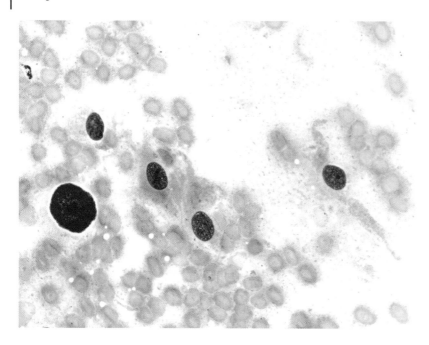

Figure 4.59 Hemangioma, dog, 50× objective. Note the bloody background, spindle cells with fine tendrils, and the mast cell (left).

- May be induced by ultraviolet exposure in poorly pigmented skin.
- Boxers are predisposed [96].

4.1.32.3 Prognosis
Excellent. Complete surgical excision is curative.

4.1.33 Hemangiosarcoma (Cutaneous)

4.1.33.1 Cytologic Features
Frequently have a densely bloody background and are variably exfoliative. Cells are spindloid, with a moderate volume of medium-blue cytoplasm. Erythrophagia may be seen in neoplastic cells and in macrophages in the background of the samples (Figure 4.60). Nuclei are ovoid with granular chromatin and prominent basophilic nucleoli. Anisocytosis/anisokaryosis are marked and N/C ratios are high (Figure 4.61). These tumors are difficult to differentiate definitively from other sarcomas cytologically.

4.1.33.2 Clinical Considerations
- Gross appearance = dermal or subcutaneous, focal or multifocal, firm and often appear deep red/purple or bruised [97, 98].

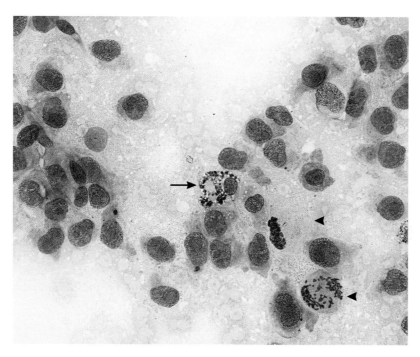

Figure 4.60 Hemangiosarcoma (cutaneous), dog, 50× objective. Note the increased mitotic figures (arrowheads) and erythrophagia/hemosiderin pigment within neoplastic cells (arrow).

Figure 4.61 Hemangiosarcoma (cutaneous), dog, 50× objective. Note the prominent nucleoli and marked anisocytosis/anisokaryosis.

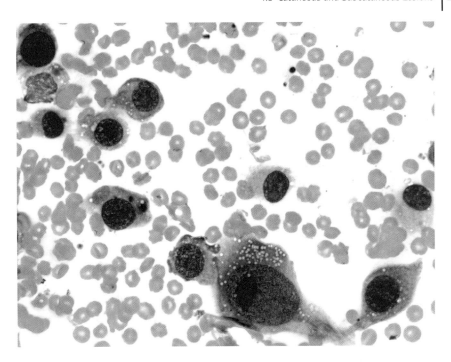

- Predilection for poorly haired skin of the ventral abdomen and preputial region (dogs) and skin of the pinna, head, and ventral abdomen (cats) [95, 98, 99].

4.1.33.3 Prognosis
Dogs = variable based on tumor stage. Stage I tumors may be treated with surgery alone and are associated with a prolonged survival time. Stage II and III tumors carry a poor prognosis [98]. Dogs with nonsolar induced dermal tumors invasive into the subcutaneous tissues have decreased survival times and increased metastatic disease compared to noninvasive solar induced dermal tumors [100].

Cats = wide surgical excision is associated with prolonged survival; however, if untreated, the prognosis is poor [99].

4.1.34 Myxoma

4.1.34.1 Cytologic Features
Myxomas have a thick, pink-stippled background of extracellular matrix, often distributing the cells in a streaming pattern (Figure 4.62). Cells are spindloid, with a scant

Figure 4.62 Myxoma, dog, 50× objective. Note the dense pink, streaming mucinous background.

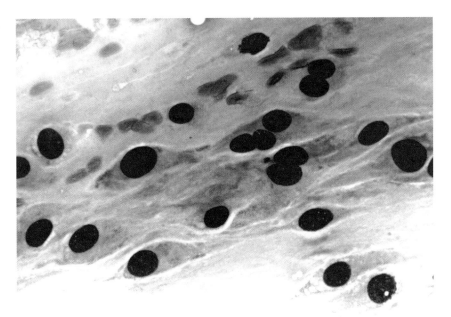

volume of pale-blue cytoplasm forming delicate wisps. Nuclei are elongated with finely granular chromatin and small basophilic nucleoli. Anisocytosis/anisokaryosis are mild and N/C ratios are high.

4.1.34.2 Clinical Considerations

- Most common in large breed, middle-aged to older dogs (Doberman Pinschers are overrepresented), but rare overall in both dogs and cats [101].
- Predilection sites = joints (especially digits and stifle) > heart and skin [101, 102].
- May be locally invasive.

4.1.34.3 Prognosis

Excellent. Prolonged survival times are reported, even in cases with incomplete excision [101].

4.1.35 Myxosarcoma

4.1.35.1 Cytologic Features

Myxosarcomas have a similar thick, pink-stippled myxoid background as myxomas. The cells have more prominent criteria for malignancy, particularly anisokaryosis and larger basophilic nucleoli (Figure 4.63).

4.1.35.2 Clinical Considerations

- Rare tumors in older dogs and cats.
- Predilection sites = trunk and limbs > joints, heart, and eye [103].
- Locally infiltrative with ill-defined margins.

4.1.35.3 Prognosis

Guarded. Recurrence is common after surgical removal, and metastasis may occur, both of which are more likely in tumors with high mitotic counts [103–105].

4.1.36 Anaplastic Sarcoma with Giant Cells

4.1.36.1 Cytologic Features

Cells are spindloid with tapering ends and have ovoid to elongated nuclei with granular chromatin and prominent nucleoli. Multinucleated giant cells may be round or spindloid with tendrils and wisps (Figure 4.64). These cells often have nuclei of varying size and shape, relative to osteoclasts (see Figure 7.4), or multinucleated macrophages (see Figure 4.74), which have multiple, regular nuclei.

4.1.36.2 Clinical Considerations

- Rare in dogs and cats.
- Previously known as malignant fibrous histiocytomas or giant cell tumors of soft tissues.
- Likely poorly differentiated sarcomas of multiple tumor types including fibrosarcoma, leiomyosarcoma, and rhabdomyosarcoma [106].
- Solitary, firm, poorly circumscribed lesions around the legs and shoulders.

4.1.36.3 Prognosis

Variable based on grade and underlying origin.

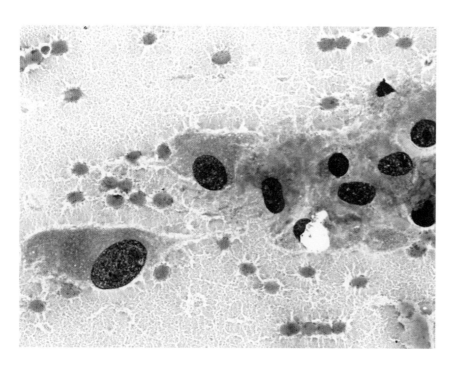

Figure 4.63 Myxosarcoma, dog, 50× objective. Note the dense pink stippled, mucinous background, and prominent anisokaryosis.

Figure 4.64 Anaplastic sarcoma with giant cells, cat, 50× objective.

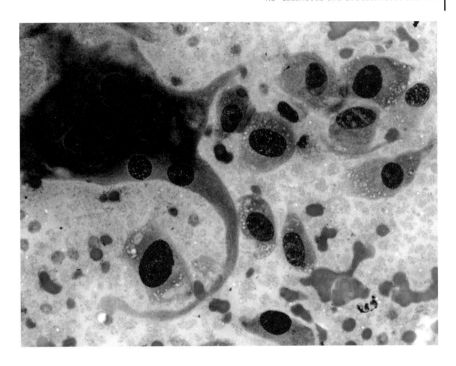

4.1.37 Lipoma

4.1.37.1 Cytologic Features

Lipomas contain large aggregates of mature adipocytes with an abundant cytoplasm that balloons with clear lipid material (Figure 4.65). Nuclei are small and condensed, with inapparent nucleoli, and frequently are pushed to the periphery of the cells. Capillaries frequently course through clusters of adipocytes (Figure 4.66), and occasional supporting stromal cells (e.g., fibroblasts) may be present. Free lipid often is present in the background of the slide.

4.1.37.2 Clinical Considerations

- Common subcutaneous tumors in middle-aged to older dogs > cats.
- Fat can dissolve with alcohol-based fixatives, and slides may be acellular.

Figure 4.65 Lipoma, dog, 4× objective.

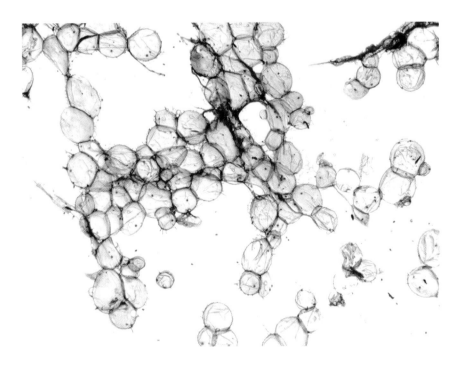

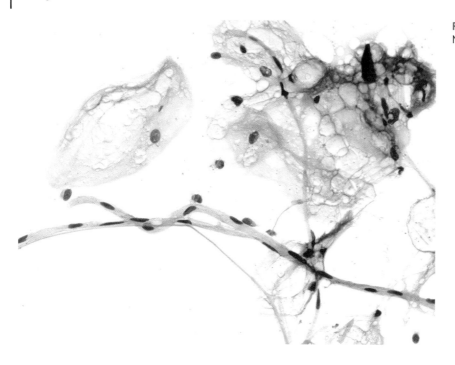

Figure 4.66 Lipoma, dog, 20× objective. Note the streaming, linear capillaries.

- Aspiration of normal adipose tissue may look similar, and interpretation should be correlated with clinical impressions.
- Infiltrative lipomas have a similar cytologic appearance. They do not metastasize but can be locally invasive/aggressive [107].

4.1.37.3 Prognosis

Excellent, with surgical excision curative. Infiltrative lipomas may require more aggressive therapy to obtain local control and have high recurrence rates [107].

4.1.38 Liposarcoma

4.1.38.1 Cytologic Features

There are numerous histologic subtypes of liposarcomas, resulting in a wide array of cytologic appearances. Well-differentiated liposarcomas (Figure 4.67) contain neoplastic cells that vaguely resemble adipocytes but are characterized by a basophilic cytoplasm with a fine lacy appearance and immature nuclei, with prominent nucleoli and moderate anisokaryosis. Poorly or dedifferentiated liposarcomas (Figure 4.68) appear somewhat cohesive and contain coarse,

Figure 4.67 Liposarcoma (well differentiated), dog, 10× objective.

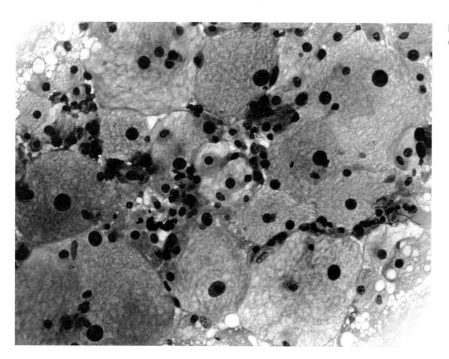

Figure 4.68 Liposarcoma (poorly differentiated), dog, 50× objective. The cells lack prominent intercellular borders and appear vaguely cohesive but contain coarse, clear lipid vacuoles. Note also the small size of the cells relative to Figure 4.67.

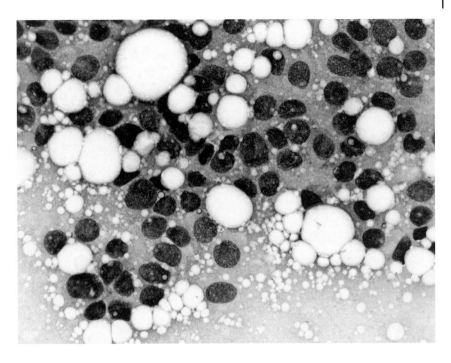

clear lipid vacuoles in their cytoplasm. Such a finding should raise a suspicion for a liposarcoma, regardless of cell shape or arrangement. Globular pink inclusions may be seen in the cytoplasm (Figure 4.69) [108]. Anisocytosis and anisokaryosis are moderate to marked and N/C ratios are variable.

4.1.38.2 Clinical Considerations
- Most common in appendicular or axial locations.
- Reported in locations other than the skin including sublingual and internal organs including the spleen [109, 110].

- Locally invasive tumors with low metastatic potential, though metastatic disease is reported [111].
- No evidence for malignant transformation from lipomas.

4.1.38.3 Prognosis
Good with wide surgical margins. Tumors with marginal excision are associated with lower median survival times. Factors not associated with survival time in one study included tumor size, location, and histological subtype [111].

Figure 4.69 Liposarcoma, dog, 50× objective. Note the prominent coarse clear vacuoles and pink globular material in the cytoplasm.

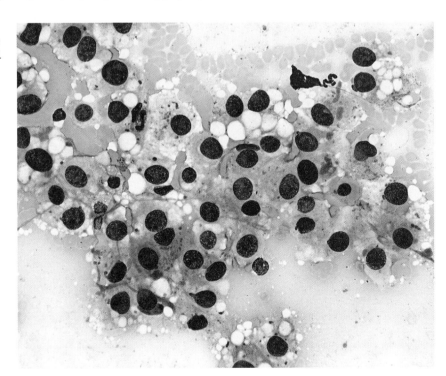

4.1.39 Xanthoma

4.1.39.1 Cytologic Features

Xanthomas exfoliate well as individualized cells that have abundant cytoplasm containing variably sized, coarse, clear vacuoles (Figure 4.70). Nuclei are round, eccentrically placed, and have finely stippled chromatin with small nucleoli. Anisocytosis is moderate and anisokaryosis is mild. Varying degrees of inflammation are seen. Cytologically, xanthomas can be difficult to differentiate from liposarcomas and reactive fibrohistiocytic nodules (compare to Figures 4.69 and 4.71).

4.1.39.2 Clinical Considerations

- Cats > dogs.
- Benign inflammatory lesions of macrophages laden with cholesterol and lipid.
- Usually multiple (rarely solitary) raised, hairless, white/yellow, plaques or nodules.
- Most common around the face and periorbital regions. Rarely disseminated [112].
- May be idiopathic [113], or manifest secondary to diseases of lipid metabolism (e.g., hyperlipidemia from diabetes mellitus or glucocorticoid therapy).

4.1.39.3 Prognosis

Excellent with surgical resection and treatment of any underlying predisposing cause.

4.1.40 Reactive Fibrohistiocytic Nodule

4.1.40.1 Cytologic Features

Reactive fibrohistiocytic nodules contain reactive macrophages seen individually and in sheets. The cells have a moderate volume of pale- to medium-blue cytoplasm that contains fine, coarse, clear vacuoles. Nuclei are round with stippled chromatin and small or inconspicuous nucleoli (Figure 4.71). Anisocytosis/anisokaryosis are mild (compared to liposarcomas). The macrophages are accompanied by a population of well-differentiated spindle cells. These lesions can appear similar to cutaneous xanthomas (compare to Figure 4.70), but generally have more fine vacuoles and are accompanied by a spindle cell population. Additionally, cutaneous xanthomas usually are multiple, while reactive fibrohistiocytic nodules are solitary.

4.1.40.2 Clinical Considerations

- Rare lesions. Seen in young dogs (aged <3 years).
- Usually single, <1 cm, haired, or partially alopecic nodules [114].
- Most common on the face and legs.

4.1.40.3 Prognosis

Excellent with surgical excision.

4.1.41 Canine Sterile Nodular Panniculitis

4.1.41.1 Cytologic Features

These lesions are characterized by a population of reactive macrophages that have abundant, vacuolated cytoplasm

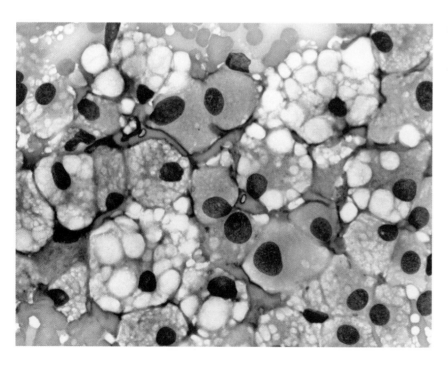

Figure 4.70 Xanthoma, dog, 50× objective. Macrophages are monomorphic and frequently contain coarse, clear vacuoles.

Figure 4.71 Reactive fibrohistiocytic nodule, dog, 50× objective. Note the reactive, vacuolated macrophages and the spindle cell (lower left).

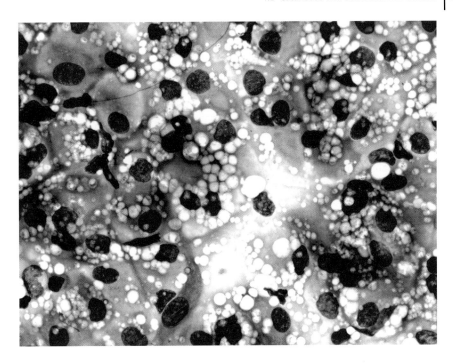

and numerous clear vacuoles in the background (Figure 4.72). Variable numbers of other inflammatory cells are present.

4.1.41.2 Clinical Considerations
- Usually multiple nodules on the trunk and neck ± ulceration or draining tracts.
- Predisposed breeds = Australian Shepherd, Brittany Spaniel, Dalmatian, Pomeranian, Chihuahua [115].

- May be associated with other inflammatory diseases, especially immune-mediated polyarthritis [115, 116].
- Rule out other causes of panniculitis (see Section 4.1.42) and histopathology required for definitive diagnosis.

4.1.41.3 Prognosis
Good. High rate of remission with appropriate therapy. Investigation for underlying systemic disease may be recommended [115, 116].

Figure 4.72 Sterile nodular panniculitis, dog, 50× objective. Note the abundant free lipid vacuoles and the multinucleated macrophage (top).

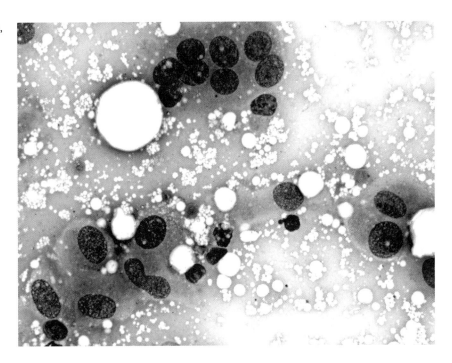

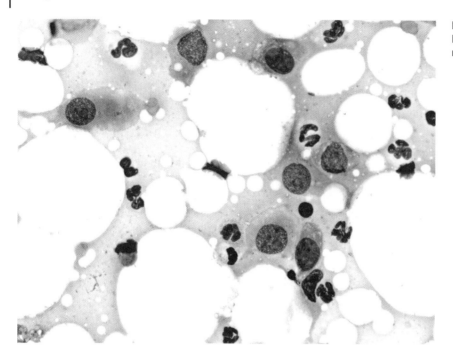

Figure 4.73 Steatitis, dog, 50× objective. Mixed inflammation is centered around numerous clear lipid vacuoles.

4.1.42 Panniculitis/Steatitis

4.1.42.1 Cytologic Features

These lesions are characterized by an inflammatory population of cells intimately associated with abundant adipose tissue (Figure 4.73). The inflammatory population ranges from neutrophilic to mononuclear, and the process may be sterile or septic.

4.1.42.2 Clinical Considerations

- May present with nodules or diffuse subcutaneous thickening.
- Infectious agents are a common cause (see Chapter 3).
- Noninfectious causes = blunt or penetrating trauma (including vaccine or injection site reactions), foreign body reactions, drug reactions, pancreatic disease, and immune-mediated causes (see canine sterile nodular panniculitis).
- Rule out inflamed/traumatized lipomas.

4.1.42.3 Prognosis

Generally good based on the underlying cause and treatment.

4.1.43 Granulomatous/Pyogranulomatous Inflammation

4.1.43.1 Cytologic Features

Granulomatous lesions are characterized by a predominance of reactive macrophages, which may be seen individually or in crowded aggregates (epithelioid macrophages). Multinucleated macrophages frequently are seen (Figure 4.74). Other inflammatory cells often are present and may include neutrophils (pyogranulomatous inflammation) or small mature lymphocytes.

4.1.43.2 Clinical Considerations

- DDx = acral lick granulomas, furunculosis, foreign body reactions, vaccine or injection site reactions, infectious agents (especially fungi and atypical bacteria such as *Mycobacterium spp.* or *Actinomyces*; see Chapter 3) or secondary to rupture of epidermal cysts.

4.1.43.3 Prognosis

Mostly good depending on treatment of the underlying cause. Some lesions are self-limiting.

4.1.44 Vaccination Reaction

4.1.44.1 Cytologic Features

Vaccination reactions mostly are characterized by a granulomatous or pyogranulomatous inflammatory response, with infiltration of lymphocytes and plasma cells in chronic lesions. The vaccine adjuvant is often (but not always) present in the background or phagocytosed by macrophages and appears as globular magenta to blue material (Figure 4.75). Reactive fibroblasts may be present, and abundant adipose tissue may be present in the background.

4.1.44.2 Clinical Considerations

- Firm, single, subcutaneous nodules in the area of injection/vaccine.
- Often delayed onset after vaccination (weeks).
- May take weeks or even months to resolve.

Figure 4.74 Pyogranulomatous inflammation, dog, 50× objective. Note the large multinucleated macrophage accompanied by neutrophils.

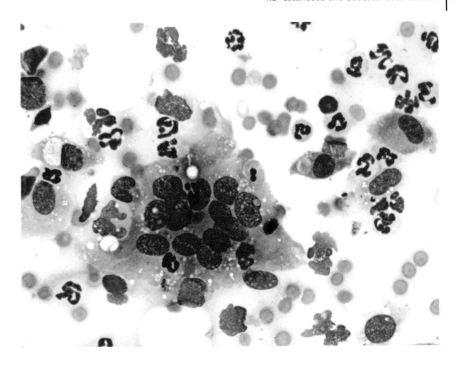

Figure 4.75 Vaccine reaction (rabies vaccine), dog, 50× objective. Note the abundant magenta granular material (adjuvant) in the background and phagocytosed by macrophages.

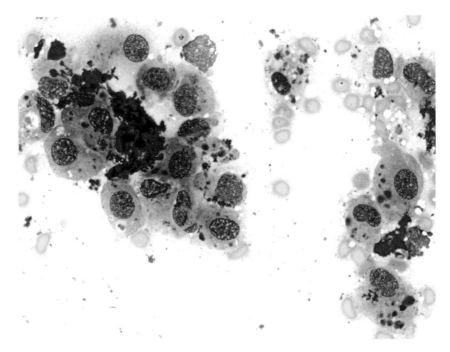

4.1.44.3 Prognosis
Excellent.

4.1.45 Abscess

4.1.45.1 Cytologic Features
Abscesses generally are characterized by large numbers of degenerative neutrophils (see Chapter 2). When these changes are seen, close evaluation for infectious organisms is warranted. Intracellular organisms confirm a septic etiology (Figure 4.76). Many different infectious organisms can cause cutaneous abscesses (see Chapter 3). Sterile abscessation is less common.

4.1.45.2 Clinical Considerations
- Lesions variably fluctuant, warm, and painful. Draining tracts may be present.
- Purulent material often aspirated.

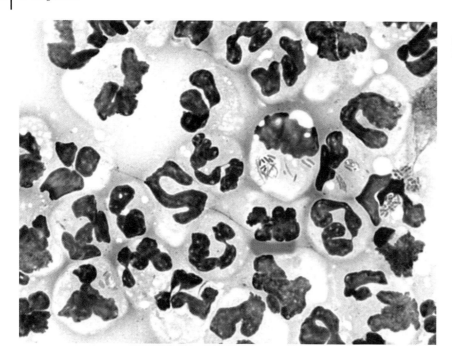

Figure 4.76 Abscess, cat, 100× objective. Neutrophils are degenerative and contain intracellular bacteria.

- Microbial culture and susceptibility testing recommended.
- May represent a primary process or secondary infection around a separate lesion.

4.1.45.3 Prognosis
Generally excellent with appropriate therapy, but variable based on the underlying cause/etiologic agent.

4.1.46 Seroma/Hygroma

4.1.46.1 Cytologic Features
Seromas typically have a variably thick, blue/purple proteinaceous background, with low numbers of inflammatory cells scattered individually (Figure 4.77). The type of inflammatory cells often reflects the time course of the lesion, dominated by nondegenerative neutrophils acutely, and macrophages in the chronic stages. There

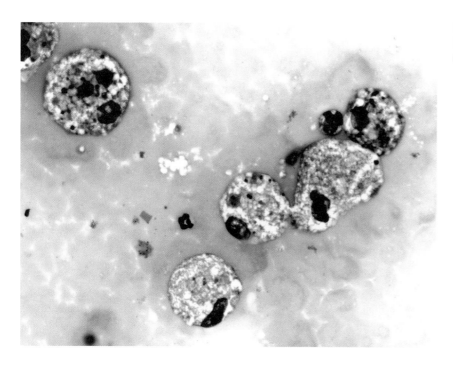

Figure 4.77 Seroma, dog, 50× objective. Macrophages contain phagocytosed proteinaceous material.

may be evidence of chronic hemorrhage including erythrophagia or heme-breakdown pigment in macrophages (see Chapter 2).

4.1.46.2 Clinical Considerations
- Soft, fluctuant, fluid-filled lesions.
- Unilateral > bilateral [117].
- Often associated with trauma or surgery.
- Hygromas form over bony prominences secondary to chronic trauma and appear similar to seromas.

4.1.46.3 Prognosis
Excellent. Spontaneous resolution is common, but drainage or surgical excision may be required which are typically curative [117].

4.1.47 Calcinosis Circumscripta

4.1.47.1 Cytologic Features
Samples have a thick purple background with abundant aggregates of refractile, crystalline material (Figure 4.78). Nucleated cells usually are present in low numbers, mostly reactive macrophages, which may contain phagocytosed mineralized debris. Grossly, the aspirated material appears milky, and stained sides have a characteristic chalky appearance (Figure 4.79).

4.1.47.2 Clinical Considerations
- Dogs > cats. German Shepherds are predisposed.
- Young animals overrepresented (88% of dogs <4 years of age in one study) [118].

- Mostly firm, gritty, solitary lesions between 0.5 and 3 cm around the joints and bony prominences of limbs. Other sites include tongue and paw pads [118].
- Pathogenesis is unknown, but dystrophic mineralization secondary to trauma has been proposed.

4.1.47.3 Prognosis
Excellent. Spontaneous regression may occur, and surgical excision generally is curative.

4.1.48 Calcinosis Cutis

4.1.48.1 Cytologic Features
Samples have a similar appearance to those of calcinosis circumscripta but usually are more cellular with greater numbers of inflammatory cells (Figure 4.80).

4.1.48.2 Clinical Considerations
- Erythematous papules or gritty plaques commonly found on the dorsal trunk and head, as well as the inguinal region and extremities [119].
- DDx = glucocorticoid exposure, hyperadrenocorticism (dogs), calcium/phosphorus imbalance, tissue trauma, and infectious disease [119, 120].
- Idiopathic calcinosis cutis occurs in young dogs (usually aged <1 year) and spontaneously resolves [121].

4.1.48.3 Prognosis
Generally good with spontaneous resolution after treatment of the underlying cause.

Figure 4.78 Calcinosis circumscripta, dog, 20× objective. Note the thick background and aggregates of refractile mineralized debris.

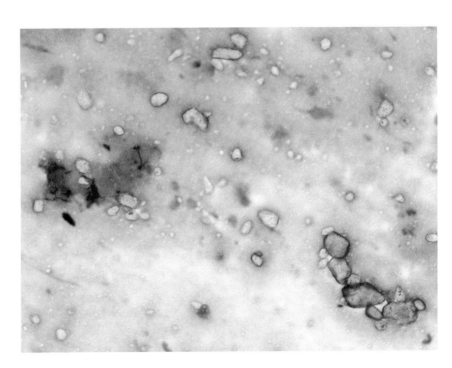

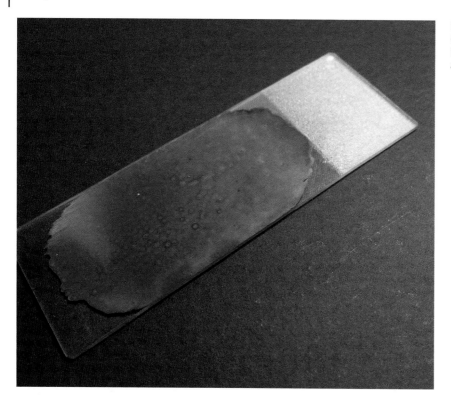

Figure 4.79 Calcinosis circumscripta (gross appearance), dog. The samples have a characteristic, thick chalky appearance.

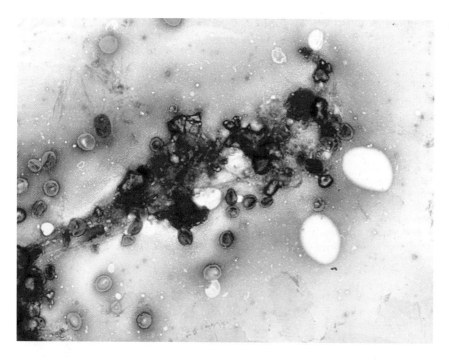

Figure 4.80 Calcinosis cutis, dog, 50× objective.

4.1.49 Hypersensitivity Reaction

4.1.49.1 Cytologic Features

Hypersensitivity reactions frequently are dominated by eosinophils, with lesser numbers of mast cells and other inflammatory cells (Figure 4.81). Differential diagnoses may include eosinophilic granuloma or mast cell tumor. Useful findings to help differentiate from mast cell tumors include individualized cells (compared to aggregates of mast cells in neoplastic lesions) and well-differentiated mast cells with many granules (compare to mast cell tumors; Sections 4.1.1 and 4.1.2).

Figure 4.81 Hypersensitivity reaction, dog, 50× objective. Note the mast cell (top left).

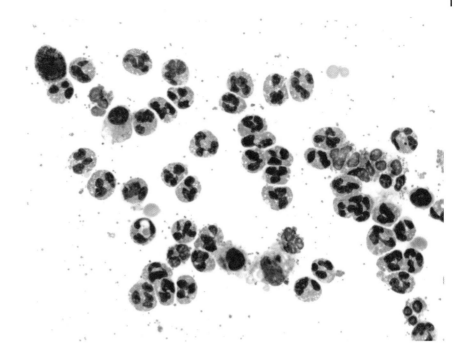

4.1.49.2 Clinical Considerations

- Acute onset of single or multiple, haired nodules.
- May be associated with arthropod bites or contact allergens.

4.1.49.3 Prognosis

Excellent. Lesions mostly spontaneously resolve, but those requiring therapy also have a good prognosis.

4.1.50 Eosinophilic Granuloma/Inflammatory Disease

4.1.50.1 Cytologic Features

Eosinophils predominate and frequently are found in aggregates. Many free eosinophil granules may be seen in the background (Figure 4.82). A variable number of other inflammatory cells may be present, with macrophages generally present in eosinophilic granulomas.

Figure 4.82 Eosinophilic granuloma, cat, 50× objective. Note the abundant eosinophil granules in the background.

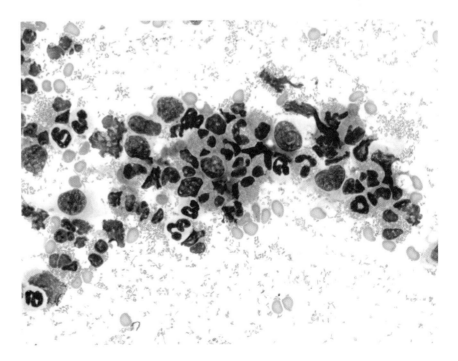

4.1.50.2 Clinical Considerations

- Eosinophilic granulomas occur in cats and dogs. Lesions are erythematous to yellow, raised nodules or linear bands most common on the inner thigh/posterior hind limbs > head and mouth.
- Eosinophilic ulcers and plaques also are common lesions in cats around the oral cavity and ventral abdomen [122].
- Rule out allergic/hypersensitivity disease, infectious agents, and immune-mediated/idiopathic.
- Concurrent sepsis is common [123].

4.1.50.3 Prognosis

Good with appropriate therapy.

4.1.51 Pemphigus Foliaceus

4.1.51.1 Cytologic Features

Pemphigus lesions are characterized by acantholytic keratinocytes. These cells are round, with an abundant cytoplasm that contains variably prominent magenta granules (keratohyaline granules) (Figures 4.83 and 4.84). They have

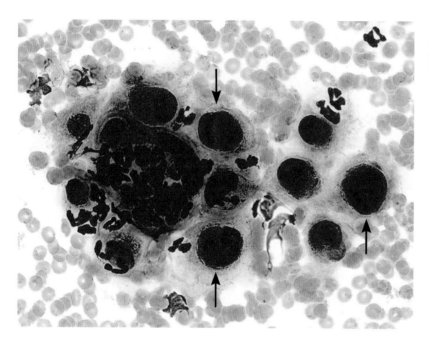

Figure 4.83 Pemphigus foliaceus, dog, 50× objective. Numerous acantholytic cells (arrows) accompany neutrophilic inflammation.

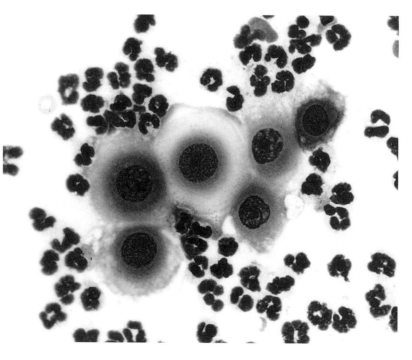

Figure 4.84 Pemphigus foliaceus, dog, 50× objective. Acantholytic cells surrounded by nondegenerative neutrophils.

large, centrally located nuclei with reticulated chromatin and variably prominent nucleoli. Neutrophils and other inflammatory cells are frequently present. Although acantholytic cells are not pathognomonic for pemphigus (and can be seen in other chronic inflammatory or immune-mediated conditions), they are most common in this disease and were present in 77% of cases in one study [124].

4.1.51.2 Clinical Considerations
- Most common autoimmune disease of skin in dogs and cats.

- May occur spontaneously or secondary to drug administration or neoplasia.
- Grossly = crusts, papules, and alopecia [124].
- Predilection sites in order of frequency = trunk, inner pinna, face, and footpads [124, 125].

4.1.51.3 Prognosis
Variable. High mortality can be seen in the early stages of the disease, but long-term survival is possible with response to therapy [124, 126].

References

1 Kiupel, M., Webster, J.D., Bailey, K.L., *et al.* (2011) Proposal of a 2-tier histologic grading system for canine cutaneous mast cell tumors to more accurately predict biological behavior. *Vet. Pathol.*, **48** (1), 147–155.

2 Camus, M.S., Priest, H.L., Koehler, J.W., *et al.* (2016) Cytologic criteria for mast cell tumor grading in dogs with evaluation of clinical outcome. *Vet. Pathol.*, **53** (6), 1117–1123.

3 Paes, P.R.O., Horta, R.S., Luza, L.C., *et al.* (2022) Inclusion of fibroblasts and collagen fibrils in the cytologic grading of canine cutaneous mast cell tumors. *Vet. Clin. Pathol.*, **51** (3), 339–348.

4 Allison, R.W., Velguth, K.E. (2010) Appearance of granulated cells in blood films stained by automated aqueous versus methanolic Romanowsky methods. *Vet. Clin. Pathol.*, **39** (1), 99–104.

5 Sabattini, S., Renzi, A., Marconato, L., *et al.* (2018) Comparison between May-Grünwald-Giemsa and rapid cytological stains in fine-needle aspirates of canine mast cell tumour: diagnostic and prognostic implications. *Vet. Comp. Oncol.*, **16** (4), 511–517.

6. de Nardi, A.B., Dos Santos Horta, R., Fonseca-Alves, C.E., et al. (2022) Diagnosis, prognosis and treatment of canine cutaneous and subcutaneous mast cell tumors. *Cells*, 11 (4), 618

7 Rigas, K., Biasoli, D., Polton, G., *et al.* (2020) Mast cell tumours in dogs less than 12 months of age: a multi-institutional retrospective study. *J. Small Anim. Pract.*, **61** (7), 449–457.

8 Yang, C., Bradley, C.W., Preziosi, D., *et al.* (2023) Cutaneous mastocytosis in 8 young dogs and review of literature. *Vet. Pathol.*, **60** (6), 849–856.

9 Mullins, M.N., Dernell, W.S., Withrow, S.J., *et al.* (2006) Evaluation of prognostic factors associated with outcome in dogs with multiple cutaneous mast cell tumors treated with surgery with and without adjuvant treatment: 54 cases (1998–2004). *J. Am. Vet. Med. Assoc.*, **228** (1), 91–95.

10 Marconato, L., Stefanello, D., Basano, F.S., *et al.* (2023) Subcutaneous mast cell tumours: a prospective multi-institutional clinicopathological and prognostic study of 43 dogs. *Vet. Rec.*, **193** (1): e2991. doi: 10.1002/vetr.2991. Last accessed October 15, 2023.

11 Cherzan, N.L., Fryer, K., Burke, B., *et al.* (2023) Factors affecting prognosis in canine subcutaneous mast cell tumors: 45 cases. *Vet. Surg.*, **52** (4), 531–537.

12 Arz, R., Chiti, L.E., Krudewig, C., *et al.* (2023) Lymph node metastasis in feline cutaneous low-grade mast cell tumours. *J. Feline Med. Surg.*, **25** (1), 1–7.

13 Ho, N.T., Smith, K.C., Dobromylskyj, M.J. (2018) Retrospective study of more than 9000 feline cutaneous tumours in the UK: 2006–2013. *J. Feline Med. Surg.*, **20** (2), 128–134.

14 Blackwood, L., Murphy, S., Buracco, P., *et al.* (2012) European consensus document on mast cell tumours in dogs and cats. *Vet. Comp. Oncol.*, **10** (3), e1–e29.

15 Sabattini, S., Bettini, G. (2019) Grading cutaneous mast cell tumors in cats. *Vet. Pathol.*, **56** (1), 43–49.

16 Litster, A.L., Sorenmo, K.U. (2006) Characterisation of the signalment, clinical and survival characteristics of 41 cats with mast cell neoplasia. *J. Feline Med. Surg.*, **8** (3), 177–183.

17 Molander-McCrary, H., Henry, C.J., Potter, K., *et al.* (1998) Cutaneous mast cell tumors in cats: 32 cases (1991–1994). *J. Am. Anim. Hosp. Assoc.*, **34** (4), 281–284.

18 Melville, K., Smith, K.C., Dobromylskyj, M.J. (2015) Feline cutaneous mast cell tumours: a UK-based study comparing signalment and histological features with long-term outcomes. *J. Feline Med. Surg.*, **17** (6), 486–493.

19 Moore, P.F., Schrenzel, M.D., Affolter, V.K., *et al.* (1996) Canine cutaneous histiocytoma is an epidermotropic Langerhans cell histiocytosis that expresses CD1 and specific beta 2-integrin molecules. *Am. J. Pathol.*, **148** (5), 1699–1708.

20 Kim, D., Dobromlskyj, M.J., O'Neill, D., *et al.* (2022) Skin masses in dogs under one year of age. *J. Small Anim. Pract.*, **63** (1), 10–15.

21 Costa, D., Ferreira, R., Prada, J., *et al.* (2020) A role for angiogenesis in canine cutaneous histiocytoma regression: insights into an old clinical enigma. *In Vivo*, **34** (6), 3279–3284.

22 Moore, P.F. (2022) Histiocytic diseases. *Vet. Clin. North Am. Small Anim. Pract.*, **53** (1), 121–140.

23 Moore, P.F. (2014) A review of histiocytic diseases of dogs and cats. *Vet. Pathol.*, **51** (1), 167–184.

24 Affolter, V.K., Moore, P.F. (2002) Localized and disseminated histiocytic sarcoma of dendritic cell origin in dogs. *Vet. Pathol.*, **39** (1), 74–83.

25 Doka, R.M., Suter, S.E., Mastromauro, M.L., *et al.* (2022) Doxorubicin for treatment of histiocytic sarcoma in dogs: 31 cases (2003–2017). *J. Am. Vet. Med. Assoc.*, **260** (14), 1827–1833.

26 Klahn, S.L., Kitchell, B.E., Dervisis, N.G. (2011) Evaluation and comparison of outcomes in dogs with periarticular and nonperiarticular histiocytic sarcoma. *J. Am. Vet. Med. Assoc.*, **239** (1), 90–96.

27 Dettwiler, M., Mauldin, E.A., Jastrebski, S., *et al.* (2023) Prognostic clinical and histopathological features of canine cutaneous epitheliotropic T-cell lymphoma. *Vet. Pathol.*, **60** (2), 162–171.

28 Fontaine, J., Heimann, M., Day, M.J. (2011) Cutaneous epitheliotropic T-cell lymphoma in the cat: a review of the literature and five new cases. *Vet. Dermatol.*, **22** (5), 454–461.

29 Affolter, V.K., Gross, T.L., Moore, P.F. (2009) Indolent cutaneous T-cell lymphoma presenting as cutaneous lymphocytosis in dogs. *Vet. Dermatol.*, **20** (5–6), 577–585.

30 van der Steen, F.E.M.M., Grinwis, G.C.M., Weerts, E.A.W.S., *et al.* (2021) Feline and canine Merkel cell carcinoma: a case series and discussion on cellular origin. *Vet. Comp. Oncol.*, **19** (2), 393–398.

31 Joiner, K.S., Smith, A.N., Henderson, R.A., *et al.* (2010) Multicentric cutaneous neuroendocrine (Merkel cell) carcinoma in a dog. *Vet. Pathol.*, **47** (6), 1090–1094.

32 Dohata, A., Chambers, J.K., Uchida, K., *et al.* (2015) Clinical and pathological study of feline Merkel cell carcinoma with immunohistochemical characterization of normal and neoplastic Merkel cells. *Vet. Pathol.*, **52** (6), 1012–1018.

33 Sumi, A., Chambers, J.K., Doi, M., *et al.* (2018) Clinical features and outcomes of Merkel cell carcinoma in 20 cats. *Vet. Comp. Oncol.*, **16** (4), 554–561.

34 Baer, K.E., Patnaik, A.K., Gilbertson, S.R., *et al.* (1989) Cutaneous plasmacytomas in dogs: a morphologic and immunohistochemical study. *Vet. Pathol.*, **26** (3), 216–221.

35 Grassinger, J.M., Floren, A., Müller, A., *et al.* (2021) Digital lesions in dogs: a statistical breed analysis of 2912 cases. *Vet. Sci.*, **8** (7), 136.

36 Boostrom, B.O., Moore, A.S., DeRegis, C.J., *et al.* (2017) Canine cutaneous plasmacytosis: 21 cases (2005-2015). *J. Vet. Intern. Med.*, **31** (4), 1074–1080.

37 Mukaratirwa, S., Gruys, E. (2003) Canine transmissible venereal tumour: cytogenetic origin, immunophenotype, and immunobiology. A review. *Vet. Q.*, **25** (3), 101–111.

38 Ganguly, B., Das, U., Das, A.K. (2016) Canine transmissible venereal tumour: a review. *Vet. Comp. Oncol.*, **14** (1), 1–12.

39 Varughese, E.E., Singla, V.K., Ratnakaran, U., *et al.* (2012) Successful management of metastatic transmissible venereal tumor to skin of mammary region. *Reprod. Domest. Anim.*, **47** (Suppl 6), 366–369.

40 Park, M.S., Kim, Y., Kang, M.S., *et al.* (2006) Disseminated transmissible venereal tumor in a dog. *J. Vet. Diagn. Investig.*, **18** (1), 130–133.

41 Smedley, R.C., Spangler, W.L., Esplin, D.G., *et al.* (2011) Prognostic markers for canine melanocytic neoplasms: a comparative review of the literature and goals for future investigation. *Vet. Pathol.*, **48** (1), 54–72.

42 Goldschmidt, M.H., Dunstan, R.W., Stannard, A.A., *et al.* (1998) Histological classification of epithelial and melanocytic neoplasms of the skin of domestic animals. In: *World Health Organization International Histological Classification of Neoplasms of Domestic Animals*, 2nd series, Vol. III. Armed Forces Institute of Pathology, Washington, DC, pp. 38–40.

43 van der Weyden, L., Brenn, T., Patton, E.E., *et al.* (2020) Spontaneously occurring melanoma in animals and their relevance to human melanoma. *J. Pathol.*, **252** (1), 4–21.

44 Spangler, W.L., Kass, P.H. (2006) The histologic and epidemiologic bases for prognostic considerations in canine melanocytic neoplasia. *Vet. Pathol.*, **43** (2), 136–149.

45 Williams, L.E., Packer, R.A. (2003) Association between lymph node size and metastasis in dogs with oral malignant melanoma: 100 cases (1987–2001). *J. Am. Vet. Med. Assoc.*, **222** (9), 1234–1236.

46 Seiler, R.J. (1982) Granular basal cell tumors in the skin of three dogs: a distinct histopathologic entity. *Vet. Pathol.*, **19** (1), 23–29.

47 Bohn, A.A., Wills, T., Caplazi, P. (2006) Basal cell tumor or cutaneous basilar epithelial neoplasm? Rethinking the cytologic diagnosis of basal cell tumors. *Vet. Clin. Pathol.*, **35** (4), 449–453.

48 Simeonov, R., Simeonova, G. (2008) Nucleomorphometric analysis of feline basal cell carcinomas. *Res. Vet. Sci.*, **84** (3), 440–443.

49 Nibe, K., Uchida, K., Itoh, T., *et al.* (2005) A case of canine apocrine sweat gland adenoma, clear cell variant. *Vet. Pathol.*, **42** (2), 215–218.

50 Kalaher, K.M., Anderson, W.I., Scott, D.W. (1990) Neoplasms of the apocrine sweat glands in 44 dogs and 10 cats. *Vet. Rec.*, **127** (16), 400–403.

51 Simko, E., Wilcock, B.P., Yager, J.A. (2003) A retrospective study of 44 canine apocrine sweat gland adenocarcinomas. *Can. Vet. J.*, **44** (1), 38–42.

52 Haziroglu, R., Haligur, M., Keles, H. (2014) Histopathological and immunohistochemical studies of apocrine sweat gland adenocarcinomas in cats. *Vet. Comp. Oncol.*, **12** (1), 85–90.

53 Jasik, A., Kycko, A., Olech, M., *et al.* (2021) Mutations of p53 gene in canine sweat gland carcinomas probably associated with UV radiation. *J. Vet. Res.*, **65** (4), 519–526.

54 Scott, D.W., Anderson, W.I. (1990) Canine sebaceous gland tumors: a retrospective analysis of 172 cases. *Canine Pract.*, **15** (1), 19–21, 24–27.

55 Sabattini, S., Bassi, P., Bettini, G. (2015) Histopathological findings and proliferative activity of canine sebaceous gland tumours with a predominant reserve cell population. *J. Comp. Pathol.*, **152** (2–3), 145–152.

56 Bettini, G., Morini, M., Mandrioli, L., *et al.* (2009) CNS and lung metastasis of sebaceous epithelioma in a dog. *Vet. Dermatol.*, **20** (4), 289–294.

57 Petterino, C., Hoffmann, I. (2019) What is your diagnosis? Subcutaneous inguinal mass in a Greyhound. *Vet. Clin. Pathol.*, **48** (4), 780–782.

58 Scott, D.W., Anderson, W.I. (1991) Feline sebaceous gland tumors: a retrospective analysis of 9 cases. *Feline Pract.*, **19**, 16–18, 20–21.

59 White, S.D., Rappaport, J., Carpenter, J.L., *et al.* (1985) Cutaneous metastases of a mammary adenocarcinoma resembling eosinophilic plaques in a cat. *Feline Pract.*, **15** (3), 27–29.

60 Reed, L.T., Knapp, D.W., Miller, M.A. (2013) Cutaneous metastasis of transitional cell carcinoma in 12 dogs. *Vet. Pathol.*, **50** (4), 676–681.

61 Favrot, C., Degorce-Rubiales, F. (2005) Cutaneous metastases of a bronchial adenocarcinoma in a cat. *Vet. Dermatol.*, **16** (3), 183–186.

62 Petterino, C., Guazzi, P., Ferro, S., *et al.* (2005) Bronchogenic adenocarcinoma in a cat: an unusual case of metastasis to the skin. *Vet. Clin. Pathol.*, **34** (4), 401–404.

63 Gould, A.P., Coyner, K.S., Trimmer, A.M., *et al.* (2021) Canine pedal papilloma identification and management: a retrospective series of 44 cases. *Vet. Dermatol.*, **32** (5), 509-e141.

64 DeBey, B.M., Bagladi-Swanson, M., Kapil, S., *et al.* (2001) Digital papillomatosis in a confined beagle. *J. Vet. Diagn. Investig.*, **13** (4), 346–348.

65 Santana, C.H., Moreira, P.R.R., Rosolem, M.C., *et al.* (2016) Relationship between the inflammatory infiltrate and the degree of differentiation of the canine cutaneous squamous cell carcinoma. *Vet. Anim. Sci.*, **1–2**, 4–8.

66 Dos Santos, A., Lamego, É.C., Eisenhardt, L.M., *et al.* (2023) Prevalence and anatomopathological characterization of cutaneous squamous cell carcinomas with regional and distant metastases in dogs and cats: 20 cases (1985–2020). *Vet. Comp. Oncol.*, **21** (2), 291–301.

67 Wobeser, B.K., Kidney, B.A., Powers, B.E., *et al.* (2007) Diagnoses and clinical outcomes associated with surgically amputated canine digits submitted to multiple veterinary diagnostic laboratories. *Vet. Pathol.*, **44** (3), 355–361.

68 Sabattini, S., Renzi, A., Rigillo, A., *et al.* (2019) Cytological differentiation between benign and malignant perianal gland proliferative lesions in dogs: a preliminary study. *J. Small Anim. Pract.*, **60** (10), 616–622.

69 Pisani, G., Millanta, F., Lorenzi, D., *et al.* (2006) Androgen receptor expression in normal, hyperplastic and neoplastic hepatoid glands in the dog. *Res. Vet. Sci.*, **81** (2), 231–236.

70 Evans, S.J.M., Connolly, S.L., Schaffer, P.A., *et al.* (2018) Basal cell enumeration does not predict malignancy in canine perianal gland tumor cytology. *Vet. Clin. Pathol.*, **47** (4), 634–637.

71 Berrocal, A., Vos, J.H., van den Ingh, T.S., *et al.* (1989) Canine perineal tumours. *J. Veterinary Med. Ser. A*, **36** (1–10), 739–749.

72 McCourt, M.R., Levine, G.M., Breshears, M.A., *et al.* (2018) Metastatic disease in a dog with a well-differentiated perianal gland tumor. *Vet. Clin. Pathol.*, **47** (4), 649–653.

73 Vail, D.M., Withrow, S.J., Schwarz, P.D., *et al.* (1990) Perianal adenocarcinoma in the canine male: a retrospective study of 41 cases. *J. Am. Anim. Hosp. Assoc.*, **26** (3), 329–334.

74 Amsellem, P.M., Cavanaugh, R.P., Chou, P.Y., *et al.* (2019) Apocrine gland anal sac adenocarcinoma in cats: 30 cases (1994–2015). *J. Am. Vet. Med. Assoc.*, **254** (6), 716–722.

75 Bennett, P.F., DeNicola, D.B., Bonney, P., *et al.* (2002) Canine anal sac adenocarcinomas: clinical presentation and response to therapy. *J. Vet. Intern. Med.*, **16** (1), 100–104.

76 Bowlt, K.L., Friend, E.J., Delisser, P., *et al.* (2013) Temporally separated bilateral anal sac gland adenocarcinomas in four dogs. *J. Small Anim. Pract.*, **54** (8), 432–436.

77 Wong, H., Byrne, S., Rasotto, R., *et al.* (2021) A retrospective study of clinical and histopathological features of 81 cases of canine apocrine gland adenocarcinoma of the anal sac: independent clinical and histopathological risk factors associated with outcome. *Animals (Basel)*, **11** (11), 3327.

78 Williams, L.E., Gliatto, J.M., Dodge, R.K., *et al.* (2003) Carcinoma of the apocrine glands of the anal sac in dogs: 113 cases (1985–1995). *J. Am. Vet. Med. Assoc.*, **223** (6), 825–831.

79 Griffin, M.A., Mayhew, P.D., Culp, W.T.N., *et al.* (2023) Short- and long-term outcomes associated with anal sacculectomy in dogs with massive apocrine gland anal sac adenocarcinoma. *J. Am. Vet. Med. Assoc.*, **261** (10), 1–8.

80 Jones, A.E., Wustefeld-Janssens, B.G. (2023) A relatively high proportion of dogs with small apocrine gland anal sac adenocarcinoma (AGASACA) primary tumours present with locoregional lymph node metastasis. *Vet. Comp. Oncol.*, **21** (2), 327–331.

81 Piviani, M., Sánchez, M.D., Patel, R.T. (2012) Cytologic features of clear cell adnexal carcinoma in 3 dogs. *Vet. Clin. Pathol.*, **41** (3), 405–411.

82 Schulman, F.Y., Lipscomb, T.P., Atkin, T.J. (2005) Canine cutaneous clear cell adnexal carcinoma: histopathology, immunohistochemistry, and biologic behavior of 26 cases. *J. Vet. Diagn. Investig.*, **17** (5), 403–411.

83 Masserdotti, C., Drigo, M. (2022) Cytologic features of reactive fibroplasia in cutaneous and subcutaneous lesions of dogs: a retrospective study. *Vet. Clin. Pathol.*, **51** (2), 244–251.

84 Miller, M.A., Nelson, S.L., Turk, J.R., *et al.* (1991) Cutaneous neoplasia in 340 cats. *Vet. Pathol.*, **28** (5), 389–395.

85 Pakhrin, B., Kang, M.S., Bae, I.H., *et al.* (2007) Retrospective study of canine cutaneous tumors in Korea. *J. Vet. Sci.*, **8** (3), 229–236.

86 Kuntz, C.A., Dernell, W.S., Powers, B.E., *et al.* (1997) Prognostic factors for surgical treatment of soft-tissue sarcomas in dogs: 75 cases (1986–1996). *J. Am. Vet. Med. Assoc.*, **211** (9), 1147–1151.

87 McKnight, J.A., Mauldin, G.N., McEntee, M.C., *et al.* (2000) Radiation treatment for incompletely resected soft-tissue sarcomas in dogs. *J. Am. Vet. Med. Assoc.*, **217** (2), 205–210.

88 Selting, K.A., Powers, B.E., Thompson, L.J., *et al.* (2005) Outcome of dogs with high-grade soft tissue sarcomas treated with and without adjuvant doxorubicin chemotherapy: 39 cases (1996–2004). *J. Am. Vet. Med. Assoc.*, **227** (9), 1442–1448.

89 Little, L.K., Goldschmidt, M. (2007) Cytologic appearance of a keloidal fibrosarcoma in a dog. *Vet. Clin. Pathol.*, **36** (4), 364–367.

90 Mikaelian, I., Gross, T.L. (2002) Keloidal fibromas and fibrosarcomas in the dog. *Vet. Pathol.*, **39** (1), 149–153.

91 Avallone, G., Helmbold, P., Caniatti, M., *et al.* (2007) The spectrum of canine cutaneous perivascular wall tumors: morphologic, phenotypic and clinical characterization. *Vet. Pathol.*, **44** (5), 607–620.

92 Dennis, M.M., McSporran, K.D., Bacon, N.J., *et al.* (2011) Prognostic factors for cutaneous and subcutaneous soft tissue sarcomas in dogs. *Vet. Pathol.*, **48** (1), 73–84.

93 Davis, A., Hosgood, G. (2023) Long-term outcome following surgical excision of large, low to intermediate grade soft tissue sarcomas in dogs. *Aust. Vet. J.*, **101** (5), 193–199.

94 Chiti, L.E., Ferrari, R., Boracchi, P., *et al.* (2021) Prognostic impact of clinical, haematological, and histopathological variables in 102 canine cutaneous perivascular wall tumours. *Vet. Comp. Oncol.*, **19** (2), 275–283.

95 García-Iglesias, M.J., Cuevas-Higuera, J.L., Bastida-Sáenz, A., *et al.* (2020) Immunohistochemical detection of p53 and pp53 Ser^{392} in canine hemangiomas and hemangiosarcomas located in the skin. *BMC Vet. Res.*, **16** (1), 239.

96 Trappler, M.C., Popovitch, C.A., Goldschmidt, M.H., *et al.* (2014) Scrotal tumors in dogs: a retrospective study of 676 cases (1986–2010). *Can. Vet. J.*, **55** (1), 1229–1233.

97 Griffin, M.A., Culp, W.T.N., Rebhun, R.B. (2021) Canine and feline haemangiosarcoma. *Vet. Rec.*, **189** (9), 585.

98 Ward, H., Fox, L.E., Calderwood-Mays, M.B., *et al.* (1994) Cutaneous hemangiosarcoma in 25 dogs: a retrospective study. *J. Vet. Intern. Med.*, **8** (5), 345–348.

99 McAbee, K.P., Ludwig, L.L., Bergman, P.J., *et al.* (2005) Feline cutaneous hemangiosarcoma: a retrospective study of 18 cases (1998–2003). *J. Am. Anim. Hosp. Assoc.*, **41** (2), 110–116.

100 Szivek, A., Burns, R., Gericota, B., *et al.* (2012) Clinical outcome in 94 cases of dermal hemangiosarcoma in dogs treated with surgical excision: 1993-2007. *Vet. Comp. Oncol.*, **10** (1), 65–73.

101 Craig, L.E., Krimer, P.M., Cooley, A.J. (2010) Canine synovial myxoma: 39 cases. *Vet. Pathol.*, **47** (5), 931–936.

102 Machida, N., Hoshi, K., Kobayashi, M., *et al.* (2003) Cardiac myxoma of the tricuspid valve in a dog. *J. Comp. Pathol.*, **129** (4), 320–324.

103 Iwaki, Y., Lindley, S., Smith, A., *et al.* (2019) Canine myxosarcomas, a retrospective analysis of 32 dogs (2003-2018). *BMC Vet. Res.*, **15** (1), 217.

104 Bostock, D.E., Dye, M.T. (1980) Prognosis after surgical excision of canine fibrous connective tissue sarcomas. *Vet. Pathol.*, **17** (5), 581–588.

105 Headley, S.A., Faria Dos Reis, A.C., Bracarense, A.P. (2011) Cutaneous myxosarcoma with pulmonary metastases in a dog. *J. Comp. Pathol.*, **145** (1), 31–34.

106 Schneider, P., Busch, U., Meister, H., *et al.* (1999) Malignant fibrous histiocytoma (MFH). A comparison of MFH in man and animals. A critical review. *Histol. Histopathol.*, **14** (3), 845–860.

107 Bergman, P.J., Withrow, S.J., Straw, R.C., *et al.* (1994) Infiltrative lipoma in dogs: 16 cases (1981–1992). *J. Am. Vet. Med. Assoc.*, **205** (2), 322–324.

108 McAloney, C.A., Brown, M.E., Martinez, M.P., *et al.* (2020) What is your diagnosis? Subcutaneous mass in a dog. *Vet. Clin. Pathol.*, **49** (1), 161–163.

109 Piseddu, E., De Lorenzi, D., Freeman, K., *et al.* (2011) Cytologic, histologic and immunohistochemical features of lingual liposarcoma in a dog. *Vet. Clin. Pathol.*, **40** (3), 393–397.

110 Gower, K.L., Liptak, J.M., Culp, W.T., *et al.* (2015) Splenic liposarcoma in dogs: 13 cases (2002–2012). *J. Am. Vet. Med. Assoc.*, **247** (12), 1404–1407.

111 Baez, J.L., Hendrick, M.J., Shofer, F.S., *et al.* (2004) Liposarcomas in dogs: 56 cases (1989–2000). *J. Am. Vet. Med. Assoc.*, **224** (6), 887–891.

112 Chanut, F., Colle, M.A., Deschamps, J.Y., *et al.* (2005) Systemic xanthomatosis associated with hyperchylomicronaemia in a cat. *J. Vet. Med. A Physiol. Pathol. Clin. Med.*, **52** (6), 272–274.

113 Banajee, K.H., Orandle, M.S., Ratterree, W., *et al.* (2011) Idiopathic solitary cutaneous xanthoma in a dog. *Vet. Clin. Pathol.*, **40** (1), 95–98.

114 Gross, T.L., Ihrke, P.J., Walder, E.J., *et al.* (2005) Histiocytic tumors. In: *Skin Diseases of the Dog and Cat: Clinical and Histopathological Diagnosis*, 2nd edn, Blackwell Science, Oxford, UK, pp. 837–840.

115 Contreary, C.L., Outerbridge, C.A., Affolter, V.K., *et al.* (2015) Canine sterile nodular panniculitis: a retrospective study of 39 dogs. *Vet. Dermatol.*, **26** (6), 451–458.

116 O'Kell, A.L., Inteeworn, N., Diaz, S.F., *et al.* (2010) Canine sterile nodular panniculitis: a retrospective study of 14 cases. *J. Vet. Intern. Med.*, **24** (2), 278–284.

117 Angelou, V., Papazoglou, L.G., Tsioli, V., *et al.* (2020) Complete surgical excision versus Penrose drainage for the treatment of elbow hygroma in 19 dogs (1997 to 2014). *J. Small Anim. Pract.*, **61** (4), 230–235.

118 Tafti, A.K., Hanna, P., Bourque, A.C. (2005) Calcinosis circumscripta in the dog: a retrospective pathological study. *J. Vet. Med. A Physiol. Pathol. Clin. Med.*, **52** (1), 13–17.

119 Tan, R.M., Stern, A.W., White, A.G., *et al.* (2013) Pathology in practice. Calcinosis cutis. *J. Am. Vet. Med. Assoc.*, **243** (3), 347–349.

120 Muller, C., Gaguère, E., Muller, A., *et al.* (2022) Localized cutaneous calcinosis associated with leptospirosis in a 4-month-old beagle puppy. *Can. Vet. J.*, **63** (10), 1027–1031.

121 Doerr, K.A., Outerbridge, C.A., White, S.D., *et al.* (2013) Calcinosis cutis in dogs: histopathological and clinical analysis of 46 cases. *Vet. Dermatol.*, **24** (3), 355–361.

122 Buckley, L., Nuttall, T. (2012) Feline eosinophilic granuloma complex(ities): some clinical clarification. *J. Feline Med. Surg.*, **14** (7), 471–481.

123 Wildermuth, B.E., Griffin, C.E., Rosenkrantz, W.S. (2012) Response of feline eosinophilic plaques and lip ulcers to amoxicillin trihydrate-clavulanate potassium therapy: a randomized, double-blind placebocontrolled prospective study. *Vet. Dermatol.*, **23** (2), 110–118.

124 Mueller, R.S., Krebs, I., Power, H.T., *et al.* (2006) Pemphigus foliaceus in 91 dogs. *J. Am. Anim. Hosp. Assoc.*, **42** (3), 189–196.

125 Bizikova, P., Linder, K.E., Mamo, L.B. (2022) Trunk-dominant and classic facial pemphigus foliaceus in dogs – comparison of anti-desmocollin-1 and anti-desmoglein-1 autoantibodies and clinical presentations. *Vet. Dermatol.*, **33** (5), 414–425.

126 Gomez, S.M., Morris, D.O., Rosenbaum, M.R., *et al.* (2004) Outcome and complications associated with treatment of pemphigus foliaceus in dogs: 43 cases (1994–2000). *J. Am. Vet. Med. Assoc.*, **224** (8), 1312–1316.

5

Hemolymphatic

5.1 Lymph Nodes

5.1.1 Normal

5.1.1.1 Cytologic Appearance
Small mature lymphocytes predominate (∼80 + %) in normal lymph nodes. These cells have nuclei with diameters approximately equal to that of a red blood cell, and mature, clumped chromatin with inapparent nucleoli. A scant amount of cytoplasm is present. Low numbers of intermediate-sized lymphocytes, rare plasma cells, and larger lymphocytes may be seen (Figures 5.1 and 5.2).

5.1.2 Reactive Lymphoid Hyperplasia

5.1.2.1 Cytologic Appearance
Reactive lymphoid hyperplasia is characterized by a heterogeneous population of lymphocytes (Figures 5.3–5.5). Small mature cells typically predominate and are admixed with variably increased numbers of plasma cells, intermediate and large reactive lymphocytes. Mitotic figures can be seen in reactive lymph nodes (Figure 5.5). Some plasma cells may accumulate immunoglobulin, seen as bright-blue or pink inclusions (Mott cells) or diffuse pink coloration (Flame cells) (see Figure 2.27E and F).

Figure 5.1 Lymph node (normal), cat, 50× objective. Small lymphocytes constitute >80% of cells and have nuclei approximately one red blood cell in diameter with clumped chromatin.

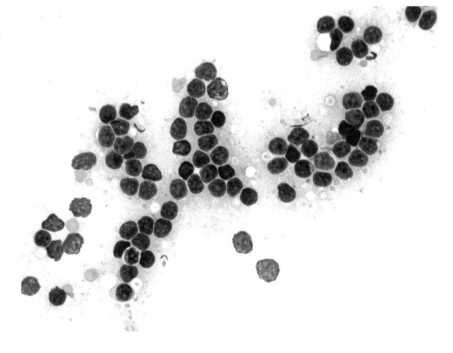

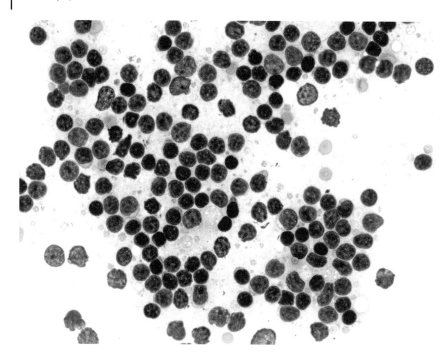

Figure 5.2 Lymph node (normal), cat, 50× objective.

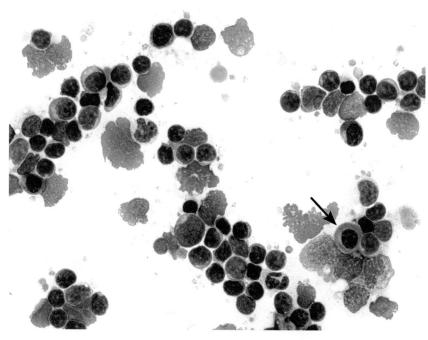

Figure 5.3 Lymph node (reactive), dog, 50× objective. Note the variation in lymphocyte size, volume and color of the cytoplasm, and the presence of plasma cells (arrow).

5.1.2.2 Clinical Considerations

- Associated with enlargement of single or multiple lymph nodes.
- Secondary to antigenic stimulation, which may be local or generalized.

5.1.2.3 Prognosis

Mostly good, but variable, based on the underlying cause.

5.1.3 Neutrophilic Lymphadenitis

5.1.3.1 Cytologic Appearance

Neutrophils should be seen in very low numbers in lymph nodes, especially in the absence of any blood. Increased numbers may indicate a sterile inflammatory process (Figure 5.6) or a septic process (Figure 5.7).

Figure 5.4 Lymph node (reactive), dog, 50× objective.

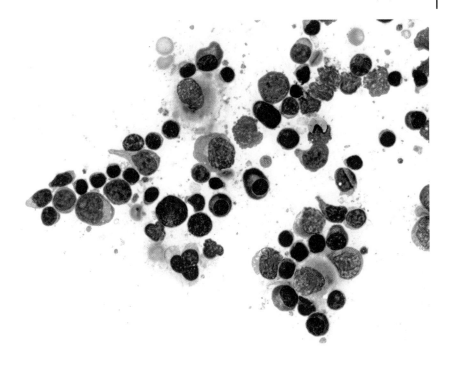

Figure 5.5 Lymph node (reactive), dog, 50× objective. Note that mitotic figures may be present in hyperplastic nodes (arrow).

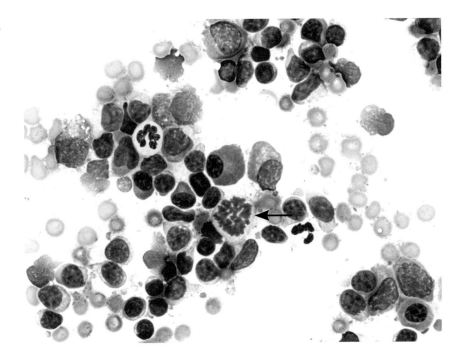

5.1.3.2 Clinical Considerations
- May be primary (lymphadenitis) or secondary (inflammation draining to the node).
- Sterile inflammatory responses may include juvenile cellulitis [1], other pyoderma, paraneoplastic, or immune-mediated disease [2].
- Sepsis (typically bacterial) may accompany neutrophilic lymphadenitis [3].

5.1.3.3 Prognosis
Mostly good, but variable with underlying diagnosis and appropriate therapy.

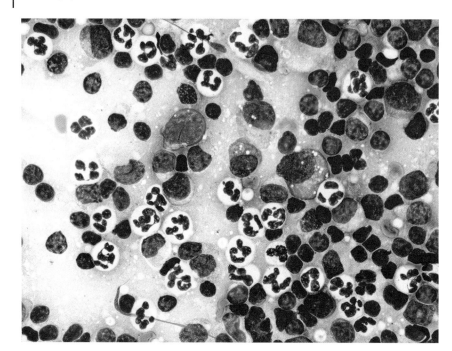

Figure 5.6 Lymph node, neutrophilic lymphadenitis from puppy with juvenile cellulitis, 50× objective.

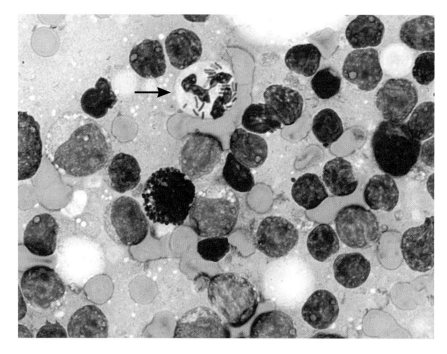

Figure 5.7 Lymph node, septic neutrophilic lymphadenitis, 100× objective. Note intracellular bacteria within a neutrophil (arrow).

5.1.4 Eosinophilic Lymphadenitis

5.1.4.1 Cytologic Appearance

Eosinophils are rare in normal lymph nodes. Increased numbers may be distributed individually or in aggregates. Evidence of chronic hemorrhage (hemosiderin in the background and within macrophages) may also be seen and is common in cases of chronic skin disease (Figure 5.8).

5.1.4.2 Clinical Considerations

- DDx = inflammation (e.g., chronic skin disease, allergic/hypersensitivity disease, and primary eosinophilic inflammatory disease) [4, 5], paraneoplastic (e.g., mast cell neoplasia and T-cell lymphoma) [6], or infectious (especially fungal or protozoal) [7].

5.1.4.3 Prognosis

Mostly good, but variable based on the underlying diagnosis (e.g., inflammatory versus paraneoplastic).

Figure 5.8 Lymph node, eosinophilic lymphadenitis, dog, 50× objective. Note the blue/green hemosiderin pigment granules in the background.

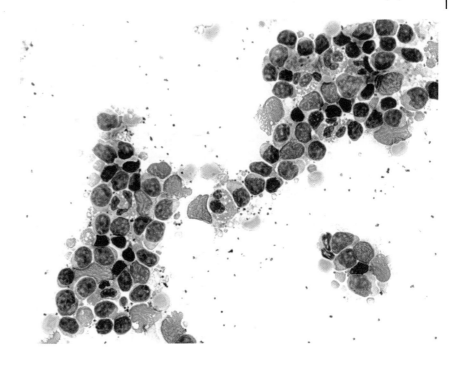

5.1.5 Infectious Organisms

Many infectious organisms may be found in lymph nodes (see Chapter 3 for detailed descriptions of common organisms). Lymph node involvement is an important manifestation of salmon poisoning disease, which is described in detail in the next section.

5.1.6 Salmon Poisoning Disease

5.1.6.1 Cytologic Appearance
Salmon poisoning disease is characterized by a granulomatous infiltrate, with macrophages containing numerous intracellular organisms ~1–2 µm in length. Organisms appear as curvilinear structures distributed individually and clumped throughout the cytoplasm (Figure 5.9). An expanded population of intermediate to large reactive lymphocytes is seen, as well as many plasma cells.

5.1.6.2 Clinical Considerations
- Dogs only. Caused by *Neorickettsia helminthoeca*.
- Seen in the Pacific Northwest of the United States and in Brazil [8, 9].
- Clinical signs = lethargy, vomiting, diarrhea, peripheral lymphadenopathy, and fever [8, 10].

5.1.6.3 Prognosis
Good with appropriate therapy early in the disease course [10]. Mortality can be up to 90% without treatment [11].

5.1.7 Lymphoma (Large-cell)

5.1.7.1 Cytologic Appearance
Large-cell lymphomas exfoliate well, with cells distributed individually and in sheets. The cells have nuclei with diameters about twofold to more than threefold that of red blood cells and have finely stippled chromatin. The nucleoli vary in prominence and number. Mitotic figures frequently are seen but vary in number. The cells mostly have a small to moderate volume of encircling deep-blue cytoplasm (see Figures 5.10–5.13). Large neoplastic cells frequently efface the lymph node, making diagnosis straightforward. As a guide, the large, neoplastic cells should constitute 30–50% of the lymphoid population for a diagnosis of lymphoma. However, emerging or early disease may result in lesser numbers, and re-sampling of a node in 1–2 weeks, or histopathology, may be required for definitive diagnosis.

5.1.7.2 Clinical Considerations
Dogs
- Multicentric lymphoma (affecting peripheral lymph nodes) is the most common form of lymphoma [12, 13].
- Generally seen in middle-aged to older dogs (median age 7–9 years), but have also been reported in dogs <1 year of age [14, 15].
- Many dog breeds affected. Overrepresented breeds include Boxers, Bull Mastiffs, Bulldogs, Bassett Hounds, and Golden Retrievers [16, 17].

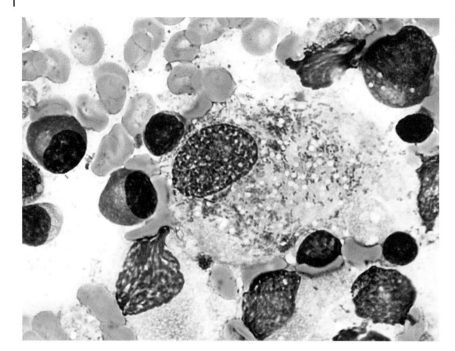

Figure 5.9 Lymph node, *Neorickettsia helminthoeca* (salmon poisoning disease), dog, 100× objective. Note the curvilinear organisms within macrophage and in the background.

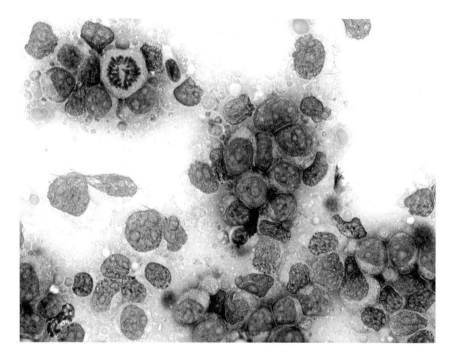

Figure 5.10 Lymph node, large-cell lymphoma, dog, 50× objective. Note the large nuclei (2-fold to 3-fold the size of red blood cells in diameter), prominent nucleoli, and mitotic figure (upper left).

- B-cell phenotype is the most common form of multicentric lymphoma involving lymph nodes (60–80% of cases). Involvement of abdominal nodes or viscera is seen in 15–20% of cases [14, 18].
- T-cell phenotype is associated with shorter remission and survival times, and is more commonly associated with hypercalcemia [18–20].

Cats
- Lymphoma limited to peripheral lymph nodes is uncommon in cats (5–19% of cases) [21, 22]; however, many other anatomic forms will involve lymph nodes.
- Nodal lymphoma is the most common form in cats <1-year old [23].
- T-cell phenotype is more common in cats [14, 24].
- FeLV and FIV increase the risk of lymphoma.

Figure 5.11 Lymph node, large-cell lymphoma, cat, 50× objective. The cells are large, monomorphic and have finely stippled chromatin.

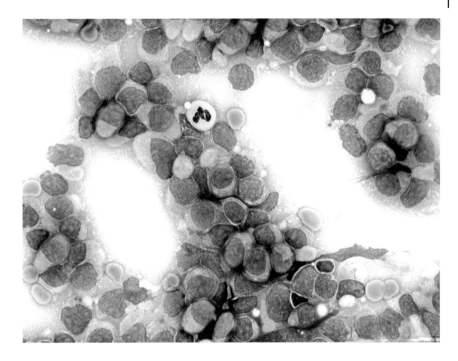

Figure 5.12 Lymph node, large-cell lymphoma, dog, 50× objective. Note the smooth pink nuclear material in the background from lysed cells.

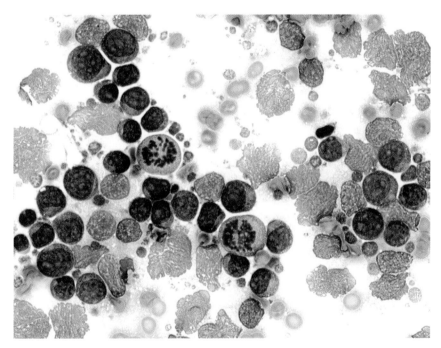

5.1.7.3 Prognosis

Highly variable, based on treatment and many prognostic factors. Without treatment, most dogs with large-cell lymphoma will die within 4–6 weeks of diagnosis; [25] similar survival times have been reported for dogs and cats treated with prednisone alone [26, 27]. Combination chemotherapeutic protocols may result in long-term clinical remission that is longer in dogs than in cats [24, 28]. Some factors contributing to poorer prognosis include T-cell phenotype,

World Health Organization (WHO) clinical stage (stage V = poor outcome), and substage b (clinically ill patients).

5.1.8 Lymphoma (Small-cell)

5.1.8.1 Cytologic Appearance

Nodal small-cell lymphomas comprise monomorphic sheets of small lymphocytes. When compared to normal small mature lymphocytes, these cells have

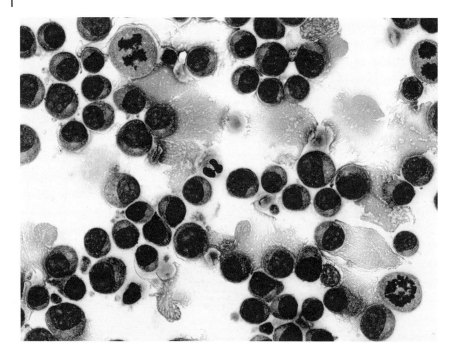

Figure 5.13 Lymph node, large-cell lymphoma, dog, 50× objective. Diff-Quik stain.

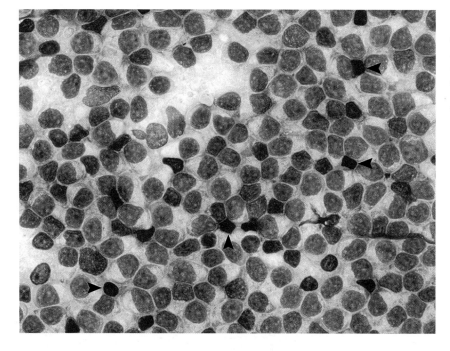

Figure 5.14 Lymph node, small-cell lymphoma, dog, 50× objective. Note the expansion of small cells (nuclei ~1.25-fold the size of red blood cells in diameter) with prominent nucleoli. These cells outnumber small mature lymphocytes with clumped chromatin (arrowheads).

slightly larger nuclei (diameter ~1.25-fold the size of a red blood cell) and more open, less-clumped chromatin, often with prominent nucleoli (Figures 5.14 and 5.15). The cells typically have an increased volume of pale-blue cytoplasm forming a unipolar cap, which may form an elongated pseudopod, giving the cells a "hand mirror" morphology, particularly common in T-zone lymphoma (Figure 5.16) [29].

Note: The "hand mirror" morphology is not pathognomonic for T-zone lymphoma, and is also commonly present in cases of reactive lymphoid hyperplasia.

5.1.8.2 Clinical Considerations

- Dogs > cats.
- T-cell phenotype more common [18, 30, 31].
- Single or multiple nodes affected.

Figure 5.15 Lymph node, small-cell lymphoma, dog, 100× objective. The more open chromatin pattern and nucleoli of neoplastic cells can be contrasted to the clumped, dark chromatin of small mature cells.

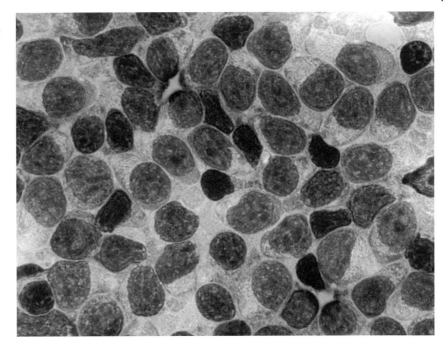

Figure 5.16 Lymph node, small-cell lymphoma (T-zone), dog, 50× objective. Note the prominent unipolar pseudopod of cytoplasm giving the cells a 'hand mirror' appearance.

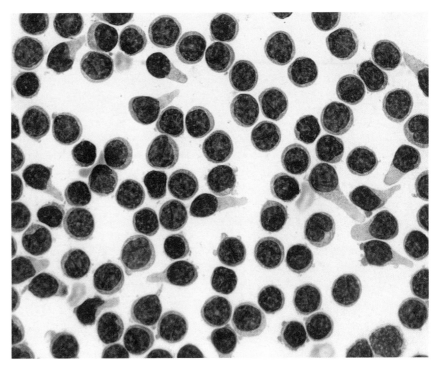

- May be associated with a lymphocytosis with small mature cells [32, 33].

5.1.8.3 Prognosis
Variable. T-cell phenotypes typically are indolent and associated with prolonged survival times (years), even in the absence of systemic therapy [30]. Small B-cell lymphomas can be high grade and associated with short survival times [31]. See Chapter 9 for discussions of small-cell lymphoma affecting the gastrointestinal tract.

5.1.9 Specific Lymphoma Types

Specific types of lymphoma can be suspected based on characteristic cytologic features; three such types are described in the following sections.

5.1.10 Lymphoma (Lymphoblastic)

5.1.10.1 Cytologic Appearance

Cells are intermediate in size, with nuclei ~1.5-fold the size of red blood cells in diameter. Nuclei frequently have subtle nuclear membrane irregularity, and finely stippled chromatin with mostly inapparent nucleoli (Figure 5.17). Many mitotic figures typically are seen (Figure 5.18). The cells have a small volume of pale-blue cytoplasm.

5.1.10.2 Clinical Considerations

- T-cell phenotype. Often present in cases of mediastinal lymphoma [34].
- Common in Boxers [35].
- Aggressive biologic behavior despite intermediate cell size [34, 35].
- Often associated with hypercalcemia [34, 35].
- Histopathology required for definitive diagnosis.

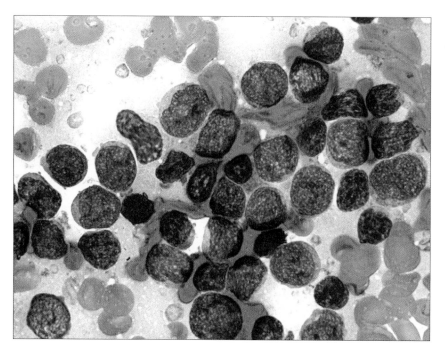

Figure 5.17 Lymph node, lymphoblastic lymphoma, dog, 60× objective. Note the finely stippled, immature chromatin, and inapparent nucleoli. Photo courtesy of Dr. Bill Vernau.

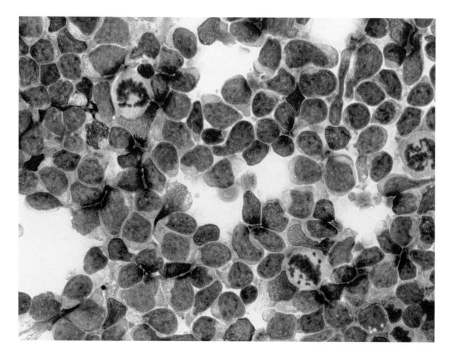

Figure 5.18 Lymph node, lymphoblastic lymphoma, dog, 50× objective. Note the irregular nuclear membranes, inapparent nucleoli, and many mitotic figures.

5.1.10.3 Prognosis

Poor. Short survival times reported, though may increase with chemotherapy [34].

5.1.11 Lymphoma (Mott Cell Differentiation)

5.1.11.1 Cytologic Appearance

Lymphoma with Mott cell differentiation is characterized by neoplastic lymphocytes that contain bright-blue (rarely pink), smooth cytoplasmic inclusions that are highly variable in size and shape (Figure 5.19) (relative to uniform inclusions in normal Mott cells; see Figure 2.27E). The cells typically have large nuclei (>2-fold the size of red blood cells in diameter) with finely stippled, immature chromatin.

5.1.11.2 Clinical Considerations

- Rare in dogs and cats.
- Miniature Dachshunds overrepresented [36, 37].
- High grade, B-cell lymphoma.
- Most commonly affects peripheral or abdominal lymph nodes/gastrointestinal tract [36, 38, 39].

5.1.11.3 Prognosis

Guarded to poor. Response to chemotherapy is mixed [38–40], but long-term survival is possible and is generally better than other high-grade gastrointestinal lymphomas [36].

5.1.12 Lymphoma (Hodgkin's-like)

5.1.12.1 Cytologic Appearance

Cases of Hodgkin's-like lymphoma are characterized by a mixed lymphoid population and the presence of (mostly rare) Reed-Sternberg cells. Reed-Sternberg cells are most commonly binucleated, but may have large single indented nuclei with stippled chromatin and large single basophilic nucleoli (Figures 5.20 and 5.21). They have a moderate volume of medium-blue cytoplasm.

5.1.12.2 Clinical Considerations

- Uncommon in cats, rare in dogs.
- Most cats >6 years old.
- Most present in a single node around the neck/mandibular region [41, 42].
- Due to the mixed nature of the lymphoid population, Hodgkin's-like lymphomas often mimic reactive lymphoid hyperplasia, necessitating histopathology for definitive diagnosis.

5.1.12.3 Prognosis

Fair to good. Hodgkin's-like lymphoma is a less aggressive neoplasm and long survival times are possible, even in the absence of treatment [41].

Figure 5.19 Lymph node, lymphoma with Mott cell differentiation, dog, 50× objective. Note the large, globular, bright-blue Russell bodies within the cytoplasm.

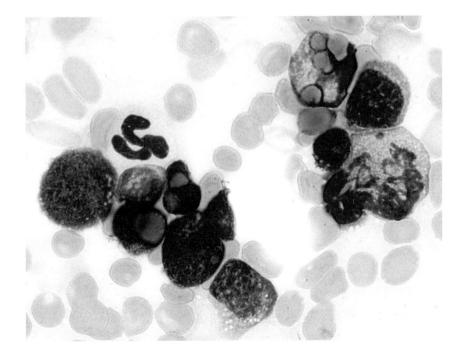

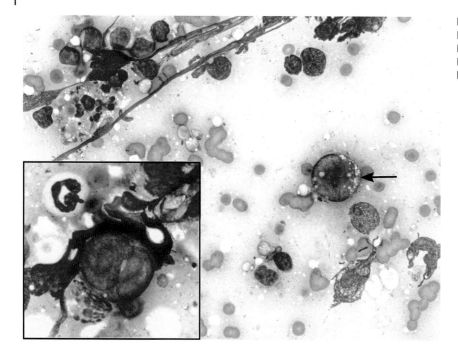

Figure 5.20 Lymph node, Hodgkin's-like lymphoma, cat, 50× objective. Most lymphocyte are small and mature (upper left), with low numbers of large, Reed-Sternberg cells (arrow and inset).

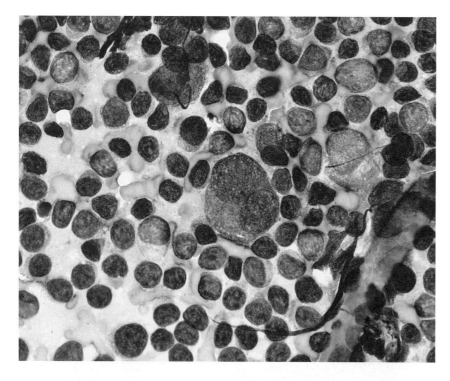

Figure 5.21 Lymph node, Hodgkin's-like lymphoma, cat, 50× objective. Note the predominance of small lymphocytes and the large, binucleated Reed-Sternberg cell with prominent nucleoli.

5.1.13 Leukemia

5.1.13.1 Cytologic Appearance

Acute leukemias can infiltrate lymph nodes. The neoplastic cells are large, with nuclei having diameters about twofold to fourfold the size of those of red blood cells, with finely stippled, immature chromatin, often with prominent nucleoli. Cytoplasm varies from scant and deep blue (lymphoid leukemia) to pale blue with fine pink granules (myeloid leukemia) or punctate clear vacuoles (myelomonocytic leukemia) (Figure 5.22). Mitotic figures often are seen in increased numbers. These can be difficult to distinguish from large-cell lymphomas – correlate with CBC findings ± bone marrow evaluation.

Figure 5.22 Lymph node, acute leukemia infiltration, dog, 60× objective. Acute myeloid (myelomonocytic) leukemia (AML-M4). Photo courtesy of Dr. Bill Vernau.

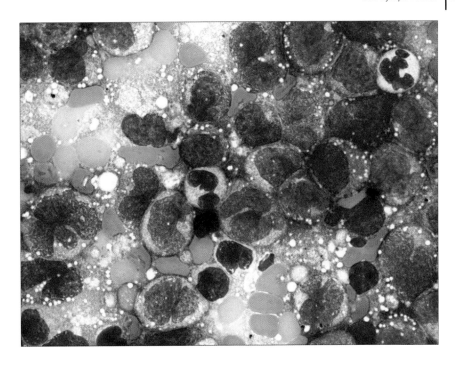

5.1.13.2 Clinical Considerations

- Commonly associated with a neoplastic leukocytosis, as well as thrombocytopenia, neutropenia, or anemia.
- Neoplastic cells usually CD34+ on immunocytochemistry [43, 44].

5.1.13.3 Prognosis

Grave.

5.1.14   Metastatic Disease

5.1.14.1 Cytologic Appearance

Metastatic neoplasia within lymph nodes is characterized by a population of cells not normally present in lymphoid tissue. Neoplasms that commonly metastasize to lymph nodes include carcinomas (e.g., squamous cell carcinoma; Figure 5.23), round cell neoplasms such as

Figure 5.23 Lymph node, metastatic squamous cell carcinoma, dog, 50× objective. Small mature lymphocytes surround a sheet of neoplastic cells with marked criteria of malignancy.

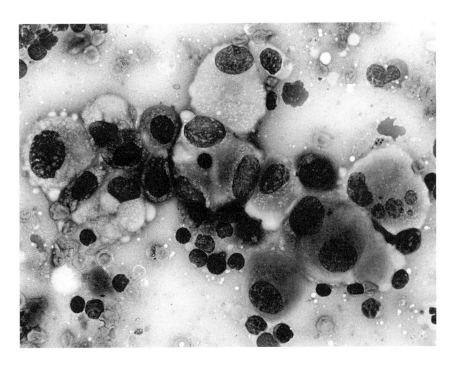

mast cell tumors (Figure 5.24), transmissible venereal tumors (Figure 5.25), and melanomas (Figure 5.26). Sarcomas metastasize less frequently to lymph nodes; however, spindloid cells are readily identified when present (Figure 5.27).

5.1.14.2 Clinical Considerations

- Metastatic disease may be focal or multifocal in the node, and the whole slide should be examined on low power (e.g., 10× objective) to avoid missing any foci of disease [45].

- Sensitivity is typically lower than specificity, and the absence of neoplastic cells does not preclude metastatic disease, especially if the sample size is small [45, 46].

- Mast cells can be seen in low numbers within normal or hyperplastic lymph nodes [47, 48], and aggregates of cells or increased pleomorphism are required to confirm metastatic disease [6].

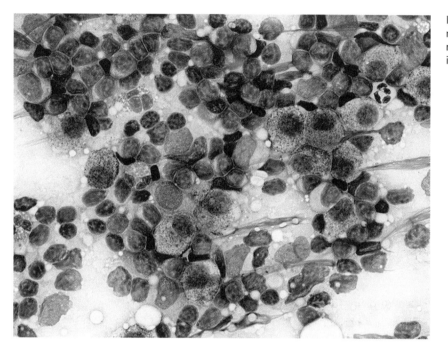

Figure 5.24 Lymph node, metastatic mast cell tumor, dog, 50× objective. The mast cells are poorly granular and seen in clusters.

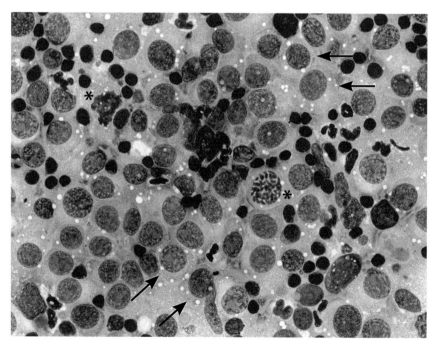

Figure 5.25 Lymph node, metastatic transmissible venereal tumor, dog, 50× objective. The neoplastic cells appear similar to lymphocytes but have an increased volume of pale-blue cytoplasm that contains fine clear vacuoles (arrows). Note the increased mitotic figures (asterisks).

Figure 5.26 Lymph node, metastatic amelanotic melanoma, dog, 50× objective.

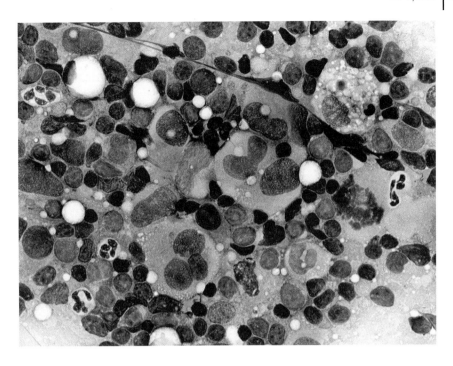

Figure 5.27 Lymph node, metastatic fibrosarcoma, dog, 50× objective.

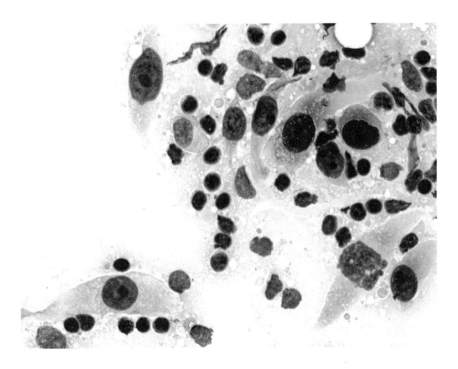

- Lymph nodes with metastatic disease are not always grossly enlarged [45, 49].

5.1.14.3 Prognosis
Guarded to poor. Metastasis to lymph nodes generally is associated with advanced disease and a poor prognosis. Correlate with specific neoplasm.

5.2 Spleen

5.2.1 Normal

5.2.1.1 Cytologic Appearance
Aspirates from normal spleen typically have a densely bloody background. Small aggregates of splenic red pulp/stroma are useful to confirm aspiration of splenic

parenchyma (Figure 5.28). Nucleated cells are predominated by small mature lymphocytes, with low numbers of plasma cells or intermediate-sized lymphocytes. Low numbers of hematopoietic cells may be seen.

5.2.2 Hyperplasia

5.2.2.1 Cytologic Appearance

Nodular hyperplastic lesions are characterized by increased numbers of stromal aggregates of splenic red pulp (Figure 5.29) and a mixed population of lymphocytes, with variably increased numbers of hematopoietic precursors (Figure 5.30).

5.2.2.2 Clinical Considerations

- Spleen mostly contains single or multiple nodules. Diffuse splenic enlargement possible [50].
- Nodules typically ~2 cm in diameter but may become large [50].
- Common incidental finding in older dogs [50].
- Lymphoid hyperplasia may reflect antigenic stimulation.

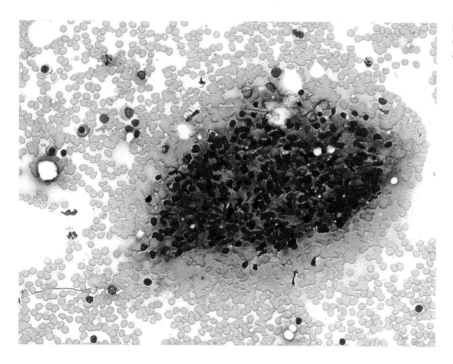

Figure 5.28 Spleen (normal), dog, 20× objective. Note the large stromal aggregate of splenic red pulp.

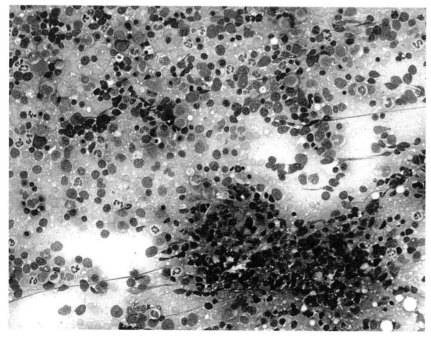

Figure 5.29 Spleen, benign nodular hyperplasia, dog, 20× objective. An aggregate of splenic red pulp is present (lower right), with many lymphoid and hematopoietic cells.

Figure 5.30 Spleen, benign nodular hyperplasia, dog, 50× objective. The mixed lymphocytes/plasma cells and hematopoietic precursors can be seen.

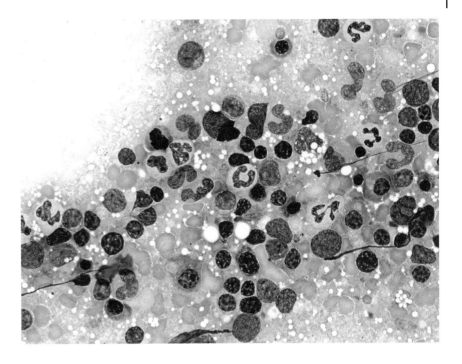

5.2.2.3 Prognosis
Generally good.

5.2.3 Extramedullary Hematopoiesis

5.2.3.1 Cytologic Appearance
Erythroid precursors tend to predominate, with lesser numbers of granulocytic and megakaryocytic precursors (Figure 5.31), though ratios may differ based on peripheral demand.

5.2.3.2 Clinical Considerations
- Seen in low numbers in normal spleen.
- Increased amounts may be seen in times of increased demand.
- May be diffuse or nodular [51].

5.2.3.3 Prognosis
Variable based on any underlying cause/disease.

Figure 5.31 Spleen, extramedullary hematopoiesis, dog, 50× objective. Erythroid precursors predominate, with rare granulocyte precursors (arrow).

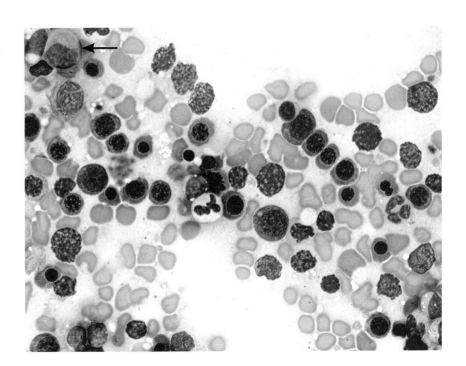

5.2.4 Myelolipoma

5.2.4.1 Cytologic Appearance

Myelolipomas contain hematopoietic precursors similar to cases of extramedullary hematopoiesis, but can be differentiated due to the concurrent presence of abundant variably sized clear lipid vacuoles (Figures 5.32 and 5.33).

5.2.4.2 Clinical Considerations

- Reported in dogs and cats, most common in the spleen, but also in the liver and omentum [52–54].
- Benign tumors, often an incidental finding [53].
- Single or multiple masses may be present [52, 54].
- Usually small (1–2 cm) masses but can be >5–10 cm [52]. Hyperechoic and not cavitated on ultrasound [53].

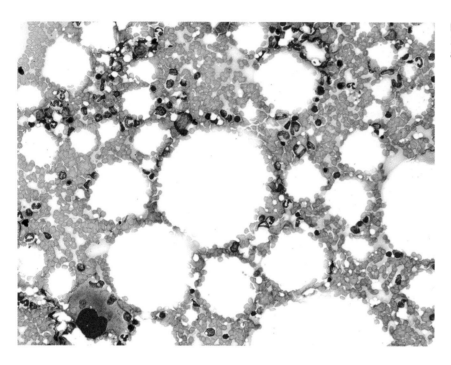

Figure 5.32 Spleen, myelolipoma, cat, 20× objective. Note the abundant lipid and the megakaryocyte (lower left).

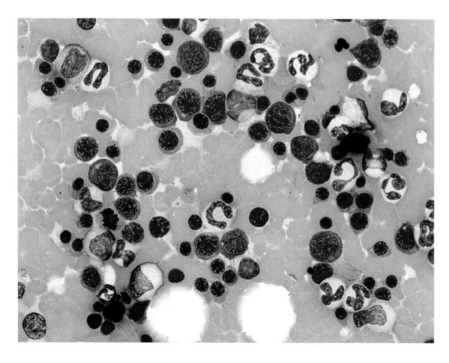

Figure 5.33 Spleen, myelolipoma, dog, 50× objective. Lipid vacuoles are seen, with many erythroid and rare granulocytic precursors.

5.2.4.3 Prognosis

Excellent.

5.2.5 Hemangiosarcoma

5.2.5.1 Cytologic Appearance

Hemangiosarcomas (HSA) exfoliate variably well as pleomorphic spindle cells seen individually or in aggregates/sheets that may form cords (Figure 5.34). The spindle cells are plump, with a moderate volume of medium-blue cytoplasm that forms tapering ends, and occasionally long tendrils (Figure 5.35). Erythrophagia by neoplastic cells is reported, but not specific to HSA [55]. Nuclei are ovoid, with finely stippled chromatin, and multiple prominent basophilic nucleoli. Multinucleation and mitotic figures are common. Anisocytosis/anisokaryosis are marked.

5.2.5.2 Clinical Considerations

- Most common malignant neoplasm in the spleen of dogs. Less common in cats [56, 57].

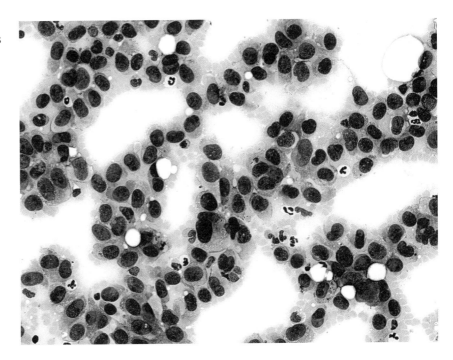

Figure 5.34 Spleen, hemangiosarcoma, dog, 20× objective. Note the spindle cells forming sticky cords.

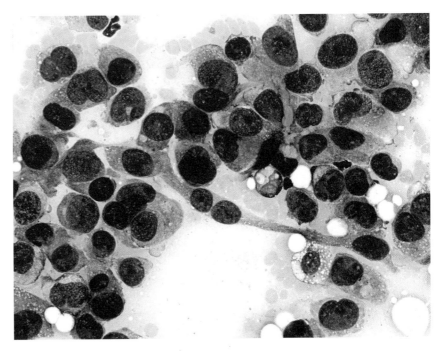

Figure 5.35 Spleen, hemangiosarcoma, dog, 40× objective.

- Often rupture, causing hemoabdomen (most common cause of non-traumatic hemoabdomen in dogs) [58].
- Metastatic disease is common at diagnosis, mostly to the liver, omentum, lungs, and bone [59–61].

5.2.5.3 Prognosis

Poor to grave, with short survival times even with surgical ± medical therapy in both dogs and cats [57, 62]. Clinical stage is the most important prognostic factor in dogs, with distant metastatic disease (stage III) associated with a grave prognosis [59]. High mitotic counts are associated with shorter survival times in cats [57].

5.2.6 Lymphoma (Large-cell)

5.2.6.1 Cytologic Appearance

Large-cell lymphoma appears similar to other organs, characterized by an expanded population of large, immature lymphocytes with nuclei having diameters about twofold to threefold the size of that of red blood cells, and with finely stippled chromatin, and many mitotic figures may be present (Figures 5.36 and 5.37). These cells should ideally be seen in large numbers in the spleen to help differentiate from a hyperplastic germinal center or florid lymphoid hyperplasia.

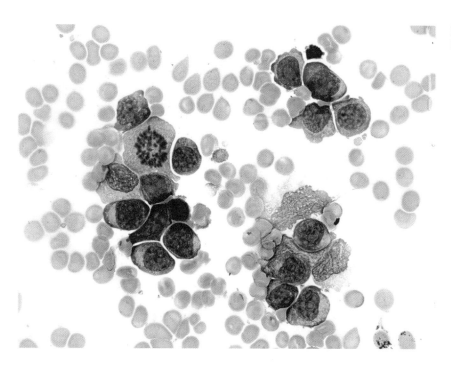

Figure 5.36 Spleen, large-cell lymphoma, dog, 50× objective.

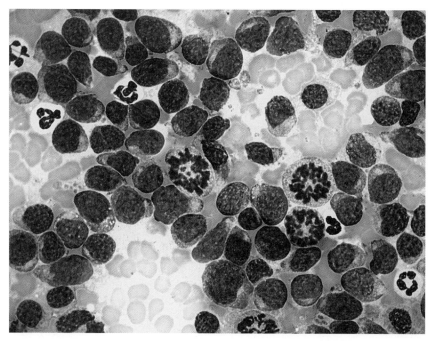

Figure 5.37 Spleen, large-cell lymphoma, dog, 50× objective. Note the numerous mitotic figures.

5.2.6.2 Clinical Considerations

- Normally part of multicentric disease.
- May present with diffuse splenic enlargement or nodules [63].

5.2.6.3 Prognosis

Similar to nodal large-cell lymphoma (see Section 5.1.7). Hemoabdomen and clinical signs of lethargy, anorexia, and abdominal distension are associated with a poor prognosis [64].

5.2.7 Lymphoma (Marginal Zone)

5.2.7.1 Cytologic Appearance

Marginal zone lymphoma (MZL) of the spleen is characterized by sheets of large lymphocytes with round nuclei approximately twofold the size of red blood cells in diameter, and a characteristic single, centrally located, prominent nucleolus (Figure 5.38) [65]. A moderate volume of pale-blue cytoplasm encircles the cells. *Note*: Large sheets of such cells should be present to raise any suspicion of neoplasia, as marginal zone hyperplasia is common in reactive lymphoid follicles secondary to antigenic stimulation.

5.2.7.2 Clinical Considerations

- Indolent form of B-cell lymphoma, often an incidental finding [65].
- Usually a single splenic nodule [66].
- Masses may rupture causing hemoabdomen [67].
- Although cytologic findings may be suggestive of MZL, a definitive diagnosis requires histopathologic assessment of the splenic architecture [66].

5.2.7.3 Prognosis

Fair to excellent. Splenectomy alone in asymptomatic dogs is associated with prolonged survival. Prognosis is less favorable in dogs with clinical signs of disease (e.g., hemoabdomen and vomiting) [67]. Disseminated disease is rare [66].

5.2.8 Lymphoma (Hepatosplenic)

5.2.8.1 Cytologic Appearance

Neoplastic lymphocytes have nuclei approximately twofold to threefold the size of red blood cells in diameter, that frequently have irregular membrane boundaries and finely stippled, immature chromatin. They have a small volume of pale-blue cytoplasm that frequently contains a perinuclear packet of faint azurophilic granules (Figure 5.39). Neoplastic cells may be erythrophagocytic. Extramedullary hematopoiesis and reactive histiocytes (often erythrophagocytic) typically are present in abundance.

5.2.8.2 Clinical Considerations

- Distinct clinical entity, separate from other lymphomas affecting spleen, liver, and bone marrow [68].
- Granular, T-cell phenotype.
- Often associated with regenerative anemia and thrombocytopenia [68, 69].
- Histopathology is required for definitive diagnosis.

5.2.8.3 Prognosis

Grave. Aggressive form of lymphoma associated with very short survival times [68–70].

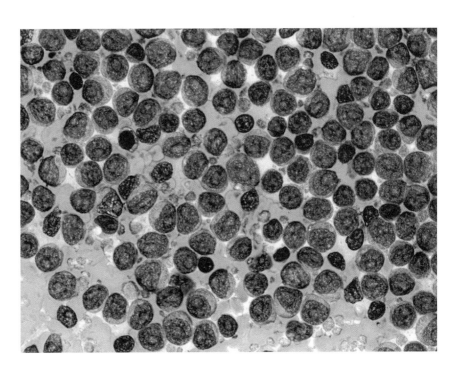

Figure 5.38 Spleen, marginal zone lymphoma, dog, 50× objective. Note the large sheet of lymphocytes with prominent, single, centrally located nucleoli.

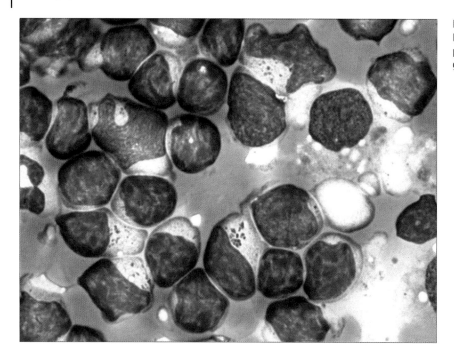

Figure 5.39 Spleen, hepatosplenic lymphoma, dog, 100× objective. Note the perinuclear, azurophilic cytoplasmic granules. Photo courtesy of Dr. Bill Vernau.

5.2.9 Acute Leukemias

5.2.9.1 Cytologic Appearance

Acute leukemias are characterized by large numbers of neoplastic cells, with nuclei about twofold to threefold the size of a red blood cell that have finely stippled, immature chromatin and mostly prominent nucleoli. Mitotic rates generally are high. The cells have a variable volume of cytoplasm, which may contain pink granules if the cells are of granulocytic origin (Figure 5.40) or may be deep blue in erythroid leukemias (Figure 5.41).

5.2.9.2 Clinical Considerations

- Neoplastic leukemia cells infiltrate the red pulp of the spleen [51].
- Normally associated with circulating neoplastic cells and cytopenias.

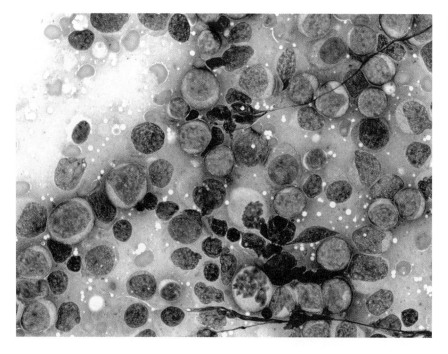

Figure 5.40 Spleen, acute granulocytic leukemia, dog, 50× objective.

Figure 5.41 Spleen, acute erythroid leukemia, cat, 50× objective. Note the deep blue cytoplasm of the cells.

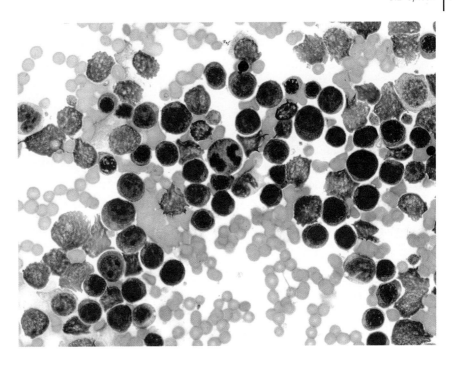

5.2.9.3 Prognosis
Grave.

5.2.10 Lymphoma (Small-cell)/Chronic Lymphocytic Leukemia

5.2.10.1 Cytologic Appearance
Small-cell lymphoma and chronic lymphocytic leukemia (CLL) are cytologically similar, characterized by sheets of a monomorphic population of small lymphocytes. When compared to normal small mature lymphocytes, these cells have slightly larger nuclei (diameter ~1.25-fold the size of a red blood cell), and more open, less-clumped chromatin, often with prominent nucleoli (Figure 5.42).

5.2.10.2 Clinical Considerations
- Affects middle-aged to older patients.
- Usually diffuse splenic enlargement [71].
- Accompanied by lymphocytosis (range in dogs = 15 000–1 600 000 cells µl^{-1}; median value in cats = 34 200 cells µl^{-1}) [44, 71].

Figure 5.42 Spleen, chronic lymphocytic leukemia (CLL), dog, 50× objective.

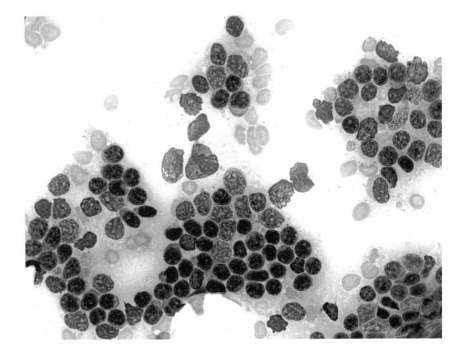

5.2.10.3 Prognosis
Good.

5.2.11 Multiple Myeloma

5.2.11.1 Cytologic Features
Multiple myeloma is characterized by large sheets and aggregates of well-differentiated plasma cells. The cells have a moderate volume of pale-blue cytoplasm, and often have a characteristic, perinuclear clear zone (Golgi zone) (Figure 5.43). The nuclei are round, eccentrically placed, and have clumped chromatin.

5.2.11.2 Clinical Considerations
- Dogs > cats.
- Other clinical features = monoclonal gammopathy, lytic bone lesions, anemia, bleeding diatheses, Bence-Jones proteinuria [72, 73].

5.2.11.3 Prognosis
Dogs = Good short-term prognosis with treatment, and long-term control is possible. Negative prognostic factors include extensive bone lysis/involvement as well as hypercalcemia and Bence-Jones proteinuria [72].

Cats = Guarded prognosis, with generally short survival times [73, 74].

5.2.12 Histiocytic Sarcoma

5.2.12.1 Cytologic Features
Histiocytic sarcoma (HS) is characterized by individualized cells with many criteria of malignancy, including marked anisocytosis and anisokaryosis, with karyomegaly a common finding. Multinucleation, nuclear fragmentation, and hyperchromasia also are common (Figure 5.44). The cytoplasm usually is vacuolated.

5.2.12.2 Clinical Considerations
- Dogs > > cats.
- Reported in many dog breeds, but Bernese Mountain Dogs, Rottweilers, Golden Retrievers, Labrador Retrievers, and Flat-Coated Retrievers are predisposed [75, 76].
- May represent primary or involvement with disseminated disease [76, 77].

5.2.12.3 Prognosis
Generally grave. Localized splenic disease treated with surgery ± chemotherapy may be associated with prolonged survival in some dogs [77].

5.2.13 Hemophagocytic Histiocytic Sarcoma

5.2.13.1 Cytologic Appearance
Hemophagocytic histiocytic sarcoma (HHS) is characterized by well-differentiated histiocytes/macrophages, seen mostly in aggregates but also individually. They have a moderate to abundant volume of medium-blue cytoplasm that may contain clear vacuoles, and cells often are erythrophagocytic (Figure 5.45). Anisocytosis/anisokaryosis are mild to moderate. *Note*: It is important to rule out causes of reactive histiocytosis.

5.2.13.2 Clinical Considerations
- Rare in dogs and cats [76].
- Predisposed breeds = Bernese Mountain Dog, Golden Retriever, Labrador Retriever.

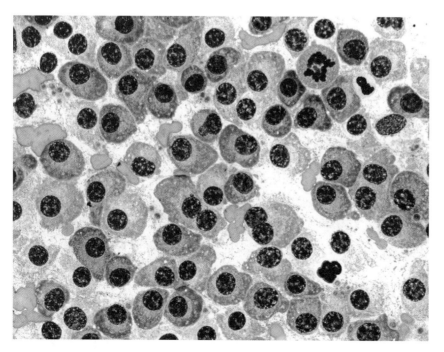

Figure 5.43 Spleen, myeloma-like disease, cat, 50× objective.

Figure 5.44 Spleen, histiocytic sarcoma, dog, 50× objective.

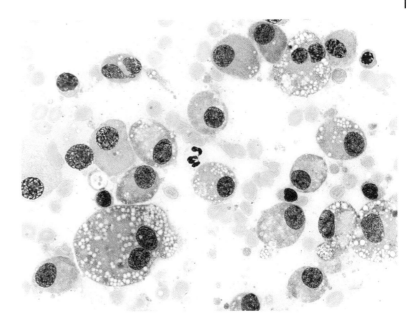

Figure 5.45 Spleen, hemophagocytic histiocytic sarcoma, dog, 50× objective. Note erythrophagia within neoplastic cells (arrow).

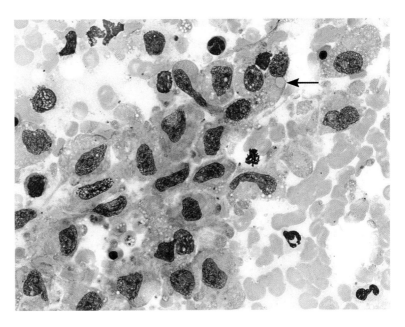

- Arises in spleen and bone marrow. May metastasize to liver and lungs [76].
- Common concurrent hematologic findings (% of cases): Coomb's negative regenerative anemia (94%), hypoalbuminemia (94%), thrombocytopenia (88%), and hypocholesterolemia (69%) [78].
- Ultrasound = diffuse splenomegaly with ill-defined masses.

5.2.13.3 Prognosis
Grave. HHS is an aggressive malignancy associated with short survival times (median survival time of 4 weeks post diagnosis), even with therapy [78, 79].

5.2.14 Feline Visceral Mast Cell Neoplasia

5.2.14.1 Cytologic Appearance
Visceral mast cell neoplasia is characterized by large sheets of mast cells (Figure 5.46). These cells have a moderate volume of cytoplasm that contains a variable number of metachromatic granules. Nuclei are centrally located and have granular chromatin with prominent nucleoli.

5.2.14.2 Clinical Considerations
- Most common cause of splenic disease in cats [80].
- Spleen may be diffusely enlarged or nodular.
- Often associated with mastocytemia (see Chapter 18) [81].
- Common metastatic sites = liver, internal lymph nodes, bone marrow, and skin.

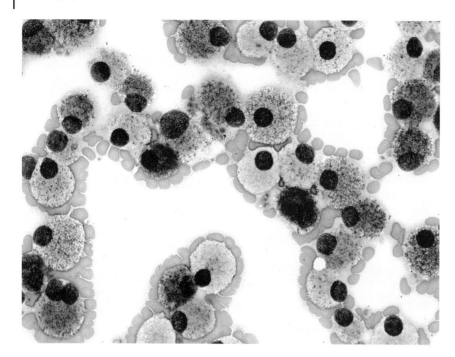

Figure 5.46 Spleen, visceral mast cell neoplasia, cat, 50× objective.

5.2.14.3 Prognosis

Prolonged survival seen if disease confined to the spleen with splenectomy ± chemotherapy [82, 83]. Variable survival times for disseminated disease [84, 85]. Metastatic disease, administration of blood products, and evidence of other historical neoplasia associated with poor prognosis [86].

5.2.15 Metastatic Disease

5.2.15.1 Cytologic Appearance

Many neoplasms metastasize to the spleen. Epithelial neoplasms are particularly apparent, as epithelial cells are not normally seen in splenic aspirates (Figure 5.47). Metastatic

mesenchymal tumors (Figure 5.48) may be difficult to differentiate from primary sarcomas of the spleen (e.g., hemangiosarcoma). Round-cell neoplasms frequently metastasize to the spleen, including mast cell neoplasia (Figure 5.49), histiocytic sarcoma (see Section 5.2.12), and lymphoma (see Section 5.2.6).

5.2.15.2 Clinical Considerations

The spleen is a common site for metastatic disease [87].

5.2.15.3 Prognosis

Poor, with metastatic disease confirming disseminated neoplasia. Dogs with metastatic cutaneous mast cell neoplasia involving the spleen have shorter survival times [88].

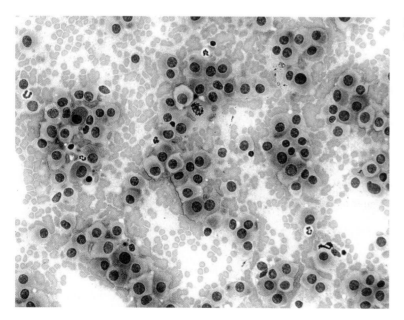

Figure 5.47 Spleen, metastatic hepatocellular carcinoma, dog, 20× objective.

Figure 5.48 Spleen, metastatic fibrosarcoma, dog, 50× objective.

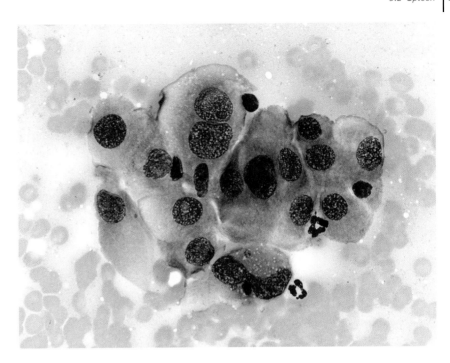

Figure 5.49 Spleen, metastatic mast cell neoplasia, dog, 50× objective.

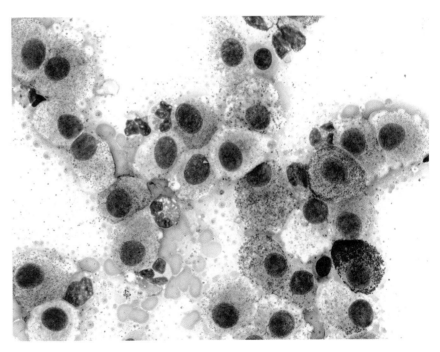

5.2.16 Amyloid

5.2.16.1 Cytologic Appearance
Amyloid is seen as smooth to fibrillar, magenta extracellular material, mostly associated with stromal aggregates of red pulp (Figure 5.50).

5.2.16.2 Clinical Considerations
- Amyloid deposition may be localized or systemic (involving kidney and liver) [89].

- Amyloid may accumulate due to a primary familial predisposition, or secondary to chronic systemic inflammation.
- Predisposed breeds = Shar Pei dogs and Abyssinian cats [90].

5.2.16.3 Prognosis
Variable based on primary or secondary, organs involved, and ability to treat any underlying disease.

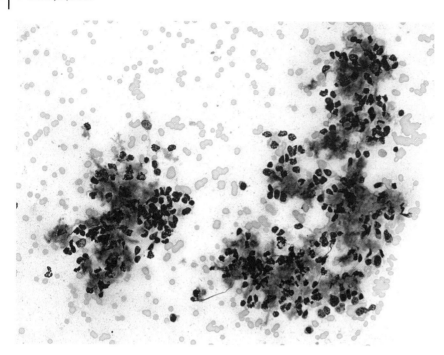

Figure 5.50 Spleen, amyloid, cat, 20× objective. Note the bright-purple fibrillar material between cells.

5.2.17 Hemophagocytic Syndrome

5.2.17.1 Cytologic Appearance

Hemophagocytic syndrome is characterized by increased numbers of macrophages that are heavily erythrophagocytic, with the cytoplasm often distended with numerous erythrocytes or erythroid precursors (Figure 5.51). These macrophages typically represent 2% to >5% of nucleated cells in the samples [91].

5.2.17.2 Clinical Considerations

- Also termed *hemophagocytic lymphohistiocytosis* [91, 92].
- Associated with fever, peripheral bi- or pancytopenia, and increased hemophagocytic macrophages in the spleen and bone marrow (see also Section 5.4.10) [91].
- Reported secondary to infectious disease, immune-mediated disease, and neoplasia including multiple myeloma and lymphoma [68, 92–94].

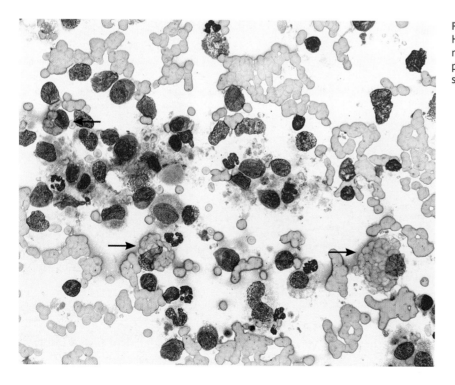

Figure 5.51 Spleen, dog, 50× objective. Hemophagocytic syndrome with numerous macrophages distended with phagocytosed erythrocytes (arrows) secondary to large-cell lymphoma.

5.2.17.3 Prognosis

Variable based on underlying disease process, but reported outcomes are frequently poor.

5.2.18 Infectious Organisms

Many infectious organisms may affect the spleen, and details of such organisms are available in Chapter 3.

5.3 Thymus

5.3.1 Thymoma

5.3.1.1 Cytologic Appearance

Cytologic samples from thymomas usually comprise mostly of resident thymic small mature lymphocytes, admixed with lesser numbers of intermediate or large lymphocytes. The neoplastic cells exfoliate as sheets of polygonal cells with moderate to abundant pale-blue cytoplasm and ovoid nuclei with reticular chromatin and variably prominent nucleoli (Figure 5.52). Anisocytosis/anisokaryosis are mild and N/C ratios are low. The neoplastic epithelial cells do not always exfoliate, which can make cytologic diagnosis of thymoma difficult. Well-differentiated mast cells are a common finding, scattered individually across samples (Figure 5.53).

5.3.1.2 Clinical Considerations

- Mostly older dogs and cats [95].
- Commonly located in the cranial mediastinum. Ectopic tumors rare [96].
- Paraneoplastic syndromes include hypercalcemia (reported in up to 34% of dogs) and myasthenia gravis [97, 98]. Thymomas may also be associated with megaesophagus and a reactive lymphocytosis that resolves with surgical excision of the tumor [95, 99].

5.3.1.3 Prognosis

Good with surgical excision, even in patients with paraneoplastic syndromes. Recurrence rate is low [97, 100]. Improved survival seen in dogs and cats with lymphocyte-rich tumors [100]. Metastatic disease and myasthenia gravis are associated with reduced survival in epithelial-rich tumors [101]. Untreated patients have short survival times [97].

5.3.2 Thymic Carcinoma

5.3.2.1 Cytologic Appearance

Thymic carcinoma cells are cohesive and have a moderate volume of cytoplasm, which may contain fine clear vacuoles. Nuclei are ovoid with finely granular chromatin, and increased numbers of mitotic figures often are seen (Figure 5.54).

5.3.2.2 Clinical Considerations

- Reported rarely in dogs [102].
- Myasthenia gravis seen as a paraneoplastic syndrome [103].

Figure 5.52 Thymus, thymoma, dog, 20× objective. Mixed lymphocytes surround loose sheets of epithelial cells with abundant pale-blue cytoplasm.

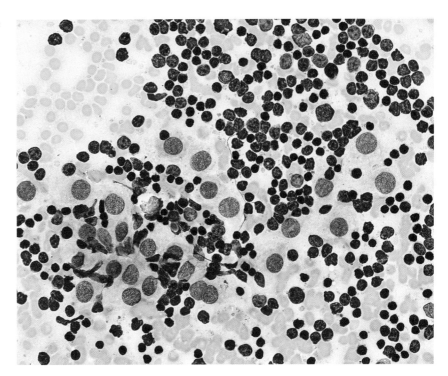

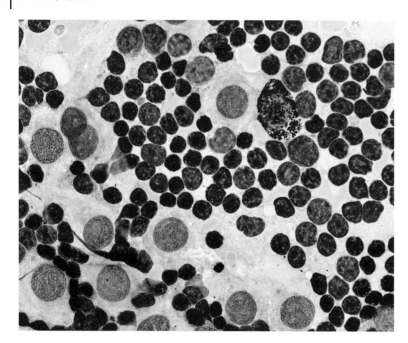

Figure 5.53 Thymus, thymoma, dog, 50× objective. Note the mixed lymphoid population, well-differentiated epithelial cells, and well-granulated mast cell (common finding in thymomas).

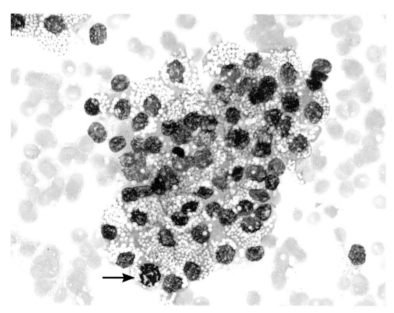

Figure 5.54 Thymus, thymic carcinoma, dog, 50× objective. The cells have a decreased volume of vacuolated cytoplasm. Note the mitotic figure (arrow).

5.3.2.3 Prognosis

Metastasis is uncommon but tends to be seen in the lungs and liver [104]. Median survival times generally are short, even with therapy [102, 103].

5.3.3 Thymic (Mediastinal) Lymphoma

5.3.3.1 Cytologic Appearance

Lymphoma of the thymus and mediastinal lymph nodes is a high-grade disease, characterized by cells with nuclei 1.5-fold to 3-fold the size of red blood cells in diameter. Nuclei often have irregular membrane boundaries, and mitotic figures are common (Figure 5.55). The cells have a small

volume of pale-blue cytoplasm. Lesser numbers of residual small mature lymphocytes may be present.

5.3.3.2 Clinical Considerations

Mediastinal lymphoma involves the mediastinal lymph nodes, thymus, or both.

Dogs
- Patients may present with respiratory distress or precaval syndrome, and pleural effusion is common [34].
- T-cell phenotype (and lymphoblastic type) most common [34, 105].
- Hypercalcemia is common (up to 43% of patients) [106].

Figure 5.55 Thymus, lymphoma, dog, 50× objective. Note the irregular nuclear membrane boundaries.

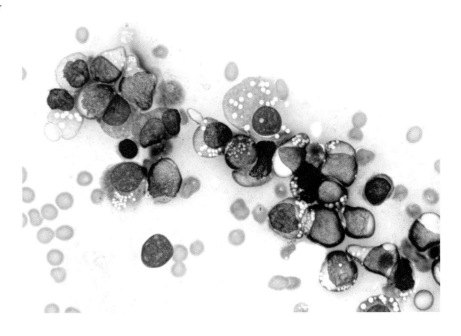

Cats
- Most common in young, FeLV-positive cats [22, 23, 95].
- Hypercalcemia is rare.

5.3.3.3 Prognosis

Guarded to poor. T-cell phenotype and high grade confer a poorer prognosis in dogs [34]. FeLV-positive cats with lymphoma have a grave prognosis.

5.3.4 Thymic Branchial Cyst

5.3.4.1 Cytologic Appearance

Samples from thymic branchial cysts have a blue proteinaceous background. Nucleated cells comprise cuboidal to columnar epithelial cells which may be ciliated (Figure 5.56).

Figure 5.56 Thymus, branchial cyst, 50× objective. Note the ciliated epithelial cells.

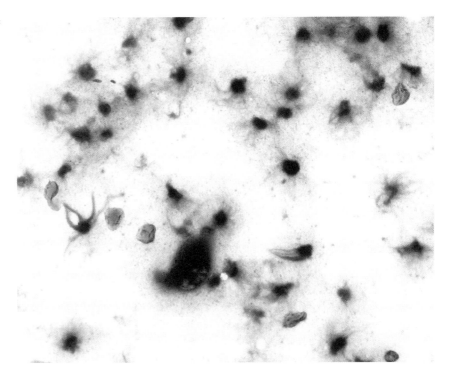

5.3.4.2 Clinical Considerations

- Uncommon in dogs and cats [95, 107].
- Clinical signs = dyspnea > lethargy, cough, inappetence [107–109].
- Malignant transformation to carcinoma has been reported [108, 109].

5.3.4.3 Prognosis

Good for animals surviving surgical resection [107].

5.4 Bone Marrow

5.4.1 Normal

5.4.1.1 Cytologic Appearance

Normal bone marrow contains a mixture of granulocytic and erythroid cells. Both lineages should have orderly maturation, with low numbers of blasts (<5%) leading to progressively greater numbers of mature cells. Stages of maturation are shown in Figures 5.57–5.59. Megakaryocytes

(A)

(B)

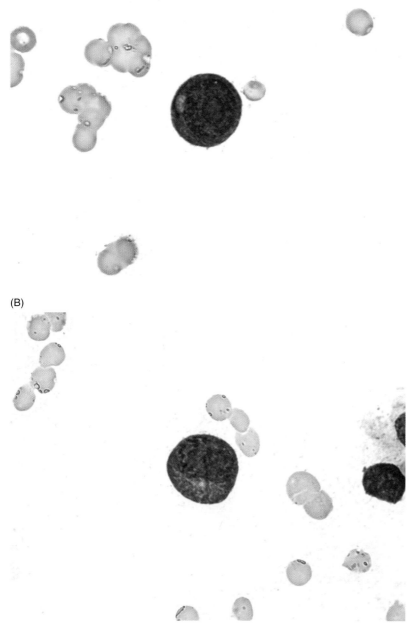

Figure 5.57 Erythroid precursor cells from youngest to most mature. (A) Rubriblast. (B) Prorubricyte.

(C)

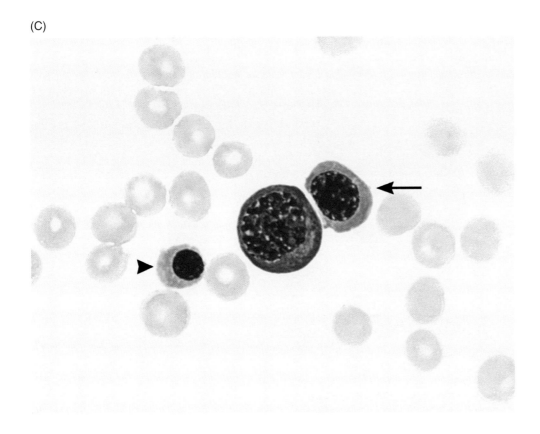

(D)

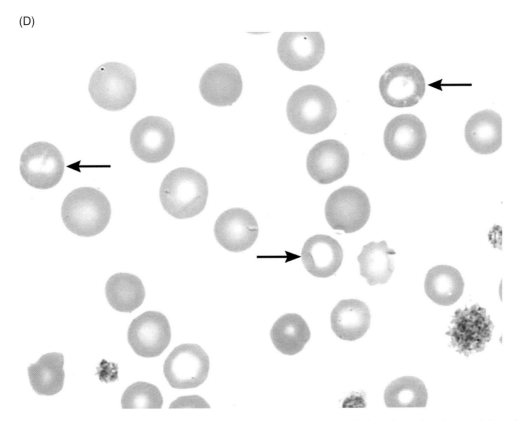

Figure 5.57 (Continued) (C) Basophilic rubricyte, polychromatophilic rubricyte (arrow) and metarubricyte (arrowhead). (D) Polychromatophils (arrows) and mature erythrocytes.

(A)

(B)

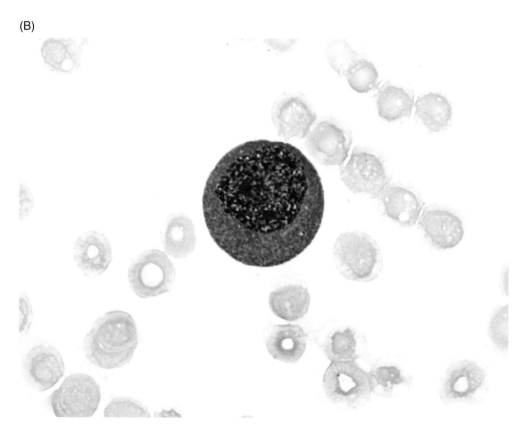

Figure 5.58 Granulocytic precursor cells from youngest to most mature. (A) Myeloblast. (B) Promyelocyte (note abundant pink cytoplasmic granules).

(C)

(D)

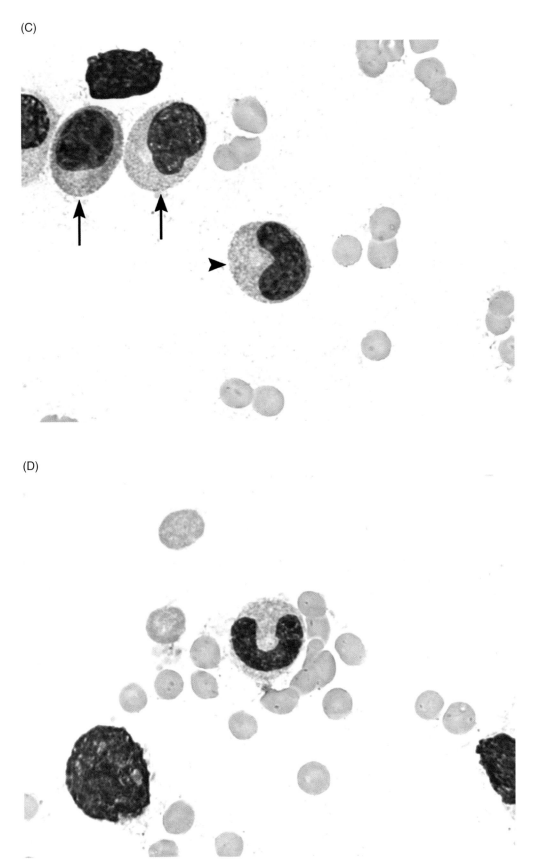

Figure 5.58 (Continued) (C) Myelocytes (arrows) and metamyelocyte (arrowhead). (D) Band neutrophil.

(E)

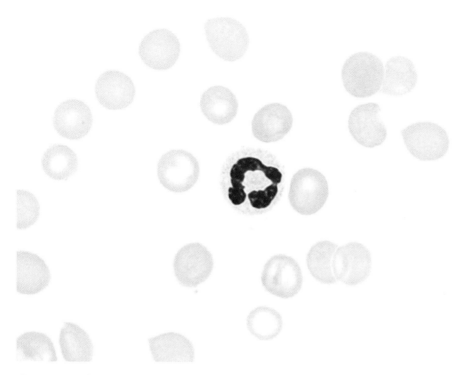

Figure 5.58 (Continued) (E) Mature neutrophil.

(A)

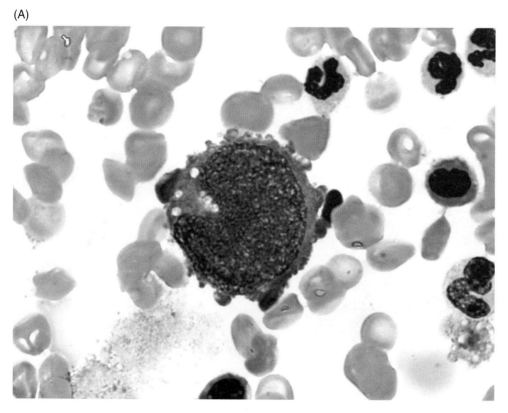

Figure 5.59 Megakaryocytic precursor cells from youngest to most mature. (A) Megakaryoblast.

(B)

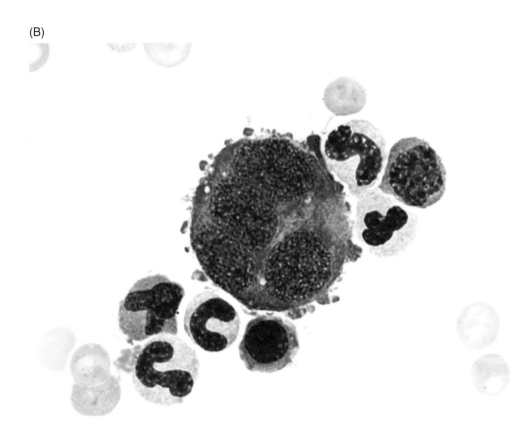

(C)

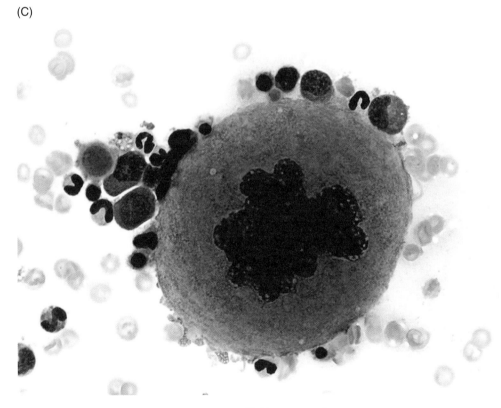

Figure 5.59 (Continued) (B) Promegakaryocyte. (C) Mature megakaryocyte.

should mostly be mature, and about three to four should be seen per unit particle.

5.4.1.2 Clinical Considerations

- Cellularity decreases with age: juveniles ~75%, adults ~50%, and geriatrics ~30% cellular relative to marrow lipid [110].
- The granulocytic to erythroid (G/E) ratio for dogs and cats is typically between 1.0 and 2.0 (range 0.45 to 2.87) [110].
- Lymphocytes are seen in low numbers (<5% dogs and <10–15% cats), as are plasma cells (<2% for both species) [110, 111].
- Moderate to heavy iron stores should be visible in unit particles from healthy dogs [112]. Iron stores are not typically noted in unit particles from healthy cats.

5.4.2 Acute Myeloid Leukemia

Acute myeloid leukemias (AMLs) may have a granulocytic, monocytic, erythroid, or megakaryocytic origin. Acute leukemias should be considered when the percentage of blasts exceeds 30% of nucleated cells (excluding lymphoid cells and macrophages) [113]. These can sometimes be distinguished based on cytomorphology (see below), but definitive diagnosis often requires special stains. Spleen, liver, and lymph nodes may be involved, and peripheral cytopenias (anemia, leukopenia, thrombocytopenia) often are present.

5.4.3 Acute Granulocytic/Monocytic Leukemia

5.4.3.1 Cytologic Appearance

Cells of granulocytic origin have a moderate volume of pale- to medium-blue cytoplasm, and often have diffuse pink granules in their cytoplasm (Figures 5.60 and 5.61). Monocytic leukemias frequently have lobulated nuclei (Figure 5.62).

5.4.3.2 Clinical Considerations

- Multiple subtypes: AML-M1 (myeloblastic leukemia without maturation); AML-M2 (myeloblastic leukemia with differentiation); AML-M3 (promyelocytic leukemia – not reported in veterinary species); AML-M4 (myelomonocytic leukemia); and AML-M5 (monocytic leukemia).
- Eosinophilic and basophilic variants reported [113, 114].

5.4.3.3 Prognosis

Grave. Short survival times reported, even with therapy [115, 116].

5.4.4 Acute Erythroid Leukemia

5.4.4.1 Cytologic Appearance

Erythroblasts have a small volume of deep-blue cytoplasm, and nuclei often have irregularly condensed chromatin (Figure 5.63).

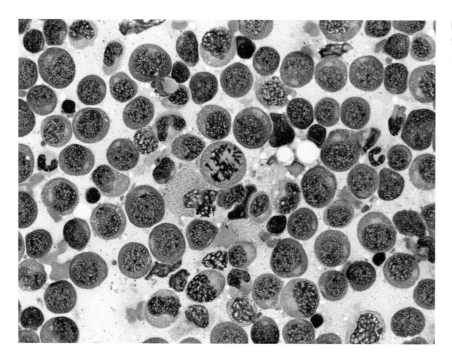

Figure 5.60 Bone marrow, acute granulocytic leukemia (AML-M2), dog, 50× objective.

Figure 5.61 Bone marrow, acute granulocytic leukemia (AML-M2; same case as Figure 5.58), dog, 100× objective. Note the diffuse, pink cytoplasmic granules.

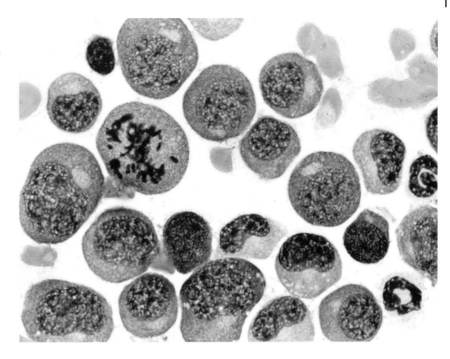

Figure 5.62 Bone marrow, acute myelomonocytic leukemia (AML-M4), dog, 50× objective. Note the indented and vaguely lobulated nuclei.

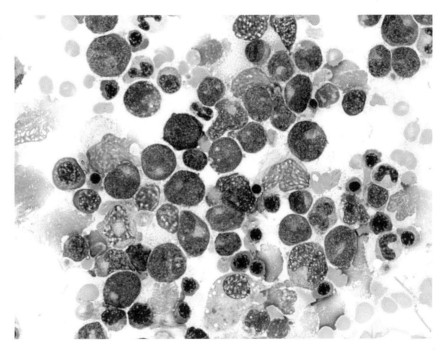

5.4.4.2 Clinical Considerations
- AML-M6/M6Er subtype.
- Cats > dogs [117].
- Associated with Feline Leukemia Virus in cats [118, 119].

5.4.4.3 Prognosis
Grave [117, 120].

5.4.5 Acute Megakaryoblastic Leukemia

5.4.5.1 Cytologic Appearance
Blast cells of megakaryocytic origin have a moderate volume of medium- to deep-blue cytoplasm, which can appear similar to erythroid leukemias. Nuclei, however, often are bilobed or multilobulated and have finely stippled chromatin with prominent basophilic nucleoli. Unique features include cytoplasmic projections and multiple discrete cytoplasmic vacuoles (Figure 5.64) [121].

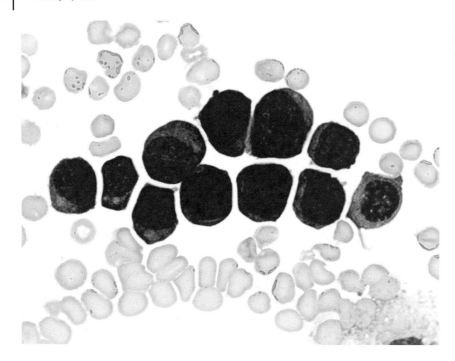

Figure 5.63 Bone marrow, acute erythroid leukemia (AML-M6Er), cat, 100× objective. Note the deep blue cytoplasm.

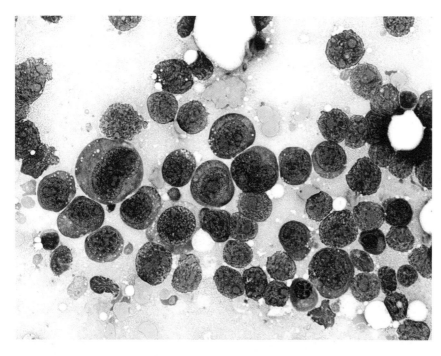

Figure 5.64 Bone marrow, acute megakaryoblastic leukemia (AML-M7), dog, 50× objective. Characteristic features include indented nuclei, binucleation, and deep blue cytoplasm with fine clear vacuoles.

5.4.5.2 Clinical Considerations

- AML-M7 subtype.
- Dogs > cats.
- May be associated with platelet dysfunction [122].
- Thrombocytopenia is common, but thrombocytosis is reported [123, 124].

5.4.5.3 Prognosis

Mostly grave with short survival times, though rare reports of prolonged survival with chemotherapy [125].

5.4.6 Acute Lymphoid Leukemia

5.4.6.1 Cytologic Appearance

Acute lymphoid leukemia (ALL) is characterized by an expanded population of lymphocytes with large nuclei, finely stippled, immature chromatin, and variably prominent nucleoli. Nuclei often have irregular nuclear margins (Figure 5.65). The cells mostly have high N/C ratios with a small volume of medium-blue cytoplasm. Differentiation from metastatic large-cell lymphoma is difficult (compare to Figure 5.66) and although number of cells may be

Figure 5.65 Bone marrow, acute lymphoid leukemia, dog, 50× objective.

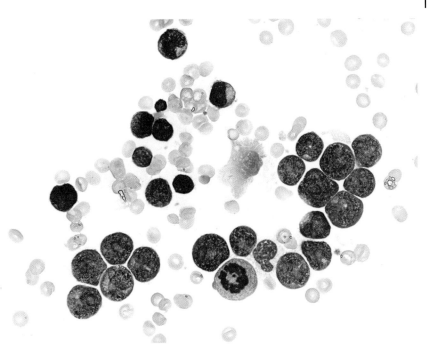

Figure 5.66 Bone marrow, metastatic large-cell lymphoma, dog, 50× objective.

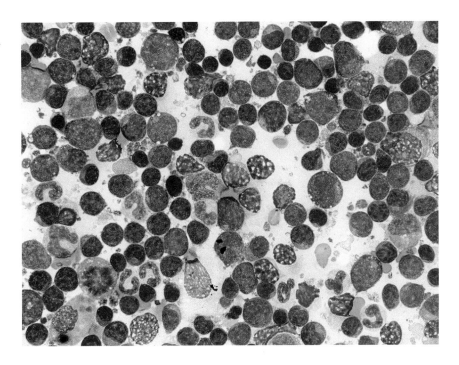

helpful, other clinical information (concurrent cytopenias, enlarged lymph nodes, etc.) is essential.

5.4.6.2 Clinical Considerations
- Dogs and cats.
- May affect bone marrow and spleen.
- B-cell phenotype more common in dogs and cats [43, 126].
- Associated with Feline Leukemia Virus infection in cats [127].

5.4.6.3 Prognosis
Grave [128].

5.4.7 Lymphoma (Large-cell)

5.4.7.1 Cytologic Appearance
Large-cell lymphoma may metastasize to the bone marrow and appear similar to ALL or other acute leukemias (Figure 5.66).

5.4.7.2 Clinical Considerations

- Associated with enlarged lymph nodes/lymphoid organs.
- Marrow involvement often associated with circulating neoplastic cells and thrombocytopenia [129].

5.4.7.3 Prognosis

Poor. >3% bone marrow infiltration associated with short survival times and poor prognosis [130].

5.4.8 Granulocytic Hyperplasia

5.4.8.1 Cytologic Appearance

Granulocytic hyperplasia is characterized by an overall orderly increase in the granulocytic series, with increased numbers of immature cells including bands, metamyelocytes, promyelocytes, and myeloblasts. Increased numbers of mitotic figures may be seen (Figure 5.67).

5.4.8.2 Clinical Considerations

- Myeloblasts are increased but comprise <20–30% of nucleated cells.
- Mature neutrophil production takes ~3–4 days [131].
- Appropriate response to increased peripheral demand or previous bone marrow insults.

5.4.8.3 Prognosis

Excellent if regenerative response is effective.

5.4.9 Erythroid Hyperplasia

5.4.9.1 Cytologic Appearance

Erythroid hyperplasia is characterized by an overall orderly increase in the erythroid series, with increased numbers of immature cells including basophilic rubricytes, prorubricytes, and rubriblasts (Figure 5.68).

5.4.9.2 Clinical Considerations

- Rubriblasts are increased but comprise <20–30% of nucleated cells.
- Erythrocyte regeneration takes ~4 days [132].
- Appropriate response to hemolysis/hemorrhage or previous bone marrow insults.
- Ineffective erythroid hyperplasia may result from iron deficiency, myeloproliferative/dysplastic diseases, and immune-mediated disease [133].

5.4.9.3 Prognosis

Guarded to excellent, based on the underlying cause.

5.4.10 Hemophagocytosis

5.4.10.1 Cytologic Appearance

Hemophagocytosis in the bone marrow is characterized by increased numbers of well-differentiated macrophages containing phagocytosed red blood cells.

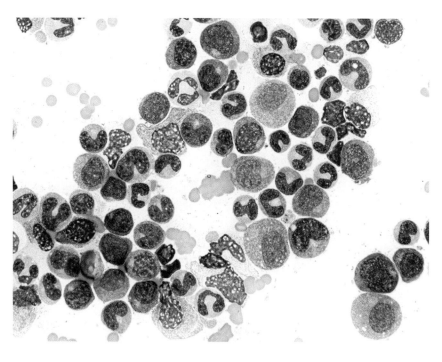

Figure 5.67 Bone marrow, granulocytic hyperplasia, cat, 50× objective. The series is left shifted, with increased numbers of bands and metamyelocytes but low numbers of promyelocytes and rare myeloblasts.

Figure 5.68 Bone marrow, erythroid hyperplasia, dog, 50× objective. Increased numbers of erythroid precursors are seen. Note the mitotic figure (arrow).

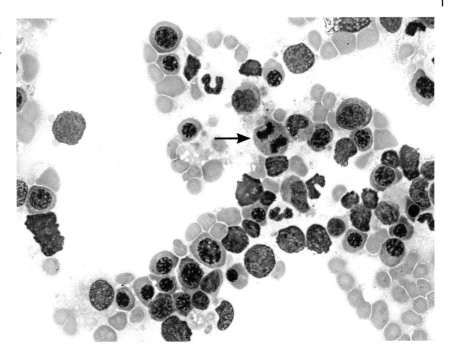

Earlier erythroid precursors may even be ingested, especially in cases of immune-mediated hemolytic anemia at the level of the bone marrow (Figure 5.69). Macrophages generally are seen individually and in lesser numbers than in cases of HHS (compare to Figure 5.70).

5.4.10.2 Clinical Considerations

- Seen secondary to immune-mediated destruction of red blood cells. Arrest at the level of destruction usually is apparent [134].
- May also be secondary to infectious, neoplastic, immune-mediated, or metabolic diseases [68, 91, 135, 136].

Figure 5.69 Bone marrow, hemophagocytosis, dog, 50× objective. Precursor-targeted immune-mediated anemia with maturational arrest at the level of basophilic rubricytes. Note the phagocytosed basophilic rubricyte (arrow).

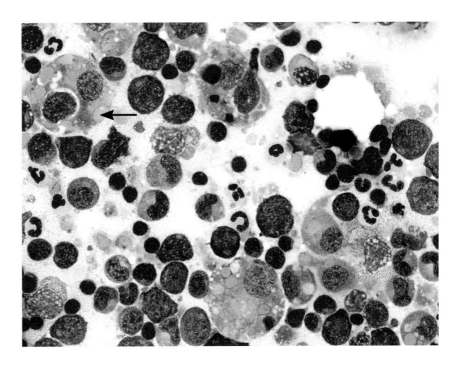

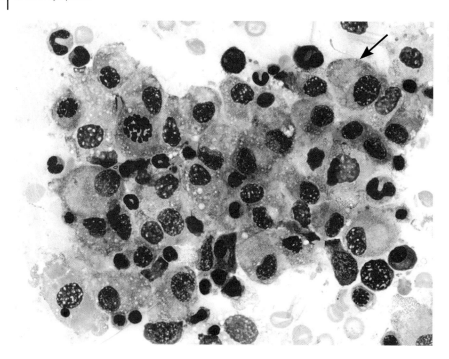

Figure 5.70 Bone marrow, hemophagocytic histiocytic sarcoma, dog, 50× objective. Note sheets of well-differentiated macrophages that are erythrophagocytic (arrow).

5.4.10.3 Prognosis
Variable, based on the underlying cause.

5.4.11 Hemophagocytic Histiocytic Sarcoma

5.4.11.1 Cytologic Appearance
Similar to that described in the spleen, HHS is characterized by well-differentiated histiocytes/macrophages, seen mostly in aggregates (Figure 5.70). Anisocytosis/anisokaryosis are mild to moderate. *Note*: It is important to rule out causes of reactive histiocytosis and erythrophagocytosis (see Section 5.4.10).

5.4.11.2 Clinical Considerations
- Rare in dogs and cats.
- Predisposed breeds = Bernese Mountain Dog, Golden Retriever, Labrador Retriever.
- Arises in bone marrow and spleen. May metastasize to liver and lungs [76].
- Common concurrent hematologic findings (% of cases): Coomb's negative regenerative anemia (94%); hypoalbuminemia (94%); thrombocytopenia (88%); hypocholesterolemia (69%) [78].

5.4.11.3 Prognosis
Grave. HHS is an aggressive malignancy associated with short survival times (median survival time of 4 weeks post diagnosis), even with therapy [78, 79].

5.4.12 Histiocytic Sarcoma

5.4.12.1 Cytologic Features
HS is characterized by individualized cells with many criteria of malignancy including marked anisocytosis and anisokaryosis, and with karyomegaly a common finding. Multinucleation, nuclear fragmentation, and hyperchromasia also are common (Figure 5.71). The cytoplasm is variably vacuolated.

5.4.12.2 Clinical Considerations
- Dogs > > cats.
- Reported in many dog breeds, but Bernese Mountain Dogs, Rottweilers, Golden Retrievers, Labrador Retrievers, and Flat-Coated Retrievers are predisposed [75].
- Other organs commonly affected by disseminated HS = spleen, liver, lungs, and lymph nodes.

5.4.12.3 Prognosis
Grave.

5.4.13 Inflammation/Infection

5.4.13.1 Cytologic Appearance
Inflammation can be difficult to diagnose in bone marrow samples due to the normal presence of neutrophils and monocytes. Plasma cells and lymphocytes should be seen in low numbers normally (see Section 5.4.1), and increased numbers may be indicative of inflammation/antigenic stimulation (Figure 5.72). The presence of infectious

Figure 5.71 Bone marrow, histiocytic sarcoma, dog, 50× objective. Note the large, bizarre neoplastic cells (arrows).

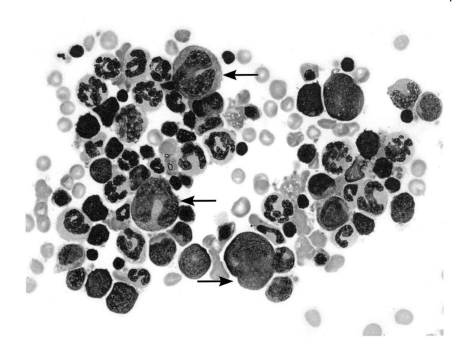

Figure 5.72 Bone marrow, plasmacytosis, dog, 50× objective. Increased numbers of plasma cells are seen (arrows).

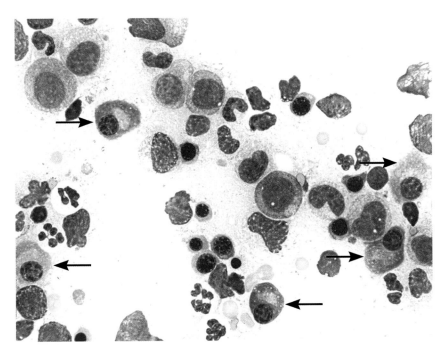

organisms confirms inflammation/infection (Figure 5.73). Many infectious organisms may affect the bone marrow (see Chapter 3 for details).

5.4.13.2 Clinical Considerations
- Reactive lymphocytosis associated with immune-mediated and inflammatory diseases [111].
- Reactive lymphocytes seen in aggregates and smaller than those of CLL [111].

5.4.13.3 Prognosis
Variable, based on the underlying cause.

5.4.14 Chronic Lymphocytic Leukemia

5.4.14.1 Cytologic Appearance
CLL is considered present when small mature lymphocytes exceed 15–30% of nucleated cells in the bone marrow [71, 137]. The cells have nuclei that are about onefold the size

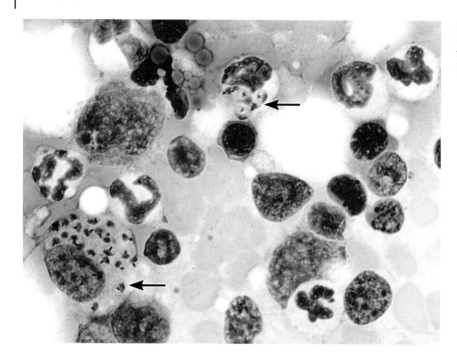

Figure 5.73 Bone marrow, Leishmaniasis, dog, 100× objective. Note the *Leishmania* organisms within macrophages (arrows).

of red blood cell in diameter, and mature, clumped chromatin with inapparent nucleoli (Figure 5.74). Hematopoietic cells may be present in normal or decreased numbers, depending on the stage of disease.

5.4.14.2 Clinical Considerations
- Dogs > cats.
- Affects middle-aged to older patients.

- Accompanied by lymphocytosis (range in dogs = 15 000–1 600 000 cells μl^{-1}; median value in cats = 34 200 cells μl^{-1}) [44, 71].

5.4.14.3 Prognosis
Generally good, with long survival times reported. Young age and the presence of anemia may confer a poorer prognosis in dogs [138].

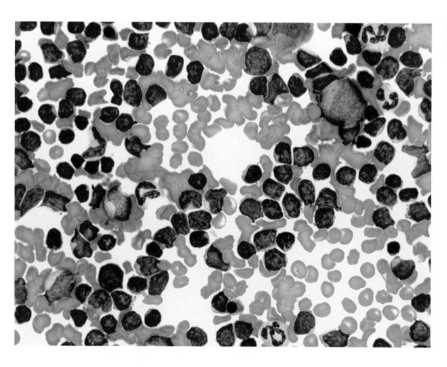

Figure 5.74 Bone marrow, chronic lymphocytic leukemia (CLL), dog, 50× objective.

5.4.15 Multiple Myeloma

5.4.15.1 Cytologic Features

Multiple myeloma is characterized by a neoplastic expansion of well-differentiated plasma cells that are seen in large sheets and aggregates. The cells have a moderate volume of pale-blue cytoplasm and often have a characteristic, perinuclear clear zone (Golgi zone) (Figure 5.75). The nuclei are round, eccentrically placed, and have clumped chromatin. Normal bone marrow elements may be replaced by neoplastic cells.

5.4.15.2 Clinical Considerations

- Dogs > cats.
- Other clinical features = monoclonal gammopathy, lytic bone lesions, anemia, bleeding diatheses, and Bence-Jones proteinuria [72, 73].

5.4.15.3 Prognosis

Dogs = good short-term prognosis with treatment, and long-term control is possible. Negative prognostic factors include extensive bone lysis/involvement as well as hypercalcemia and Bence-Jones proteinuria [72].

Cats = guarded prognosis, with generally short survival times [73, 74].

5.4.16 Metastatic Disease

5.4.16.1 Cytologic Appearance

Metastatic disease is characterized by a population of cells not normally present within the bone marrow. Carcinoma cells (Figures 5.76 and 5.77) and round cell neoplasms such as mast cell neoplasia (Figure 5.78) may be seen.

5.4.16.2 Clinical Considerations

- Rare in dogs and cats, though true incidence unknown [139].
- Epithelial tumors most common [140].
- Mast cells are seen in extremely low numbers in normal bone marrow [47].

5.4.16.3 Prognosis

Poor to grave.

5.4.17 Marrow Hypoplasia/Aplasia

5.4.17.1 Cytologic Appearance

Hypocellular bone marrow is characterized by unit particles with >75% lipid in adults (Figure 5.79). Hypoplasia may be due to one or more cell lines being decreased. Aplasia is seen when all cell lines are decreased.

5.4.17.2 Clinical Considerations

- DDx = drug/toxin exposure (e.g., estrogen, phenylbutazone, phenobarbital), infectious agents (e.g., parvovirus, FeLV), and myelofibrosis [141, 142].

5.4.17.3 Prognosis

Variable, based on the underlying cause and ability for reversal.

Figure 5.75 Bone marrow, multiple myeloma, dog, 50× objective.

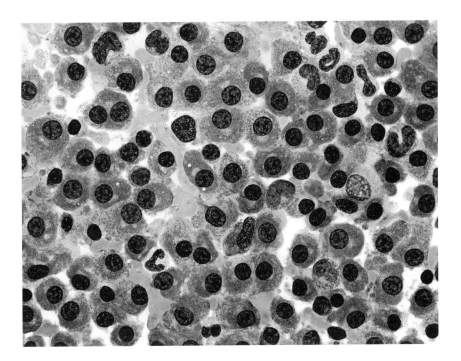

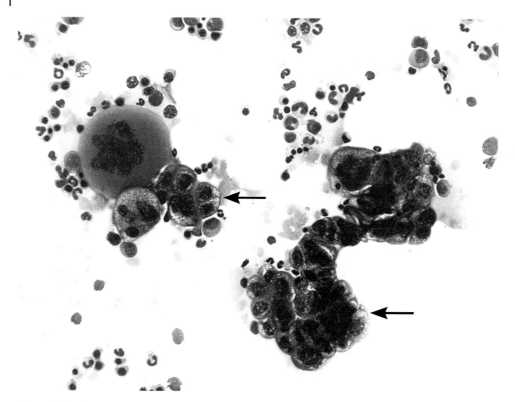

Figure 5.76 Bone marrow, metastatic carcinoma (prostatic), dog, 20× objective. Note the sheets of cohesive neoplastic cells (arrows).

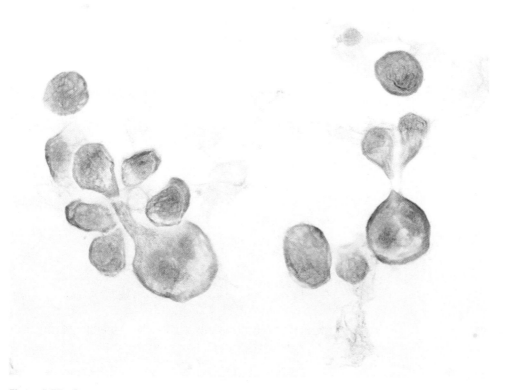

Figure 5.77 Bone marrow, metastatic carcinoma (prostatic), dog, 50× objective. Same case as Figure 5.74 stained with immunocytochemical stain PanCK, with positive stain confirming epithelial origin.

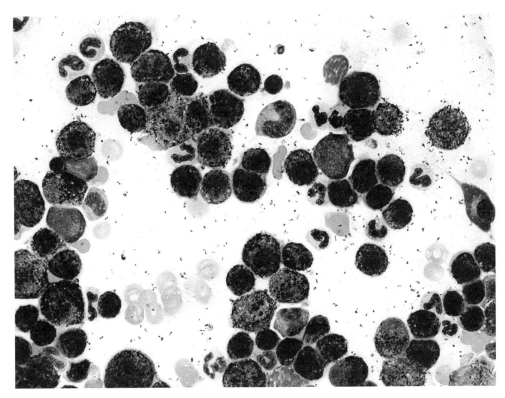

Figure 5.78   Bone marrow, metastatic mast cell neoplasia, dog, 50× objective.

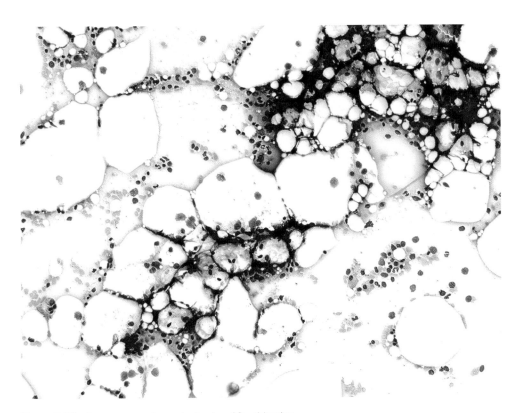

Figure 5.79   Bone marrow, hypoplasia, dog, 10× objective.

References

1 White, S.D., Rosychuk, R.A., Stewart, L.J., *et al.* (1989) Juvenile cellulitis in dogs: 15 cases (1979–1988). *J. Am. Vet. Med. Assoc.*, **195** (11), 1609–1611.

2 Ribas Latre, A., McPartland, A., Cain, D., *et al.* (2019) Canine sterile steroid-responsive lymphadenitis in 49 dogs. *J. Small Anim. Pract.*, **60** (5), 280–290.

3 Wong, S.W., Fernandez, N.J., Cosford, K., *et al.* (2022) What is your diagnosis? Septic peritonitis, lymphadenitis, and lymph node abscesses in a dog. *Vet. Clin. Pathol.*, **51** (2), 276–278.

4 James, F.E., Mansfield, C.S. (2009) Clinical remission of idiopathic hypereosinophilic syndrome in a Rottweiler. *Aust. Vet. J.*, **87** (8), 330–333.

5 Wu, C.Y., Ramos, S.J., Watanabe, T.T.N., *et al.* (2022) Pathology in practice. *J. Am. Vet. Med. Assoc.*, **259** (S2), 1–4.

6 Krick, E.L., Billings, A.P., Shofer, A.S., *et al.* (2009) Cytological lymph node evaluation in dogs with mast cell tumours: association with grade and survival. *Vet. Comp. Oncol.*, **7** (2), 130–138.

7 Costa, S.F., Trivellato, G.F., Rebech, G.T., *et al.* (2018) Eosinophilic inflammation in lymph nodes of dogs with visceral leishmaniasis. *Parasite Immunol.*, **40** (8), e12567. doi: 10.1111/pim.12567. Last accessed October 15, 2023.

8 Sykes, J.E., Marks, S.L., Mapes, S., *et al.* (2010) Salmon poisoning disease in dogs: 29 cases. *J. Vet. Intern. Med.*, **24** (3), 504–513.

9 Headley, S.A., Kano, F.S., Scorpio, D.G., *et al.* (2009) *Neorickettsia helminthoeca* in Brazilian dogs: a cytopathological, histopathological and immunohistochemical study. *Clin. Microbiol. Infect.*, **15**, 21–23.

10 Furtado, A.P., Cohen, H., Handa, A., *et al.* (2022) Salmon poisoning disease in dogs: clinical presentation, diagnosis and treatment. *Br. J. Vet. Med.*, **44**, e004822. doi: 10.29374/2527-2179.bjvm004822. Last accessed October 15, 2023.

11 Johns, J.L. (2011) Salmon poisoning in dogs: a satisfying diagnosis. *Vet. J.*, **187** (2), 149–150.

12 Valli, V.E., San Myint, M., Barthel, A., *et al.* (2011) Classification of canine malignant lymphomas according to the World Health Organization criteria. *Vet. Pathol.*, **48** (1), 198–211.

13 Seelig, D.M., Avery, A.C., Ehrhart, E.J., *et al.* (2016) The comparative diagnostic features of canine and human lymphoma. *Vet. Sci.*, **3** (2), 11. doi: 10.3390/vetsci3020011. Last accessed October 15, 2023.

14 Vezzali, E., Parodi, A.L., Marcato, P.S., *et al.* (2010) Histopathologic classification of 171 cases of canine and feline non-Hodgkin lymphoma according to the WHO. *Vet. Comp. Oncol.*, **8** (1), 38–49.

15 Merlo, D.F., Rossi, L., Pellegrino, C., *et al.* (2008) Cancer incidence in pet dogs: findings of the Animal Tumor Registry of Genoa, Italy. *J. Vet. Intern. Med.*, **22** (4), 976–984.

16 Edwards, D.S., Henley, W.E., Harding, E.F., *et al.* (2003) Breed incidence of lymphoma in a UK population of insured dogs. *Vet. Comp. Oncol.*, **1** (4), 200–206.

17 Dobson, J.M. Breed-predispositions to cancer in pedigree dogs. *ISRN Vet. Sci.*, **2013**, 941275. doi: 10.1155/2013/941275. Last accessed January 2, 2017.

18 Valli, V.E., Kass, P.H., San Myint, M., *et al.* (2013) Canine lymphomas: association of classification type, disease stage, tumor subtype, mitotic rate, and treatment with survival. *Vet. Pathol.*, **50** (5), 738–748.

19 Kiupel, M., Teske, E., Bostock, D. (1999) Prognostic factors for treated canine malignant lymphoma. *Vet. Pathol.*, **36** (4), 292–300.

20 Purzycka, K., Peters, L.M., Desmas, I., *et al.* (2020) Clinicopathological characteristics and prognostic factors for canine multicentric, non-indolent T-cell lymphoma: 107 cases. *Vet. Comp. Oncol.*, **18** (4), 656–663.

21 Vail, D.M., Moore, A.S., Ogilvie, G.K., *et al.* (1998) Feline lymphoma (145 cases): proliferation indices, cluster of differentiation 3 immunoreactivity, and their association with prognosis in 90 cats. *J. Vet. Intern. Med.*, **12** (5), 349–354.

22 Louwerens, M., London, C.A., Pedersen, N.C., *et al.* (2005) Feline lymphoma in the post-feline leukemia virus era. *J. Vet. Intern. Med.*, **19** (3), 329–335.

23 Schmidt, J.M., North, S.M., Freeman, K.P., *et al.* (2010) Feline paediatric oncology: retrospective assessment of 233 tumours from cats up to one year (1993 to 2008). *J. Small Anim. Pract.*, **51** (6), 306–311.

24 Wolfesberger, B., Skor, O., Hammer, S.E., *et al.* (2017) Does categorisation of lymphoma subtypes according to the World Health Organization classification predict clinical outcome in cats? *J. Feline Med. Surg.*, **19** (8), 897–906.

25 MacEwen, E.G., Patnaik, A.K., Wilkins, R.J. (1977) Diagnosis and treatment of canine hematopoietic neoplasms. *Vet. Clin. North Am.*, **7** (1), 105–118.

26 Rassnick, K.M., Bailey, D.B., Kamstock, D.A., *et al.* (2021) Survival times for dogs with previously untreated, peripheral nodal, intermediate- or large-cell lymphoma treated with prednisone alone: the canine lymphoma steroid only trial. *J. Am. Vet. Med. Assoc.*, **259** (1), 62–71.

27 Brick, J.O., Roenigk, W.J., Wilson, G.P. (1968) Chemotherapy of malignant lymphoma in dogs and cats. *J. Am. Vet. Med. Assoc.*, **153** (1), 47–52.

28 Rassnick, K.M., McEntee, M.C., Erb, H.N., *et al.* (2007) Comparison of 3 protocols for treatment after induction of remission in dogs with lymphoma. *J. Vet. Intern. Med.* **21**, 1364–1373.

29 Mizutani, N., Goto-Koshino, Y., Takahashi, M., *et al.* (2016) Clinical and histopathological evaluation of 16 dogs with T-zone lymphoma. *J. Vet. Med. Sci.*, **78** (8), 1237–1244.

30 Flood-Knapik, K.E., Durham, A.C., Gregor, T.P., *et al.* (2013) Clinical, histopathological and immunohistochemical characterization of canine indolent lymphoma. *Vet. Comp. Oncol.*, **11** (4), 272–286.

31 Hughes, K.L., Ehrhart, E.J., Rout, E.D., *et al.* (2021) Diffuse small B-cell lymphoma: a high grade malignancy. *Vet. Pathol.*, **58** (5), 912–922.

32 Seelig, D.M., Avery, P., Webb, T., *et al.* (2014) Canine T-zone lymphoma: unique immunophenotypic features, outcome, and population characteristics. *J. Vet. Intern. Med.*, **28** (3), 878–886.

33 Williams, M.J., Avery, A.C., Lana, S.E., *et al.* (2008) Canine lymphoproliferative disease characterized by lymphocytosis: immunophenotypic markers of prognosis. *J. Vet. Intern. Med.*, **22** (3), 596–601.

34 Moore, E.L., Vernau, W., Rebhun, R.B., *et al.* (2018) Patient characteristics, prognostic factors and outcome of dogs with high-grade primary mediastinal lymphoma. *Vet. Comp. Oncol.*, **16** (1), E45–E51.

35 Lurie, D.M., Milner, R.J., Suter, S.E., *et al.* (2008) Immunophenotypic and cytomorphologic subclassification of T-cell lymphoma in the boxer breed. *Vet. Immunol. Immunopathol.*, **125** (1–2), 102–110.

36 Ohmi, A., Tanaka, M., Rinno, J., *et al.* (2023) Clinical characteristics and outcomes of Mott cell lymphoma in nine miniature Dachshunds. *Vet. Med. Sci.*, **9** (2), 609–617.

37 Rimpo, K., Hirabayashi, M., Tanaka, A. (2022) Lymphoma in Miniature Dachshunds: a retrospective multicenter study of 108 cases (2006-2018) in Japan. *J. Vet. Intern. Med.*, **36** (4), 1390–1397.

38 Kol, A., Christopher, M.M., Skorupski, K.A., *et al.* (2013) B-cell lymphoma with plasmacytoid differentiation, atypical cytoplasmic inclusions, and secondary leukemia in a dog. *Vet. Clin. Pathol.*, **42** (1), 40–46.

39 Stacy, N.I., Nabity, M.B., Hackendahl, N., *et al.* (2009) B-cell lymphoma with Mott cell differentiation in two young adult dogs. *Vet. Clin. Pathol.*, **38** (1), 113–120.

40 Seelig, D.M., Perry, J.A., Zaks, K., *et al.* (2011) Monoclonal immunoglobulin protein production in two dogs with secretory B-cell lymphoma with Mott cell differentiation. *J. Am. Vet. Med. Assoc.*, **239** (11), 1477–1482.

41 Walton, R.M., Hendrick, M.J. (2001) Feline Hodgkin's-like lymphoma: 20 cases (1992–1999). *Vet. Pathol.*, **38** (5), 504–511.

42 Steinberg, J.D., Keating, J.H. (2008) What is your diagnosis? Cervical mass in a cat. *Vet. Clin. Pathol.*, **37** (3), 323–327.

43 Tasca, S., Carli, E., Caldin, M., *et al.* (2009) Hematologic abnormalities and flow cytometric immunophenotyping results in dogs with hematopoietic neoplasia: 210 cases (2002-2006). *Vet. Clin. Pathol.*, **38** (1), 2–12.

44 Vernau, W., Moore, P.F. (1999) An immunophenotypic study of canine leukemias and preliminary assessment of clonality by polymerase chain reaction. *Vet. Immunol. Immunopathol.*, **69** (2–4), 145–164.

45 Fournier, Q., Cazzini, P., Bavcar, S., *et al.* (2018) Investigation of the utility of lymph node fine-needle aspiration cytology for the staging of malignant solid tumors in dogs. *Vet. Clin. Pathol.*, **47** (3), 489–500.

46 Ku, C.K., Kass, P.H., Christopher, M.M. (2017) Cytologic-histologic concordance in the diagnosis of neoplasia in canine and feline lymph nodes: a retrospective study of 367 cases. *Vet. Comp. Oncol.*, **15** (4), 1206–1217.

47 Bookbinder, P.F., Butt, M.T., Harvey, H.J. (1992) Determination of the number of mast cells in lymph node, bone marrow, and buffy coat cytologic specimens from dogs. *J. Am. Vet. Med. Assoc.*, **200** (11), 1648–1650.

48 Mutz, M.L., Boudreaux, B.B., Royal, A., *et al.* (2017) Cytologic comparison of the percentage of mast cells in lymph node aspirate samples from clinically normal dogs versus dogs with allergic dermatologic disease and dogs with cutaneous mast cell tumors. *J. Am. Vet. Med. Assoc.*, **251** (4), 421–428.

49 Williams, L.E., Packer, R.A. (2003) Association between lymph node size and metastasis in dogs with oral malignant melanoma: 100 cases (1987–2001). *J. Am. Vet. Med. Assoc.*, **222** (9), 1234–1236.

50 Sabattini, S., Lopparelli, R.M., Rigillo, A., *et al.* (2018) Canine splenic nodular lymphoid lesions: immunophenotyping, proliferative activity, and clonality assessment. *Vet. Pathol.*, **55** (5), 645–653.

51 Christopher, M.M. (2003) Cytology of the spleen. *Vet. Clin. North Am. Small Anim. Pract.*, **33** (1), 135–152.

52 Thomas, R.M., Fischetti, A.J. (2012) What is your diagnosis? Myelolipoma. *J. Am. Vet. Med. Assoc.*, **241** (7), 881–883.

53 Schwarz, L.A., Penninck, D.G., Gliatto, J. (2001) Canine splenic myelolipomas. *Vet. Radiol. Ultrasound*, **42** (4), 347–348.

54 Kamiie, J., Fueki, K., Amagi, H., *et al.* (2009) Multicentric myelolipoma in a dog. *J. Vet. Med. Sci.*, **71** (3), 371–373.

55 Barger, A.M., Skowronski, M.C., MacNeill, A.L. (2012) Cytologic identification of erythrophagocytic neoplasms in dogs. *Vet. Clin. Pathol.*, **41** (4), 587–589.

56 Griffin, M.A., Culp, W.T.N., Rebhun, R.B. (2021) Canine and feline haemangiosarcoma. *Vet. Rec.*, **189** (9), 585.

57 Johannes, C.M., Henry, C.J., Turnquist, S.E., *et al.* (2007) Hemangiosarcoma in cats: 53 cases (1992-2002). *J. Am. Vet. Med. Assoc.*, **231** (12), 1851–1856.

58 Schick, A.R., Grimes, J.A. (2022) Evaluation of the validity of the double two-thirds rule for diagnosing hemangiosarcoma in dogs with nontraumatic hemoperitoneum due to a ruptured splenic mass: a systematic review. *J. Am. Vet. Med. Assoc.*, **261** (1), 69–73.

59 Wendelburg, K.M., Price, L.L., Burgess, K.E., *et al.* (2015) Survival time of dogs with splenic hemangiosarcoma treated by splenectomy with or without adjuvant chemotherapy: 208 cases (2001–2012). *J. Am. Vet. Med. Assoc.*, **247** (4), 393–403.

60 Clifford, C.A., Mackin, A.J., Henry, C.J. (2000) Treatment of canine hemangiosarcoma: 2000 and beyond. *J. Vet. Intern. Med.*, **14** (5), 479–485.

61 Agnoli, C., Sabattini, S., Ubiali, A., *et al.* (2023) A retrospective study on bone metastasis in dogs with advanced-stage solid cancer. *J. Small Anim. Pract.*, **64** (9), 561–567.

62 Faroni, E., Sabattini, S., Guerra, D., *et al.* (2023) Timely adjuvant chemotherapy improves outcome in dogs with non-metastatic splenic hemangiosarcoma undergoing splenectomy. *Vet. Comp. Oncol.*, **21** (1), 123–130.

63 Quinci, M., Sabattini, S., Agnoli, C., *et al.* (2020) Ultrasonographic honeycomb pattern of the spleen in cats: correlation with pathological diagnosis in 33 cases. *J. Feline Med. Surg.*, **22** (8), 800–804.

64 van Stee, L.L., Boston, S.E., Singh, A., *et al.* (2015) Outcome and prognostic factors for canine splenic lymphoma treated by splenectomy (1995–2011). *Vet. Surg.*, **44** (8), 976–982.

65 Stein, L., Bacmeister, C., Ylaya, K., *et al.* (2019) Immunophenotypic characterization of canine splenic follicular-derived B-cell lymphoma. *Vet. Pathol.*, **56** (3), 350–357.

66 O'Brien, D., Moore, P.F., Vernau, W., *et al.* (2013) Clinical characteristics and outcome in dogs with splenic marginal zone lymphoma. *J. Vet. Intern. Med.*, **27** (4), 949–954.

67 Stefanello, D., Valenti, P., Zini, E., *et al.* (2011) Splenic marginal zone lymphoma in 5 dogs (2001-2008). *J. Vet. Intern. Med.*, **25** (1), 90–93.

68 Keller, S.M., Vernau, W., Hodges, J., *et al.* (2013) Hepatosplenic and hepatocytotropic T-cell lymphoma: two distinct types of T-cell lymphoma in dogs. *Vet. Pathol.*, **50** (2), 281–290.

69 Fry, M.M., Vernau, W., Pesavento, P.A., *et al.* (2003) Hepatosplenic lymphoma in a dog. *Vet. Pathol.*, **40** (5), 556–562.

70 Deravi, N., Berke, O., Woods, J.P., *et al.* (2017) Specific immunotypes of canine T cell lymphoma are associated with different outcomes. *Vet. Immunol. Immunopathol.*, **191**, 5–13.

71 Campbell, M.W., Hess, P.R., Williams, L.E. (2013) Chronic lymphocytic leukaemia in the cat: 18 cases (2000–2010). *Vet. Comp. Oncol.*, **11** (4), 256–264.

72 Matus, R.E., Leifer, C.E., MacEwen, E.G., *et al.* (1986) Prognostic factors for multiple myeloma in the dog. *J. Am. Vet. Med. Assoc.*, **188** (11), 1288–1292.

73 Patel, R.T., Caceres, A., French, A.F., *et al.* (2005) Multiple myeloma in 16 cats: a retrospective study. *Vet. Clin. Pathol.*, **34** (4), 341–352.

74 Hanna, F. (2005) Multiple myelomas in cats. *J. Feline Med. Surg.*, **7** (5), 275–287.

75 Affolter, V.K., Moore, P.F. (2002) Localized and disseminated histiocytic sarcoma of dendritic cell origin in dogs. *Vet. Pathol.*, **39** (1), 74–83.

76 Moore, P.F. (2023) Histiocytic diseases. *Vet. Clin. North Am. Small Anim. Pract.*, **53** (1), 121–140.

77 Latifi, M., Tuohy, J.L., Coutermarsh-Ott, S.L., *et al.* (2020) Clinical outcomes in dogs with localized splenic histiocytic sarcoma treated with splenectomy with or without adjuvant chemotherapy. *J. Vet. Intern. Med.*, **34** (6), 2645–2650.

78 Moore, P.F., Affolter, V.K., Vernau, W. (2006) Canine hemophagocytic histiocytic sarcoma: a proliferative disorder of CD11d+ macrophages. *Vet. Pathol.*, **43** (5), 632–645.

79 Elliott, J. (2018) Lomustine chemotherapy for the treatment of presumptive haemophagocytic histiocytic sarcoma in Flat-coated Retrievers. *Aust. Vet. J.*, **96** (12), 502–507.

80 Spangler, W.L., Culbertson, M.R. (1992) Prevalence and type of splenic diseases in cats: 455 cases (1985–1991). *J. Am. Vet. Med. Assoc.*, **201** (5), 773–776.

81 Piviani, M., Walton, R.M., Patel, R.T. (2013) Significance of mastocytemia in cats. *Vet. Clin. Pathol.*, **42** (1), 4–10.

82 Evans, B.J., O'Brien, D., Allstadt, S.D., *et al.* (2018) Treatment outcomes and prognostic factors of feline splenic mast cell tumours: a multi-institutional retrospective study of 64 cases. *Vet. Comp. Oncol.*, **16** (1), 20–27.

83 Sabattini, S., Barzon, G., Giantin, M., *et al.* (2016) Kit receptor tyrosine kinase dysregulations in feline splenic mast cell tumours. *Vet. Comp. Oncol.* 2016; doi: 10.1111/vco.12246. Epub ahead of print. Last accessed May 1, 2017.

84 Gordon, S.S., McClaran, J.K., Bergman, P.J., *et al.* (2010) Outcome following splenectomy in cats. *J. Feline Med. Surg.*, **12** (4), 256–261.

85 Liska, W.D., MacEwen, E.G., Zaki, F.A., *et al.* (1979) Feline systemic mastocytosis: a review and results of splenectomy in 7 cases. *J. Am. Anim. Hosp. Assoc.*, **15** (5), 589–597.

86 Kraus, K.A., Clifford, C.A., Davis, G.J., *et al.* (2015) Outcome and prognostic indicators in cats undergoing splenectomy for splenic mast cell tumors. *J. Am. Anim. Hosp. Assoc.*, **51** (4), 231–238.

87 Rossi, F., Aresu, L., Vignoli, M., *et al.* (2015) Metastatic cancer of unknown primary in 21 dogs. *Vet. Comp. Oncol.*, **13** (1), 11–19.

88 Stefanello, D., Valenti, P., Faverzani, S., *et al.* (2009) Ultrasound-guided cytology of spleen and liver: a prognostic tool in canine cutaneous mast cell tumor. *J. Vet. Intern. Med.*, **23** (5), 1051–1057.

89 Flatland, B., Moore, R.R., Wolf, C.M., *et al.* (2007) Liver aspirate from a Shar Pei dog. *Vet. Clin. Pathol.*, **36** (1), 105–108.

90 DiBartola, S.P., Tarr, M.J., Benson, M.D. (1986) Tissue distribution of amyloid deposits in Abyssinian cats with familial amyloidosis. *J. Comp. Pathol.*, **96** (4), 387–398.

91 Strandberg, N.J., Tang, K.M., dos Santos, A.P. (2023) Hemophagocytic syndrome in a cat with *Mycoplasma haemofelis* infection. *Vet. Clin. Pathol.*, **52** (2), 320–323.

92 Tagawa, M., Aoki, M., Uemura, A., *et al.* (2023) Hemophagocytic syndrome in a cat with immune-mediated hemolytic anemia. *Vet. Clin. Pathol.*, **52** (2), 313–319.

93 Schaefer, D.M.W., Rizzi, T.E., Royal, A.B. (2019) Hemophagocytosis and histoplasma-like fungal infection in 32 cats. *Vet. Clin. Pathol.*, **48** (2), 250–254.

94 Dunbar, M.D., Lyles, S. (2013) Hemophagocytic syndrome in a cat with multiple myeloma. *Vet. Clin. Pathol.*, **42** (1), 55–60.

95 Day, M.J. (1997) Review of thymic pathology in 30 cats and 36 dogs. *J. Small Anim. Pract.*, **38** (9), 393–403.

96 Lara-Garcia, A., Wellman, M., Burkhard, M.J., *et al.* (2008) Cervical thymoma originating in ectopic thymic tissue in a cat. *Vet. Clin. Pathol.*, **37** (4), 397–402.

97 Robat, C.S., Cesario, L., Gaeta, R., *et al.* (2013) Clinical features, treatment options, and outcome in dogs with thymoma: 116 cases (1999–2010). *J. Am. Vet. Med. Assoc.*, **243** (10), 1448–1454.

98 Hague, D.W., Humphries, H.D., Mitchell, M.A., *et al.* (2015) Risk factors and outcomes in cats with acquired myasthenia gravis (2001-2012). *J. Vet. Intern. Med.*, **29** (5), 1307–1312.

99 Burton, A.G., Borjesson, D.L., Vernau, W. (2014) Thymoma-associated lymphocytosis in a dog. *Vet. Clin. Pathol.*, **43** (4), 584–588.

100 Zitz, J.C., Birchard, S.J., Couto, G.C., *et al.* (2008) Results of excision of thymoma in cats and dogs: 20 cases (1984–2005). *J. Am. Vet. Med. Assoc.*, **232** (8), 1186–1192.

101 Yale, A.D., Priestnall, S.L., Pittaway, R., *et al.* (2022) Thymic epithelial tumours in 51 dogs: Histopathologic and clinicopathologic findings. *Vet. Comp. Oncol.*, **20** (1), 50–58.

102 Martano, M., Buracco, P., Morello, E.M. (2021) Canine epithelial thymic tumors: outcome in 28 dogs treated by surgery. *Animals (Basel)*, **11** (12), 3444.

103 Burgess, K.E., DeRegis, C.J., Brown, F.S., *et al.* (2016) Histologic and immunohistochemical characterization of thymic epithelial tumours in the dog. *Vet. Comp. Oncol.*, **14** (2), 113–121.

104 Bellah, J.R., Stiff, M.E., Russell, R.G. (1983) Thymoma in the dog: two case reports and review of 20 additional cases. *J. Am. Vet. Med. Assoc.*, **183** (3), 306–311.

105 Ruslander, D.A., Gebhard, D.H., Tompkins, M.B., *et al.* (1997) Immunophenotypic characterization of canine lymphoproliferative disorders. *In Vivo*, **11** (2), 169–172.

106 Rosenberg, M.P., Matus, R.E., Patnaik, A.K. (1991) Prognostic factors in dogs with lymphoma and associated hypercalcemia. *J. Vet. Intern. Med.*, **5** (5), 268–271.

107 Liu, S., Patnaik, A.K., Burk, R.L. (1983) Thymic branchial cysts in the dog and cat. *J. Am. Vet. Med. Assoc.*, **182** (10), 1095–1098.

108 Levien, A.S., Summers, B.A., Szladovits, B., *et al.* (2010) Transformation of a thymic branchial cyst to a carcinoma with pulmonary metastasis in a dog. *J. Small Anim. Pract.*, **51** (11), 604–608.

109 Sano, Y., Seki, K., Miyoshi, K., *et al.* (2021) Mediastinal basloid carcinoma arising from thymic cysts in two dogs. *J. Vet. Med. Sci.*, **83** (5), 876–880.

110 Mischke, R., Busse, L. (2002) Reference values for the bone marrow aspirates in adult dogs. *J. Vet. Med. A Physiol. Pathol. Clin. Med.*, **49** (10), 499–502.

111 Weiss, D.J. (2005) Differentiating benign and malignant causes of lymphocytosis in feline bone marrow. *J. Vet. Intern. Med.*, **19** (6), 855–859.

112 Pawsat, G.A., Fry, M.M., Behling-Kelly, E., *et al.* (2023) Bone marrow iron scoring in healthy and clinically ill dogs with and without evidence of iron-restricted erythropoiesis. *Vet. Clin. Pathol.*, **52** (2), 243–251.

113 Jain, N.C., Blue, J.T., Grindem, C.B., *et al.* (1991) Proposed criteria for classification of acute myeloid leukemia in dogs and cats. *Vet. Clin. Pathol.*, **20** (3), 63–82.

114 Bounous, D.I., Latimer, K.S., Campagnoli, R.P., *et al.* (1994) Acute myeloid leukemia with basophilic differentiation (AML, M-2B) in a cat. *Vet. Clin. Pathol.*, **23** (1), 15–18.

115 Juopperi, T.A., Bienzle, D., Bernreuter, D.C., *et al.* (2011) Prognostic markers for myeloid neoplasms: a comparative review of the literature and goals for future investigation. *Vet. Pathol.*, **48** (1), 182–197.

116 Davis, L.L., Hume, K.R., Stokol, T. (2018) A retrospective review of acute myeloid leukaemia in 35 dogs diagnosed by a combination of morphologic findings, flow cytometric immunophenotyping and cytochemical staining results (2007-2015). *Vet. Comp. Oncol.*, **18** (2), 268–275.

117 Tomiyasu, H., Fujino, Y., Takahashi, M., *et al.* (2011) Spontaneous acute erythroblastic leukaemia (AMLM6Er) in a dog. *J. Small Anim. Pract.*, **52** (8), 445–447.

118 Rolph, K.E., Cavanaugh, R.P. (2022) Infectious causes of neoplasia in the domestic cat. *Vet. Sci.*, **9** (9), 467.

119 Comazzi, S., Paltrinieri, S., Caniatti, M., *et al.* (2000) Erythremic myelosis (AML6er) in a cat. *J. Feline Med. Surg.*, **2** (4), 213–215.

120 Park, D.S., Lee, J., Song, K.H., *et al.* (2022) Treatment of acute erythroleukemia with high dose cytarabine in a cat with feline leukemia virus infection. *Vet. Med. Sci.*, **8** (1), 9–13.

121 Bolon, B., Buergelt, C.D., Harvey, J.W., *et al.* (1989) Megakaryoblastic leukemia in a dog. *Vet. Clin. Pathol.*, **18** (3), 69–74.

122 Cain, G.R., Feldman, B.F., Kawakami, T.G., *et al.* (1986) Platelet dysplasia associated with megakaryoblastic leukemia in a dog. *J. Am. Vet. Med. Assoc.*, **188** (5), 529–530.

123 Comazzi, S., Gelain, M.E., Bonfanti, U., *et al.* (2010) Acute megakaryoblastic leukemia in dogs: a report of three cases and review of the literature. *J. Am. Anim. Hosp. Assoc.*, **46** (5), 327–335.

124 Rochel, D., Abadie, J., Robveille, C., *et al.* (2018) Thrombocytosis and central nervous system involvement in a case of canine acute megakaryoblastic leukemia. *Vet. Clin. Pathol.*, **47** (3), 363–367.

125 Willmann, M., Müllauer, L., Schwendenwein, I., *et al.* (2009) Chemotherapy in canine acute megakaryoblastic leukemia: a case report and review of the literature. *In Vivo*, **23** (6), 911–918.

126 Tomiyasu, H., Doi, A., Chambers, J.K., *et al.* (2018) Clinical and clinicopathological characteristics of acute lymphoblastic leukemia in six cats. *J. Small Anim. Pract.*, **59** (12), 742–746.

127 Essex, M.E. (1982) Feline leukemia: a naturally occurring cancer of infectious origin. *Epidemiol. Rev.*, **4**, 189–203.

128 Matus, R.E., Leifer, C.E., MacEwen, E.G. (1983) Acute lymphoblastic leukemia in the dog: a review of 30 cases. *J. Am. Vet. Med. Assoc.*, **183** (8), 859–862.

129 Graff, E.C., Spangler, E.A., Smith, A., *et al.* (2014) Hematologic findings predictive of bone marrow disease in dogs with multicentric large-cell lymphoma. *Vet. Clin. Pathol.*, **43** (4), 505–512.

130 Marconato, L., Martini, V., Aresu, L., *et al.* (2013) Assessment of bone marrow infiltration diagnosed by flow cytometry in canine large B cell lymphoma: prognostic significance and proposal of a cut-off value. *Vet. J.*, **197** (3), 776–781.

131 Deubelbeiss, K.A., Dancey, J.T., Harker, L.A., *et al.* (1975) Neutrophil kinetics in the dog. *J. Clin. Invest.*, **55** (4), 833–839.

132 Smith, J.E., Agar, N.S. (1975) The effect of phlebotomy on canine erythrocyte metabolism. *Res. Vet. Sci.*, **18** (3), 231–236.

133 Grimes, C.N., Fry, M.M. (2015) Nonregenerative anemia: mechanisms of decreased or ineffective erythropoiesis. *Vet. Pathol.*, **52** (2), 298–311.

134 Assenmacher, T.D., Jutkowitz, L.A., Koenigshof, A.M., *et al.* (2019) Clinical features of precursor-targeted immune-mediated anemia in dogs: 66 cases (2004-2013). *J. Am. Vet. Med. Assoc.*, **255** (3), 366–376.

135 Walton, R.M., Modiano, J.F., Thrall, M.A., *et al.* (1996) Bone marrow cytological findings in 4 dogs and a cat with hemophagocytic syndrome. *J. Vet. Intern. Med.*, **10** (1), 7–14.

136 Fonseca, J., Silveira, J., Faísca, P., *et al.* (2023) Presumptive hemophagocytic syndrome associated with coinfections with FIV, *Toxoplasma gondii*, and Canditus mycoplasma haemominutum in an adult cat. *Vet. Clin. Pathol.*, **52** (2), 324–333.

137 Leifer, C.E., Matus, R.E. (1986) Chronic lymphocytic leukemia in the dog: 22 cases (1974–1984). *J. Am. Vet. Med. Assoc.*, **189** (2), 214–217.

138 Comazzi, S., Gelain, M.E., Martini, V., *et al.* (2011) Immunophenotype predicts survival time in dogs with chronic lymphocytic leukemia. *J. Vet. Intern. Med.*, **25** (1), 100–106.

139 Turinelli, V., Gavazza, A., Stock, G., *et al.* (2015) Canine bone marrow cytological examination, classification and reference values: a retrospective study of 295 cases. *Res. Vet. Sci.*, **103**, 224–230.

140 Taylor, B.E., Leibman, N.F., Luong, R., *et al.* (2013) Detection of carcinoma micrometastases in bone marrow of dogs and cats using conventional and cell block cytology. *Vet. Clin. Pathol.*, **42** (1), 85–91.

141 Withers, S.S., Lawson, C.M., Burton, A.G., *et al.* (2016) Management of an invasive and metastatic Sertoli cell tumor with associated myelotoxicosis in a dog. *Can. Vet. J.*, **57** (3), 299–304.

142 Scott, T.N., Bailin, H.G., Jutkowitz, L.A., *et al.* (2021). Bone marrow, blood, and clinical findings in dogs treated with phenobarbital. *Vet. Clin. Pathol.*, **50** (1), 122–131.

6

Body Cavity Fluids

6.1 General Classification

Body cavity fluids often are classified broadly as transudates (low and high protein), and exudates based on cell concentration and protein concentration. While these categories can be clinically helpful, they do not always accurately reflect the underlying pathophysiology of the effusion and should be considered as guidelines only, and interpreted with other clinical and diagnostic findings.

6.1.1 Low Protein Transudate

6.1.1.1 Cytologic Appearance
Low protein transudates have a clear background and usually contain only rare erythrocytes. Nucleated cells are seen in very low numbers and comprise mostly variably reactive macrophages (Figure 6.1). Low numbers of small mature lymphocytes and nondegenerative neutrophils ± reactive mesothelial cells also may be seen.

6.1.1.2 Clinical Considerations
- Also known as *pure transudate*.
- Cell concentration typically <1500 cells μl^{-1}; protein concentration <2.5 $g\,dl^{-1}$ [1, 2].
- Classically associated with decreased oncotic pressure from hypoalbuminemia (<1.5 $g\,dl^{-1}$), though albumin concentrations may be higher [2].
- DDx = decreased production of albumin (liver failure), loss of protein (e.g., protein-losing nephropathy/enteropathy, and exudation), or decreased protein intake.
- Uroabdomen may appear similar with low protein, though neutrophils are typically increased, and further testing may be required for differentiation (see Section 6.2.5) [1].

6.1.1.3 Prognosis
Variable, based on the underlying cause.

6.1.2 High Protein Transudate

6.1.2.1 Cytologic Appearance
High protein transudates may have a pale-blue background due to the increased concentration of protein. Red blood cells usually are present in low numbers. Cells also are seen in low to moderate numbers and typically comprise a mixture of nondegenerative neutrophils and variably reactive macrophages. Reactive mesothelial cells may be present.

6.1.2.2 Clinical Considerations
- Also known as *modified transudate*.
- Cell concentration typically between 1500 and 5000 cells μl^{-1}; protein concentration typically between 2.5 and 3.5 $g\,dl^{-1}$ [1, 2].
- Neutrophil percentage of limited value to differentiate from exudates, as neutrophils often exceed 50% of the differential in transudates [1].
- Classically associated with increased intravascular hydrostatic pressure.
- DDx = cardiac disease, liver disease, space-occupying lesions (non-exfoliating neoplasia, granuloma, organ enlargement), or early inflammatory disease [3].

6.1.2.3 Prognosis
Variable, based on the underlying cause.

6.1.3 Exudate

Exudates form secondary to increased vessel permeability, most notably in response to inflammation, but may also be associated with vasculitis or anaphylaxis [3–5]. Consequently, these typically have elevated cell concentrations (5000+ cells μl^{-1}) and protein concentrations (>4.0 $g\,dl^{-1}$). Common etiologies leading to exudate formation are discussed in the following sections.

Clinical Atlas of Small Animal Cytology and Hematology, Second Edition. Andrew G. Burton.
© 2024 John Wiley & Sons, Inc. Published 2024 by John Wiley & Sons, Inc.

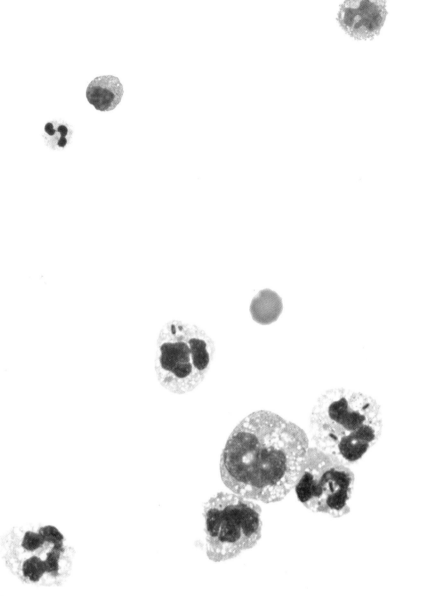

Figure 6.1 Low protein transudate, dog, 50× objective.

Figure 6.2 Septic exudate (bacterial peritonitis), dog, 100× objective. Note the degenerative neutrophils and intracellular bacterial rods.

6.1.4 Exudate: Septic

6.1.4.1 Cytologic Appearance

Septic effusions often are highly cellular with cell concentrations >5000 cells μl^{-1}, and often exceeding 100 000 cells μl^{-1}, especially in cats with pyothorax that have significantly higher cell concentrations than dogs [6]. Septic exudates also have an elevated total protein, typically >4.0 g dl^{-1}, but may be lower [1, 6]. They most commonly are associated with degenerative neutrophils (see Chapter 2). The presence of intracellular/phagocytosed organisms confirms sepsis, though some organisms may be present extracellularly. Bacteria are most common (Figure 6.2), but many fungal, protozoal, and parasitic agents (especially *Mesocestoides*) have been reported (see Chapter 3).

6.1.4.2 Clinical Considerations

- Reported in the abdomen (septic peritonitis), thorax (pyothorax), and pericardial sac (septic pericarditis).
- Septic peritonitis most commonly associated with gastrointestinal pathology/rupture in dogs and cats [7, 8].
- Pyothorax commonly associated with penetrating wounds (including trauma, bite wounds, and foreign body migration) but may also be associated with pulmonary parenchymal disease [6].

6.1.4.3 Confirmation

- Intracellular organisms confirm sepsis. Microbial culture and susceptibility testing or fungal culture and identification are recommended.
- When organisms are not seen but there is a clinical suspicion of bacterial sepsis, a blood-to-fluid glucose difference >20 $mg\,dl^{-1}$ was 100% specific for septic peritoneal effusion in dogs and cats, and 100% and 86% sensitive in dogs and cats, respectively [9]. False negative results have also been reported by other investigators [10].

6.1.4.4 Prognosis

Guarded. Septic effusions can be associated with high mortality rates [8] and are an independent risk factor for mortality in hospitalized dogs [11]. Cats tend to have a better prognosis for pyothorax than dogs [12, 13]. Septic shock confers a poor prognosis, though early antimicrobial therapy increases survival [14].

6.1.5 Exudate: Sterile (Neutrophilic)

6.1.5.1 Cytologic Appearance

Neutrophilic exudates may be caused by noninfectious etiologies. Neutrophils typically are nondegenerative or even pyknotic/apoptotic (see Chapter 2). Variable numbers of other inflammatory cells may be present, particularly if the inflammatory process is chronic (e.g., increased small mature lymphocytes).

6.1.5.2 Clinical Considerations

- Pancreatitis is a common cause of neutrophilic exudates in the abdomen of dogs and cats. Neutrophils may contain coarse clear vacuoles of lipids in their cytoplasm (Figure 6.3).
- Other differentials include inflammation of other viscera, vasculitis, or non-exfoliating neoplasia (inflammation or paraneoplastic).
- Microbial culture and susceptibility testing may be warranted to rule out incipient infectious disease.

6.1.5.3 Prognosis

Variable, based on the underlying cause.

6.1.6 Exudate: Sterile (Eosinophilic)

6.1.6.1 Cytologic Appearance

Eosinophilic exudates are characterized by an increased percentage of eosinophils, which frequently predominate (Figure 6.4). Other inflammatory cells are seen to varying

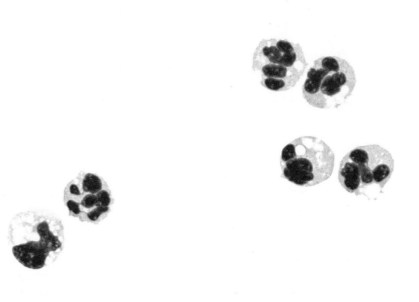

Figure 6.3 Sterile neutrophilic exudate from dog with pancreatitis, 100× objective. Note the clear lipid vacuoles within the cytoplasm.

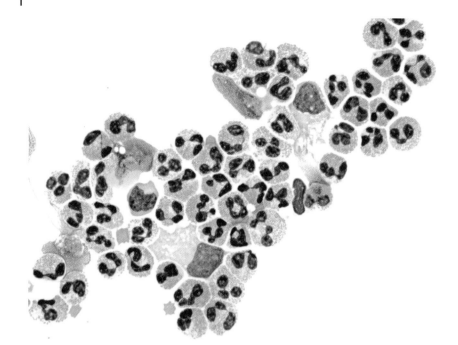

Figure 6.4 Eosinophilic exudate, cat, 50× objective.

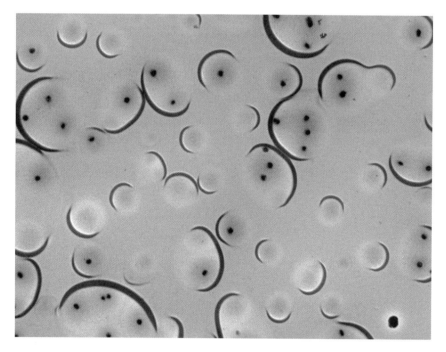

Figure 6.5 High protein exudate, cat, 10× objective. Note the thick, proteinaceous, and scalloped background with low numbers of red blood cells.

degrees, and neoplastic cells or infectious agents may be present, depending on the underlying etiology.

6.1.6.2 Clinical Considerations

- Reported in the pleural, abdominal, and pericardial spaces [15, 16].
- Neoplasia is the most common cause (e.g., mast cell neoplasia or lymphoma) [15].
- Other rule-outs include infectious organisms (parasitic disease and fungal disease) [17], allergic/hypersensitivity disease, and primary eosinophilic inflammatory disease.

6.1.6.3 Prognosis

Variable, based on the underlying cause.

6.1.7 Exudate: High Protein

6.1.7.1 Cytologic Appearance

Exudates with high protein concentrations ($>5\,g\,dl^{-1}$) often have a thick blue/purple, scalloped proteinaceous background (Figure 6.5). The cell concentrations and differentials in these fluids are variable.

6.1.7.2 Clinical Considerations

- Feline infectious peritonitis (FIP) is a common cause of high protein exudates, typically in young cats (aged <2 years) [18].
- In one study, 90% of cats with FIP had protein >5.0 g dl (range 3.0–7.8 g dl^{-1}) [18].
- Other rule-outs may include fulminant inflammation of viscera (e.g., pancreatitis), other causes of vasculitis (immune-mediated and neoplasia), and incipient infectious disease.

6.1.7.3 Prognosis

Variable, based on the underlying cause. The prognosis for FIP remains poor, though promising treatment options are being investigated [19, 20].

6.2 Specific Effusions

Many body cavity fluids have characteristic diagnostic and cytologic features, allowing a more specific diagnosis to be made.

6.2.1 Bile Peritonitis

6.2.1.1 Cytologic Features

Bile peritonitis is characterized by aggregates of yellow/green bile pigment that are seen both extracellularly and phagocytosed by macrophages or neutrophils (Figure 6.6). Bile peritonitis is frequently accompanied by a marked inflammatory response.

6.2.1.2 Clinical Considerations

- Dogs > cats.
- Mostly associated with trauma to the biliary tract or necrotizing cholecystitis.
- May be septic or sterile.
- Serum bilirubin concentration may be elevated but is often normal [21].
- Bilothorax is rare and is associated with bile peritonitis with or without an intact diaphragm [22, 23].

6.2.1.3 Confirmation

- Compare the concentration of bilirubin in serum and fluid collected at the same time: a bilirubin concentration twofold or more than that of serum is consistent with bile peritonitis [24].

6.2.1.4 Prognosis

Bile peritonitis is a surgical emergency. Prognosis is excellent for sterile effusions but poorer for septic bile peritonitis [24].

6.2.2 White Bile Peritonitis

6.2.2.1 Cytologic Features

White bile appears as amorphous pools of smooth, pale-blue material and can readily be differentiated from the yellow/green aggregates of classic bile peritonitis (compare Figures 6.7 and 6.6). The amount of white bile present is variable, and a close examination of inflammatory effusions is warranted.

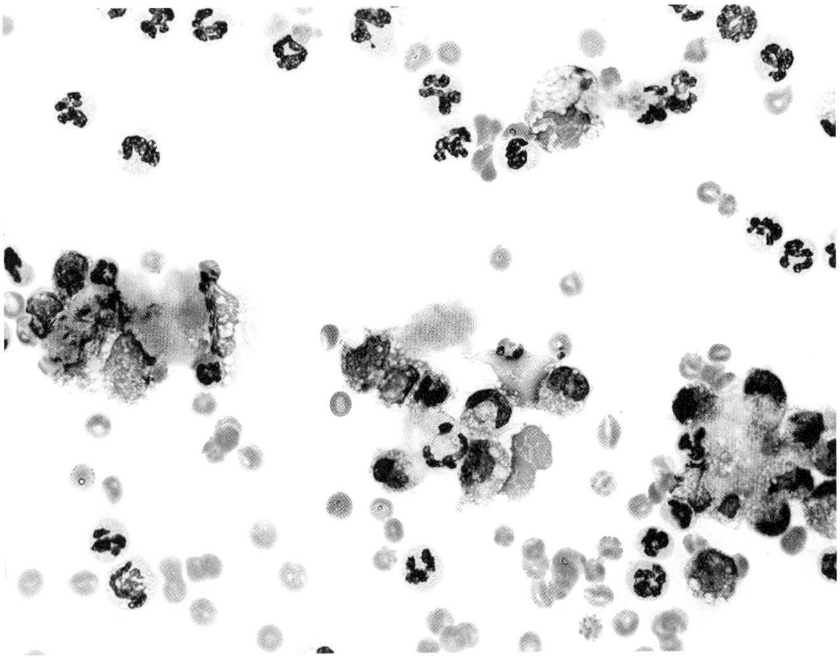

Figure 6.6 Bile peritonitis, dog, 50× objective. Note the aggregates of green/yellow bile.

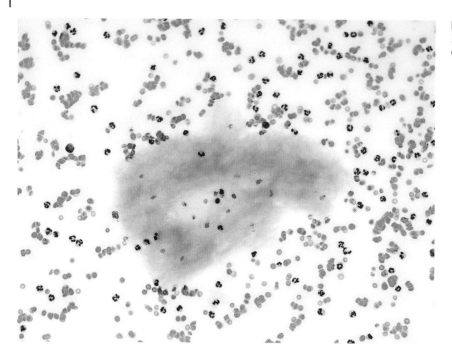

Figure 6.7 White bile peritonitis, dog, 20× objective. Note the large aggregates of smooth, pale-blue mucinous material.

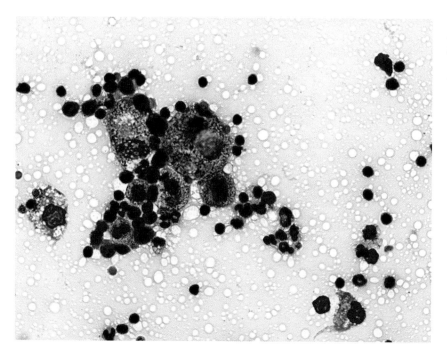

Figure 6.8 Chylous effusion, cat, 50× objective. Note the abundant, variably sized clear lipid vacuoles and predominance of small mature lymphocytes.

6.2.2.2 Clinical Considerations

- Only reported in dogs [21, 25].
- White bile comprises mucinous material from the gallbladder [25].

6.2.2.3 Prognosis

White bile peritonitis represents a variant of classic bile peritonitis, and the prognosis is similar.

6.2.3 Chylous Effusion

6.2.3.1 Cytologic Features

Chylous effusions are characterized by variably sized clear lipid vacuoles in the background of the sample (Figure 6.8). Small mature lymphocytes usually predominate. Increased neutrophils may be seen in chronic effusions. Evidence of chronic hemorrhage may be present.

6.2.3.2 Clinical Considerations

- Gross appearance is milky or opaque.
- May be seen in the pleural cavity (chylothorax), abdominal cavity (chyloabdomen), or both [26, 27].
- Chylothorax DDx = Congestive heart failure, heart worm disease, mediastinal masses (neoplasia, granuloma, enlarged lymph nodes), trauma to the thoracic duct, thrombi in the vena cava, diaphragmatic hernia, and idiopathic [26, 28].
- Chyloabdomen DDx = Abdominal masses (neoplasia, granuloma), lymphangiectasia, pancreatitis, and FIP [27, 29, 30].

6.2.3.3 Confirmation

- Measure concentrations of triglycerides and cholesterol in the fluid. A triglyceride concentration >100 mg dl^{-1} is supportive of chylous effusion [31]. Additionally, the cholesterol-to-triglyceride ratio (Chol:TG) is <1 in chylous effusions and usually >1 in non-chylous effusions.

6.2.3.4 Prognosis

Variable, based on the underlying cause. Patients with chyloabdomen often have a poor prognosis, likely due to a high association with malignant neoplasia [27].

6.2.4 Lymphocyte-rich Effusion

6.2.4.1 Cytologic Appearance

Lymphocyte-rich effusions contain a predominance of small or mixed lymphocytes, with no lipid vacuoles seen in the background of the samples (Figure 6.9). *Note*: Lipid is not always seen in chylous fluid samples, and measuring triglyceride and cholesterol concentrations is recommended to further rule out a chylous effusion.

6.2.4.2 Clinical Considerations

- Gross appearance is typically clear.
- Fluid has either triglyceride concentration <100 mg dl^{-1} and/or a cholesterol-to-triglyceride ratio (Chol:TG) >1.
- Cardiac disease is the most common cause. Consider also space-occupying masses in the thorax and chronic inflammation [32].

6.2.4.3 Prognosis

Variable, based on the underlying cause.

6.2.5 Uroabdomen

6.2.5.1 Cytologic Appearance

Fluid from cases of uroabdomen can vary from a transudate to exudate with components of hemorrhage or sepsis (Figure 6.10) based on the original composition of urine, etiology, and duration of fluid accumulation [33]. Urine is a chemical irritant, and inflammation develops over time.

6.2.5.2 Clinical Considerations

- Fluid may smell like ammonia.
- Uroabdomen commonly presents with a low protein, high neutrophil exudate [1].
- Rupture most common in the bladder but may occur at any level of the urinary tract [34].

Figure 6.9 Lymphocyte-rich effusion, cat, 50× objective. Note the variation in cell size with a predominance of small mature cells.

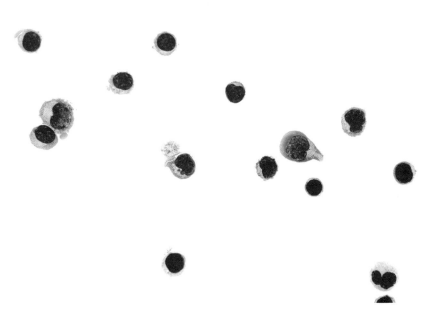

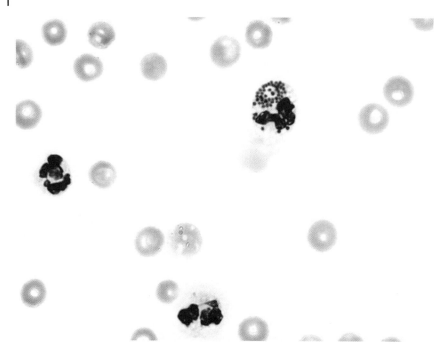

Figure 6.10 Uroabdomen, septic, dog, 100× objective.

- DDx = trauma, obstruction, neoplasia, iatrogenic (bladder expression, catheterization, or post cystotomy) [34–36].
- Urothorax is rare and may accompany cases of uroabdomen, particularly secondary to trauma, with or without evidence of diaphragmatic rupture [37–39].

6.2.5.3 Confirmation

- In one study, a fluid-to-serum potassium ratio >1.4 to 1 had 100% sensitivity and specificity for uroabdomen [40]. *Note*: an elevated fluid-to-serum potassium ratio (>2.67) has been reported in a case of gastric rupture [41]. A fluid-to-serum creatinine ratio >2 to 1 had a 100% specificity and 86% sensitivity for diagnosis of uroabdomen [40].

6.2.5.4 Prognosis

Variable, based on the underlying cause and therapy; however, high survival rates are reported for both dogs and cats with appropriate medical or surgical therapy [34, 42].

6.2.6 Hemorrhagic Effusion

6.2.6.1 Cytologic Appearance

Hemorrhagic effusions are characterized by a dense background of erythrocytes. Platelets may be present if acute hemorrhage has occurred but may also indicate iatrogenic hemorrhage at the time of sampling. Chronic hemorrhage is confirmed by the presence of reactive macrophages that contain heme-breakdown pigments such as hemosiderin or hematoidin crystals (Figure 6.11). Erythrophagocytosis may also support chronic hemorrhage; however, this can occur *in vitro* in stored samples.

6.2.6.2 Clinical Considerations

- PCV of peripheral blood and the effusion often are similar [43].
- DDx = coagulopathies, trauma, ruptured mass (neoplasia/hematomas), bleeding gastrointestinal ulcers, anaphylaxis, lung lobe torsion, and idiopathic (common for pericardial) [43–46].
- Nontraumatic hemoabdomen secondary to ruptured splenic mass most commonly due to malignant neoplasia (73%) and specifically hemangiosarcoma (87.3% of malignant tumors) [47].
- Common finding in pericardial effusions, often accompanied by mesothelial hyperplasia (see Section 6.2.7).

6.2.6.3 Prognosis

Variable, based on the underlying cause and site. Rodenticide toxicity, anaphylaxis, and trauma generally carry a favorable prognosis with appropriate therapy. Hemoperitoneum secondary to rupture of hemangiosarcoma confers a poor prognosis [48]. Surgery prolongs survival in cases of canine nontraumatic hemoadbomen, but the prognosis is still poor [49]. Cats with hemoperitoneum typically have a poor prognosis [43].

6.2.7 Reactive Mesothelial Hyperplasia

6.2.7.1 Cytologic Appearance

Reactive/hyperplastic mesothelial cells vary in appearance from readily to poorly recognizable. They may be seen individually or in variably sized cohesive sheets. Classic features of mesothelium include a pink fringe

Figure 6.11 Hemorrhagic effusion, dog, 50× objective. Reactive macrophages contain phagocytosed red blood cells and heme-breakdown pigment including hemosiderin (green/blue) and hematoidin (golden/orange).

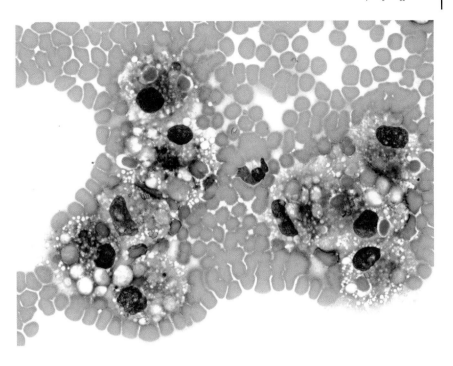

Figure 6.12 Reactive mesothelial cell, dog, 50× objective. Classic features of cytoplasmic blebbing and a pink fringe border are seen.

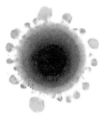

border and peripheralized blebbing of the cytoplasm (Figure 6.12). They occasionally have a perinuclear ring of small clear vacuoles. Highly reactive cells may lose these features and assume many criteria of malignancy, including moderate to marked anisocytosis/anisokaryosis, multinucleation, and prominent nucleoli (Figures 6.13 and 6.14).

6.2.7.2 Clinical Considerations

- Common finding in effusions, particularly chronic effusions.
- More common, greater numbers, and more pleomorphism in dogs than cats.
- Marked mesothelial hyperplasia may be difficult to distinguish from neoplastic effusions (see Sections 6.2.8 and 6.2.9).

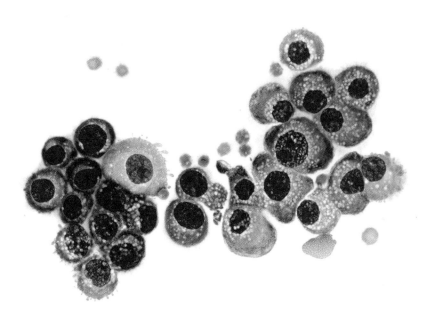

Figure 6.13 Reactive mesothelial hyperplasia, dog, 50× objective. Note the fine clear, perinuclear vacuoles, cytoplasmic blebbing, and faint pink fringe border.

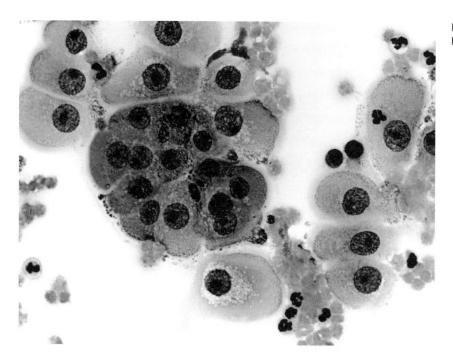

Figure 6.14 Reactive mesothelial hyperplasia, dog, 50× objective.

6.2.8 Neoplastic Effusion: Mesothelioma

6.2.8.1 Cytologic Appearance

Mesothelioma exfoliates in large sheets, which frequently have a papillary arrangement. Marked criteria of malignancy are present, including anisokaryosis and karyomegaly, multinucleation, and even cell cannibalism (Figure 6.15). Cannibalism is also reported in other malignancies [50]. Neoplastic mesothelial cells may be erythrophagocytic or contain heme-breakdown pigments (hematoidin crystals seen in Figure 6.16). Differentiation of mesothelioma from carcinoma or even florid mesothelial hyperplasia is difficult with cytology alone (compare to Figures 6.14 and 6.18). Useful cytomorphologic criteria in human mesothelioma cases include the presence of microvesicles in the cytoplasm, dense cytoplasm, and angulated cell shape (Figure 6.17) [51].

Figure 6.15 Mesothelioma, dog, 50× objective. Note the neoplastic cell that has been phagocytosed by another neoplastic cell (cell cannibalism, arrow).

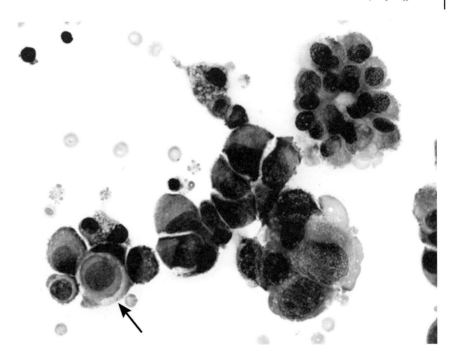

Figure 6.16 Mesothelioma, dog, 50× objective. Neoplastic cells contain golden hematoidin crystals.

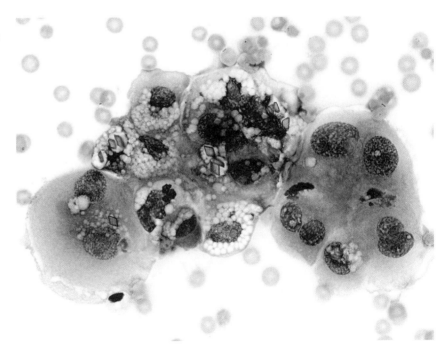

6.2.8.2 Clinical Considerations
- Rare in dogs and cats.
- Can arise from the pleura (most common), pericardium, peritoneum, or tunica vaginalis [52, 53].
- Usually multinodular and disseminated throughout the affected cavity.

- Often highly effusive, with a large amount of fluid present that returns quickly after drainage.

6.2.8.3 Prognosis
Grave without therapy. Therapy may prolong survival times in dogs, though long-term survival is poor [54].

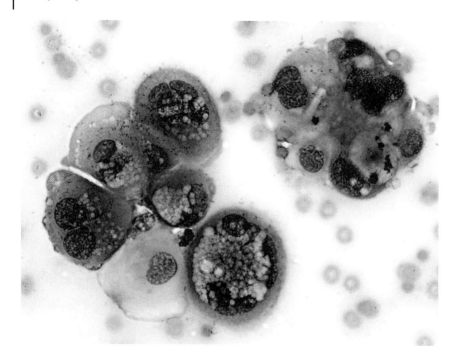

Figure 6.17 Mesothelioma, dog, 50× objective. Note the angular cell shape and microvesicles within the cytoplasm.

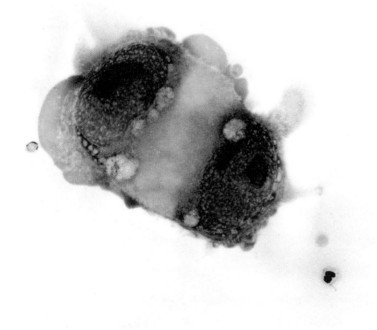

Figure 6.18 Carcinoma, abdominal fluid, cat, 20× objective. Note the enormous size of the neoplastic cells relative to the neutrophil and red blood cells.

6.2.9 Neoplastic Effusion: Carcinoma

6.2.9.1 Cytologic Appearance

Carcinoma cells frequently exfoliate in large numbers, often in a papillary or acinar arrangement. Cells are mostly round/ovoid, with a variable volume of cytoplasm that may balloon with abundant secretory material (Figure 6.18). Nuclei often have the greatest pleomorphism, and common criteria of malignancy include multinucleation, anisokaryosis (both within and between cells), mitotic figures, and multiple, large basophilic nucleoli (Figures 6.19 and 6.20). Carcinomas can be difficult to differentiate from reactive mesothelial hyperplasia or mesothelioma.

6.2.9.2 Clinical Considerations

- May arise from tumors within the cavity or be metastatic.
- Hepatocellular carcinoma is a common cause in abdominal fluid [3].
- Inflammatory cells may be present (concurrent inflammation or paraneoplastic).

Figure 6.19 Carcinoma, pleural fluid, cat, 50× objective. There is a bizarre mitotic figure and marked anisokaryosis.

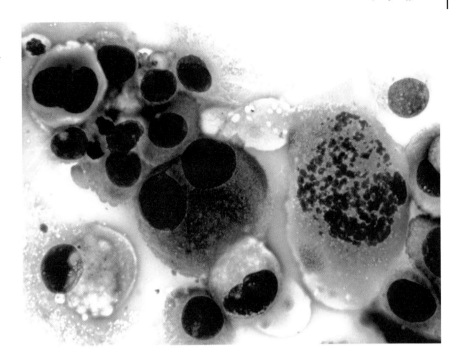

Figure 6.20 Carcinoma, pleural fluid, cat, 50× objective. Note the multinucleated cells with anisokaryosis and nuclear fragmentation within the same cell.

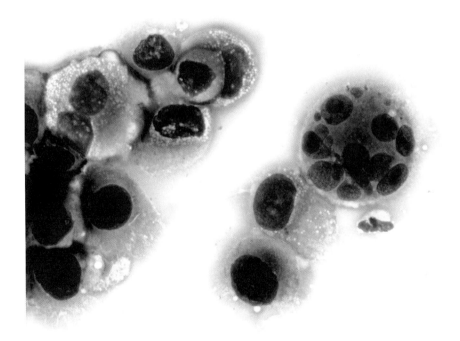

6.2.9.3 Prognosis

Poor.

6.2.10 Neoplastic Effusion: Lymphoma

6.2.10.1 Cytologic Appearance

Effusions secondary to lymphoma are most commonly associated with large-cell, high-grade disease. The neoplastic cells are large, with nuclear diameter more than two red blood cells, and finely stippled or reticulated chromatin. Nucleoli are variably prominent. The cells have a small to moderate volume of medium-blue cytoplasm that may contain fine clear vacuoles (Figure 6.21) or granules. Increased mitotic figures may be seen. Lymphoma may appear similar to histiocytic sarcoma (compare to Figure 6.22).

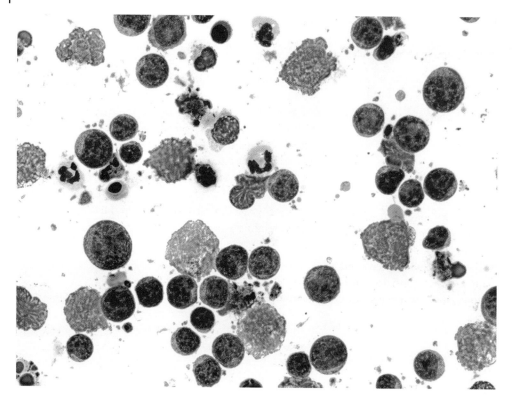

Figure 6.21 Lymphoma, pleural effusion, dog, 50× objective.

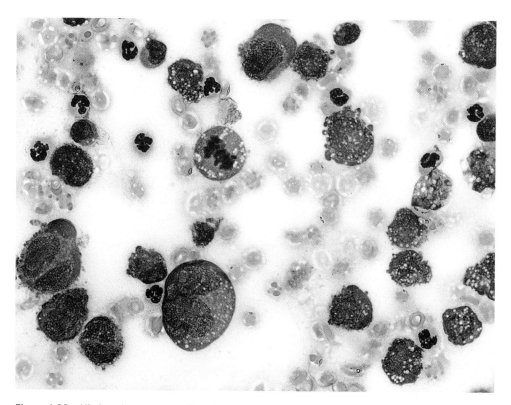

Figure 6.22 Histiocytic sarcoma, pericardial effusion, dog, 50× objective.

6.2.10.2 Clinical Considerations

- Dogs and cats.
- Reported in pleural, abdominal, and pericardial effusions [46, 55, 56].

6.2.10.3 Prognosis

Lymphoma within effusions confirms stage V disease, and the prognosis is guarded to poor.

6.2.11 Neoplastic Effusion: Histiocytic Sarcoma

6.2.11.1 Cytologic Appearance

Histiocytic sarcoma may exfoliate into body cavities and appears as round, individualized cells. Nuclei are ovoid to amoeboid and frequently have irregular or festooning borders. Binucleation or multinucleation may be seen, and mitotic figures are common (Figure 6.22). Cells have a variable volume of medium-blue cytoplasm that often contains clear vacuoles.

6.2.11.2 Clinical Considerations

- Reported rarely in pleural and pericardial fluid in dogs [46, 57].
- May appear similar to other round-cell neoplasms (e.g., lymphoma; compare to Figure 6.21), and further diagnostics may be required.

6.2.11.3 Prognosis

Grave.

6.2.12 Neoplastic Effusion: Mast Cell Neoplasia

6.2.12.1 Cytologic Appearance

Neoplastic mast cell effusions contain an expanded population of mast cells that have a moderate to abundant volume of cytoplasm that contains a variable number of metachromatic granules. Nuclei have stippled chromatin with often prominent nucleoli. Multinucleated cells and mitotic figures are often present in increased numbers (Figure 6.23). Anisocytosis/anisokaryosis are moderate to marked. Effusions often contain a prominent eosinophilic component (Figure 6.24). Mast cells may predominate, comprising >50% of nucleated cells in the fluid, or may be seen in relatively low numbers but have marked criteria of malignancy [58, 59].

6.2.12.2 Clinical Considerations

- Reported in canine patients secondary to cutaneous mast cell neoplasia [60], visceral mast cell neoplasia [61], and with systemic mastocytosis [58, 59].
- Reported in pleural, abdominal, and pericardial effusions.
- Low numbers of well-granulated mast cells are seen in many different effusions and should not raise a suspicion for underlying mast cell neoplasia.

6.2.12.3 Prognosis

Poor. Reported cases are associated with advanced or aggressive disease.

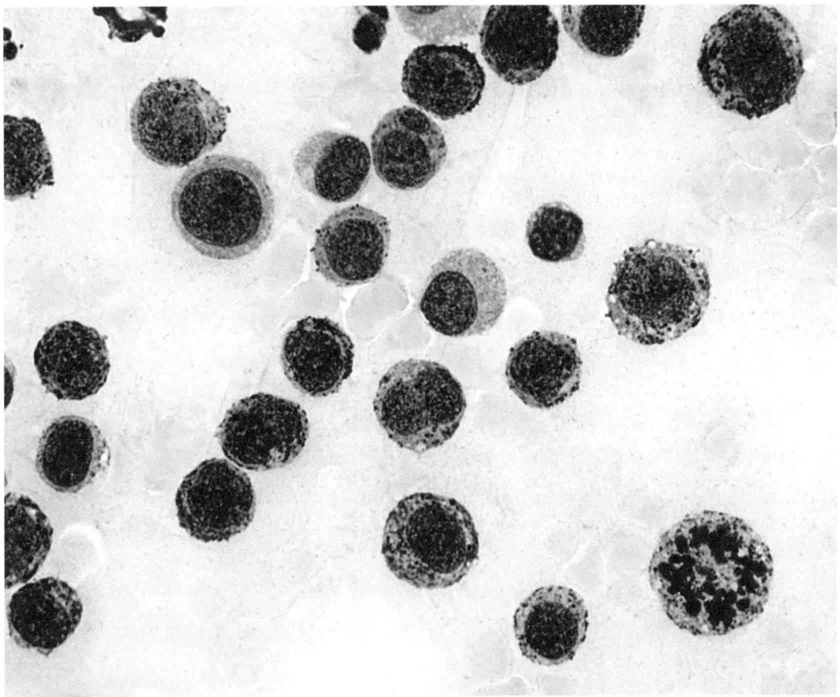

Figure 6.23 Mast cell neoplasia, abdominal fluid, dog, 50× objective. Note the poor granulation of the cells and the mitotic figure (lower right).

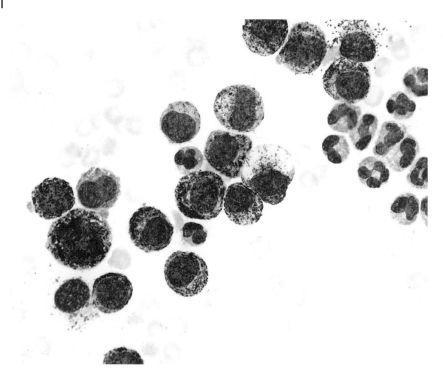

Figure 6.24 Mast cell neoplasia, pleural fluid, dog, 50× objective. The numerous mast cells are accompanied by many eosinophils.

References

1 Alonso, F.H., Christopher, M.M., Paes, P.R.O. (2021) The predominance and diagnostic value of neutrophils in differentiating transudates and exudates in dogs. *Vet. Clin. Pathol.*, **50** (3), 384–393.

2 Bohn, A.A. (2017) Analysis of canine peritoneal fluid analysis. *Vet. Clin. North Am. Small Anim. Pract.*, **47** (1), 123–133.

3 Parsley, A.L., Schnelle, A.M., Gruber, E.K., *et al.* (2022) Total protein concentration as a predictor of neoplastic peritoneal and pleural effusions of dogs. *Vet. Clin. Pathol.*, **51** (3), 391–397.

4 Addie, D., Belák, S., Boucraut-Baralon, C., *et al.* (2009) Feline infectious peritonitis. ABCD guidelines on prevention and management. *J. Feline Med. Surg.*, **11** (7), 594–604.

5 Walters, A.M., O'Brien, M.A., Selmic, L.E., *et al.* (2017) Comparison of clinical findings between dogs with suspected anaphylaxis and dogs with confirmed sepsis. *J. Am. Vet. Med. Assoc.*, **251** (6), 681–688.

6 Johnson, L.R., Epstein, S.E., Reagan, K.L. (2023) Etiology and effusion characteristics in 29 cats and 60 dogs with pyothorax (2010–2020). *J. Vet. Intern. Med.*, **37** (3), 1155–1165.

7 Costello, M.F., Drobatz, K.J., Aronson, L.R., *et al.* (2004) Underlying cause, pathophysiologic abnormalities, and response to treatment in cats with septic peritonitis: 51 cases (1990–2001). *J. Am. Vet. Med. Assoc.*, **225** (6), 897–902.

8 Bentley, A.M., Otto, C.M., Shofer, F.S. (2007) Comparison of dogs with septic peritonitis: 1988–1993 versus 1999–2003. *J. Vet. Emerg. Crit. Care*, **17** (4), 391–398.

9 Bonczynski, J.J., Ludwig, L.L., Barton, L.J., *et al.* (2003) Comparison of peritoneal fluid and peripheral blood pH, bicarbonate, glucose, and lactate concentration as a diagnostic tool for septic peritonitis in dogs and cats. *Vet. Surg.*, **32** (2), 161–166.

10 Shipov, A., Lenchner, I, Milgram, J., *et al.* (2023) Aetiology, clinical parameters and outcome in 113 dogs surgically treated for septic peritonitis (2004–2020). *Vet. Rec.*, **192** (6), e2134. doi: 10.1002/vetr.2134. Last accessed October 15, 2023.

11 Burton, A.G., Harris, L.A., Owens, S.D., *et al.* (2013) The prognostic utility of degenerative left shifts in dogs. *J. Vet. Intern. Med.*, **27** (6), 1517–1522.

12 Demetriou, J.L., Foale, R.D., Ladlow, J., *et al.* (2002) Canine and feline pyothorax: a retrospective study of 50 cases in the UK and Ireland. *J. Small Anim. Pract.*, **43** (9), 388–394.

13 Boothe, H.W., Howe, L.M., Boothe, D.M., *et al.* (2010) Evaluation of outcomes in dogs treated for pyothorax: 46 cases (1983–2001). *J. Am. Vet. Med. Assoc.*, **236** (6), 657–663.

14 Summers, A.M., Vezzi, N., Gravelyn, T., *et al.* (2021) Clinical features and outcome of septic shock in dogs: 37 cases (2008–2015). *J. Vet. Emerg. Crit. Care*, **31** (3), 360–370.

15 Fossum, T.W., Wellman, M., Relford, R.L., *et al.* (1993) Eosinophilic pleural or peritoneal effusions in dogs and cats: 14 cases (1986–1992). *J. Am. Vet. Med. Assoc.*, **202** (11), 1873–1876.

16 Prado Checa, I., Woods, G.A., Oikonomidis, I.L., *et al.* (2021) Eosinophilic pericardial effusion in a cat with complex systemic disease and associated peripheral eosinophilia. *J. Vet. Cardiol.*, **35**, 55–62.

17 Piech, T.L., Jaffey, J.A., Hostnik, E.T., *et al.* (2020) Bicavitary eosinophilic effusion in a dog with coccidiomycosis. *J. Vet. Intern. Med.*, **34** (4), 1582–1586.

18 Norris, J.M., Bosward, K.L., White, J.D., *et al.* (2005) Clinicopathological findings associated with feline infectious peritonitis in Sydney, Australia: 42 cases (1990–2002). *Aust. Vet. J.*, **83** (11), 666–673.

19 Kennedy, M.A. (2020) Feline infectious peritonitis: update on pathogenesis, diagnostics, and treatment. *Vet. Clin. North Am. Small Anim. Pract.*, **50** (5), 1001–1011.

20 Krentz, D., Zwicklbauer, K., Felten, S., *et al.* (2022) Clinical follow-up and postmortem findings in a cat that was cured of feline infectious peritonitis with an oral antiviral drug containing GS-441524. *Viruses*, **14** (9), 2040. doi: 10.3390/v14092040. Last accessed October 15, 2023.

21 Wilson, K., Powers, D., Grasperge, B., *et al.* (2021) Dogs with biliary rupture based on ultrasound findings may have normal total serum bilirubin values. *Vet. Radiol. Ultrasound*, **62** (2), 236–245.

22 Angelou, V.N., Patsikas, M.N., Kazakos, G.M., *et al.* (2020) Bilothorax associated with bile peritonitis in a dog with no diaphragmatic disruption: a case report. *Top. Companion Anim. Med.*, **40**, 100453. doi: 10.1016/j.tcam.2020.100453. Last accessed October 15, 2023

23 Murgia, D. (2013) A case of combined bilothorax and bile peritonitis secondary to gunshot wounds in a cat. *J. Feline Med. Surg.*, **15** (6), 513–516.

24 Ludwig, L.L., McLoughlin, M.A., Graves, T.K., *et al.* (1997) Surgical treatment of bile peritonitis in 24 dogs and 2 cats: a retrospective study (1987–1994). *Vet. Surg.*, **26** (2), 90–98.

25 Owens, S.D., Gossett, R., McElhaney, M.R., *et al.* (2003) Three cases of canine bile peritonitis with mucinous material in abdominal fluid as the prominent cytologic finding. *Vet. Clin. Pathol.*, **32** (3), 114–120.

26 Fossum, T.W., Forrester, S.D., Swenson, C.L., *et al.* (1991) Chylothorax in cats: 37 cases (1969–1989). *J. Am. Vet. Med. Assoc.*, **198** (4), 672–678.

27 Hatch, A., Jandrey, K.J., Tenwolde, M.C., *et al.* (2018) Incidence of chyloabdomen diagnosis in dogs and cats and corresponding clinical signs, clinicopathologic test results, and outcomes: 53 cases (1984–2014). *J. Am. Vet. Med. Assoc.*, **253** (7), 886–892.

28 Hung, L., Hopper, B.J., Lenard. Z. (2022) Retrospective analysis of radiographic signs in feline pleural effusions to predict disease aetiology. *BMC Vet. Res.*, **18** (1), 118.

29 Miguel-Garcés, M., Destri, A., Kelly, D., *et al.* (2023) Resolution of chyloabdomen following the removal of a projectile causing a granuloma. *Vet. Med. Sci.*, **9** (2), 579–583.

30 Savary, K.C., Sellon, R.K., Law, J.M. (2001) Chylous abdominal effusion in a cat with feline infectious peritonitis. *J. Am. Anim. Hosp. Assoc.*, **37** (1), 35–40.

31 Waddle, J.R., Giger, U. (1990) Lipoprotein electrophoresis differentiation of chylous and nonchylous pleural effusions in dogs and cats and its correlation with pleural effusion triglyceride concentration. *Vet. Clin. Pathol.*, **19** (3), 80–85.

32 Probo, M., Valenti, V., Venco, L., *et al.* (2018) Pleural lymphocyte-rich transudates in cats. *J. Feline Med. Surg.*, **20** (8), 767–771.

33 Connally, H.E. (2003) Cytology and fluid analysis of the acute abdomen. *Clin. Tech. Small Anim. Pract.*, **18** (1), 39–44.

34 Grimes, J.A., Fletcher, J.M., Schmiedt, C.W. (2018) Outcomes in dogs with uroabdomen: 43 cases (2006-2015). *J. Am. Vet. Med. Assoc.*, **252** (1), 92–97.

35 Aumann, M., Worth, L.T., Drobatz, K.J. (1998) Uroperitoneum in cats: 26 cases (1986–1995). *J. Am. Anim. Hosp. Assoc.*, **34** (4), 315–324.

36 Stafford, J.R., Bartges, J. W. (2013) A clinical review of pathophysiology, diagnosis, and treatment of uroabdomen in the dog and cat. *J. Vet. Emerg. Crit. Care*, **23** (2), 216–229.

37 Klainbart, S., Merchav, R., Ohad, D.G. (2011) Traumatic urothorax in a dog: a case report. *J. Small Anim. Pract.*, **52** (10), 544–546.

38 Tsompanidou, P.P., Anagnostou, T.L., Kazakos, G.M., *et al.* (2015) Urothorax associated with uroperitoneum in a dog without diaphragmatic disruption. *J. Am. Anim. Hosp. Assoc.*, **51** (4), 256–259.

39 Störk, C.K., Hamaide, A.J., Schwedes, C., *et al.* (2003) Hemiurothorax following diaphragmatic hernia and kidney prolapse in a cat. *J. Feline Med. Surg.*, **5** (2), 91–96.

40 Schmiedt, C., Tobias, K.M., Otto, C.M. (2001) Evaluation of abdominal fluid: peripheral blood creatinine and potassium ratios for diagnosis of uroperitoneum in dogs. *J. Vet. Emerg. Crit. Care*, **11** (4), 275–280.

41 Ben Oz, J., Aroch, I, Segev, G. (2016) Increased ratio of peritoneal effusion-to-serum potassium concentration in a dog with gastric perforation. *J. Vet. Emerg. Crit. Care*, **26** 6), 793–797.

42 Hornsey, S.J., Halfacree, Z., Kulendra, E., *et al.* (2021) Factors affecting survival to discharge in 53 cats

diagnosed with uroabdomen: a single-centre retrospective analysis. *J. Feline Med. Surg.*, **23** (2), 115–120.

43 Culp, W.T., Weisse, C., Kellogg, M.E., *et al.* (2010) Spontaneous hemoperitoneum in cats: 65 cases (1994–2006). *J. Am. Vet. Med. Assoc.*, **236** (9), 978–982.

44 Nakamura, R.K., Rozanski, E.A., Rush, J.E. (2008) Non-coagulopathic spontaneous hemothorax in dogs. *J. Vet. Emerg. Crit. Care*, **18** (3), 292–297.

45 Hnatusko, A.L., Gicking, J.C., Liscinandro, G.R. (2021) Anaphylaxis-related hemoperitoneum in 11 dogs. *J. Vet. Emerg. Crit. Care*, **31** (1), 80–85.

46 Cagle, L.A., Epstein, S.E., Owens, S.D., *et al.* (2014) Diagnostic yield of cytologic analysis of pericardial effusion in dogs. *J. Vet. Intern. Med.*, **28** (1), 66–71.

47 Schick, A.R., Grimes, J.A. (2022) Evaluation of the validity of the double two-thirds rule for diagnosing hemangiosarcoma in dogs with nontraumatic hemoperitoneum due to a ruptured splenic mass: a systematic review. *J. Am. Vet. Med. Assoc.*, **261** (1), 69–73.

48 Aronsohn, M.G., Dubiel, B., Roberts, B., *et al.* (2009) Prognosis for acute nontraumatic hemoperitoneum in the dog: a retrospective analysis of 60 cases (2003–2006). *J. Am. Anim. Hosp. Assoc.*, **45** (2), 72–77.

49 Menard, J.V., Sylvester, S.R., Lopez, D.J. (2023) Assessing major influences on decision-making and outcome for dogs presenting emergently with non-traumatic hemoabdomen. *J. Am. Vet. Med. Assoc.*, **261** (7), 980–988.

50 Ferreira, F.C., Soares, M.J., Carvalho, S., *et al.* (2015) Four cases of cell cannibalism in highly malignant feline and canine tumors. *Diagn. Pathol.*, **10**, 199.

51 Paintal, A., Raparia, K., Nayar, R. (2016) Cytomorphologic findings of malignant mesothelioma in FNA biopsies and touch preps of core biopsies. *Diagn. Cytopathol.*, **44** (1), 14–19.

52 Espino, L., Vazquez, S., Failde, D., *et al.* (2010) Localized pleural mesothelioma causing cranial vena cava syndrome in a dog. *J. Vet. Diagn. Investig.*, **22** (2), 309–312.

53 Vascellari, M., Carminato, A., Camali, G., *et al.* (2011) Malignant mesothelioma of the tunica vaginalis testis in a dog: histological and immunohistochemical characterization. *J. Vet. Diagn. Investig.*, **23** (1), 135–139.

54 Moberg, H.L., Gramer, I., Schofield, I., et al. (2022) Clinical presentation, treatment and outcome of canine malignant mesothelioma: a retrospective study of 34 cases. *Vet. Comp. Oncol.*, **20** (1), 304–312.

55 Bauer, N., Moritz, A. (2005) Flow cytometric analysis of effusions in dogs and cats with the automated haematology analyser ADVIA 120. *Vet. Rec.*, **156** (21), 674–678.

56 Vasilatis, D.M., Vernau, W. (2022) Pericardial effusion in a dog due to T-cell lymphoma of granular lymphocyte type. *Vet. Med. Sci.*, **8** (5), 1877–1880.

57 Tsai, S., Sutherland-Smith, J., Burgess, K., *et al.* (2012) Imaging characteristics of intrathoracic histiocytic sarcoma in dogs. *Vet. Radiol. Ultrasound*, **53** (1), 21–27.

58 Ramdass, K., Lunardon, T., Etzioni, A.L. (2021) An uncommon occurrence of bicavitary effusion due to mast cell neoplasia in a 12-year-old mixed breed dog. *Vet. Clin. Pathol.*, **50** (4), 593–596.

59 Cowgill, E., Neel, J. (2003) Pleural fluid from a dog with marked eosinophilia. *Vet. Clin. Pathol.*, **32** (3), 147–149.

60 Yale, A.D., Szladovits, B., Stell, A.J., *et al.* (2020) High-grade cutaneous mast cell tumour with widespread intrathoracic metastasis and neoplastic pericardial effusion in a dog. *J. Comp. Pathol.*, **180**, 29–34.

61 de Souza, M.L., Torres, L.F., Rocha, N.S., *et al.* (2001) Peritoneal effusion in a dog secondary to visceral mast cell tumor. A case report. *Acta. Cytol.*, **45** (1), 89–92.

7

Musculoskeletal

7.1 Bone

7.1.1 Osteoma

7.1.1.1 Cytologic Features
Osteomas comprise well-differentiated osteoblastic cells that are ovoid with abundant medium-blue cytoplasm that often contains a faint perinuclear clear zone. Nuclei are round, eccentrically placed, and often appear to be 'falling out' of the cell (Figure 7.1). They have finely granular chromatin with single nucleoli. Anisocytosis/anisokaryosis are mild and N/C ratios are low. The cells appear similar or indistinguishable from normal or reactive osteoblasts.

7.1.1.2 Clinical Considerations
- Rare tumors in cats and dogs.
- Commonly arise from the mandible and maxillofacial region, but also from the long bones and extraskeletal sites [1–4].
- Smooth proliferative lesions with well-defined borders and no bone lysis.

7.1.1.3 Prognosis
Good with surgical excision of the mass [1, 5]. The insidious growth and location of many tumors can make surgical treatment more difficult, and prognosis may be more guarded in such cases, though recurrence is low even with surgical debulking [1, 2].

7.1.2 Osteosarcoma

7.1.2.1 Cytologic Features
Osteosarcomas frequently are highly cellular and associated with a bright pink, fibrillar extracellular matrix (osteoid) (Figure 7.2). Cells are distributed individually and in aggregates, and range from ovoid to fusiform. Their cytoplasm may contain fine clear vacuoles or fine pink granules. Nuclei are round to ovoid and often eccentrically placed, with the appearance of 'falling out' of the cell (see Figure 2.33). They have finely granular chromatin with multiple basophilic nucleoli, and hyperchromasia is common (see Figure 2.48). Marked criteria of malignancy often are present (Figure 7.3), including multinucleated giant cells, though these should not be confused with resident osteoclasts (Figure 7.4). *Note*: subtypes of osteosarcoma exist, including chondroblastic and fibroblastic, which can make differentiation from chondrosarcomas and fibrosarcomas difficult.

7.1.2.2 Clinical Considerations
- Most common primary bone tumor in dogs. Rare in cats.
- Large breed dogs predisposed. Bimodal age distribution: mostly middle-aged to older dogs, but a small peak in frequency for dogs 18–24 months of age [6, 7].
- Seen most frequently in the metaphyseal region of the appendicular skeleton, with tumors twice as likely in the front limbs [6, 8].
- Primary osteosarcomas are seen rarely in extraskeletal sites, and can metastasize to extraskeletal sites.
- Metallic implants may increase the risk of osteosarcoma, which is significantly more likely to involve the diaphysis [9].
- Early metastasis to the lungs is common (but is often subclinical at the time of diagnosis). Metastatic disease to lymph nodes is rare and is associated with a poor prognosis [10].
- ALP staining on cytology samples may assist in differentiating osteosarcoma from other sarcomas with high sensitivity and specificity [11, 12]. Other tumors that may stain positively include amelanotic melanoma, chondrosarcoma, multilobular osteochondrosarcoma, and gastrointestinal stromal tumors.

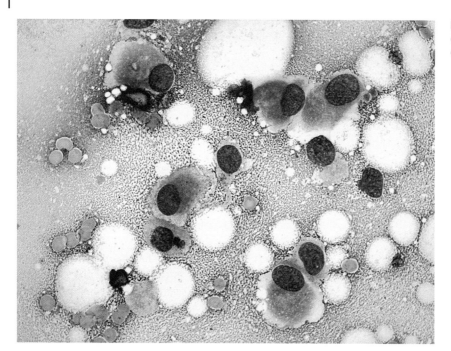

Figure 7.1 Bone, osteoma, cat, 50× objective. Numerous well-differentiated osteoblasts are present.

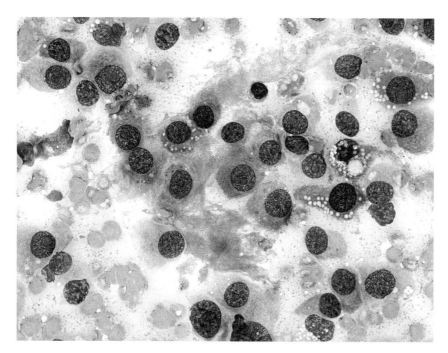

Figure 7.2 Bone, osteosarcoma, dog, 50× objective. Note the smooth to fibrillar pink osteoid between cells.

7.1.2.3 Prognosis

Osteosarcomas are highly aggressive malignancies with high rates of metastatic disease and prognosis is guarded to poor [13]. Factors contributing to a poor outcome include tumor size and histologic grade. Elevated serum ALP and proximal humeral location have been reported as negative prognosticators in a meta-analysis of dogs [14], and humeral location is associated with a higher incidence of metastatic disease in cats [15]. Metastatic disease also confers a poor prognosis, with median survival times of 2 months compared to 12 months for dogs without evidence of metastases [16]. Tumors affecting flat bones may have a better prognosis [17].

7.1.3 Chondrosarcoma

7.1.3.1 Cytologic Features

Chondrosarcomas are characterized by dense, metachromatic extracellular chondroid (Figure 7.5) in

Figure 7.3 Bone, osteosarcoma, dog, 50× objective. Many criteria of malignancy are present including multinucleation, marked anisokaryosis, and mitotic figures (arrow).

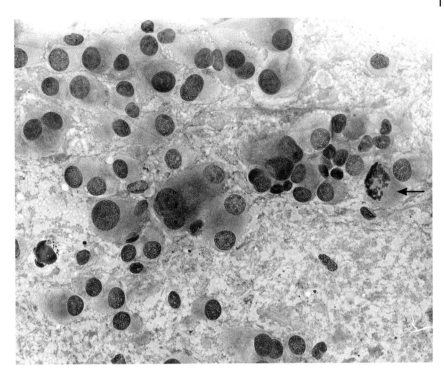

Figure 7.4 Bone, osteosarcoma, dog, 100× objective. Note the ovoid, neoplastic osteoblasts associated with pink osteoid (right) and the large multinucleated osteoclast (upper left).

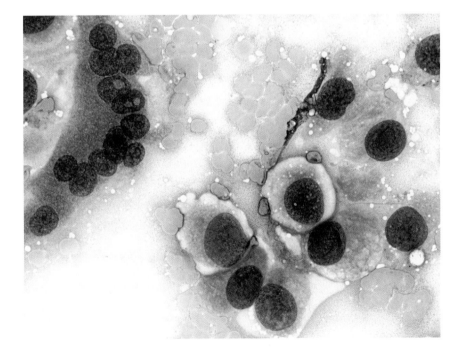

which cells may be embedded, forming lacunae. Cells mostly are round but can be spindloid and have a pale-blue cytoplasm that often contains diffuse, fine pink granules. Unlike osteosarcomas, nuclei are more often centrally placed within the cell, but also have finely stippled chromatin and multiple basophilic nucleoli.

7.1.3.2 Clinical Considerations

- Second most common bone tumor in dogs. Rare in cats [18].
- Predilection sites = nasal cavity > ribs, scapula, and other flat bones [19].
- Occurs in extraosseous sites, including mammary gland tissue [18].

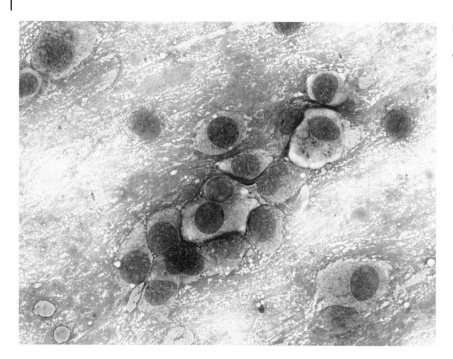

Figure 7.5 Bone, chondrosarcoma, dog, 50× objective. Neoplastic cells are embedded within thick chondroid.

- Metastatic disease is not a feature of nasal chondrosarcomas, and extra-nasal tumors are generally slow to metastasize [18, 19].

7.1.3.3 Prognosis
Variable. Nasal chondrosarcomas carry a poor prognosis, though radiation therapy may increase survival times [19]. Dedifferentiated chondrosarcomas have high metastatic rates and also impart a poor prognosis [20]. Wide surgical excision of extra-nasal chondrosarcomas in dogs significantly improves survival time and can be associated with long-term survival [21].

7.1.4 Multilobular Osteochondrosarcoma

7.1.4.1 Cytologic Features
Cytologic samples from multilobular osteochondrosarcoma (MLO) are highly variable, as tumors are composed of cartilaginous, osseous, and spindle cells (the latter predominate in Figure 7.6). Multiple such components, together with clinical considerations (see Section 7.1.4.2), should raise suspicion of these tumors.

7.1.4.2 Clinical Considerations
- Synonyms = multilobular tumor of bone, chondroma rodens, multilobular osteoma.
- Dogs > > cats.
- Affects flat bones, particularly of the skull > ribs, pelvis, os penis [22, 23].
- Moderately metastatic, generally to lungs [24].

7.1.4.3 Prognosis
Long-term survival is expected with complete resection. Incomplete resection dramatically decreases survival times [24]. Recurrence and metastatic rates are linked to histologic grade [24].

7.1.5 Hemangiosarcoma

7.1.5.1 Cytologic Features
Hemangiosarcomas of bone may exfoliate poorly, and samples may be very bloody. When present, cells are ovoid to spindloid and may be seen in aggregates/epithelioid sheets. The cells have a small to moderate volume of medium-blue cytoplasm that may form streaming cytoplasmic wisps. Nuclei are ovoid to occasionally amoeboid and have finely granular chromatin with prominent, often large, basophilic nucleoli. Mitotic figures and hyperchromasia of nuclei are common (Figure 7.7). Anisocytosis/anisokaryosis are marked and N/C ratios mostly are high.

7.1.5.2 Clinical Considerations
- Rare primary tumors of bone [25].
- May be primary or metastatic [25, 26].
- Radiography = marked lysis (often accompanied by pathologic fracture) and minimal or no periosteal new bone formation [27].
- Tibia most commonly affected [28].

7.1.5.3 Prognosis
Poor to grave. Even if confined to a single bony lesion at the time of diagnosis [27], these are aggressive tumors with high rates of metastatic disease [28]. Younger age

Figure 7.6 Bone, multilobular osteochondrosarcoma, dog, 50× objective.

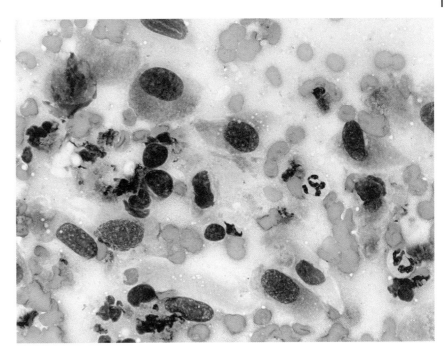

Figure 7.7 Bone, hemangiosarcoma, dog, 50× objective.

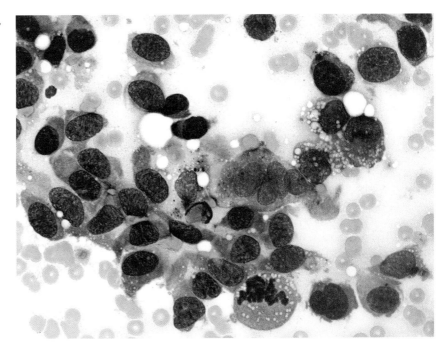

and more aggressive therapy associated with longer survival times [28].

7.1.6 Fibrosarcoma

7.1.6.1 Cytologic Features

Fibrosarcomas of bone are characterized by a population of spindloid cells with a small to moderate volume of pale-blue cytoplasm that form bipolar tapering ends. Nuclei are round to ovoid, with finely granular chromatin and multiple prominent nucleoli. Anisocytosis/anisokaryosis

are moderate to marked (Figure 7.8). Care should be taken to differentiate these from reactive fibroplasia, and histopathology is required to differentiate from the fibroblastic variant of osteosarcoma and MLO (compare to Figure 7.6).

7.1.6.2 Clinical Considerations

- Rare primary tumors of bone [25, 29].
- Most commonly affects the skull > appendicular bones [17, 29].
- May be primary or metastatic [30].

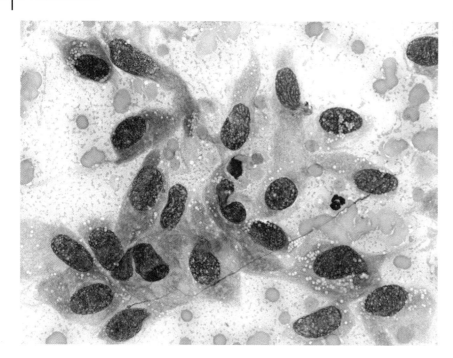

Figure 7.8 Bone, fibrosarcoma, dog, 50× objective.

7.1.6.3 Prognosis

Variable, based on location and presence of metastatic disease, with the latter conferring a poor prognosis [31]. Long-term survival is possible with appropriate therapy [17], and complete surgical excision of a single tumor may be curative [9, 31].

7.1.7 Histiocytic Sarcoma

7.1.7.1 Cytologic Features

Histiocytic sarcoma cells are round and discrete, which can make them difficult to distinguish from osteosarcoma (compare to Figure 7.4). Distinguishing features may include vacuolation of the cytoplasm and lack of pink granules. Differentiation from osteosarcoma is more straightforward when criteria of malignancy are marked, as karyomegaly and prominent nucleoli are more common in histiocytic sarcoma (Figure 7.9).

7.1.7.2 Clinical Considerations

- May be localized to bone or part of disseminated disease.
- Sites of predilection = periarticular bones, vertebrae, proximal humerus [32].
- Predisposed breeds = Rottweilers and Golden Retrievers [32, 33].
- Have been associated with metallic implants in dogs [9].

7.1.7.3 Prognosis

Poor to grave.

7.1.8 Multiple Myeloma

7.1.8.1 Cytologic Features

Multiple myeloma is characterized by a neoplastic expansion of mostly well-differentiated plasma cells seen in large sheets. The cells have a moderate volume of pale-blue cytoplasm and often have a characteristic, perinuclear clear zone (Golgi zone). Some cells may contain bright-pink material within the periphery of the cytoplasm, representing the production of immunoglobulins (flame cells) (Figure 7.10). Nuclei are round, eccentrically placed, and have clumped chromatin.

7.1.8.2 Clinical Considerations

- Dogs > cats.
- Other clinical findings = monoclonal gammopathy, bone marrow plasmacytosis, anemia, bleeding diatheses, Bence-Jones proteinuria, and multicentric osteolysis [34, 35].

7.1.8.3 Prognosis

Dogs = Good short-term prognosis with treatment, and long-term control is possible. Negative prognostic factors include extensive bone lysis/involvement, hypercalcemia, and Bence-Jones proteinuria [34].

Cats = Guarded prognosis, with generally short survival times [35, 36].

7.1.9 Metastatic Neoplasia to Bone

7.1.9.1 Cytologic Features

Metastatic bone tumors will appear cytologically similar to the primary tumor, often with marked criteria of malignancy. Mildly pleomorphic, reactive osteoblasts or osteoclasts may accompany neoplastic cells (Figure 7.11).

Figure 7.9   Bone, histiocytic sarcoma, dog, 50× objective.

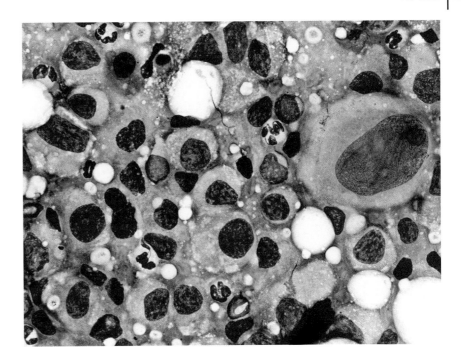

Figure 7.10   Bone, multiple myeloma, dog, 100× objective. Lytic lesion in spinal process. Note the bright-pink immunoglobulin accumulation within the cytoplasm (flame cells).

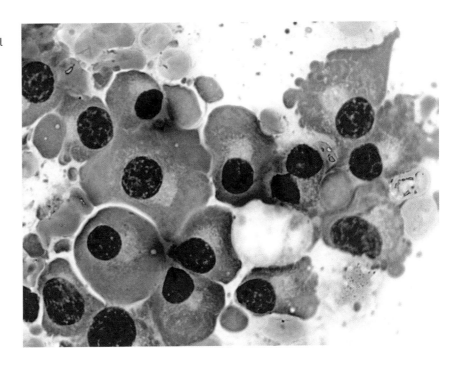

7.1.9.2   Clinical Considerations

- Most common in the axial skeleton (particularly vertebrae) and proximal appendicular bones (particularly the humerus) [30, 37].
- Often affect multiple bones.
- Carcinomas are most common, and mammary gland is the most frequent origin, but hemangiosarcoma from the spleen is also common [17, 26, 37, 38].

7.1.9.3   Prognosis

Grave.

7.1.10   Osteomyelitis

7.1.10.1   Cytologic Features

Osteomyelitis is characterized by an infiltration of inflammatory cells, the type of which will vary with the

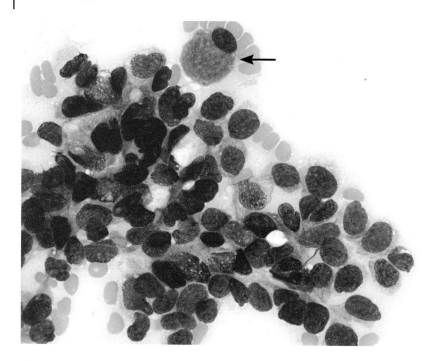

Figure 7.11 Bone, metastatic mammary carcinoma, dog, 50× objective. Note the cytologically normal osteoblast (arrow).

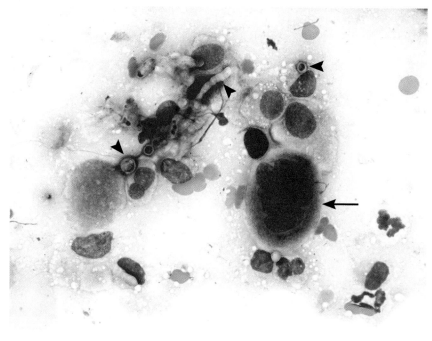

Figure 7.12 Bone, osteomyelitis, dog, 50× objective. Fungal organisms are seen budding and forming hyphae (arrowheads), and an osteoclast is present (arrow).

underlying infectious agent. Granulomatous inflammation generally accompanies fungal agents, while neutrophils are seen with bacterial osteomyelitis. Osteoblasts or osteoclasts may be seen, confirming involvement of bone (Figure 7.12).

7.1.10.2 Clinical Considerations

- May be associated with puncture wounds/trauma, hematogenous spread, or orthopedic procedures [39–41].
- Aerobic bacteria most common with bacterial osteomyelitis. Anaerobes seen secondary to bite/puncture wounds or tooth root abscess [39, 42].

- Common fungal agents = *Blastomyces*, *Coccidioides*, *Histoplasma*, *Cryptococcus*, *Aspergillus* (see Chapter 3 for details) [43].

7.1.10.3 Prognosis

Bacterial osteomyelitis generally carries a favorable prognosis with appropriate therapy. Fungal osteomyelitis is more guarded, based on the extent of disease, with disseminated disease or CNS involvement carrying a grave prognosis [44].

7.2 Joints

7.2.1 Normal Synovial Fluid

7.2.1.1 Cytologic Features

Synovial fluid from normal joints has a variably thick, pink stippled, mucinous background (Figure 7.13). Erythrocytes should be absent or seen in very low numbers. Nucleated cells are seen individually in low numbers and should comprise almost exclusively quiescent large mononuclear cells (macrophages or synoviocytes that look cytologically similar). Rare small mature lymphocytes may be seen. Neutrophils should be absent or extremely rare.

7.2.1.2 Clinical Considerations

- Grossly, fluid should be clear and viscous.
- Cell count: Generally <1500 cells μl^{-1}. Stifle joints often have higher cell counts, up to 3000 cells μl^{-1} [45, 46].

7.2.2 Mononuclear Reactivity/Inflammation

7.2.2.1 Cytologic Features

Mononuclear reactive changes may be seen with either a normal or an elevated cell count. Relative to quiescent macrophages/synoviocytes, the cells are larger and have a greater volume of cytoplasm that frequently becomes vacuolated (compare Figures 7.14 and 7.13). These mononuclear cells may form sheets or dense aggregates, suggestive of synovial hyperplasia.

7.2.2.2 Clinical Considerations

- Classically seen with degenerative diseases of the joint.
- DDx = osteoarthritis, ligament/meniscal disease, chronic irritation/trauma to the joint, chronic orthopedic disease (e.g., osteochondritis dissecans).
- Cytologic abnormalities may precede radiographic changes [47].

7.2.2.3 Prognosis

Disease is seldom reversible, but progression is variable with underlying cause.

7.2.3 Neutrophilic Inflammation (Bacterial Sepsis)

7.2.3.1 Cytologic Features

Bacterial septic arthritis is associated with a markedly elevated cell count, predominated by neutrophils. Neutrophils frequently are non-degenerative. Bacteria may be seen in neutrophil phagolysosomes (Figure 7.15) but are not always seen in cases of septic arthritis. Care should be taken to differentiate bacteria from phagocytosed immunoglobulin, which can be seen in immune-mediated disease (compare to Figure 7.18).

7.2.3.2 Clinical Considerations

- Dogs > Cats [48, 49].
- Bacteria may not be seen cytologically, and microbial culture is recommended, though it may not yield growth [50].
- Common isolates include *Staphylococcus* spp., *Streptococcus* spp., *Pasteurella* spp., *Bacillus* spp., and *Pseudomonas aeruginosa* [50, 51].

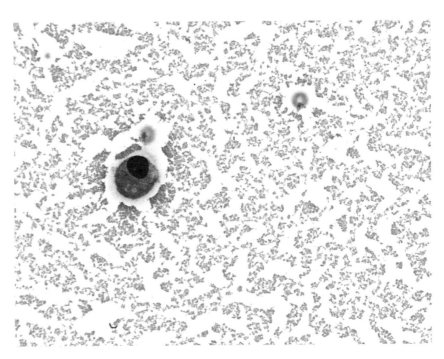

Figure 7.13 Synovial fluid (normal), dog, 50× objective. There is a medium-pink stippled background, rare erythrocytes and a single, quiescent macrophage/synoviocyte.

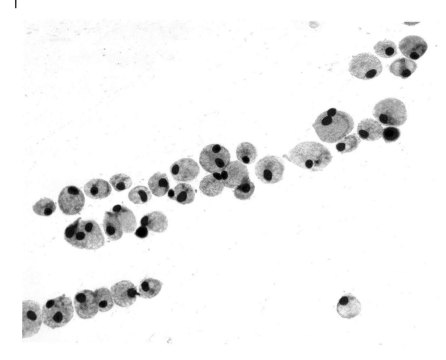

Figure 7.14 Synovial fluid, dog, 20× objective. Mononuclear inflammation and reactive changes.

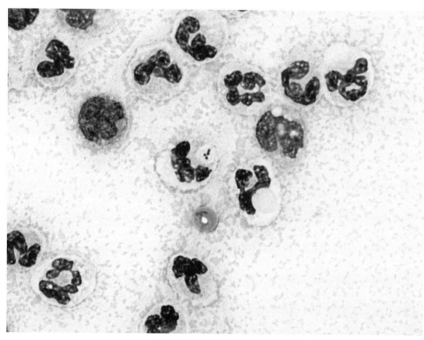

Figure 7.15 Synovial fluid, dog, 100× objective. Septic arthritis. Note bacterial cocci within a phagolysosome in the neutrophil.

- Stifle and elbow joints most commonly affected [48, 52].
- May be secondary to surgical procedures, hematogenous spread, penetrating wounds or spontaneous [48, 52, 53].
- Preexisting osteoarthritis is common and is associated with recurrence [48].

7.2.3.3 Prognosis
Generally good with appropriate therapy. Successful outcomes are more likely with early treatment and in cases of direct penetration or spontaneous infection [48]. Full joint function may not be restored [52, 53]. Recurrence more likely in dogs >30 kg [48].

7.2.4 Neutrophilic Inflammation (Rickettsial Sepsis)

7.2.4.1 Cytologic Appearance
Neutrophilic arthritis is seen with Rickettsial infections (see Chapter 3 for details). Organisms may be visible within neutrophils in synovial fluid, often in low numbers, and

Figure 7.16 Synovial fluid, dog, 100× objective. Rickettsial infection. Note the morula of *Anaplasma phagocytophilum* in the neutrophil on the right.

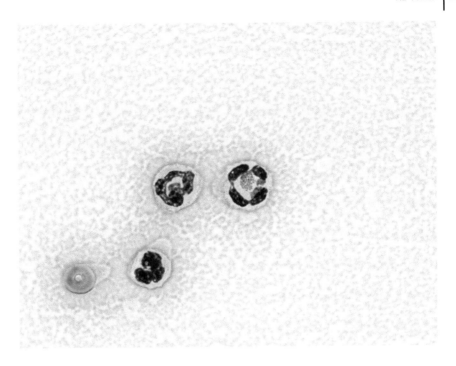

careful examination of many neutrophils is recommended. The bacteria form round aggregates known as morulae (Figure 7.16).

7.2.4.2 Clinical Considerations
- Polyarthropathy is most commonly due to infection with *Ehrlichia ewingii* or *Anaplasma phagocytophilum* [54].
- Absence of organisms does not rule out underlying Rickettsial disease [55].

7.2.4.3 Prognosis
Good with appropriate therapy.

7.2.5 Neutrophilic Inflammation (Noninfectious)

7.2.5.1 Cytologic Features
Noninfectious neutrophilic inflammation is characterized by variably increased numbers of neutrophils that are non-degenerate (Figure 7.17). In cases of immune-mediated polyarthritis (IMPA), neutrophils may rarely contain numerous, variably sized cytoplasmic inclusions that are pink to purple and irregularly shaped (Figure 7.18). These represent phagocytosed immune complexes or nuclear remnants. These cells are called 'ragocytes' when unstained. These inclusions can be distinguished from ingested bacteria, the latter being uniform in size, staining, and shape (compare to Figure 7.15).

7.2.5.2 Clinical Considerations
- Clinical signs = shifting limb lameness, fever, joint pain [56].
- May be primary autoimmune, or secondary to other pathology (e.g., neoplasia or infectious organisms such as Rickettsial agents).
- An increased number of small lymphocytes may accompany the neutrophilic inflammation in cases of erosive IMPA [57].

7.2.5.3 Prognosis
Primary IMPA has a good prognosis with appropriate therapy [58]. Prognosis variable for secondary cases based on the underlying disease.

7.2.6 Systemic Lupus Erythematosus

7.2.6.1 Cytologic Features
Patients with systemic lupus erythematosus (SLE) often have polyarthritis, characterized by large numbers of non-degenerate neutrophils. In addition, a (rare) characteristic finding is the presence of lupus erythematosus (LE) cells. LE cells are neutrophils that have large, round, homogeneous pink inclusions with a smooth border, representing phagocytosis of nuclear material (Figure 7.19).

7.2.6.2 Clinical Considerations
- LE cells are rare but, when present, strongly support a diagnosis of SLE [45].
- Rare disease in dogs and cats.
- Further confirmation of SLE should include the presence of other signs including a positive antinuclear antibody (ANA) test; dermatopathy; glomerulonephritis; hemolytic anemia [59].

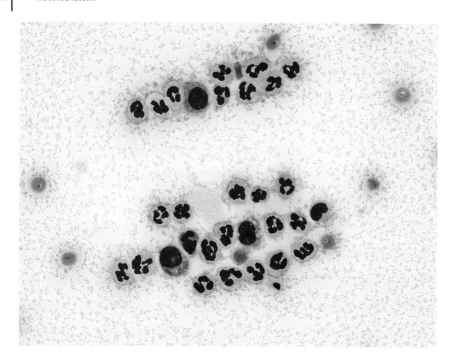

Figure 7.17 Synovial fluid, dog, 50× objective. Sterile neutrophilic inflammation (IMPA).

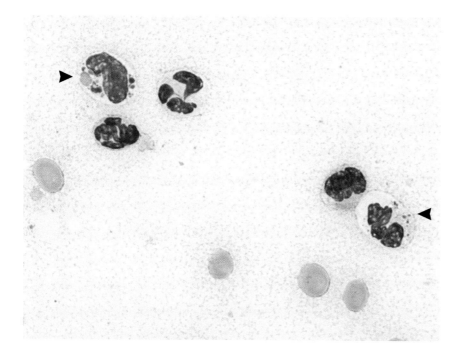

Figure 7.18 Synovial fluid, dog, 100× objective. IMPA with ragocytes. Note the amorphous, pink/purple inclusions within the cytoplasm of some neutrophils.

7.2.6.3 Prognosis
Variable, based on disease severity and organ systems involved.

7.2.7 Metastatic Neoplasia

7.2.7.1 Cytologic Features
Rarely, neoplastic cells may be seen in synovial fluid, and their appearance will reflect the tumor of origin. They often display marked criteria of malignancy (see Chapter 2 for details), such as anisokaryosis and prominent nucleoli. Cells may be present in low numbers, and examination of sedimented or cytocentrifuged samples may be necessary.

7.2.7.2 Clinical Considerations
- Neoplasia may invade from around the joint (e.g., histiocytic sarcoma; Figure 7.20) or metastasize to the joint (e.g., bronchogenic carcinoma; Figure 7.21) [60].

Figure 7.19 Synovial fluid, dog, 100× objective. Systemic lupus erythematosus. Note the bright pink, spherical inclusion within the neutrophil or lupus erythematosus (LE) cell.

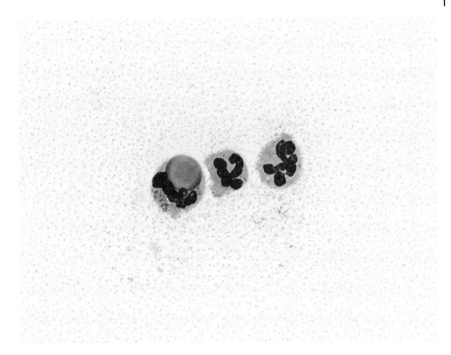

Figure 7.20 Synovial fluid, dog, 50× objective. Metastatic histiocytic sarcoma.

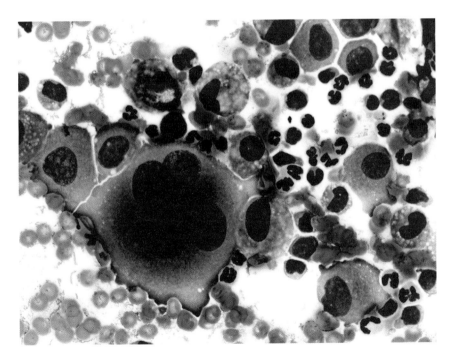

7.2.7.3 Prognosis
Poor.

7.2.8 Hemarthrosis

7.2.8.1 Cytologic Features
Erythrocytes within synovial fluid can pose a diagnostic challenge to distinguish between iatrogenic hemorrhage from sampling and true hemorrhage (hemarthrosis). Prior hemorrhage is confirmed by visualizing erythrophagia or heme-breakdown pigments within mononuclear cells (Figure 7.22). Iatrogenic hemorrhage is often associated with platelets [45].

7.2.8.2 Clinical Considerations
- DDx = iatrogenic, trauma, coagulopathy, neoplasia [45].
- Clearance of erythrocytes occurs quickly after the onset of hemorrhage [61].

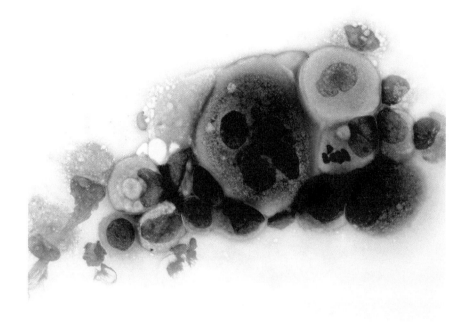

Figure 7.21 Synovial fluid, dog, 50× objective. Metastatic bronchogenic carcinoma.

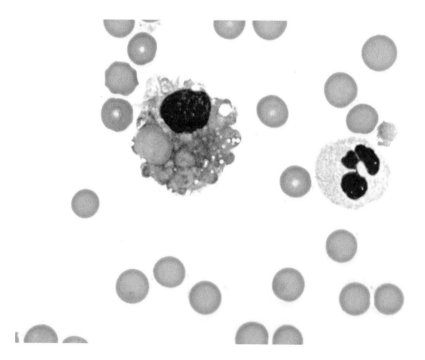

Figure 7.22 Synovial fluid, dog, 100× objective. Hemarthrosis. Note the blood in the background and the red blood cell phagocytosed by the macrophage.

7.2.8.3 Prognosis
Generally excellent.

7.2.9 Synovial Cyst

7.2.9.1 Cytologic Features
Synovial cysts frequently have a similar pink stippled, mucinous background to normal synovial fluid; however, a clear background may be present. Cellularity generally is low and comprises reactive macrophages/

synoviocytes. Cholesterol crystals may also be seen (Figure 7.23).

7.2.9.2 Clinical Considerations
- Fluid-filled, variably fluctuant lesions around joints.
- Unilateral elbow lesions most common in cats [62, 63].
- Chronic lesions often associated with underlying degenerative joint disease [62, 63].
- Often have acute onset in dogs and may be associated with trauma or underlying joint disease [64].

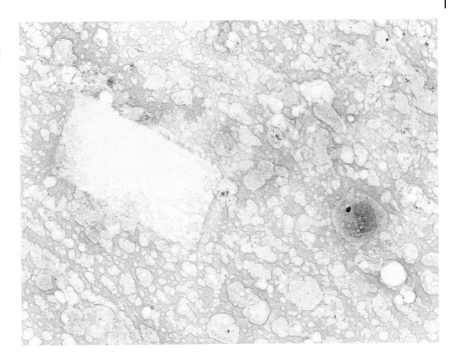

Figure 7.23 Synovial cyst, dog, 50× objective. Note the thick pink mucinous background, cholesterol crystal (left) and macrophage/synoviocyte (right).

7.2.9.3 Prognosis

Excellent. Recurrence is common with drainage [63]. Some cysts in cats may transform into synovial myxomas [62].

7.2.10 Synovial Cell Sarcoma

7.2.10.1 Cytologic Features

Synovial cell sarcomas frequently are associated with a thick, pink stippled background, and cells may be seen in a streaming or windrowing distribution. This can make differentiation from myxosarcomas difficult (compare to Figure 4.63). Cells are seen individually and in cohesive sheets, which may be intimately associated with capillaries [65]. They are polygonal to spindloid and have a moderate volume of medium-blue cytoplasm that forms bipolar tendrils and wisps and may contain fine pink granules or fine clear vacuoles. Nuclei are ovoid with coarsely granular chromatin and multiple, prominent, basophilic nucleoli (Figure 7.24). Anisocytosis/anisokaryosis are moderate and N/C ratios are high.

7.2.10.2 Clinical Considerations
- Dogs > > cats [66].
- More common in larger joints (particularly stifle) in middle-aged to older, large breed dogs [33].
- Locally aggressive and moderate metastatic potential (linked to tumor grade) with metastatic disease detected in ~25% of dogs at the time of diagnosis [33, 67].
- Bone involvement common in dogs, rare in cats [67, 68].

7.2.10.3 Prognosis

Variable, based on clinical stage and histologic grade. Complete surgical removal of tumors without metastatic disease can carry a good long-term prognosis [33, 67]. Metastatic disease at the time of diagnosis confers a poor prognosis.

7.2.11 Histiocytic Sarcoma (Periarticular)

7.2.11.1 Cytologic Features

Periarticular histiocytic sarcomas contain discrete cells with marked criteria of malignancy including anisokaryosis, karyomegaly, multinucleation, and high mitotic rates (Figure 7.25). Cells usually are vacuolated.

7.2.11.2 Clinical Considerations
- Most common synovial tumor in dogs [33].
- Bernese Mountain Dogs and Rottweilers appear to be predisposed [69].
- There is a relation between previous traumatic injury to joints (especially cranial cruciate ligament rupture) and the development of periarticular histiocytic sarcoma [33, 69, 70].

7.2.11.3 Prognosis

While prognosis is still poor even with therapy [71], periarticular histiocytic sarcoma appears to carry a better prognosis than non-periarticular sites, even in the presence of metastatic disease [72].

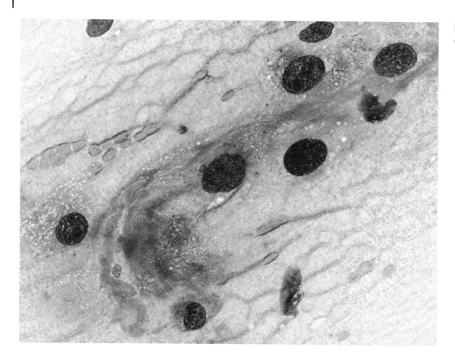

Figure 7.24 Synovial sarcoma, dog, 50× objective.

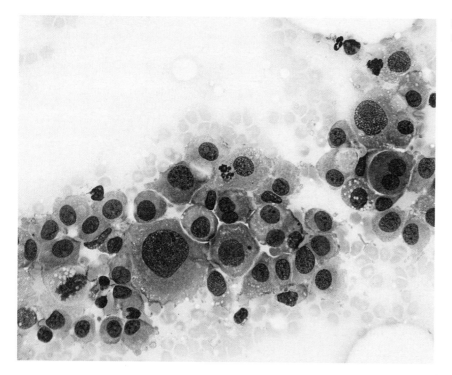

Figure 7.25 Periarticular histiocytic sarcoma, dog, 50× objective.

7.3 Muscle

7.3.1 Rhabdomyoma

7.3.1.1 Cytologic Features

Rhabdomyomas contain round to polygonal cells seen individually and in loose aggregates. They have abundant pale-blue cytoplasm that often has a faint pink granular appearance (due to abundant mitochondria) (Figure 7.26) and may contain cytoplasmic vacuolation [73, 74]. Nuclei are round, centrally located, and have coarsely granular chromatin with small, single nucleoli. Anisocytosis/ anisokaryosis are mild and N/C ratios are low.

7.3.1.2 Clinical Considerations

- Rare tumors. Dog > cat.
- Most commonly reported in the heart and larynx, as well as the tongue in dogs [73–76]. Reported on the pinna in cats [77].
- DDx = granular cell tumor, liposarcoma, balloon cell melanoma, and oncocytoma [74].

Figure 7.26 Rhabdomyoma, dog larynx, 50× objective. Note the faint pink granular appearance of the cytoplasm of some cells.

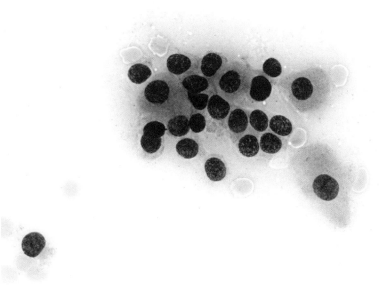

7.3.1.3 Prognosis

Good. Dogs with laryngeal rhabdomyomas have long survival times, with no evidence of recurrence or metastatic disease [73].

7.3.2 Rhabdomyosarcoma

7.3.2.1 Cytologic Features

Cytologic appearance of rhabdomyosarcomas is highly variable based on the degree of differentiation of the cells. Rhabdomyoblasts (in embryonal rhabdomyosarcomas) are round, individualized cells with a small volume of medium-blue cytoplasm that contains fine clear vacuoles. Nuclei frequently are indented or bilobed (Figure 7.27). These rhabdomyoblasts may be difficult to differentiate from lymphoma (see Chapter 5). More differentiated rhabdomyosarcomas have a polygonal appearance with abundant medium-blue cytoplasm that may have fine pink granules (Figure 7.28) and perinuclear clearing (Figure 7.29). Nuclei are ovoid and have prominent single nucleoli. Linear cells with nuclei in rows (strap cells) and cytoplasmic striations may be seen in very well-differentiated tumors.

7.3.2.2 Clinical Considerations

- Rare tumors. Dogs > cats.
- Often affects younger patients [78, 79].
- Mostly single but may be multiple masses [80, 81].
- Predilection sites = oral cavity, urinary bladder, vagina, skin, and retrobulbar [78, 80, 82, 83].
- Locally invasive with moderate to high metastatic potential (regional lymph nodes, lungs, spleen) [78]. Local recurrence may occur [80, 82].

7.3.2.3 Prognosis

Variable. Metastatic disease confers a poor prognosis and is often associated with short survival times [78]. Embryonal variants appear to have a more aggressive clinical course [78, 79]. Prolonged survival is possible in the absence of metastatic disease, even with recurrence of the tumor [82].

7.3.3 Leiomyoma

7.3.3.1 Cytologic Features

Leiomyomas exfoliate variably well and comprise well-differentiated spindle cells seen individually and in aggregates. The cells have a scant volume of pale cytoplasm forming bipolar tendrils and wisps, and elongated nuclei with finely granular chromatin and small basophilic nucleoli (Figure 7.30). Anisocytosis/anisokaryosis are mild and N/C ratios are high. May look similar to fibromas or gastrointestinal stromal tumors (compare to Figures 4.52 and 9.17).

7.3.3.2 Clinical Considerations

- Benign neoplasms of smooth muscle origin in dogs and cats.
- Predilection sites = vagina, uterus, gastrointestinal tract, and gall bladder [84–86].
- Usually small, solitary, and well-encapsulated. Vaginal leiomyomas often are pedunculated.
- May be associated with paraneoplastic hypercalcemia [87].

7.3.3.3 Prognosis

Excellent. Vaginal leiomyomas may spontaneously regress after ovariohysterectomy [88].

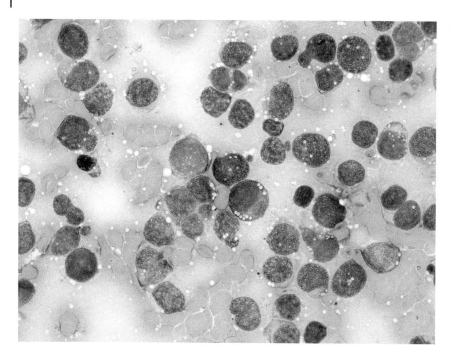

Figure 7.27 Rhabdomyosarcoma (embryonal), dog, 50× objective.

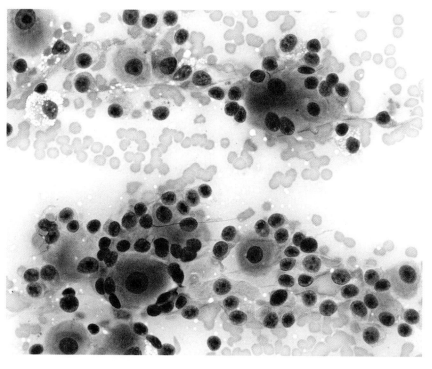

Figure 7.28 Rhabdomyosarcoma (differentiated), dog, 20× objective. Note the faint pink granular appearance of the cytoplasm and the prominent single nucleoli.

7.3.4 Leiomyosarcoma

7.3.4.1 Cytologic Features

Leiomyosarcomas exfoliate variably well in loose aggregates and individually. They comprise plump spindle cells with a moderate volume of medium-blue cytoplasm forming short bipolar tapering ends and may contain fine clear vacuoles. Nuclei are ovoid with coarsely granular chromatin and prominent basophilic nucleoli. Anisocytosis/ anisokaryosis are variable and N/C ratios are moderate to high (Figure 7.31).

7.3.4.2 Clinical Considerations

- Malignant tumors arising from smooth muscle cells.
- Older dogs and cats.
- Predilection sites = gastrointestinal tract (see Chapter 9) > spleen, genitourinary tract, liver, blood vessel walls, and subcutaneous tissues [84, 89–92].

Figure 7.29 Rhabdomyosarcoma (differentiated), dog, 50× objective. Many cells have a faint pink granular appearance to their cytoplasm.

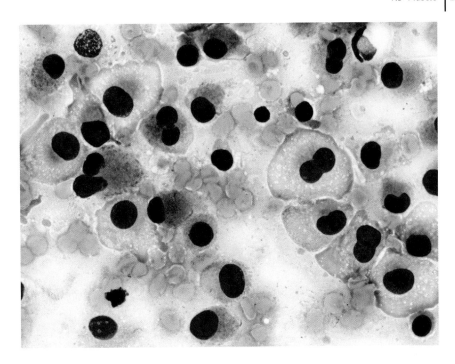

Figure 7.30 Leiomyoma, dog, vagina, 50× objective.

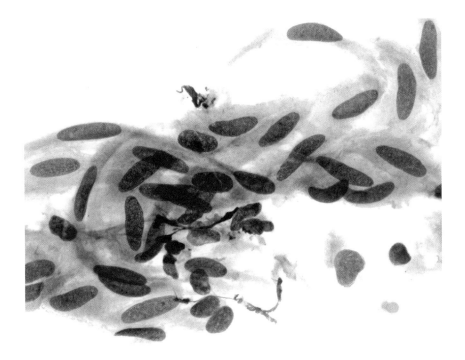

- May be associated with paraneoplastic syndromes such as hypoglycemia and nephrogenic diabetes insipidus [89].

7.3.4.3 Prognosis

Variable, based on location. Neoplasms in the liver have a grave prognosis, with 100% metastatic rate [90]. The metastatic rate for other abdominal locations is approximately 50%, and dermal tumors are not reported to metastasize [89, 93]. Surgical excision may be curative, and moderate to long-term survival is possible with surgical removal, even with concurrent metastatic disease [89].

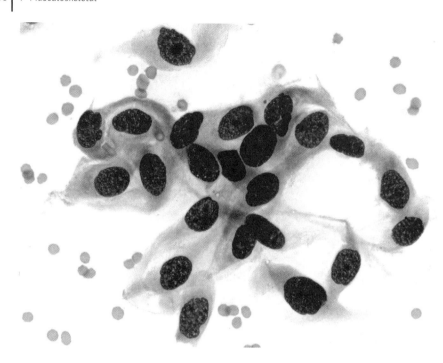

Figure 7.31 Leiomyosarcoma, cat, stomach, 50× objective.

References

1 Fiani, N., Arzi, B., Johnson, E.G., *et al.* (2011) Osteoma of the oral and maxillofacial regions in cats: 7 cases (1999–2009). *J. Am. Vet. Med. Assoc.*, **238** (11), 1470–1475.

2 Volker, M.K., Luskin, I.R. (2014) Oral osteoma in 6 dogs. *J. Vet. Dent.*, **31** (2), 88–91.

3 Haynes, K.H., Cavanaugh, R.P., Steinheimer, D. (2012) What is your diagnosis? Osteoma in a cat. *J. Am. Vet. Med. Assoc.*, **241** (11), 1433–1444.

4 Jabara, A.G., Paton, J.S. (1984) Extraskeletal osteoma in a cat. *Aust. Vet. J.*, **61** (12), 405–407.

5 Maas, C.P.H.J., Theyse, L.F.H. (2007) Temperomandibular joint ankylosis in cats and dogs. A report of 10 cases. *Vet. Comp. Orthop. Traumatol.*, **20** (3), 192–197.

6 Beck, J., Ren, L., Huang, S., *et al.* (2022) Canine and murine models of osteosarcoma. *Vet. Pathol.*, **59** (3), 399–414.

7 Spodnick, G.J., Berg, J., Rand, W.M., *et al.* (1992) Prognosis for dogs with appendicular osteosarcoma treated by amputation alone: 162 cases (1978–1988). *J. Am. Vet. Med. Assoc.*, **200** (7), 995–999.

8 Knecht, C.D., Priester, W.A. (1978) Musculoskeletal tumors in dogs. *J. Am. Vet. Med. Assoc.*, **172** (1), 72–74.

9 Burton, A.G., Johnson, E.G., Vernau, W., *et al.* (2015) Implant-associated neoplasia in dogs: 16 cases (1983–2013). *J. Am. Vet. Med. Assoc.*, **247** (7), 778–785.

10 Hillers, K.R., Dernell, W.S., Lafferty, M.H., *et al.* (2005) Incidence and prognostic importance of lymph node metastases in dogs with appendicular osteosarcoma: 228 cases (1986–2003). *J. Am. Vet. Med. Assoc.*, **226** (8), 1364–1367.

11 Barger, A., Graca, R., Bailey, K., *et al.* (2005) Use of alkaline phosphatase staining to differentiate canine osteosarcoma from other vimentin-positive tumors. *Vet. Pathol.*, **42** (2). 161–165.

12 Ryseff, J.K., Bohn, A.A. (2012) Detection of alkaline phosphatase in canine cells previously stained with Wright-Giemsa and its utility in differentiating osteosarcoma from other mesenchymal tumors. *Vet. Clin. Pathol.*, **41** (3), 391–395.

13 Szewczyk, M., Lechowski, R., Zabielska, K. (2015) What do we know about canine osteosarcoma treatment? Review. *Vet. Res. Commun.*, **39** (1), 61–67.

14 Boerman, I., Selvarajah, G.T., Nielen, M., *et al.* (2012) Prognostic factors in canine appendicular osteosarcoma – a meta-analysis. *BMC Vet. Res.*, 8, 56. doi: 10.1186/1746-6148-8-56. Last accessed May 1, 2017.

15 Nakano, Y., Kagawa, Y., Shimoyama, Y., *et al.* (2021) Outcome of appendicular or scapular osteosarcoma treated by limb amputation in cats: 67 cases (1997–2018). *J. Am. Vet. Med. Assoc.*, **260** (S1), S24–S28.

16 Liptak, J.M., Dernell, W.S., Ehrhart, N., *et al.* (2004) Canine appendicular osteosarcoma: diagnosis and palliative treatment. *Compend. Contin. Educ. Pract. Vet.*, **26**, 172–183.

17 Liptak, J.M., Thatcher, G.P., Mestrinho, L.A., *et al.* (2021) Outcomes of cats treated with maxillectomy: 60 cases. A

Veterinary Society of Surgical Oncology retrospective study. *Vet. Comp. Oncol.*, **19** (4), 641–650.

18 Durham, A.C., Popovitch, C.A., Goldschmidt, M.H. (2008) Feline chondrosarcoma: a retrospective study of 67 cats (1987–2005). *J. Am. Anim. Hosp. Assoc.*, **44** (3), 124–130.

19 Sones, E., Smith, A., Schleis, S., *et al.* (2013) Survival times for canine intranasal sarcomas treated with radiation therapy: 86 cases (1996–2011). *Vet. Radiol. Ultrasound*, **54** (2), 194–201.

20 Vinayak, A., Worley, D.R., Withrow, S.J., *et al.* (2018) Dedifferentiated chondrosarcoma in the dog and cat: a case series and review of the literature. *J. Am. Anim. Hosp. Assoc.*, **54** (1), 50–59.

21 Waltman, S.S., Seguin, B., Cooper, B.J., *et al.* (2007) Clinical outcome of non-nasal chondrosarcoma in dogs: thirty-one cases (1986–2003). *Vet. Surg.*, **36** (3), 266–271.

22 Holmes, M.E., Keyerleber, M.A., Faissler, D. (2019) Prolonged survival after craniectomy with skull reconstruction and adjuvant definitive radiation therapy in three dogs with multilobular osteochondrosarcoma. *Vet. Radiol. Ultrasound*, **60** (4), 447–455.

23 Webb, J.A., Liptak, J.M., Hewitt, S.A., *et al.* Multilobular osteochondrosarcoma of the os penis in a dog. *Can. Vet. J.*, **50** (1), 81–84.

24 Dernell, W.S., Straw, R.C., Cooper, M.F., *et al.* (1998) Multilobular osteochondrosarcoma in 39 dogs: 1979–1993. *J. Am. Anim. Hosp. Assoc.*, **34** (1), 11–18.

25 Liu, S.-K., Dorfman, H.D., Hurvitz, A.I., *et al.* (1977) Primary and secondary bone tumours in the dog. *J. Small Anim. Pract.*, **18** (5), 313–326.

26 Agnoli, C., Sabattini, S., Ubiali, A., *et al.* (2023) A retrospective study on bone metastasis in dogs with advanced-stage solid cancer. *J. Small Anim. Pract.*, **64** (9), 561–567.

27 Hidaka, Y., Hagio, M., Uchida, K., *et al.* (2006) Primary hemangiosarcoma of the humerus in a Maltese dog. *J. Vet. Med. Sci.*, **66** (8), 895–898.

28 Giuffrida, M.A., Kamstock, D.A., Selmic, L.E., *et al.* (2018) Primary appendicular hemangiosarcoma and telangiectatic osteosarcoma in 70 dogs: a Veterinary Society of Surgical Oncology retrospective study. *Vet. Surg.*, **47** (6), 774–783.

29 Upchurch, D.A., Saile, K., Rademacher, N. (2014) What is your diagnosis? Medullary fibrosarcoma with cortical bone destruction. *J. Am. Vet. Med. Assoc.*, **244** (5), 531–533.

30 Trost, M.E., Inkelmann, M.A., Galiza, G.J., *et al.* (2014) Occurrence of tumors metastatic to bones and multicentric tumors with skeletal involvement in dogs. *J. Comp. Pathol.*, **150** (1), 8–17.

31 Wesselhoeft-Albin, L.A., Berg, J., Schelling, S.H. (1991) Fibrosarcoma of the canine appendicular skeleton. *J. Am. Anim. Hosp. Assoc.*, **27**, 303–309.

32 Schultz, R.M., Puchalski, S.M., Kent, M., *et al.* (2007) Skeletal lesions of histiocytic sarcoma in nineteen dogs. *Vet. Radiol. Ultrasound*, **48** (6), 539–543.

33 Craig, L.E., Julian, M.E., Ferracone, J.D. (2002) The diagnosis and prognosis of synovial tumors in dogs: 35 cases. *Vet. Pathol.*, **39** (1), 66–73.

34 Matus, R.E., Leifer, C.E., MacEwen, E.G., *et al.* (1986) Prognostic factors for multiple myeloma in the dog. *J. Am. Vet. Med. Assoc.*, **188** (11), 1288–1292.

35 Patel, R.T., Caceres, A., French, A.F., *et al.* (2005) Multiple myeloma in 16 cats: a retrospective study. *Vet. Clin. Pathol.*, **34** (4), 341–352.

36 Hanna, F. (2005) Multiple myelomas in cats. *J. Feline Med. Surg.*, **7** (5), 275–287.

37 Cooley, D.M., Waters, D.J. (1998) Skeletal metastasis as the initial clinical manifestation of metastatic carcinoma in 19 dogs. *J. Vet. Intern. Med.*, **12** (4), 288–293.

38 Renzi, A., Sabattini, S., D'Annunzio, G., *et al.* (2023) Multiorgan metastases with massive bone involvement of a medullary thyroid carcinoma in a dog. *Vet. Clin. Pathol.*, **52** (2), 341–345.

39 Bubenik, L.J. (2005) Infections of the skeletal system. *Vet. Clin. North Am. Small Anim. Pract.*, **35** (5), 1093–1109.

40 Bergh, M.S., Peirone, B. (2012) Complications of tibial plateau leveling osteotomy in dogs. *Vet. Comp. Orthop. Traumatol.*, **25** (5), 349–358.

41 Gieling, F., Peters, S., Erichsen, C., *et al.* (2019) Bacterial osteomyelitis in veterinary orthopaedics: pathophysiology, clinical presentation and advances in treatment across multiple species. *Vet. J.*, **250**, 44–54.

42 Muir, P., Johnson, K.A. (1992) Anaerobic bacteria isolated from osteomyelitis in dogs and cats. *Vet. Surg.*, **21** (6), 463–466.

43 Hakamata, M., Kano, R., Kondo, H., *et al.* (2019) Canine fungal osteomyelitis. *Mycopathologica*, **184** (5), 707–708.

44 Mamone, C.M., Rademacher, N., Grooters, A.M., *et al.* (2014) What is your diagnosis? Fungal osteomyelitis. *J. Am. Vet. Med. Assoc.*, **244** (12), 1373–1375.

45 MacWilliams, P.S., Friedrichs, K.R. (2003) Laboratory evaluation and interpretation of synovial fluid. *Vet. Clin. North Am. Small Anim. Pract.*, **33** (1), 153–178.

46 Pacchiana, P.D., Gilley, R.S., Wallace, L.J., *et al.* (2004) Absolute and relative cell counts for synovial fluid from clinically normal shoulder and stifle joints in cats. *J. Am. Vet. Med. Assoc.*, **225** (12), 1866–1870.

47 Lewis, D.D., Goring, R.L., Parker, R.B., *et al.* (1987) A comparison of diagnostic methods used in the evaluation of early degenerative joint disease in the dog. *J. Am. Anim. Hosp. Assoc.*, **23** (3), 305–315.

48 Phillips, T.F., Bleyaert, H.F. (2022) Retrospective evaluation of 103 cases of septic arthritis in dogs. *Vet. Rec.*, **190** (5), e938.

49 Lemetayer, J., Taylor, S. (2014) Inflammatory joint disease in cats: diagnostic approach and treatment. *J. Feline Med. Surg.*, **16** (7), 547–562.

50 Scharf, V.F., Lewis, S.T., Wellehan, J.F., *et al.* (2015) Retrospective evaluation of the efficacy of isolating bacteria from synovial fluid in dogs with suspected septic arthritis. *Aust. Vet. J.*, **93** (6), 200–203.

51 Fitch, R.B., Hogan, T.C., Kudnig, S.T. (2003) Hematogenous septic arthritis in the dog: results of five patients treated nonsurgically with antibiotics. *J. Am. Anim. Hosp. Assoc.*, **39** (6), 563–566.

52 Clements, D.N., Owen, M.R., Mosley, J.R., *et al.* (2005) Retrospective study of bacterial infective arthritis in 31 dogs. *J. Small Anim. Pract.*, **46** (4), 171–176.

53 Marchevsky, A.M., Read, R.A. (1999) Bacterial septic arthritis in 19 dogs. *Aust. Vet. J.*, **77** (4), 233–237.

54 Allison, R.W., Little, S.E. (2013) Diagnosis of rickettsial diseases in dogs and cats. *Vet. Clin. Pathol.*, **42** (2), 127–144.

55 Theodorou, K., Leontides, L., Siarkou, V.I., *et al.* (2015) Synovial fluid cytology in experimental acute canine monocytic ehrlichiosis (*Ehrlichia canis*). *Vet. Microbiol.*, **177** (1–2), 224–227.

56 Rondeau, M.P., Walton, R.M., Bissett, S., *et al.* (2005) Suppurative, nonseptic, polyarthropathy in dogs. *J. Vet. Intern. Med.*, **19** (5), 654–662.

57 Shaughnessy, M.L., Sample, S.J., Abicht, C., *et al.* (2016) Clinical features and pathological joint changes in dogs with erosive immune-mediated polyarthritis: 13 cases (2004–2012). *J. Am. Vet. Med. Assoc.*, **249** (10), 1156–1164.

58 Rhoades, A.C., Vernau, W., Kass, P.H., *et al.* (2016) Comparison of the efficacy of prednisone and cyclosporine for treatment of dogs with primary immune-mediated polyarthritis. *J. Am. Vet. Med. Assoc.*, **248** (4), 395–404.

59 Smee, N.M., Harkin, K.R., Wilkerson, M.J. (2007) Measurement of serum antinuclear antibody titer in dogs with and without systemic lupus erythematosus: 120 cases (1997–2005). *J. Am. Vet. Med. Assoc.*, **230** (8), 1180–1183.

60 Colledge, S.L., Raskin, R.E., Messick, J.B., *et al.* (2013) Multiple joint metastasis of a transitional cell carcinoma in a dog. *Vet. Clin. Pathol.*, **42** (2), 216–220.

61 Jansen, N.W., Roosendaal, G., Wenting, M.J., *et al.* (2009) Very rapid clearance after a joint bleed in the canine knee cannot prevent adverse effects on cartilage and synovial tissue. *Osteoarthr. Cartil.*, **17** (4), 433–440.

62 Craig, L.E., Krimer, P.M., O'Toole, A.D. (2020) Synovial cysts and myxomas in 16 cats. *Vet. Pathol.*, **57** (4), 554–558.

63 Kligman, K.C., Kim, S.E., Winter, M.D., *et al.* (2009) What is your diagnosis? Synovial cysts. *J. Am. Vet. Med. Assoc.*, **235** (8), 945–946.

64 Franklin, A.D., Havlicek, M., Krockenberger, M.B. (2011) Stifle synovial cyst in a Labrador Retriever with concurrent cranial cruciate ligament deficiency. *Vet. Comp. Orthop. Traumatol.*, **24** (2), 157–160.

65 Monti, P., Barnes, D., Adrian, A.M., *et al.* (2018) Synovial cell sarcoma in a dog: a misnomer – cytologic and histologic findings and review of the literature. *Vet. Clin. Pathol.*, **47** (2), 181–185.

66 Cazzini, P., Frontera-Acevedo, K., Garner, B., *et al.* (2015) Morphologic, molecular, and ultrastructural characterization of a feline synovial cell sarcoma and derived cell line. *J. Vet. Diagn. Investig.*, **27** (3), 369–376.

67 Vail, D.M., Powers, B.E., Getzy, D.M., *et al.* (1994) Evaluation of prognostic factors for dogs with synovial sarcoma: 36 cases (1986–1991). *J. Am. Vet. Med. Assoc.*, **205** (9), 1300–1307.

68 Liptak, J.M., Withrow, S.J., Macy, D.W., *et al.* (2004) Metastatic synovial cell sarcoma in two cats. *Vet. Comp. Oncol.*, **2** (3), 164–170.

69 Manor, E.K., Craig, L.E., Sun, X., *et al.* (2018) Prior joint disease is associated with increased risk of periarticular histiocytic sarcoma in dogs. *Vet. Comp. Oncol.*, **16** (1), E83–E88.

70 van Kuijk, L., van Ginkel, K., de Vos, J.P., *et al.* (2013) Peri-articular histiocytic sarcoma and previous joint disease in Bernese Mountain Dogs. *J. Vet. Intern. Med.*, **27** (2), 293–299.

71 Marconato, L., Sabattini, S., Buchholz, J., *et al.* (2020) Outcome comparison between radiation therapy and surgery as primary treatment for dogs with periarticular histiocytic sarcoma: an Italian Society of Veterinary Oncology study. *Vet. Comp. Oncol.*, **18** (4), 778–786.

72 Klahn, S.L., Kitchell, B.E., Dervisis, N.G. (2011) Evaluation and comparison of outcomes in dogs with periarticular and nonperiarticular histiocytic sarcoma. *J. Am. Vet. Med. Assoc.*, **239** (1), 90–96.

73 Meuten, D.J., Calderwood Mays, M.B., Dillman, R.C., *et al.* (1985) Canine laryngeal rhabdomyoma. *Vet. Pathol.*, **22** (6), 533–539.

74 Sebastian, K.N., Magestro, L., Kiupel, M., *et al.* (2021) What is your diagnosis? Lingual mass aspirate from a dog. *Vet. Clin. Pathol.*, **50** (4), 615–617.

75 Radi, Z.A., Metz, A. (2009) Canine cardiac rhabdomyoma. *Toxicol. Pathol.*, **37** (3), 348–350.

76 Dunbar, M.D., Ginn, P., Winter, M., *et al.* (2012) Laryngeal rhabdomyoma in a dog. *Vet. Clin. Pathol.*, **41** (4), 590–593.

77 Roth, L. (1990) Rhabdomyoma of the ear pinna in four cats. *J. Comp. Pathol.*, **103** (2), 237–240.

78 Connell, D.R., Rodriguez, C.O. Jr., Sternberg, R.A., *et al.* (2020) Biological behavior and ezrin expression in canine rhabdomyosarcomas: 25 cases (1990–2012). *Vet. Comp. Oncol.*, **18** (4), 675–682.

79 Miller, A.D., Steffey, M., Alcaraz, A., *et al.* (2009) Embryonal rhabdomyosarcoma in a young Maine coon cat. *J. Am. Anim. Hosp. Assoc.*, **45** (1), 43–47.

80 Brockus, C.W., Myers, R.K. (2004) Multifocal rhabdomyosarcomas within the tongue and oral cavity of a dog. *Vet. Pathol.*, **41** (3), 273–274.

81 Spugnini, E.P., Filipponi, M., Romani, L., *et al.* (2010) Electrochemotherapy treatment for bilateral pleomorphic rhabdomyosarcoma in a cat. *J. Small Anim. Pract.*, **51** (6), 330–332.

82 Avallone, G., Pinto da Cunha, N., Palmieri, C., *et al.* (2010) Subcutaneous embryonal rhabdomyosarcoma in a dog: cytologic, immunocytochemical, histologic, and ultrastructural features. *Vet. Clin. Pathol.*, **39** (4), 499–504.

83 Kuwamura, M., Yoshida, H., Yamate, J., *et al.* (1998) Urinary bladder rhabdomyosarcoma (sarcoma botryoides) in a young Newfoundland dog. *J. Vet. Med. Sci.*, **60** (5), 619–621.

84 Avallone, G., Pelligrino, V., Muscatello, L.V., *et al.* (2022) Canine smooth muscle tumors: a clinicopathological study. *Vet. Pathol.*, **59** (2), 244–255.

85 Ogden, J.A., Selmic, L.E., Liptak, J.M., *et al.* (2020) Outcomes associated with vaginectomy and vulvovaginectomy in 21 dogs. *Vet. Surg.*, **49** (6), 1132–1143.

86 MacLeod, A.N., Reichle, J.K., Szabo, D., *et al.* (2023) Ultrasonographic appearance of gall bladder neoplasia in 14 dogs and 1 cat. *Vet. Radiol. Ultrasound*, **64** (3), 537–545.

87 Stiver, S., Laukkanen, C., Luong, R. (2019) Suspected hypercalcemia of benignancy associated with canine vaginal leiomyoma. *J. Am. Anim. Hosp. Assoc.*, **55** (2), e55205. doi: 10.5326/JAAHA-MS-6828. Last accessed October 15, 2023.

88 Sathya, S., Linn, K. (2014) Regression of a vaginal leiomyoma after ovariohysterectomy in a dog: a case report. *J. Am. Anim. Hosp. Assoc.*, **50** (6), 424–428.

89 Cohen, M., Post, G.S., Wright, J.C. (2003) Gastrointestinal leiomyosarcoma in 14 dogs. *J. Vet. Intern. Med.*, **17** (1), 107–110.

90 Kapatkin, A.S., Mullen, H.S., Matthiesen, D.T., *et al.* (1992) Leiomyosarcoma in dogs: 44 cases (1983–1988). *J. Am. Vet. Med. Assoc.*, **201** (7), 1077–1079.

91 Miller, M.A., Ramos-Vara, J.A., Dickerson, M.F., *et al.* (2003) Uterine neoplasia in 13 cats. *J. Vet. Diagn. Investig.*, **15** (6), 515–522.

92 Brady, R.V., Rebhun, R.B., Skorupski, K.A., *et al.* (2022) Retrospective immunohistochemical investigation of suspected non-visceral leiomyosarcoma in dogs. *J. Vet. Diagn. Investig.*, **34** (3), 465–473.

93 Liu, S.M., Mikaelian, I. (2003) Cutaneous smooth muscle tumors in the dog and cat. *Vet. Pathol.*, **40** (6), 685–692.

8

Hepatobiliary

8.1 Liver

8.1.1 Normal Hepatocytes

8.1.1.1 Cytologic Appearance
Normal hepatocytes may exfoliate in large numbers, unlike cells from many other normal tissues. They are seen mostly in cohesive sheets and have a large volume of pale-blue cytoplasm. The cytoplasm may contain lipofuscin pigment, especially in older patients (see Section 8.1.15). Nuclei are round, centrally located, and have granular to reticulated chromatin with single, prominent, centrally located nucleoli. Anisocytosis/anisokaryosis are mild (Figure 8.1). Binucleation may be seen in low numbers of cells, especially in older patients [1]. Rectangular, crystalline nuclear inclusions may also be seen and are of no clinical significance (Figure 8.2).

8.1.2 Vacuolar Hepatopathy (Non-lipid)

8.1.2.1 Cytologic Appearance
Accumulation of glycogen or water in the cytoplasm of hepatocytes gives them a lacy/feathery/rarefied vacuolar appearance with poorly defined areas of clearing (Figure 8.3). Nuclei mostly stay centrally placed.

8.1.2.2 Clinical Considerations
- Dogs > cats.
- Most commonly associated with exposure to exogenous or endogenous corticosteroids (steroid hepatopathy) [2].
- Also nonspecific change with hepatocellular damage (hypoxia, drug/toxin exposure, inflammation, proliferation, and acute liver failure) [3, 4].
- Lack of changes in cytology samples does not preclude underlying vacuolar hepatopathy [5].

8.1.2.3 Prognosis
Generally good, but variable based on the underlying cause.

8.1.3 Vacuolar Hepatopathy (Lipid)

8.1.3.1 Cytologic Appearance
Lipid appears as coarse, clear vacuoles of varying size within the cytoplasm. Small numbers may be present, or (as in feline hepatic lipidosis) they may be abundant and distend the cytoplasm of hepatocytes, pushing the nuclei to the periphery and making hepatocytes almost unrecognizable (Figures 8.4 and 8.5).

8.1.3.2 Clinical Considerations
- Small lipid vacuoles may represent a nonspecific marker of hepatocellular dysfunction.
- Cats > dogs.
- Feline hepatic lipidosis:
  - Overweight/obese cats at increased risk.
  - Disease preceded by inappetence/anorexia and may be associated with many underlying conditions [6].
  - Associated with increased liver enzymes; however, GGT is commonly within the reference interval [7].
- Often seen in dogs with acute liver failure [4].

8.1.3.3 Prognosis
Variable, based on the presence of underlying disease. Recovery rates can be high in primary feline hepatic lipidosis with appropriate therapy, especially when treated early [7, 8].

8.1.4 Nodular Hyperplasia

8.1.4.1 Cytologic Appearance
Hepatocytes in nodular hyperplastic lesions may be indistinguishable from normal cells (or even hepatomas; see Section 8.1.5), and histopathology is required for definitive characterization. Mild crowding of cells can be seen, and mild, non-lipid vacuolar changes frequently are present multifocally (Figure 8.6).

Clinical Atlas of Small Animal Cytology and Hematology, Second Edition. Andrew G. Burton.
© 2024 John Wiley & Sons, Inc. Published 2024 by John Wiley & Sons, Inc.

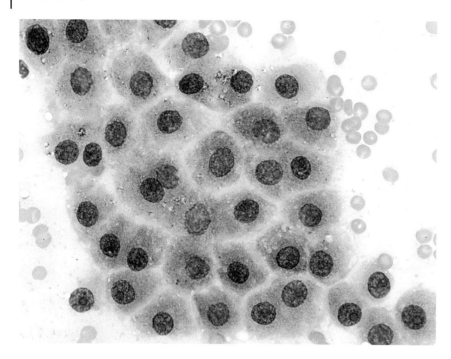

Figure 8.1 Normal hepatocytes, dog, 50× objective.

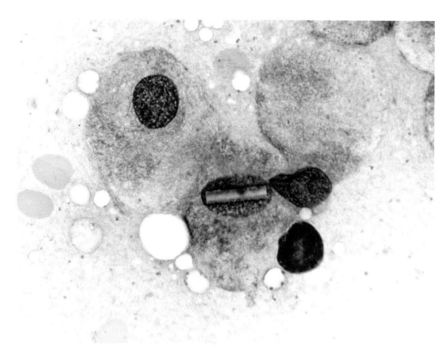

Figure 8.2 Normal hepatocytes, dog, 100× objective. Note the rectangular crystalline structure within the nucleus.

8.1.4.2 Clinical Considerations

- Older dogs > cats [9, 10].
- May be single, but usually multiple, small (typically 2–3 cm or less), well-demarcated nodules.
- There is a good correlation between cytologic and histopathologic analysis of hepatic masses, particularly benign processes such as nodular hyperplasia [11].

8.1.4.3 Prognosis

Excellent.

8.1.5 Hepatoma

8.1.5.1 Cytologic Appearance

Hepatomas comprise sheets of well-differentiated hepatocytes; however, relative to normal hepatocytes, they frequently have a mildly decreased volume of cytoplasm

Figure 8.3 Non-lipid (glycogen) vacuolar hepatopathy, dog, 50× objective.

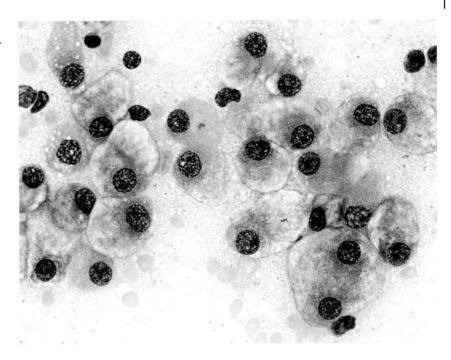

Figure 8.4 Hepatic lipidosis, cat, 20× objective.

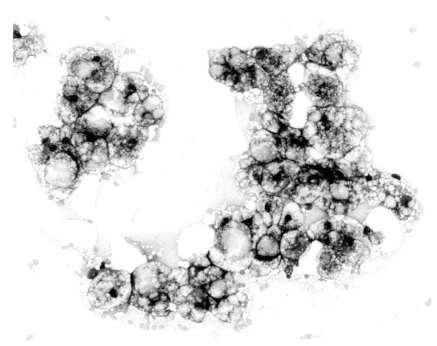

that is more basophilic and may have non-lipid vacuolar changes (Figure 8.7). There is an increasing degree of anisocytosis/anisokaryosis and cell piling relative to normal cells and those in nodular hyperplastic nodules.

8.1.5.2 Clinical Considerations

- Usually a single mass (compared to nodular hyperplasia) involving one liver lobe and often large (ranging from 2 to >10 cm).

- More common than hepatocellular carcinomas (HCCs) [12].
- Malignant transformation to well-differentiated HCC may occur [13].
- Histopathology is required for further characterization, especially to differentiate from well-differentiated HCCs (see Section 8.1.7).

8.1.5.3 Prognosis

Excellent.

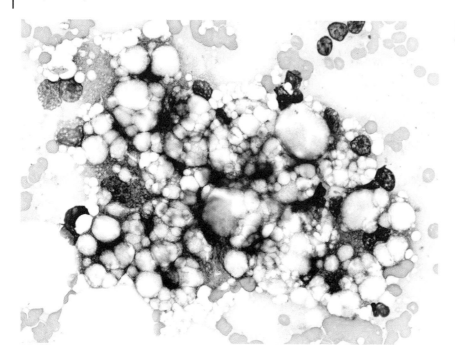

Figure 8.5 Hepatic lipidosis, cat, 50× objective.

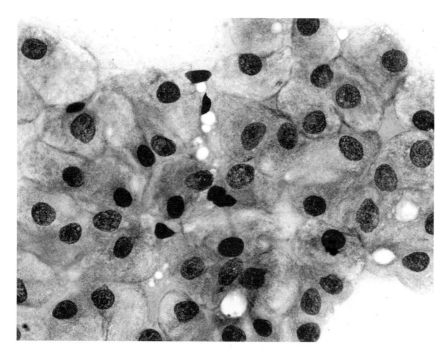

Figure 8.6 Liver, dog, 50× objective. Nodular hyperplasia.

8.1.6 Hepatocellular Carcinomas

The morphologic appearance of hepatocytes in HCC is highly variable. While highly anaplastic tumors are readily diagnosed as malignant, well-differentiated variants can be difficult to distinguish from benign processes, even with histopathology. The two ends of this diagnostic spectrum are discussed separately below to highlight morphologic and prognostic differences.

8.1.7 Hepatocellular Carcinoma (Well-differentiated)

8.1.7.1 Cytologic Appearance

Well-differentiated HCCs comprise sheets of well-differentiated hepatocytes that can be difficult to distinguish from hepatomas/nodular hyperplasia. Cytologic features reported to be useful in differentiating these from benign lesions include individualized hepatocytes, acinar or palisading arrangement of cells, and the presence of

Figure 8.7 Hepatoma, dog, 50× objective.

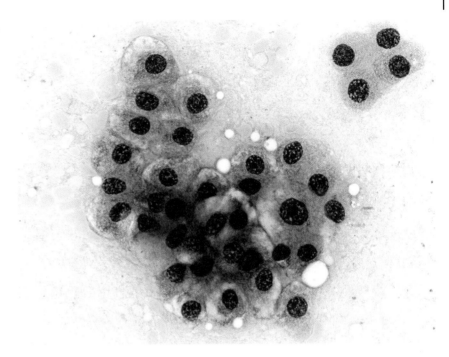

capillaries [14]. When comparing these tumors to hepatomas, the cells frequently have higher N/C ratios and a greater degree of anisocytosis/anisokaryosis (compare Figures 8.8 and 8.9 with 8.7).

8.1.7.2 Clinical Considerations
- Mostly associated with a trabecular subtype of HCC and grossly appear as well-circumscribed, single lesions [3].
- May rupture and cause hemoabdomen [15].

8.1.7.3 Prognosis
Good. Well-differentiated HCCs are almost always associated with solitary lesions that have low metastatic potential [16]. Lymphopenia may be associated with reduced survival [17].

8.1.8 Hepatocellular Carcinoma (High-grade)

8.1.8.1 Cytologic Appearance
Anaplastic or high-grade HCCs comprise highly pleomorphic hepatocytes that frequently are seen individually or are only loosely cohesive. They have a decreased volume of more deeply basophilic cytoplasm (high N/C ratios) and large nuclei with marked criteria of malignancy including anisokaryosis, karyomegaly, and multiple basophilic nucleoli of varying size and shape (Figure 8.10).

8.1.8.2 Clinical Considerations
- Three morphologic types exist: massive, nodular, and diffuse, in decreasing order of frequency [16, 18].

- Nodular and diffuse forms are more likely to have an anaplastic morphology and a poor prognosis [18].
- The left liver lobes are more commonly affected by massive HCC than the right lobes [16, 18, 19].
- Elevated ALT and AST may be seen and if present confer a poorer prognosis and may indicate tumor recurrence [18, 19].

8.1.8.3 Prognosis
Surgical excision for massive HCC in dogs provides excellent long-term control, whereas dogs treated conservatively had short survival times and were 15.4-fold more likely to die of tumor-related disease [19]. The prognosis for nodular and diffuse forms is poor due to a lack of resectability and a high metastatic potential [16, 20].

8.1.9 Carcinoid (Hepatic)

8.1.9.1 Cytologic Appearance
Carcinoids have a classic neuroendocrine appearance, with sheets of epithelial cells that have poorly defined intercellular borders. They have a moderate volume of pale-blue cytoplasm and round nuclei with finely stippled chromatin and variably prominent, single nucleoli. Anisocytosis/anisokaryosis typically are mild to moderate (Figure 8.11).

8.1.9.2 Clinical Considerations
- Rare tumors in dogs and cats [16, 21].
- Tend to occur at a younger age relative to other hepatobiliary neoplasms.

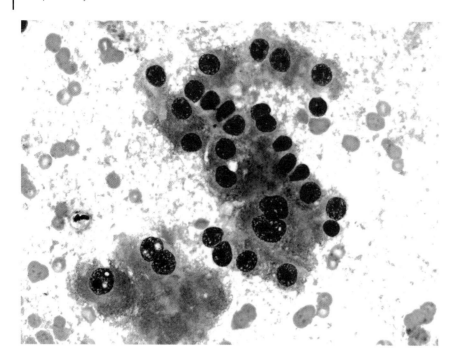

Figure 8.8 Hepatocellular carcinoma (well differentiated), dog, 50× objective. The hepatocytes have higher N/C ratios and moderate anisocytosis/anisokaryosis.

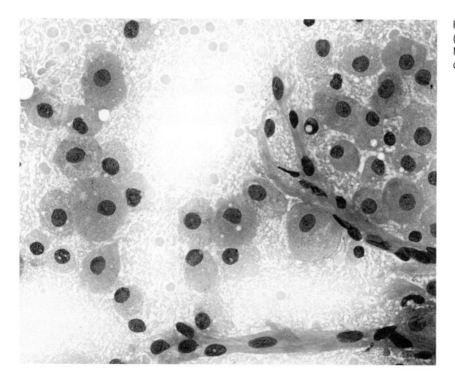

Figure 8.9 Hepatocellular carcinoma (well differentiated), dog, 50× objective. Note the streaming linear capillaries and dissociated hepatocytes.

- All liver lobes usually affected. In dogs, about two-thirds are diffuse with small coalescing nodules, and one-third have a well-circumscribed nodular appearance [21].
- Hypoglycemia and seizure activity rarely reported [22].
- Carcinoid of the gallbladder has rarely been described [23].

8.1.9.3 Prognosis
Grave. Despite mild cytologic criteria of malignancy, these tumors have an aggressive biologic behavior, with an early, high metastatic rate to the local lymph nodes and peritoneum and less commonly to other distant locations [21].

Figure 8.10 Hepatocellular carcinoma (high grade), dog, 50× objective.

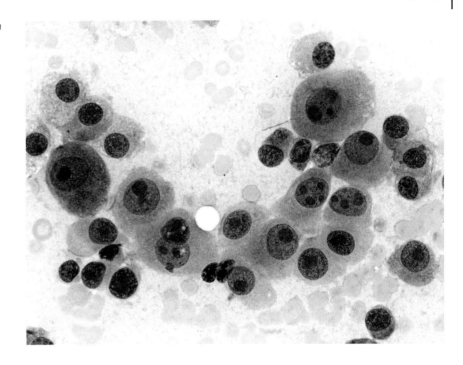

Figure 8.11 Liver, carcinoid, dog, 50× objective.

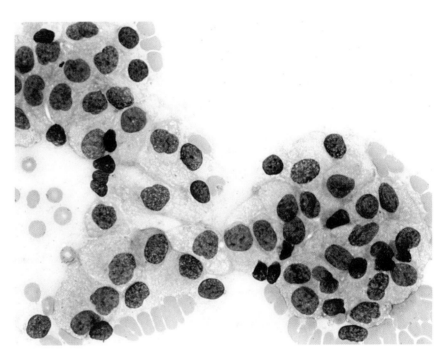

8.1.10 Metastatic Neoplasia

8.1.10.1 Cytologic Appearance

A myriad of neoplasms may metastasize to the liver. Round-cell neoplasia (Figure 8.12) and carcinomas (Figure 8.13) are most common, but sarcomas may also be seen (Figure 8.14). Neoplastic mesenchymal cells should be differentiated from primary hepatic neoplasia (e.g., hemangiosarcoma or fibrosarcoma arising in the liver).

8.1.10.2 Clinical Considerations

- Metastatic carcinomas may be difficult to differentiate from primary hepatic neoplasms such as carcinoids and biliary carcinomas.

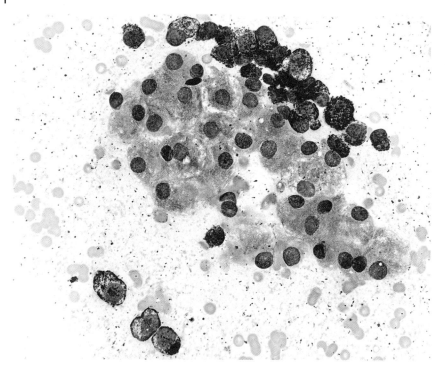

Figure 8.12 Liver, metastatic mast cell neoplasia, dog, 50× objective. The mast cells are seen in crowded aggregates and are intimately associated with hepatocytes.

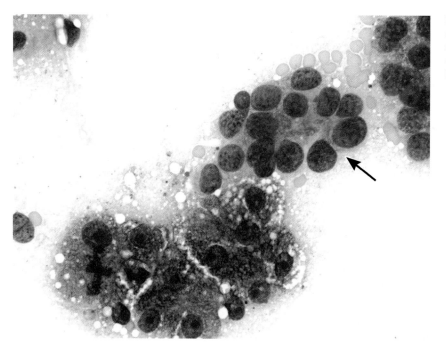

Figure 8.13 Liver, metastatic mammary carcinoma, cat, 50× objective. Note the acinar arrangement of the neoplastic cells (arrow) and the sheet of hepatocytes (lower left).

8.1.10.3 Prognosis
Poor.

8.1.11 Lymphoma (Large-cell)

8.1.11.1 Cytologic Appearance
Large-cell lymphomas typically exfoliate in large numbers and may efface hepatic parenchyma. The cells have large nuclei, about 2-fold to 3-fold the size of red blood cells in diameter,

with finely stippled chromatin, variably prominent nucleoli, and mitotic figures may be seen (Figure 8.15). They have a variable volume of pale-blue cytoplasm that may contain clear vacuoles (Figure 8.16).

8.1.11.2 Clinical Considerations
- Most commonly part of generalized disease, but may be primary [24, 25].

Figure 8.14   Liver, metastatic fibrosarcoma, dog, 50× objective.

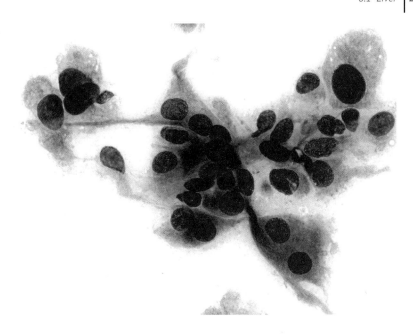

Figure 8.15   Liver, lymphoma (large-cell), dog, 50× objective. Large lymphocytes crowd sheets of well-differentiated hepatocytes. Note the mitotic figure (lower center).

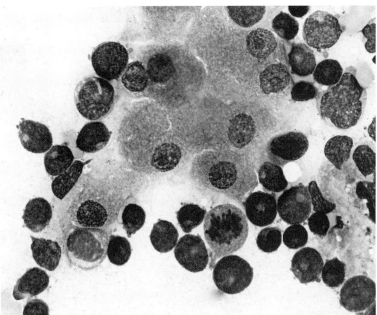

8.1.11.3   Prognosis
- Variable, based on the lymphoma type. Primary lymphomas of the liver carry a poor to grave prognosis [24].

8.1.12   Lymphoma (Small-cell)/Chronic Lymphocytic Leukemia

8.1.12.1   Cytologic Appearance
Small-cell lymphoma and chronic lymphocytic leukemia (CLL) may involve the liver. The cells have small nuclei, about 1-fold to 1.25-fold the size of red blood cells in diameter, and a small cap of pale-blue cytoplasm that may contain azurophilic granules (Figure 8.17). The maturity of the cells can make differentiation from lymphocytic inflammation difficult (compare to Figure 8.18). Features of malignancy include monomorphism of the population, more open chromatin, prominent nucleoli, and typically a greater number of cells.

8.1.12.2   Clinical Considerations
- Affects middle-aged to older dogs and cats.
- Commonly represents liver involvement with generalized disease [25].
- May be accompanied by mature lymphocytosis in peripheral blood.

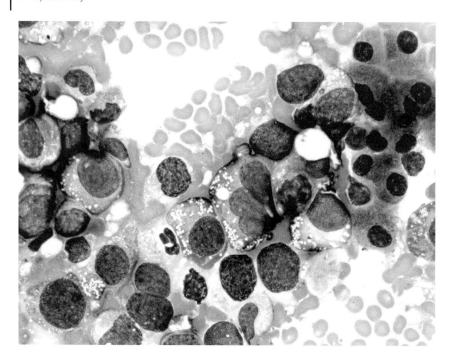

Figure 8.16 Liver, lymphoma (large-cell), dog, 50× objective. Note the fine clear vacuoles in the cytoplasm.

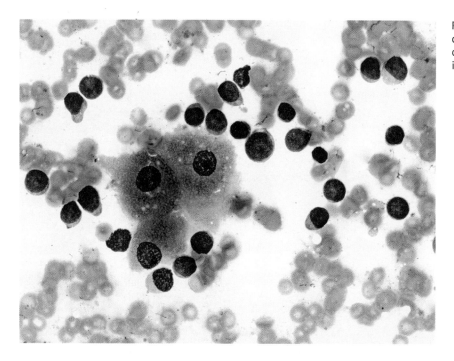

Figure 8.17 Liver, lymphoma (small-cell), dog, 50× objective. Compare the open, stippled chromatin to that of inflammatory lymphocytes in Figure 8.18.

8.1.12.3 Prognosis
Generally good, with long survival times reported.

8.1.13 Inflammation: Lymphoplasmacytic

8.1.13.1 Cytologic Appearance
Increased numbers of lymphocytes (Figure 8.18) and plasma cells (Figure 8.19) are embedded in sheets of hepatocytes and scattered across the background. The population usually is heterogeneous, and the cells have mature, clumped chromatin, which can help differentiate from a neoplastic process, though this can be difficult (compare to Figure 8.17).

8.1.13.2 Clinical Considerations
- Rare small mature lymphocytes are present in samples from healthy dogs [1].

Figure 8.18 Liver, inflammation (lymphocytic), cat, 50× objective.

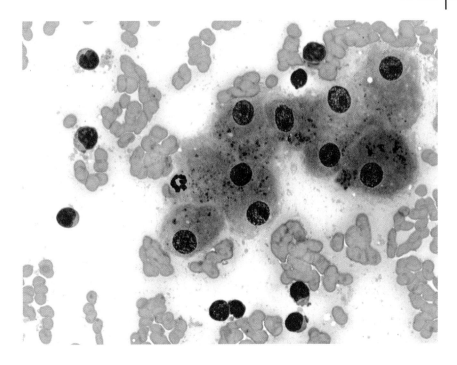

Figure 8.19 Liver, inflammation (lymphoplasmacytic), cat, 50× objective. Many plasma cells (arrowheads) and fewer small to intermediate lymphocytes (arrow) are seen. Note the concurrent hepatic lipidosis.

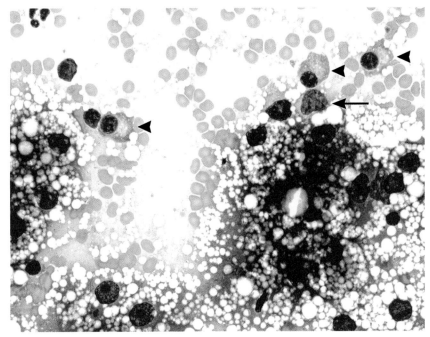

- Inflammation may be primary (e.g., lymphocytic portal hepatitis/cholangiohepatitis in cats or chronic progressive hepatitis in dogs) or secondary to inflammation in adjacent organs (e.g., pancreatitis or gastroenteritis) [26, 27].
- Histopathology is required to assess the location and extent of inflammation.

8.1.13.3 Prognosis
Variable, based on the underlying cause.

8.1.14 Inflammation: Neutrophilic

8.1.14.1 Cytologic Appearance
Increased numbers of neutrophils associated with hepatocytes are consistent with neutrophilic inflammation. Finding neutrophils in aggregates across the slide, embedded within sheets of hepatocytes or with a left shift or degenerative changes, can help differentiate inflammation from blood-associated leukocytes (Figure 8.20).

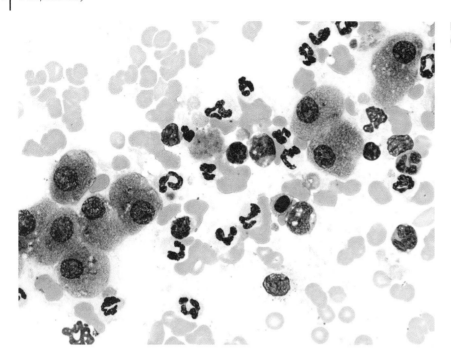

Figure 8.20 Liver, inflammation (neutrophilic), dog, 50× objective.

8.1.14.2 Clinical Considerations

- Inflammation may be sterile, but investigation for infectious organisms is warranted (see Chapter 3).
- Histopathology is required to assess the location of inflammation (e.g., hepatitis versus cholangitis) [26, 27].
- ≥6 neutrophils counted per 200 hepatocytes has high specificity for neutrophilic inflammation in dogs [28].
- Absence of cytologic evidence does not rule out underlying inflammation [29].
- Cautious interpretation is warranted with concurrent neutrophilia if blood contamination is present.

8.1.14.3 Prognosis

Variable, based on the underlying cause.

8.1.15 Lipofuscin Pigment

8.1.15.1 Cytologic Appearance

Lipofuscin pigment appears as variably chunky blue-green granular material within the cytoplasm of hepatocytes (Figure 8.21). It can be difficult to differentiate from bile (compare to Figure 8.22).

8.1.15.2 Clinical Considerations

- Most common pigment of hepatocytes, especially in older patients.
- Accumulates over time in lysosomes as a normal product of cellular aging.

8.1.15.3 Prognosis

Excellent – no pathologic significance.

8.1.16 Cholestasis/Bilirubin Pigment

8.1.16.1 Cytologic Appearance

Cholestasis manifests most commonly as green/black tubular structures coursing between hepatocytes, reflecting bile plugging of biliary canaliculi (Figure 8.22). Granular green/black pigment may also be seen within the cytoplasm of hepatocytes.

8.1.16.2 Clinical Considerations

- Disease may be prehepatic (hemolysis), hepatic (inflammation, neoplasia, etc.), or posthepatic (bile duct obstruction).
- Cytologic changes may precede hyperbilirubinemia.

8.1.16.3 Prognosis

Variable, based on the underlying cause.

8.1.17 Hemosiderin Pigment

8.1.17.1 Cytologic Appearance

Hemosiderin pigment appears mostly as golden brown, to occasionally brown/black, variably coarse granular material in the cytoplasm of hepatocytes (Figure 8.23). It may be accompanied by evidence of erythrophagia or heme-breakdown pigment in macrophages in the liver.

Figure 8.21 Lipofuscin pigment, dog, 50× objective. Note the diffuse, blue-green granular pigment in the cytoplasm.

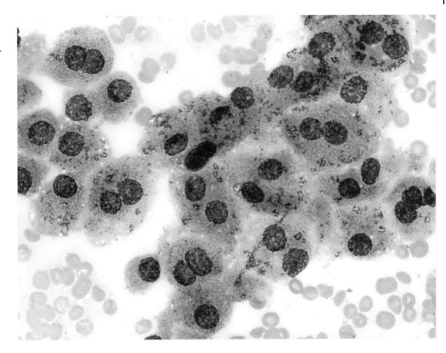

Figure 8.22 Cholestasis and bile pigment, dog, 50× objective. Note the green/black tubular structures coursing between hepatocytes (bile plugging of biliary canaliculi).

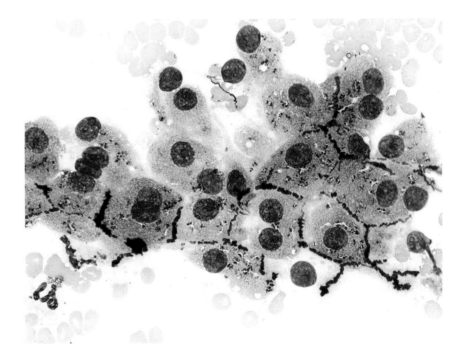

8.1.17.2 Clinical Considerations

- May be associated with hemolytic diseases, repeat blood transfusions, or iron administration [30].

8.1.17.3 Prognosis

Variable, based on the underlying cause.

8.1.18 Copper Accumulation

8.1.18.1 Cytologic Appearance

Copper pigment can be seen with routine cytologic stains as small, aquamarine crystalline aggregates in the cytoplasm of hepatocytes (Figure 8.24). It is best visualized with a 100× oil objective. Copper pigment

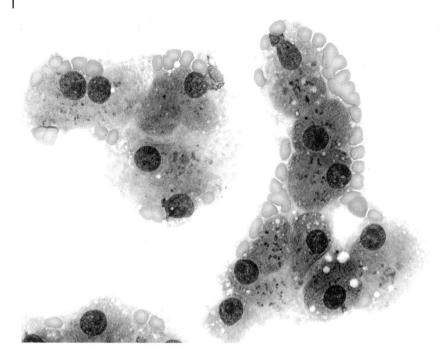

Figure 8.23 Hemosiderin pigment, dog, 50× objective. Note the golden-brown and rarely basophilic pigment.

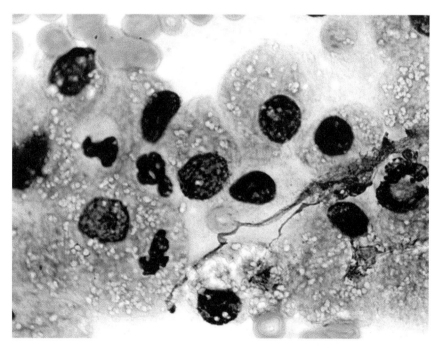

Figure 8.24 Copper pigment, dog, 100× objective. The pigment is refractile and aquamarine, scattered diffusely throughout the cytoplasm.

can be confirmed with special stains such as rhodanine (Figure 8.25).

8.1.18.2 Clinical Considerations

- Copper accumulation may be a primary cause of disease (copper storage disease) and Bedlington Terriers, Doberman Pinschers, Labrador Retrievers, Skye Terriers, Dalmatians, and West Highland White Terriers are predisposed [31, 32].

- Small amounts of copper can be seen secondary to cholestasis, chronic inflammation, or hepatic injury in both dogs and cats [33–36].
- Histopathology is required to distinguish between primary and secondary copper accumulation.

8.1.18.3 Prognosis

Variable. Copper storage disease may respond to therapy but can cause fatal hepatic failure [37]. Accumulation

Figure 8.25 Rhodanine stain highlighting copper pigment in hepatocytes, dog, 100× objective.

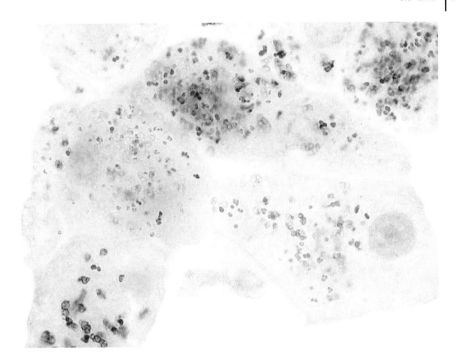

secondary to cholestasis or inflammation may have a better prognosis.

8.1.19 Amyloid

8.1.19.1 Cytologic Appearance

Amyloid is seen as smooth to fibrillar, magenta extracellular material, intimately associated with hepatocytes (Figure 8.26).

8.1.19.2 Clinical Considerations

- Amyloid deposition may be localized or systemic (involving the kidney and spleen) [38].
- Amyloid may accumulate due to a primary familial predisposition or secondary to chronic, extrahepatic/systemic inflammation [3, 38].
- Predisposed breeds = Shar Pei dogs; Siamese and Abyssinian cats [38, 39].

Figure 8.26 Amyloid, dog, 50× objective. Note the bright magenta, fibrillar amyloid material intimately associated with hepatocytes. Slide courtesy of Dr. Ida Piperisova.

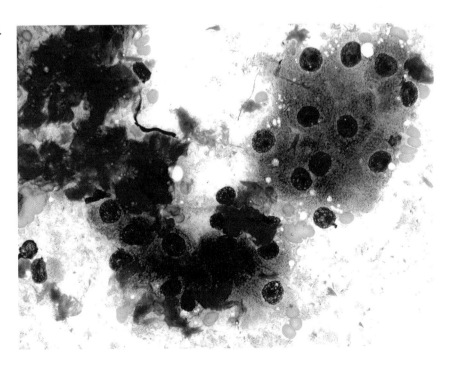

8.1.19.3 Prognosis

Variable, based on primary or secondary, organs involved and ability to treat any underlying disease.

8.2 Biliary Tract

8.2.1 Biliary Hyperplasia

8.2.1.1 Cytologic Appearance

Hyperplastic biliary epithelium is seen as sheets of minimally pleomorphic cuboidal epithelial cells in papillary arrangements (Figure 8.27). The cells have a small to moderate volume of pale-blue cytoplasm that may contain clear vacuoles and round nuclei with stippled chromatin and small nucleoli. Hyperplastic tissue cannot reliably be distinguished cytologically from normal tissue, which may be sampled incidentally during aspiration of the liver [1].

8.2.1.2 Clinical Considerations

- Biliary hyperplasia usually is seen secondary to cystic lesions or cholangitis/cholangiohepatitis.

8.2.1.3 Prognosis

Variable, based on the underlying cause of the hyperplasia, but generally good.

8.2.2 Bile Duct Adenoma/Biliary Cystadenoma

8.2.2.1 Cytologic Appearance

Bile duct adenomas/cystadenomas comprise sheets of cuboidal epithelial cells, often accompanied by pools of smooth blue mucinous material in the background (Figure 8.28). Cellular crowding often is seen, and anisocytosis/anisokaryosis and N/C ratios are increased relative to hyperplastic epithelium.

8.2.2.2 Clinical Considerations

- Cats > dogs, and male cats may be predisposed [40].
- Biliary cystadenomas may be single or multiple and variably sized [40, 41].
- Non-cystic bile duct adenomas normally are small and solitary.
- Often incidental findings but may cause compression of adjacent organs if large [42].

8.2.2.3 Prognosis

Excellent. Surgical excision (if required) is curative [42].

8.2.3 Bile Duct Carcinoma (Cholangiocarcinoma)

8.2.3.1 Cytologic Appearance

Bile duct carcinomas mostly are highly cellular, characterized by cohesive sheets of cuboidal epithelial cells, often in palisading or acinar arrangements (Figure 8.29). The cells have a small volume of medium-blue cytoplasm, which

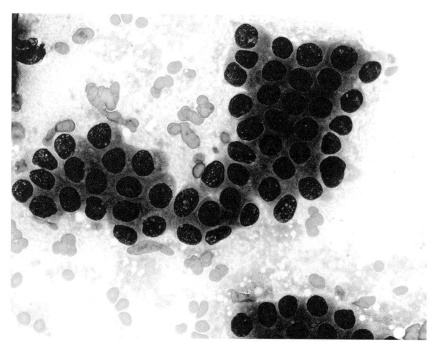

Figure 8.27 Biliary epithelial hyperplasia, cat, 50× objective.

Figure 8.28 Biliary cystadenoma, cat, 20× objective. Note the abundant smooth blue mucinous material.

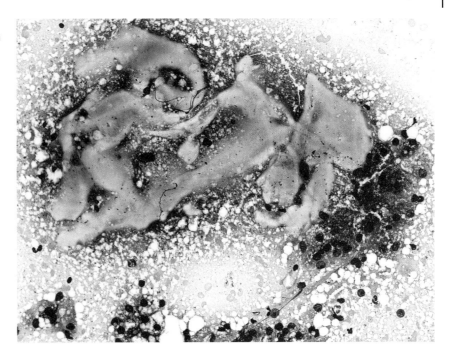

Figure 8.29 Bile duct carcinoma (cholangiocarcinoma), cat, 50× objective. Note the prominent acinar arrangement of the cells.

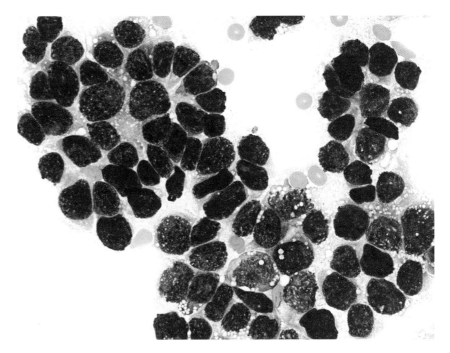

may contain small, clear vacuoles. Nuclei are round with clumped chromatin and mostly single, prominent, basophilic nucleoli. Anisocytosis/anisokaryosis are moderate to occasionally marked.

8.2.3.2 Clinical Considerations
- Most common malignant hepatobiliary tumor in cats [20].
- Massive, nodular, and diffuse variants [43].

- Tumors may be intra- or extrahepatic. Intrahepatic tumors are more common in dogs, whereas there is an equal distribution in cats [12, 20, 44].
- Combined hepatocellular-cholangiocarcinoma is also reported in dogs [45].

8.2.3.3 Prognosis
Guarded to poor. Bile duct carcinomas are aggressive, highly metastatic malignancies. Prolonged survival is

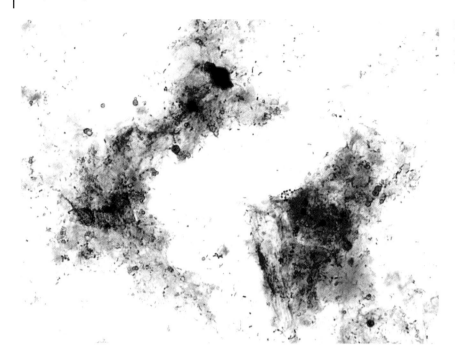

Figure 8.30 Bactibilia, dog, 50× objective. Numerous small, blue bacterial cocci are noted around aggregates of yellow/orange bile and pale-blue mucin.

possible in dogs with localized, completely resected tumors in the absence of metastatic disease [46].

8.2.4 Cholecystitis

8.2.4.1 Cytologic Appearance

Bile has a yellow/green appearance, and pale-blue mucinous material may also be present. Cholecystitis is associated with an overgrowth of infectious agents ± inflammatory cells. Bacteria are the most common infectious agent identified (bactibilia; Figure 8.30), but fungal and protozoal agents also have been reported [47–49].

8.2.4.2 Clinical Considerations

- Dogs and cats. Dachshunds may be overrepresented [47].
- Presence of infectious agents more commonly found by cytology than microbial culture [48].
- Common bacterial isolates = *Escherichia coli*, *Enterococcus* spp. [47, 48]
- Subclinical bactibilia may be present in clinically healthy dogs [50].
- Cholecystocentesis associated with low complication rate [48].

8.2.4.3 Prognosis

Good with appropriate therapy. Gallbladder rupture and cholangiohepatitis can result if untreated [47, 51].

References

1 Stockhaus, C., Teske, E., Van Den Ingh, T., *et al.* (2002) The influence of age on the cytology of the liver in healthy dogs. *Vet. Pathol.*, **39** (1), 154–158.

2 Sepesy, L.M., Center, S.A., Randolph, J.F., *et al.* (2006) Vacuolar hepatopathy in dogs: 336 cases (1993–2005). *J. Am. Vet. Med. Assoc.*, **229** (2), 246–252.

3 Cullen, J.M. (2009) Summary of the World Small Animal Veterinary Association standardization committee guide to classification of liver disease in dogs and cats. *Vet. Clin. North Am. Small Anim. Pract.*, **39** (3), 395–418.

4 Lester, C., Cooper, J., Peters, R.M., *et al.* (2016) Retrospective evaluation of acute liver failure in dogs (1995-2012): 49 cases. *J. Vet. Emerg. Crit. Care*, **26** (4), 559–567.

5 Bahr, K.L., Sharkey, L.C., Murakami, T., *et al.* (2013) Accuracy of US-guided FNA of focal liver lesions in dogs: 140 cases (2005-2008). *J. Am. Anim. Hosp. Assoc.*, **49** (3), 190–196.

6 Center, S.A. (2005) Feline hepatic lipidosis. *Vet. Clin. North Am. Small Anim. Pract.*, **35** (1), 225–269.

7 Center, S.A., Crawford, M.A., Guida, L., *et al.* (1993) A retrospective study of 77 cats with severe hepatic lipidosis: 1975–1990. *J. Vet. Intern. Med.*, **7** (6), 349–359.

8 Webb, C.B. (2018) Hepatic lipidosis: clinical review drawn from collective effort. *J. Feline Med. Surg.*, **20** (3), 217–227.

9 van Sprundel, R.G., van den Ingh, T.S., Guscetti, F., *et al.* (2013) Classification of primary hepatic tumours in the dog. *Vet. J.*, **197** (3), 596–606.

10 van Sprundel, R.G., van den Ingh, T.S., Guscetti, F., *et al.* (2014) Classification of primary hepatic tumours in the cat. *Vet. J.*, **202** (2), 255–266.

11 Lodi, M., Chinosi, S., Faverzani, S., *et al.* (2007) Clinical and ultrasonographic features of the canine hepatocellular carcinoma (CHC). *Vet. Res. Commun.*, **31** (Suppl. 1), 293–295.

12 Patnaik, A.K. (1992) A morphologic and immunocytochemical study of hepatic neoplasms in cats. *Vet. Pathol.*, **29** (5), 405–415.

13 Jornet-Rius, O., Agulla, B., López, M.C., *et al.* (2023) Needle tract seeding and malignant transformation of hepatocellular adenoma into well-differentiated hepatocellular carcinoma in a dog. *Vet. Clin. Pathol.*, **52** (3), 507–513.

14 Masserdotti, C., Drigo, M. (2012) Retrospective study of cytologic features of well-differentiated hepatocellular carcinoma in dogs. *Vet. Clin. Pathol.*, **41** (3), 382–390.

15 Reist, A.M., Reagan, J.K., Fujita, S.K., *et al.* (2022) Histopathologic findings and survival outcomes of dogs undergoing liver lobectomy as treatment for spontaneous hemoabdomen secondary to a ruptured liver mass: retrospective analysis of 200 cases (2012-2020). *J. Am. Vet. Med. Assoc.*, **261** (2), 237–245.

16 Patnaik, A.K., Hurvitz, A.I., Lieberman, P.H. (1980) Canine hepatic neoplasms: a clinicopathologic study. *Vet. Pathol.*, **17** (5), 553–564.

17 Suarez-Rodriguez, J.I., Liu, C.C., Dehghanpir, S., *et al.* (2023) Lymphopenia predicts reduced survival in canine hepatocellular carcinoma. *J. Vet. Sci.*, **24** (3), e36.

18 Lapsley, J.M., Wavreille, V., Barry, S., *et al.* (2022) Risk factors and outcome in dogs with recurrent massive hepatocellular carcinoma: a Veterinary Society of Surgical Oncology case-control study. *Vet. Comp. Oncol.*, **20** (3), 697–709.

19 Liptak, J.M., Dernell, W.S., Monnet, E., *et al.* (2004) Massive hepatocellular carcinoma in dogs: 48 cases (1992–2002). *J. Am. Vet. Med. Assoc.*, **225** (8), 1225–1230.

20 Lawrence, H.J., Erb, H.N., Harvey, H.J. (1994) Nonlymphomatous hepatobiliary masses in cats: 41 cases (1972–1991). *Vet. Surg.*, **23** (5), 365–368.

21 Patnaik, A.K., Lieberman, P.H., Hurvitz, A.I., *et al.* (1981) Canine hepatic carcinoids. *Vet. Pathol.*, **18** (4), 445–453.

22 Dorn, A.R., Brower, A., Turner, H., *et al.* (2021) Hypoglycemia and seizures associated with canine primary hepatic neuroendocrine carcinoma. *J. Vet. Diagn. Investig.*, **33** (4), 749–752.

23 Lippo, N.J., Williams, J.E., Brawer, R.S., *et al.* (2008) Acute hemobilia and hemocholecyst in 2 dogs with gallbladder carcinoid. *J. Vet. Intern. Med.*, **22** (5), 1249–1252.

24 Keller, S.M., Vernau, W., Hodges, J., *et al.* (2013) Hepatosplenic and hepatocytotropic T-cell lymphoma: two distinct types of T-cell lymphoma in dogs. *Vet. Pathol.*, **50** (2), 281–290.

25 Aresu, L., Martini, V., Rossi, F., *et al.* (2015) Canine indolent and aggressive lymphoma: clinical spectrum with histologic correlation. *Vet. Comp. Oncol.*, **13** (4), 348–362.

26 Gagne, J.M., Armstrong, P.J., Weiss, D.J., *et al.* (1999) Clinical features of inflammatory liver disease in cats: 41 cases (1983–1993). *J. Am. Vet. Med. Assoc.*, **214** (4), 513–516.

27 Hirose, N., Uchida, K., Kanemoto, H., *et al.* (2014) A retrospective histopathological survey on canine and feline liver diseases at the University of Tokyo between 2006 and 2012. *J. Vet. Med. Sci.*, **76** (7), 1015–1020.

28 Gardner, R.H., Castillo, D., Constantino-Casas, F., *et al.* (2022) Can the neutrophil count from hepatic fine-needle aspirate cytology be used to diagnose hepatitis in dogs? A pilot study. *Vet. Clin. Pathol.*, **51** (2), 237–243.

29 Roth, L. (2001) Comparison of liver cytology and biopsy diagnoses in dogs and cats: 56 cases. *Vet. Clin. Pathol.*, **30** (1), 35–38.

30 Bohn, A.A. (2013) Diagnosis of disorders of iron metabolism in dogs and cats. *Vet. Clin. North Am. Small Anim. Pract.*, **43** (6), 1319–1330.

31 Hoffmann, G. (2009) Copper-associated liver diseases. *Vet. Clin. North Am. Small Anim. Pract.*, **39** (3), 489–511.

32 Ullal, T.V., Lakin, S., Gallagher, B., *et al.* (2022) Demographic and histopathologic features of dogs with abnormally high concentrations of hepatic copper. *J. Vet. Intern. Med.*, **36** (6), 2016–2027.

33 Johnston, A.N., Center, S.A., McDonough, S.P., *et al.* (2013) Hepatic copper concentrations in Labrador Retrievers with and without chronic hepatitis: 72 cases (1980–2010). *J. Am. Vet. Med. Assoc.*, **242** (3), 372–380.

34 Vince, A.R., Hayes, M.A., Jefferson, B.J., *et al.* (2014) Hepatic injury correlates with apoptosis, regeneration, and nitric oxide synthase expression in canine chronic liver disease. *Vet. Pathol.*, **51** (5), 932–945.

35 Spee, B., Arends, B., van den Ingh, T.S., *et al.* (2006) Copper metabolism and oxidative stress in chronic inflammatory and cholestatic liver diseases in dogs. *J. Vet. Intern. Med.*, **20** (5), 1085–1092.

36 Whittemore, J.C., Newkirk, K.M., Reel, D.M., *et al.* (2012) Hepatic copper and iron accumulation and histologic findings in 104 feline liver biopsies. *J. Vet. Diagn. Investig.*, **24** (4), 656–661.

37 Noaker, L.J., Washabau, R.J., Detrisac, C.J., *et al.* (1999) Copper associated acute hepatic failure in a dog. *J. Am. Vet. Med. Assoc.*, **214** (10), 1502–1506.

38 Flatland, B., Moore, R.R., Wolf, C.M., *et al.* (2007) Liver aspirate from a Shar Pei dog. *Vet. Clin. Pathol.*, **36** (1), 105–108.

39 Niewold, T.A., van der Linde-Sipman, J.S., Murphy, C., *et al.* (1999) Familial amyloidosis in cats: Siamese and Abyssinian AA proteins differ in primary sequence and pattern of deposition. *Amyloid*, **6** (3), 205–209.

40 Adler, R., Wilson, D.W. (1995) Biliary cystadenoma of cats. *Vet. Pathol.*, **32** (4), 415–418.

41 Nyland, T.G., Koblik, P.D., Tellyer, S.E. (1999) Ultrasonographic evaluation of biliary cystadenomas in cats. *Vet. Radiol. Ultrasound*, **40** (3), 300–306.

42 Kristick, K.L., Ranck, R.S., Fink, M. (2010) What is your diagnosis? Biliary cystadenoma of the liver causing deviation of the stomach to the left. *J. Am. Vet. Med. Assoc.*, **236** (10), 1065–1066.

43 Patnaik, A.K., Hurvitz, A.I., Lieberman, P.H., *et al.* (1981) Canine bile duct carcinoma. *Vet. Pathol.*, **18** (4), 439–444.

44 Hayes, H.M., Jr, Morin, M.M., Rubenstein, D.A. (1983) Canine biliary carcinoma: epidemiological comparisons with man. *J. Comp. Pathol.*, **93** (1), 99–107.

45 Terai, K., Ishigaki, K., Kagawa, Y., *et al.* (2022) Clinical, diagnostic, and pathological features and surgical outcomes of combined hepatocellular-cholangiocarcinoma in dogs: 14 cases (2009-2021). *J. Am. Vet. Med. Assoc.*, **260** (13), 1668–1674.

46 Maeda, A., Goto, S., Iwasaki, R., *et al.* (2022) Outcome of localized bile duct carcinoma in six dogs treated with liver lobectomy. *J. Am. Anim. Hosp. Assoc.*, **58** (4), 189–193.

47 Lawrence, Y.A., Ruaux, C.G., Nemanic, S., *et al.* (2015) Characterization, treatment, and outcome of bacterial cholecystitis and bactibilia in dogs. *J. Am. Vet. Med. Assoc.*, **246** (9), 982–989.

48 Peters, L.M., Glanemann, B., Garden, O.A., *et al.* (2016) Cytological findings of 140 bile samples from dogs and cats and associated clinical pathological data. *J. Vet. Intern. Med.*, **30** (1), 123–131.

49 Neel, J.A., Tarigo, J., Grindem, C.B. (2006) Gall bladder aspirate from a dog. *Vet. Clin. Pathol.*, **35** (4), 467–470.

50 Verwey, E., Gal, A., Kettner, F., *et al.* (2021) Prevalence of subclinical bactibilia in apparently healthy shelter dogs. *J. Small Anim. Pract.*, **62** (11), 948–958.

51 Neer, T.M. (1992) A review of disorders of the gallbladder and extrahepatic biliary tract in the dog and cat. *J. Vet. Intern. Med.*, **6** (3), 186–192.

9

Digestive System

9.1 Salivary Glands

9.1.1 Salivary Gland (Normal)

9.1.1.1 Cytologic Features

Sample backgrounds contain streaming blue/purple mucin, distributing erythrocytes and cells in a prominent windrowing pattern. Salivary glandular epithelium exfoliates as tight, cohesive sheets of cells that mostly have abundant foamy cytoplasm and round, pyknotic nuclei (Figure 9.1). Anisocytosis/anisokaryosis are mild and N/C ratios are low.

9.1.1.2 Clinical Considerations

- Often an incidental or inadvertent finding when sampling mandibular lymph nodes.
- Normal salivary epithelium may be present in cases of sialadenitis and salivary mucoceles (see Figure 9.5).
- May indicate idiopathic sialadenosis [1].

9.1.2 Salivary Gland Adenoma

9.1.2.1 Cytologic Features

Salivary gland adenomas exfoliate as cohesive sheets of cells with a papillary- or an acinar-like arrangement. The cells mostly are well-differentiated, which can make differentiating these from normal or hyperplastic tissue difficult. Features include crowded sheets (with cellular piling), higher N/C ratios, and less-vacuolated cells than normal epithelium (compare Figures 9.2 and 9.1).

9.1.2.2 Clinical Considerations

- Rare in dogs and cats; they comprise <5% of salivary tumors [2, 3].
- Histopathology is required for confirmation of diagnosis.

9.1.2.3 Prognosis

Excellent. May require surgical removal if causing clinical signs.

9.1.3 Salivary Gland Adenocarcinoma

9.1.3.1 Cytologic Features

Salivary gland adenocarcinomas exfoliate in cohesive sheets and may retain a papillary- or an acinar-like arrangement. More anaplastic tumors lose features of salivary differentiation (Figure 9.3). They have a variable volume of mid-blue cytoplasm that may contain clear vacuoles. Nuclei are round with smudged chromatin and prominent basophilic nucleoli. Anisocytosis/anisokaryosis may be marked and N/C ratios high, though well-differentiated tumors are common and lack prominent criteria of malignancy [4].

9.1.3.2 Clinical Considerations

- Most common salivary gland tumor in dogs and cats [3, 5].
- Found most frequently in the mandibular gland (cats) and parotid gland (dogs) [5].
- Clinical signs = palpable mass, halitosis, exophthalmos, and Horner's syndrome.

9.1.3.3 Prognosis

Prognosis varies greatly in the literature; however, cats universally have a poorer prognosis than dogs. One study found long-term survival with surgery ± radiation therapy, but others report high metastatic rates and short survival times [5–7].

9.1.4 Sialocele (Salivary Mucocele)

9.1.4.1 Cytologic Features

Sialoceles have a distinctive background that contains numerous pools of smooth, pale-blue/lavender mucinous material (Figure 9.4). Embedded within this material are inflammatory cells. Reactive macrophages usually predominate and frequently contain hematoidin crystals (see Figures 2.3 and 9.4) or other heme-breakdown pigments.

Clinical Atlas of Small Animal Cytology and Hematology, Second Edition. Andrew G. Burton.
© 2024 John Wiley & Sons, Inc. Published 2024 by John Wiley & Sons, Inc.

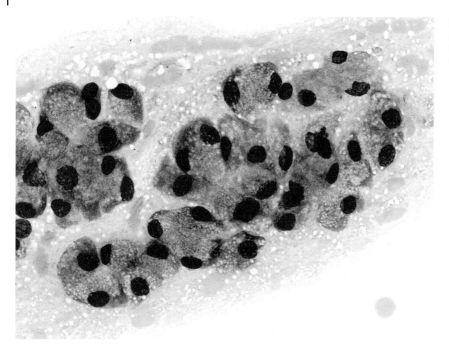

Figure 9.1 Normal salivary gland epithelium, dog, 50× objective. Note the tightly cohesive lobules of ovoid cells with lacy vacuolation.

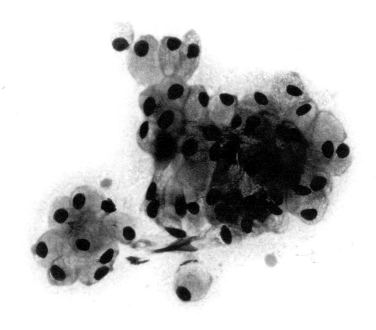

Figure 9.2 Salivary gland adenoma, dog, 40× objective. Note the higher N/C ratios and less vacuolation compared to cells in Figure 9.1. Slide courtesy of Dr. Connie Wu Siegfried.

Neutrophils and small mature lymphocytes may also be present. Normal salivary gland epithelium is variably present.

9.1.4.2 Clinical Considerations

- Dogs > cats [3, 8].
- Common in young dogs, but any age affected.
- Unilateral >> bilateral [8–10].

- Clinical signs = swelling/mass lesion, dysphagia, ptyalism, decreased appetite, and oral bleeding [8, 11].
- Idiopathic cases very common. May also be secondary to trauma or duct obstruction (calculi, neoplasia, foreign body) [9, 10].
- May also occur under the tongue (ranula) or in the pharynx [12].

Figure 9.3 Salivary gland adenocarcinoma, cat, 50× objective.

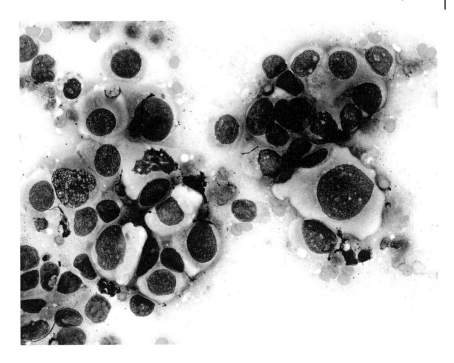

Figure 9.4 Sialocoele, dog, 20× objective. Note the smooth pools of pale-blue mucin and numerous macrophages that often contain golden hematoidin crystals.

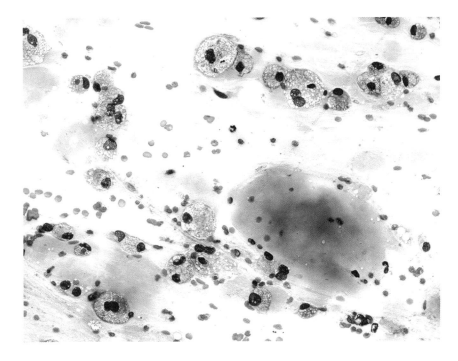

9.1.4.3 Prognosis

Excellent. Some lesions are self-limiting. Surgical excision generally is curative, with low rates of recurrence [8, 11, 13].

9.1.5 Sialadenitis

9.1.5.1 Cytologic Features

Inflammation may be seen in the salivary gland in the absence of a cystic component, though variable amounts of mucin may still be seen (Figure 9.5). The types of nucleated cells vary with the primary pathologic process and may comprise neutrophils (more common in bacterial etiologies) or small mature lymphocytes (chronic, viral, or immune-mediated causes). Infectious agents may be present.

9.1.5.2 Clinical Considerations

• Responsible for ~25% of cases of salivary gland pathology in one study [3].

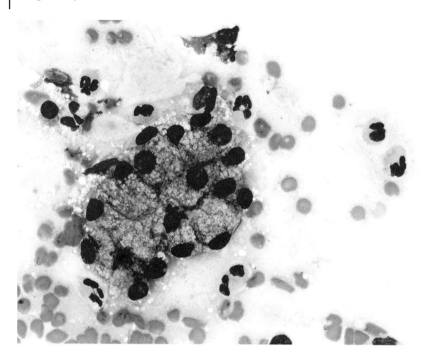

Figure 9.5 Sialadenitis, dog, 50× objective.

- May be primary (penetrating wounds, ascending infection from oral cavity, infarction) or secondary to systemic disease (e.g., viral) [14].

9.1.5.3 Prognosis
Generally good, based on the underlying etiology of the inflammation.

9.2 Stomach/Intestines

9.2.1 Inflammation

9.2.1.1 Cytologic Features
Inflammatory lesions in the gastrointestinal tract are categorized by the predominant cell type. Lymphoplasmacytic inflammation is common, often associated with inflammatory bowel disease (IBD) [15]. The lymphoid population is mixed, with plasma cells often present (Figure 9.6), helping distinguish it from small-cell lymphoma (compare to Figures 9.7 and 9.8). Eosinophils may also be present in cases of IBD, but may also indicate underlying hypersensitivity disease, parasitic disease, neoplasia (e.g., mast cell neoplasia), or feline gastrointestinal eosinophilic sclerosing fibroplasia (FGESF). When neutrophilic or granulomatous inflammation is present, careful assessment for infectious organisms is warranted (see Chapter 3 for details).

9.2.1.2 Clinical Considerations
- Cats and dogs. IBD more common in cats.
- May affect any age. IBD most common in middle-aged to older patients.

- Clinical signs = vomiting, diarrhea, weight loss, and lethargy [15].
- Histopathology required for definitive diagnosis [15].

9.2.1.3 Prognosis
Variable, based on etiology. IBD generally is associated with prolonged survival with appropriate therapy, though clinical signs may wax and wane [16, 17].

9.2.2 Lymphoma (Small-cell)

9.2.2.1 Cytologic Features
Characterized by a monomorphic population of small lymphocytes, with nuclei about 1-fold to 1.25-fold the size of red blood cells in diameter, and a unipolar cap of pale-blue cytoplasm (Figures 9.7 and 9.8). Relative to normal or reactive lymphocytes, they have more open chromatin and variably prominent nucleoli. Plasma cells generally are absent or seen in low numbers.

9.2.2.2 Clinical Considerations
- Cats > > dogs [18].
- Small intestine > > stomach. Other organs rarely concurrently involved [19].
- Diffuse thickening of intestine > discrete mass [20, 21].
- Clinical signs = diarrhea, vomiting, and weight loss [18, 22].

9.2.2.3 Prognosis
Typically good. Long-term remission and survival are common [18, 23]. Infiltration of the mucosal epithelium with

Figure 9.6 Intestine, lymphoplasmacytic inflammation, cat, 100× objective.

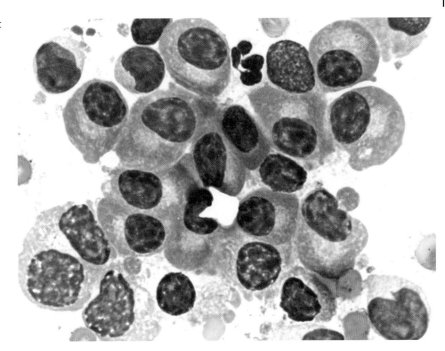

Figure 9.7 Intestine, lymphoma (small-cell), dog, 50× objective.

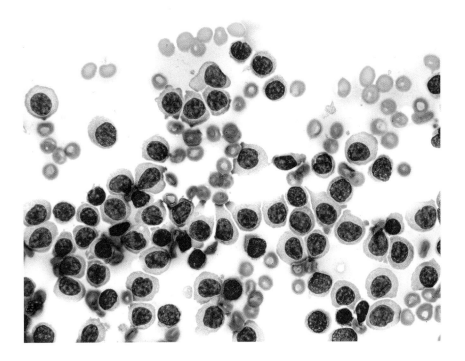

cytotoxic T-cells is a poor prognostic indicator [24]. Anemia and weight loss in dogs at the time of diagnosis may also confer a poor prognosis [20].

9.2.3 *Lymphoma (Large-cell)*

9.2.3.1 Cytologic Features
Discrete, round cells with large nuclei, ranging from 2-fold to 4-fold the size of red blood cells in diameter, with finely stippled chromatin and variably prominent nucleoli

(Figure 9.9). The cells have a small to moderate volume of medium-blue cytoplasm that may contain vacuoles. Large granular lymphoma (LGL) contains variably chunky azurophilic granules in the cytoplasm (Figure 9.10).

9.2.3.2 Clinical Considerations
Cats
- Most frequent primary site of lymphoma [25].
- Discrete mass > diffuse thickening [26].
- Small intestine and stomach > large intestine [27].

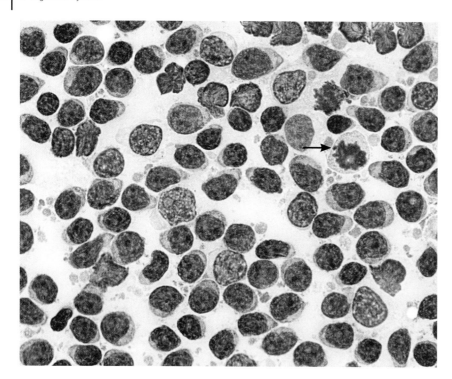

Figure 9.8 Intestine, lymphoma (small-cell), cat, 50× objective. The cells have stippled chromatin, and occasional mitotic figures are seen (arrow).

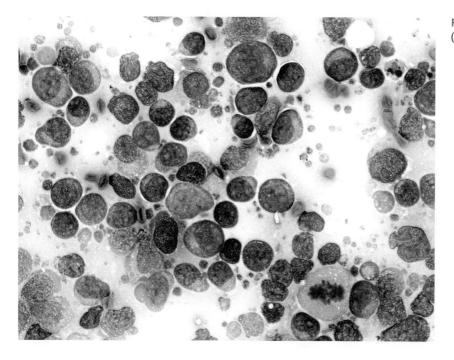

Figure 9.9 Intestine, lymphoma (large-cell), dog, 50× objective.

Dogs

- Primary disease less common than multicentric.
- Discrete mass > diffuse thickening [28].
- Often affects multiple segments but may be focal. Thickening of the wall and mucosal ulceration are common [29, 30].

9.2.3.3 Prognosis

Guarded to grave in both cats and dogs [31, 32]. LGL especially is rapidly progressive, poorly responsive to therapy, and carries a grave prognosis [33, 34].

Figure 9.10 Intestine, lymphoma (large granular), cat, 100× objective.

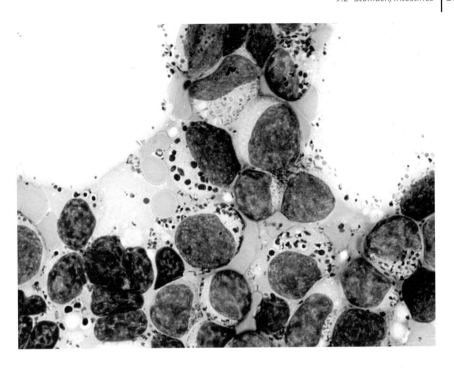

Figure 9.11 Colon, plasmacytoma, dog, 50× objective.

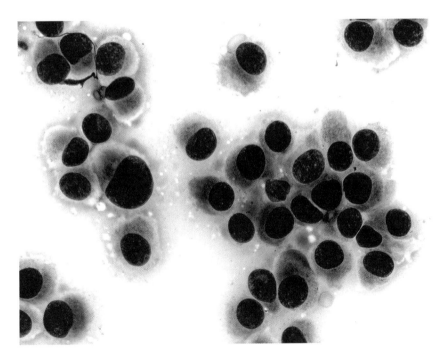

9.2.4 Plasmacytoma

9.2.4.1 Cytologic Features

Extramedullary plasmacytomas of the gastrointestinal tract exfoliate as discrete round cells. Differentiation is variable, ranging from well-differentiated cells with a Golgi zone and eccentric, round nuclei (Figure 9.11) to highly pleomorphic cells seen in crowded sheets with multinucleation and prominent nucleoli.

9.2.4.2 Clinical Considerations
- Dogs > cats.
- Rectum and colon most common sites [35].
- Usually solitary, but multiple masses may occur [36, 37].
- Clinical signs = tenesmus, hematochezia, and rectal prolapse.

9.2.4.3 Prognosis

Generally good with complete excision of solitary tumors [36]. Metastatic spread is rare [37].

9.2.5 Mast Cell Neoplasia

9.2.5.1 Cytologic Features

Discrete, round cells are seen both individually and in crowded sheets. Mast cells in the gastrointestinal tract frequently are less well granulated than those from other organs, and the cytoplasm often contains clear vacuoles (Figure 9.12). Nuclei are round, centrally located, and have granular chromatin.

9.2.5.2 Clinical Considerations

- Cats > dogs. Third most common intestinal tumor in cats [38].
- Tumors mostly are in the intestine or ileocecocolic junction; rare in the colon [39, 40].
- Mostly focal tumors, but may present with diffuse thickening [39].

9.2.5.3 Prognosis

Guarded. Metastatic disease is common and often confers a poor prognosis [41]. Poor differentiation and high mitotic rates are associated with decreased survival times [40]. Some cats respond well to medical therapy alone, and prolonged survival is possible in some patients [42].

9.2.6 Adenoma/Polyp

9.2.6.1 Cytologic Features

Adenomatous polyps exfoliate in organized, cohesive sheets, often with prominent intercellular borders. Cells are round to columnar, with a moderate volume of medium-blue cytoplasm (Figure 9.13). Nuclei are round, centrally to eccentrically placed, and have finely stippled chromatin with small or inapparent nucleoli. Anisocytosis/anisokaryosis are mild.

9.2.6.2 Clinical Considerations

- Most common in rectum (dogs) and intestine/colon (cats) [27, 43, 44].
- Solitary > multiple or diffuse [45].
- Clinical signs = hematochezia, tenesmus, rectal prolapse, increased mucus in feces (dogs) vomiting, and hematemesis (cats) [43–46].
- Histopathology required to differentiate adenomatous polyps from carcinoma *in situ*.

9.2.6.3 Prognosis

Generally good with surgical resection [44]. Polyps >1 cm may be more likely to recur or undergo malignant transformation [46].

9.2.7 Adenocarcinoma

9.2.7.1 Cytologic Features

Neoplastic cells are seen in variably sized cohesive sheets that frequently are crowded or piled, with greater disorganization than polyps (compare Figures 9.14 and 9.13). The cytoplasm may contain vacuoles, which can be large and coarse, particularly in adenocarcinomas of the colon (Figure 9.15). Nuclei may be centrally or eccentrically placed. Anisocytosis/anisokaryosis are variable, but often moderate to marked.

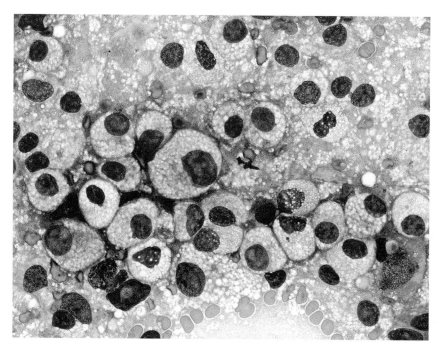

Figure 9.12 Intestine, mast cell tumor, cat, 50× objective. The fine vacuolation of the cytoplasm is characteristic of many intestinal mast cell tumors in cats.

Figure 9.13 Colon, polyp, dog, 50× objective.

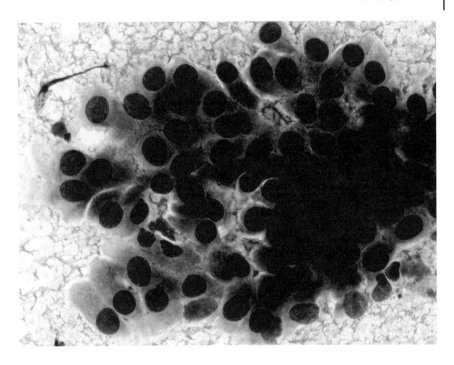

Figure 9.14 Intestine, adenocarcinoma, cat, 50× objective.

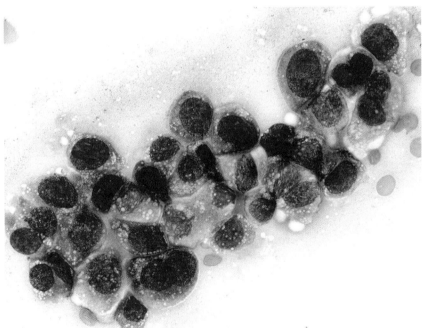

9.2.7.2 Clinical Considerations

- Second most common neoplasm of the gastrointestinal tract in cats and dogs (behind lymphoma) [27].
- Siamese cats predisposed [38].
- Most common in the small intestine (cats) and the large intestine/colon (dogs) [47, 48].

9.2.7.3 Prognosis

Variable. Prognosis is grave if untreated, with short survival times reported especially in cats [49]. Metastatic disease is common including lymph nodes and carcinomatosis, and is a poor prognostic factor in cats [47, 49]. Presence of metastatic disease may not affect survival times in dogs, and prolonged survival time reported with surgical excision [50].

9.2.8 Carcinoid (Intestinal)

9.2.8.1 Cytologic Features

Intestinal carcinoids exfoliate well in variably cohesive sheets, often with poor intercellular boundaries and many bare nuclei, which can help differentiate these from adeno-carcinomas (compare Figures 9.16 and 9.14). Intact cells

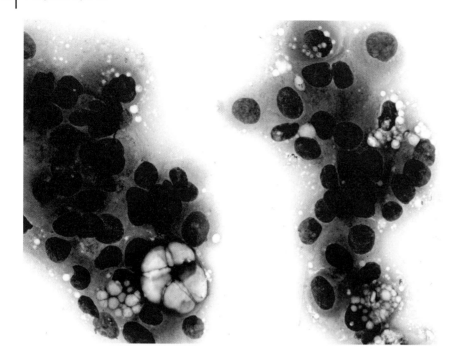

Figure 9.15 Colon, adenocarcinoma, dog, 50× objective.

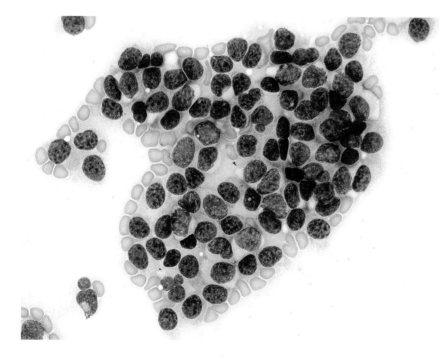

Figure 9.16 Intestine, carcinoid, dog, 50× objective.

are round, with a moderate volume of medium-blue cytoplasm. Nuclei are round, with finely stippled chromatin and multiple, small, basophilic nucleoli. Hyperchromasia is a common finding. Anisocytosis/anisokaryosis and N/C ratios generally are moderate.

9.2.8.2 Clinical Considerations

- Malignant tumors arising from enterochromaffin cells of the intestinal mucosa [51].

- May occur in the small or large intestine.
- Clinical signs = hematemesis, melena [52].

9.2.8.3 Prognosis

Guarded to poor. Some patients may experience prolonged survival with surgical and medical therapy [53]. Tumors frequently metastasize, mostly to the liver [51]. Rectal location has a favorable prognosis in humans, and may also confer a better prognosis in dogs [54].

9.2.9 Gastrointestinal Stromal Tumor

9.2.9.1 Cytologic Features

Gastrointestinal stromal tumors (GISTs) frequently are highly exfoliative, comprising spindloid cells in tight, crowded aggregates. The cells have a scant volume of pale-blue cytoplasm forming long delicate tendrils and wisps. Nuclei are elongated or 'cigar-shaped' with coarsely granular chromatin and mostly inapparent nucleoli (Figure 9.17). Anisocytosis/anisokaryosis are mild and N/C ratios are high. GISTs appear cytologically similar to leiomyomas and leiomyosarcomas (compare to Figure 9.18) and require histopathology for definitive characterization.

9.2.9.2 Clinical Considerations

- Dogs > > cats (extremely rare) [55–57].
- Originate from interstitial cells of Cajal.
- Older patients (mean age 11 years) [55].

Figure 9.17 Colon, gastrointestinal stromal tumor (GIST), dog, 50× objective.

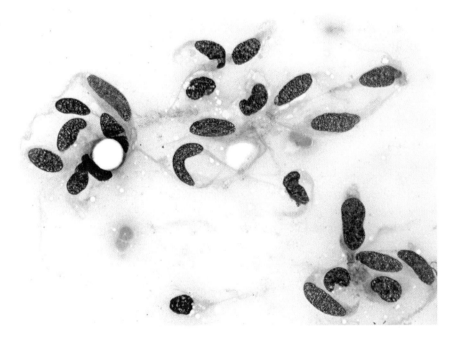

Figure 9.18 Stomach, leiomyosarcoma, cat, 50× objective.

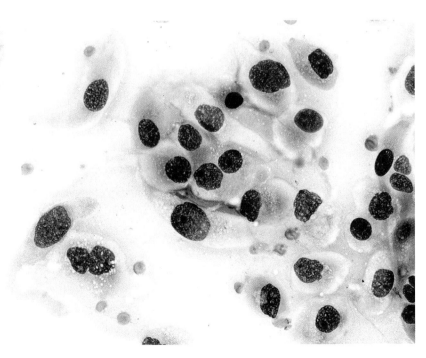

- Most common in the large intestine and cecum (>50% of cases), less common in the small intestine and stomach [55, 56].
- Often clinically silent [58], but may cause vomiting, inappetence, and melena.
- Paraneoplastic leukocytosis (predominantly neutrophilic) reported [59].

9.2.9.3 Prognosis

Metastatic disease is seen in ~30% of cases, in the liver, abdominal cavity, and spleen [55]. Patients without metastatic disease and surviving surgical removal can have a good prognosis [56, 60]. Small intestinal location is associated with shorter survival times [61].

9.2.10 Leiomyosarcoma

9.2.10.1 Cytologic Features

Leiomyosarcomas exfoliate variably well in loose aggregates and individually. They comprise plump spindle cells with a moderate volume of medium-blue cytoplasm forming short bipolar tapering ends and may contain fine clear vacuoles. Nuclei are ovoid with coarsely granular chromatin and prominent basophilic nucleoli. Anisocytosis/anisokaryosis are marked and N/C ratios are moderate to high (Figure 9.18). Well-differentiated tumors may mimic GISTs; however, leiomyosarcoma cells generally are more plump and have greater criteria of malignancy (compare to Figure 9.17).

9.2.10.2 Clinical Considerations

- Dogs > cats [27, 62, 63].
- Malignant tumors arising from smooth muscle cells [62].
- Predilection for jejunum and stomach but may affect any segment of the gastrointestinal tract [56, 62–65].
- May be associated with paraneoplastic syndromes such as hypoglycemia and nephrogenic diabetes insipidus [65].

9.2.10.3 Prognosis

Variable. Long-term survival can be seen in dogs surviving surgical resection of masses, even in the presence of metastatic disease [62, 65]. Recurrence is associated with a poor prognosis [62].

9.2.11 Feline Gastrointestinal Eosinophilic Sclerosing Fibroplasia

9.2.11.1 Cytologic Features

FGESF is characterized by an infiltrate of eosinophils, accompanied by a population of mesenchymal cells that are typically plump, spindloid cells with a moderate volume of pale-blue cytoplasm forming tendrils and wisps, with mild to moderate anisocytosis/anisokaryosis (Figure 9.19). Other inflammatory cells including neutrophils and small lymphocytes may be present, as well as bright pink ribbons of collagen. Bacterial sepsis is also common [66, 67]. *Note*: It is critical to examine closely for the presence and morphology of mast cells (see Figure 9.12), as eosinophilic inflammation and fibroplasia

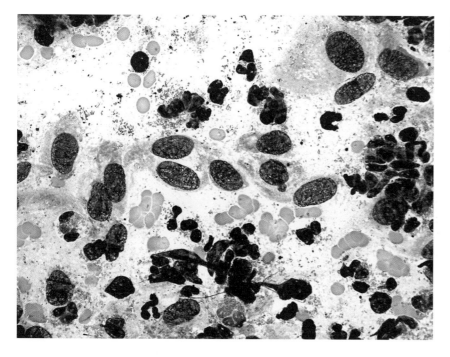

Figure 9.19 Intestine, cat, 50× objective. Feline gastrointestinal eosinophilic sclerosing fibroplasia.

are commonly present in mast cell tumors, and rare mast cells may be present in samples from FGESF.

9.2.11.2 Clinical Considerations

- Inflammatory process characterized by mass lesions; mostly solitary but may be multiple [66, 68].
- Lesions most common at the pyloric sphincter, ileocolic junction, or colon [66, 67, 69].
- Lymph nodes may be involved, and lesions have also been described in the mesentery and liver [66, 68, 70].
- Masses often feel 'gritty' on needle aspiration [67].
- Peripheral eosinophilia is variably present [66, 69].

9.2.11.3 Prognosis

Variable. Many cats have long survival times, especially with early surgical or medical therapy [66–69, 71]. Cats diagnosed late in the disease process often have poor outcomes [66, 67].

9.3 Feces

9.3.1 Normal

9.3.1.1 Cytologic Features

Normal flora within feces is predominated by a polymorphic population of mostly rod-shaped bacteria (Figure 9.20) [72]. Cocci should rarely be seen. Additionally, rare spiral bacteria and rare spore-forming bacteria may be present. Small enteric yeasts (Figure 9.21) are common in low to moderate numbers, and *Cyniclomyces guttulatus* may be an incidental finding (see Chapter 3). Well-differentiated columnar epithelial cells may be present in samples from rectal scrapes.

9.3.1.2 Clinical Considerations

- Digital collection or rectal scraping are more sensitive than rectal lavage in detecting neutrophils and epithelial cells and are the recommended sampling techniques to create dry-mount cytology slides [73].

9.3.2 Inflammation/Infection

9.3.2.1 Cytologic Features

Inflammatory cells may be seen in feces, indicative of gastroenteritis, or colitis (Figure 9.22). Evidence of infection may be seen by a monomorphic expansion of bacteria (Figure 9.23), including spore-forming bacteria or spiral-shaped bacteria (e.g., *Clostridium* spp. and *Campylobacter* spp.; see Chapter 3 for details). Additionally, many important gastrointestinal pathogens may be identified, including protozoa (e.g., *Giardia, Cryptosporidium*), algae (e.g., *Prototheca*), or fungi (e.g., *Histoplasma, Pythiosis*). The reader is referred to Chapter 3 for details of these organisms.

9.3.2.2 Clinical Considerations

- Plasma cells and lymphocytes may be seen in cases of IBD.
- Bacterial overgrowth may be primary or secondary to antibiotic therapy, exocrine pancreatic insufficiency, or IBD [74].

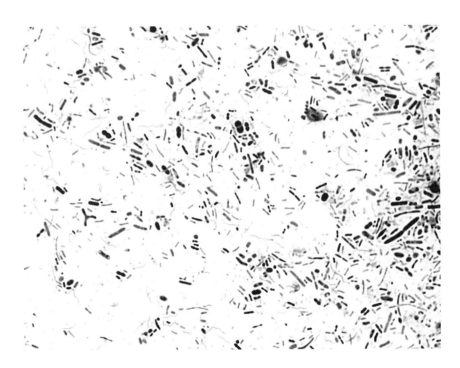

Figure 9.20 Feces, normal, dog, 100× objective. Note the mixed population of bacteria, dominated by rods.

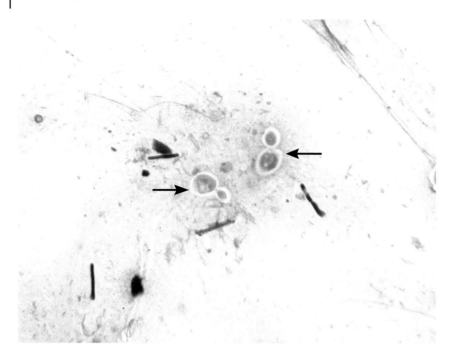

Figure 9.21 Feces, normal, dog, 100× objective. Small, encapsulated enteric yeast are seen (arrows), accompanied by rod-shaped bacteria.

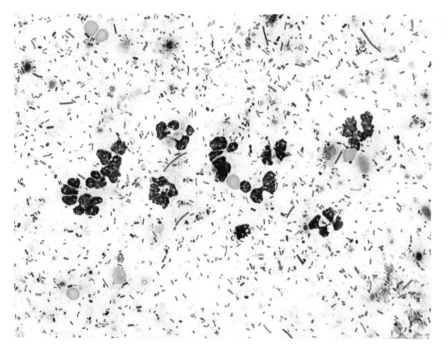

Figure 9.22 Feces, neutrophilic inflammation, dog, 50× objective.

9.3.2.3 Prognosis

Variable, based on the underlying cause of inflammation.

9.3.3 Parasite Ova: Roundworm

9.3.3.1 Cytologic Features

Eggs from roundworms are round, and ~65–90 μm in diameter. They have a characteristic rough outer shell wall. Eggs passed in feces are unlarvated and have a large, dark brown, and round embryo (Figure 9.24).

9.3.3.2 Clinical Considerations

- Most common species = *Toxocara canis* (dog), *Toxocara cati* (cats), and *Toxascaris leonina* (dog and cat).
- Zoonotic potential.

9.3.3.3 Prognosis

Good with treatment. Untreated *T. canis* can result in intussusception, obstruction, or rupture of the intestines and may be fatal. Pneumonia from parasite migration may also be fatal [75].

Figure 9.23 Feces, bacterial overgrowth (cocci), dog, 100× objective.

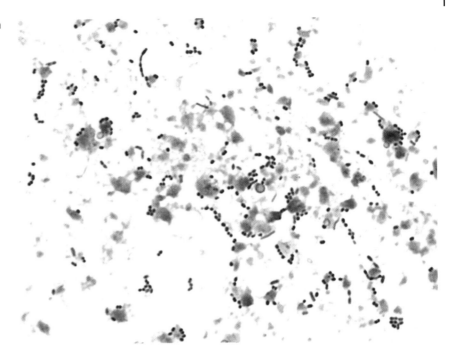

Figure 9.24 Feces, *Toxocara canis* (roundworm) ova, dog, 50× objective.

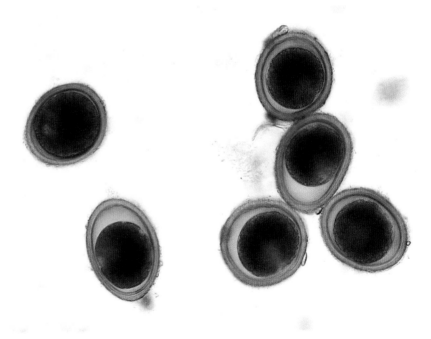

9.3.4 Parasite Ova: Hookworm

9.3.4.1 Cytologic Features

These eggs are ellipsoidal, ~50–75 μm in length and 30–50 μm wide. They have a smooth, clear shell, and contain an embryo in the morula stage of development that may have variable divisions (Figure 9.25).

9.3.4.2 Clinical Considerations

- Dogs > cats. *Ancylostoma* spp. more common than *Uncinaria* spp. [76]
- Eggs detected in feces after onset of clinical signs [75]. Common in feces of dogs with parasites present in feces [77].

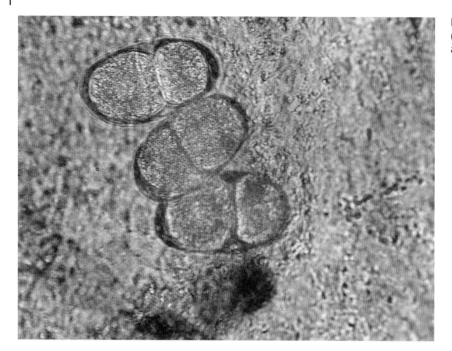

Figure 9.25 Feces, *Ancylostoma caninum* (hookworm), dog, 100× objective. Note abundant blood in the background.

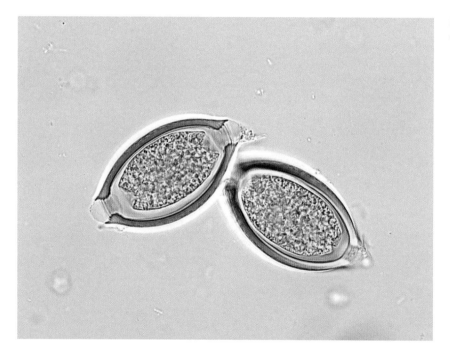

Figure 9.26 Feces, *Trichuris vulpis* (whipworm), dog, 50× objective.

- *Ancylostom caninum* associated with severe, possibly fatal anemia.
- Zoonotic potential.

9.3.4.3 Prognosis
Guarded. Poor without treatment.

9.3.5 Parasite Ova: Whipworm

9.3.5.1 Cytologic Features
Eggs are lemon-shaped with distinct bipolar plugs (Figure 9.26). Each egg contains a single cell. They generally are >75 μm in length.

9.3.5.2 Clinical Considerations

- Dogs >> cats. Infection in cats rare and incidental.
- *Trichuris vulpis* common in dogs of all ages [76].
- Most canine infections are asymptomatic but may cause intermittent mucoid diarrhea flecked with blood [75].

9.3.5.3 Prognosis

Excellent.

9.3.6 Parasite Ova: Tapeworm

9.3.6.1 Cytologic Features

Dipylidium caninum eggs often are seen in an egg capsule ~100–200 μm that contains 5–30 eggs (Figure 9.27). Individual eggs are round, ~30–50 μm in diameter, and have a thick, radially striated embryophore, containing an embryo with three pairs of hooks (Figure 9.28).

Figure 9.27 Feces, *Dipylidium caninum*, egg capsule, dog, 20× objective.

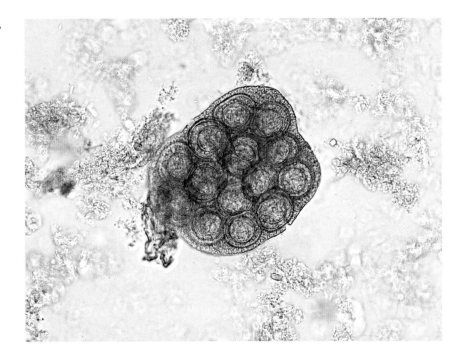

Figure 9.28 Feces, *Dipylidium caninum*, dog, 100× objective. Note individualized eggs that contain small hooks (arrows).

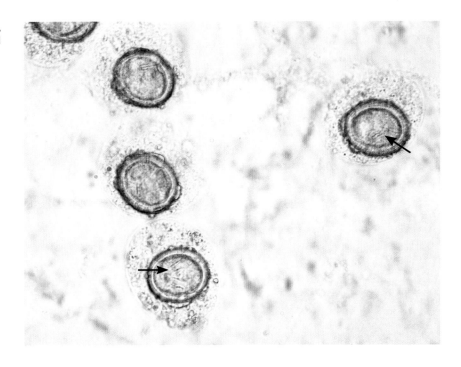

9.3.6.2 Clinical Considerations
- Common in dogs and cats, but incidence is declining [78].
- Eggs do not consistently float and may not be seen in fecal floats [79].
- Clinical disease rare. Perianal irritation most common.
- Zoonotic potential.

9.3.6.3 Prognosis
Excellent with therapy, including control of intermediate hosts (e.g., fleas).

9.3.7 Parasite Ova: Coccidia

9.3.7.1 Cytologic Features
Non-sporulated oocysts are detected in feces. These are ovoid, ~30–40 µm in length, and have a thin, double-layered outer wall encasing a small amount of clear cytoplasm and a single, or occasionally double, cell (sporont) (Figure 9.29).

9.3.7.2 Clinical Considerations
- *Cystoisospora* spp. (formerly *Isospora*) common in young dogs and cats [80, 81].
- High prevalence in crowded or unsanitary environments.
- Disease may be subclinical or self-resolving.
- Clinical signs = diarrhea, weight loss, and dehydration.

9.3.7.3 Prognosis
Excellent.

9.4 Pancreas

9.4.1 Pancreatic Nodular Hyperplasia

9.4.1.1 Cytologic Features
Nodular hyperplasia is characterized by cohesive sheets of epithelial cells with prominent intercellular borders, and cells do not overlap. Acinar or tubular arrangements are common. The cells have abundant cytoplasm that frequently contains fine clear vacuoles (Figure 9.30). Nuclei are round, with finely stippled chromatin and small basophilic nucleoli. Anisocytosis/anisokaryosis are mild and N/C ratios are low. Differentiation from adenomas or well-differentiated adenocarcinomas can be difficult (compare to Figure 9.31).

9.4.1.2 Clinical Considerations
- Common, incidental finding in older cats and dogs.
- Arise from hyperplasia of acinar cells of the exocrine pancreas.
- Mostly multiple nodules, though single masses may be present [82].
- Typically small lesions (<2 cm in cats) [82].

9.4.1.3 Prognosis
Excellent.

9.4.2 Pancreatic Adenoma

9.4.2.1 Cytologic Features
Pancreatic adenomas exfoliate in cohesive sheets of cuboidal to columnar cells that form acinar and tubular arrangements (Figure 9.31). The cells have a moderate

Figure 9.29 Feces, Cystoisospora spp. ova, cat, 100× objective.

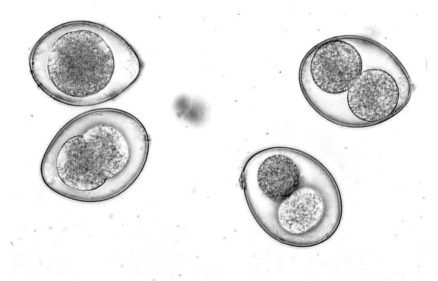

Figure 9.30 Pancreas, nodular hyperplasia, cat, 50× objective.

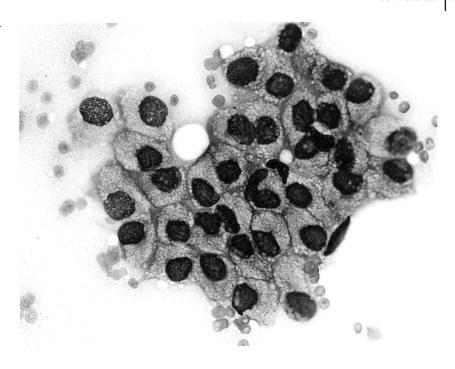

Figure 9.31 Pancreas, adenoma, dog, 50× objective.

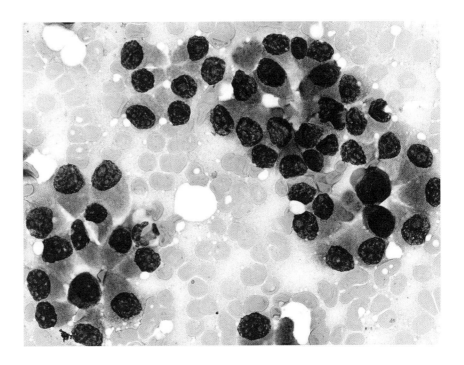

volume of medium-blue cytoplasm and round nuclei with single nucleoli. Anisocytosis/anisokaryosis are mild. These lesions may mimic well-differentiated adenocarcinomas (see Section 9.4.3 for distinguishing features).

9.4.2.2 Clinical Considerations

- Rare tumors, less common than adenocarcinomas and nodular hyperplastic lesions [83].
- Usually an incidental finding [84].

- Mostly solitary, solid, and well-encapsulated, but may be cystic [83].
- May be ductular or acinar in origin.

9.4.2.3 Prognosis

Good to excellent.

9.4.3 Pancreatic Adenocarcinoma: Well-differentiated

9.4.3.1 Cytologic Features

Well-differentiated pancreatic adenocarcinomas often are highly cellular and exfoliate in acinar or tubular arrangements that can make them difficult to differentiate from adenomas or nodular hyperplasia (Figure 9.32). Reliable distinguishing features from benign lesions are established for humans and include nuclear enlargement, nuclear membrane irregularity, anisonucleosis, and nuclear crowding/overlapping [85]. These features are seen by comparing Figures 9.30–9.34, which highlight the increasing spectrum of malignancy in pancreatic masses.

9.4.3.2 Clinical Considerations

- May be ductular or acinar in origin.
- A single mass >2 cm in diameter is more likely to represent malignant neoplasia than benign hyperplasia in cats [82].
- Cytologic analysis of pancreatic masses correlates well with histologic analysis in human and veterinary medicine when performed by experienced cytopathologists [85, 86].

9.4.3.3 Prognosis

Poor to grave. Despite a well-differentiated appearance, 85% of dogs and cats have evidence of metastatic disease at the time of diagnosis, most commonly in the liver [87].

9.4.4 Pancreatic Adenocarcinoma: Poorly Differentiated

9.4.4.1 Cytologic Features

Poorly differentiated pancreatic adenocarcinomas have marked criteria of malignancy (Figure 9.33) and may lose differentiating features of pancreatic epithelium. Anisocytosis/anisokaryosis are marked, cells may dissociate from sheets, and mitotic figures often are seen (Figure 9.34).

9.4.4.2 Clinical Considerations

- May be acinar (more common) or ductular in origin [88, 89].
- Most commonly a single mass but can be multinodular or diffuse thickening of the pancreas [89].
- Older patients (mean age 9 and 10 years for dogs and cats, respectively) [87].
- Often associated with concurrent pancreatitis [88].

9.4.4.3 Prognosis

Prognosis is similar to well-differentiated carcinomas, and is poor to grave, with high rates of metastatic disease and short survival times [90].

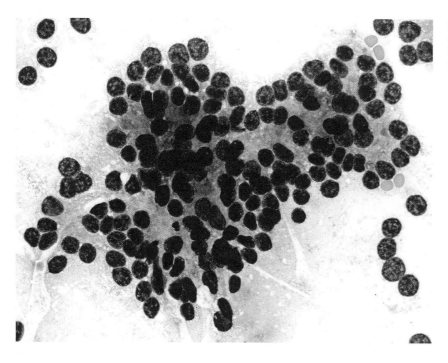

Figure 9.32 Pancreas, adenocarcinoma (well differentiated), dog, 50× objective. Note the increased cell piling and crowding compared to Figure 9.31.

Figure 9.33 Pancreas, adenocarcinoma (poorly differentiated), cat, 50× objective.

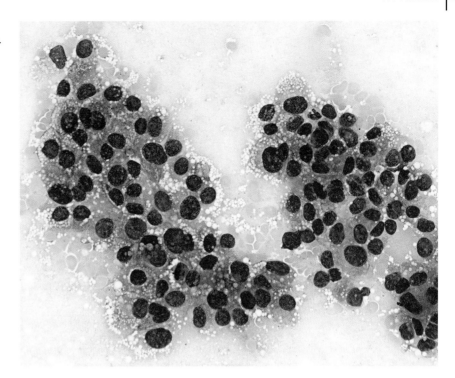

Figure 9.34 Pancreas, adenocarcinoma, (poorly differentiated), dog, 50× objective.

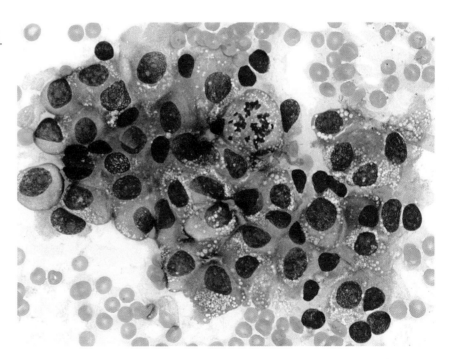

9.4.5 Insulinoma (Pancreatic Beta Islet Cell Tumors)

9.4.5.1 Cytologic Features

Insulinomas frequently are highly cellular. However, many cells may rupture creating a homogeneous blue background with many bare nuclei, typical of tumors of neuroendocrine origin. Intact cells are seen individually and in loosely cohesive sheets. They are round, with a moderate volume of medium-blue cytoplasm. Nuclear features are distinctive, with many reniform, indented, or cleaved variants (Figure 9.35). They have stippled chromatin with multiple small nucleoli. Anisocytosis/anisokaryosis are mild to moderate and N/C ratios are moderate to high. They appear similar to other tumors of neuroendocrine origin of the pancreas including gastrinoma (see Figure 9.36) and glucagonoma.

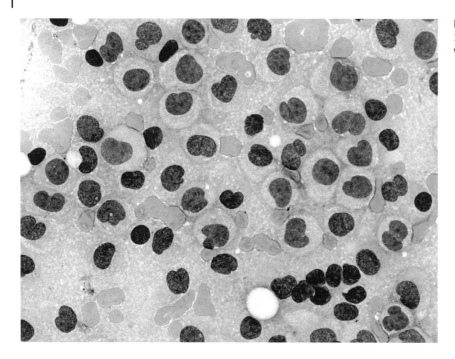

Figure 9.35 Pancreas, insulinoma, dog, 50× objective. Note the discrete cells with characteristic cleaved nuclei.

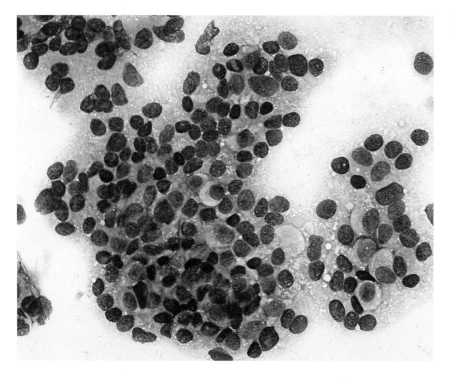

Figure 9.36 Pancreas, gastrinoma, dog, 50× objective.

9.4.5.2 Clinical Considerations
- Arise from neoplastic transformation of pancreatic beta cells.
- Dogs > cats, usually older patients.
- Often functional and associated with hypoglycemia despite a normal or elevated serum insulin concentration [91, 92].
- Clinical signs = seizures, weakness, change in behavior, and collapse [93, 94].

- Metastatic disease present at the time of diagnosis in ~50% of dogs, mostly in liver and lymph nodes [93].

9.4.5.3 Prognosis
Good short-term control is possible, but long-term prognosis is guarded to poor. Medical therapy alone and distant metastatic disease are associated with a poor prognosis in dogs [93–95]. Young age, low serum glucose concentration, metastatic disease at the time of surgery, tumor invasion,

and shorter time to euglycemia are poor prognostic factors in cats [91]. Surgical therapy ± medical therapy may result in prolonged survival times [95, 96].

9.4.6 Gastrinoma

9.4.6.1 Cytologic Features

Gastrinomas are characterized by variably cohesive sheets of round to ovoid cells that often appear discrete. They have a moderate to abundant volume of pale pink cytoplasm that may contain punctate clear vacuoles (Figure 9.36). Nuclei are ovoid with finely stippled chromatin with variably prominent nucleoli. Anisocytosis/anisokaryosis are moderate, and N/C ratios are moderate to low. They may appear similar to other tumors of neuroendocrine origin of the pancreas including insulinomas (see Figure 9.35).

9.4.6.2 Clinical Considerations

- Rare tumors in dogs and cats.
- Arise from malignant transformation of somatostatin-secreting delta cells of the endocrine pancreas to gastrin-producing cells [97].
- May also arise in other locations including duodenum, liver, and mesentery [98].
- Often associated with gastric and duodenal ulcers and Zollinger-Ellison syndrome [98, 99].

9.4.6.3 Prognosis

Guarded. Associated with high rates of metastatic disease, which confers a poor prognosis. Patients without metastatic disease treated with surgical and medical therapy can experience prolonged survival [100].

9.4.7 Non-epithelial Neoplasia

9.4.7.1 Cytologic Findings

Non-epithelial pancreatic tumors are rare [82, 86]. Lymphoma is one of the most common neoplasms identified (Figure 9.37), with other reported neoplasms including gastric carcinoma and histiocytic sarcoma [101, 102].

9.4.7.2 Clinical Considerations

- Correlate with clinical findings and other diagnostic test results in the patient.

9.4.7.3 Prognosis

Guarded to poor. Most non-epithelial neoplastic processes in the pancreas represent a wide dissemination of the underlying disease.

9.4.8 Pancreatitis

9.4.8.1 Cytologic Features

Samples usually contain both inflammatory cells and epithelial sheets. Inflammatory cells may comprise mostly non-degenerative neutrophils (acute pancreatitis) or lymphocytes/plasma cells (chronic pancreatitis). Epithelial cells generally are uniform, but they may have reactive changes such as a decreased volume of cytoplasm that is more basophilic (Figure 9.38).

Figure 9.37 Pancreas, metastatic large granular lymphoma, cat, 100× objective.

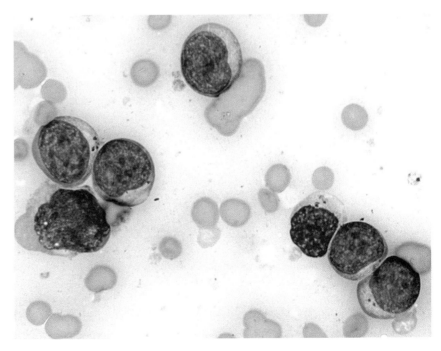

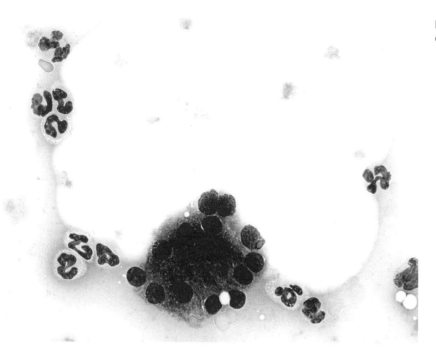

Figure 9.38 Pancreatitis, cat, 50× objective.

9.4.8.2 Clinical Considerations

- Cytologic analysis of pancreatic inflammatory disorders correlates well with histologic analysis [86].
- Careful evaluation for any infectious organisms and correlation with clinical and imaging findings are essential to differentiate neutrophilic pancreatitis from pancreatic abscesses (see Section 9.4.9).

9.4.8.3 Prognosis

Variable, based on the extent of inflammation and other comorbidities. Severe acute pancreatitis is associated with increased mortality rates, especially with concurrent abscess formation [103].

9.4.9 Pancreatic Abscess

9.4.9.1 Cytologic Features

Samples from pancreatic abscesses are dominated by variably degenerative neutrophils. Lesions may be sterile or septic and, if present, intracellular bacteria confirm septic inflammation (Figure 9.39). Reactive macrophages and small mature lymphocytes also may be present. Pancreatic epithelium may exfoliate and, if present, confirms pancreatic origin.

9.4.9.2 Clinical Considerations

- Rare in dogs and cats, and most develop as a sequela to pancreatitis.
- May be sterile or septic [104–106].
- Most present as single masses, but infection may be diffuse [107].

- Bacteria may not be seen, and microbial cultures frequently are negative [107, 108].
- Elevated BUN, ALP and rising HCO_3^- associated with poor outcome in dogs [107].

9.4.9.3 Prognosis

Guarded. Short-term mortality rates are high for dogs and cats (71% in a large retrospective study in dogs), but patients surviving surgery may do well [103, 107–109].

9.4.10 Pancreatic Cyst

9.4.10.1 Cytologic Features

Pancreatic cysts appear similar to cystic lesions in other locations and have a thick pink stippled to purple/blue proteinaceous background. Cellularity generally is low, and rare reactive macrophages or other inflammatory cells may be seen. Abundant crystalline debris often is present in pancreatic cysts, and cholesterol crystals may be present (Figure 9.40).

9.4.10.2 Clinical Considerations

- Rare findings in dogs and cats [110].
- Commonly contain pancreatic enzymes and debris, and likely form secondary to chronic pancreatitis [110].
- Congenital cysts are rare [111].
- Cytology useful to rule out other fluid-filled lesions (e.g., pancreatic abscess and cystic neoplasia) [106].

9.4.10.3 Prognosis

Mostly good with drainage. Underlying disease likely more important for prognosis.

Figure 9.39 Pancreatic abscess, cat, 50× objective. Sheets of well-differentiated pancreatic epithelium are surrounded by neutrophils. Bacterial cocci are seen in the background and within neutrophils (arrows).

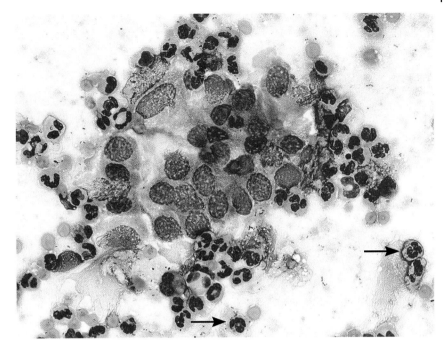

Figure 9.40 Pancreas, cyst, cat, 20× objective. Note the cholesterol crystals.

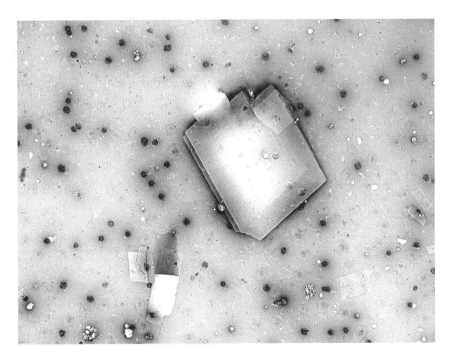

References

1 Boydell, P., Pike, R., Crossley, D., *et al.* (2000) Sialadenosis in dogs. *J. Am. Vet. Med. Assoc.*, **216** (6), 872–874.

2 Carberry, C.A., Flanders, J.A., Harvey, H.J., *et al.* (1988) Salivary gland tumors in dogs and cats: a literature and case review. *J. Am. Anim. Hosp. Assoc.*, **24**, 561–567.

3 Spangler, W.L., Culbertson, M.R. (1991) Salivary gland disease in dogs and cats: 245 cases (1985–1988). *J. Am. Vet. Med. Assoc.*, **198** (3), 465–469.

4 Lieske, D.E., Rissi, D.R. (2020) A retrospective study of salivary gland diseases in 179 dogs (2010-2018). *J. Vet. Diagn. Investig.*, **32** (4), 604–610.

5 Hammer, A., Getzy, D., Ogilivie, G., *et al.* (2001) Salivary gland neoplasia in the dog and cat: survival times and prognostic factors. *J. Am. Anim. Hosp. Assoc.*, **37** (5), 478–482.

6 Volmer, C., Benal, Y., Caplier, L., *et al.* (2009) Atypical vimentin expression in a feline salivary gland

adenocarcinoma with widespread metastases. *J. Vet. Med. Sci.*, **71** (12), 1681–1684.

7 Wong, V.M., Trageser, E.E., Luong, R.H. (2019) Pathology in practice. *J. Am. Vet. Med. Assoc.*, **254** (4), 475–477.

8 Bobis-Villagrá, D., Rossanese, M., Murgia, D., *et al.* (2022) Feline sialocoele: clinical presentation, treatment and outcome in 19 cats. *J. Feline Med. Surg.*, **24** (8), 754–758.

9 Bellenger, C.R., Simpson, D.J. (1992) Canine sialoceles – 60 cases. *J. Small Anim. Pract.*, **33** (8), 376–380.

10 Ritter, M.J., von Pfeil, D.J.F., Stanley, B.J., *et al.* (2006) Mandibular and sublingual sialocoeles in the dog: a retrospective evaluation of 41 cases using the ventral approach for treatment. *N. Z. Vet. J.*, **54** (6), 333–337.

11 Swieton, N., Oblak, M.L., Brisson, B.A., *et al.* (2022) Multi-institutional study of long-term outcomes of a ventral versus lateral approach for mandibular and sublingual sialoadenectomy in dogs with unilateral sialocele: 46 cases (1999-2019). *J. Am. Vet. Med. Assoc.*, **260** (6), 634–642.

12 Benjamino, K.P., Birchard, S.J., Niles, J.D., *et al.* (2012) Pharyngeal mucoceles in dogs: 14 cases. *J. Am. Anim. Hosp. Assoc.*, **48** (1), 31–35.

13 Tsioli, V., Papazoglou, L.G., Basdani, E., *et al.* (2013) Surgical management of recurrent cervical sialoceles in four dogs. *J. Small Anim. Pract.*, **54** (6), 331–333.

14 Brown, N.O. (1989) Salivary gland diseases. Diagnosis, treatment, and associated problems. *Probl. Vet. Med.*, **1** (2), 281–294.

15 Marsilio, S., Freiche, V., Johnson, E., *et al.* (2023) ACVIM consensus statement guidelines on diagnosing and distinguishing low-grade neoplastic from inflammatory lymphocytic chronic enteropathies in cats. *J. Vet. Intern. Med.*, **37** (3), 794–816.

16 Jergens, A.E. (2012) Feline idiopathic inflammatory bowel disease: what we know and what remains to be unraveled. *J. Feline Med. Surg.*, **14** (7), 445–458.

17 Bandara, Y., Priestnall, S.L., Chang, Y.M., *et al.* (2023) Outcome of chronic inflammatory enteropathy in cats: 65 ases (2011-2021). *J. Small Anim. Pract.*, **64** (3), 121–129.

18 Lane, J., Price, J., Moore, A., *et al.* (2018) Low-grade gastrointestinal lymphoma in dogs: 20 cases (2010-2016). *J. Small Anim. Pract.*, **59** (3), 147–153.

19 Kiselow, M.A., Rassnick, K.M., McDonough, S.P., *et al.* (2008) Outcome of cats with low-grade lymphocytic lymphoma: 41 cases (1995–2005). *J. Am. Vet. Med. Assoc.*, **232** (3), 405–410.

20 Couto, K.M., Moore, P.F., Zwingenberger, A.L., *et al.* (2018) Clinical characteristics and outcome in dogs with small cell T-cell intestinal lymphoma. *Vet. Comp. Oncol.*, **16** (3), 337–343.

21 Daniaux, L.A., Laurenson, M.P., Marks, S.L., *et al.* (2014) Ultrasonographic thickening of the muscularis propria in feline small intestinal small cell T-cell lymphoma and inflammatory bowel disease. *J. Feline Med. Surg.*, **16** (2), 89–98.

22 Freiche, V., Cordonnier, N., Paulin, M.V., *et al.* (2021) Feline low-grade intestinal T cell lymphoma: a unique natural model of human indolent T cell lymphoproliferative disorder of the gastrointestinal tract. *Lab. Investig.*, **101** (6), 794–804.

23 Stein, T.J., Pellin, M., Steinberg, H., *et al.* (2010) Treatment of feline gastrointestinal small-cell lymphoma with chlorambucil and glucocorticoids. *J. Am. Anim. Hosp. Assoc.*, **46** (6), 413–417.

24 Li, T., Chambers, J.K., Nakashima, K., *et al.* (2022) Intraepithelial cytotoxic lymphocytes are associated with a poor prognosis in feline intestinal T-cell lymphoma. *Vet. Pathol.*, **59** (6), 931–939.

25 Gieger, T. (2011) Alimentary lymphoma in cats and dogs. *Vet. Clin. North Am. Small Anim. Pract.*, **41** (2), 419–432.

26 Tidd, K.S., Durham, A.C., Brown, D.C., *et al.* (2019) Outcomes in 40 cats with discrete intermediate- or large-cell gastrointestinal lymphoma masses treated with surgical mass resection (2005-2015). *Vet. Surg.*, **48** (7), 1218–1228.

27 Kehl, A., Törner, K., Jordan, A., *et al.* (2022) Pathological findings in gastrointestinal neoplasms and polyps in 860 cats and a pilot study on miRNA analyses. *Vet. Sci.*, **9** (9), 477.

28 Stranahan, L.W., Whitley, D., Thaiwong, T., *et al.* (2019) Anaplastic large T-cell lymphoma in the intestine of dogs. *Vet. Pathol.*, **56** (6), 878–884.

29 Couto, C.G., Rutgers, H.C., Sherding, R.G., *et al.* (1989) Gastrointestinal lymphoma in 20 dogs. A retrospective study. *J. Vet. Intern. Med.*, **3** (2), 73–78.

30 Ozaki, K., Yamagami, T., Nomura, K., *et al.* (2006) T-cell lymphoma with eosinophilic infiltration involving the intestinal tract in 11 dogs. *Vet. Pathol.*, **43** (3), 339–344.

31 Gouldin, E.D., Mullin, C., Morges, M., *et al.* (2015) Feline discrete high-grade gastrointestinal lymphoma treated with surgical resection and adjuvant CHOP-based chemotherapy: retrospective study of 20 cases. *Vet. Comp. Oncol.*, **15** (2), 328–335.

32 Frank, J.D., Reimer, S.B., Kass, P.H., *et al.* (2007) Clinical outcomes of 30 cases (1997–2004) of canine gastrointestinal lymphoma. *J. Am. Anim. Hosp. Assoc.*, **43** (6), 313–321.

33 Krick, E.L., Little, L., Patel, R., *et al.* (2008) Description of clinical and pathological findings, treatment and outcome of feline large granular lymphocyte lymphoma (1996–2004). *Vet. Comp. Oncol.*, **6** (2), 102–110.

34 Snead, E.C. (2007) Large granular intestinal lymphosarcoma and leukemia in a dog. *Can. Vet. J.*, **48** (8), 848–851.

35 Ramos-Vara, J.A., Takahashi, M., Ishihara, T., *et al.* (1998) Intestinal extramedullary plasmacytoma associated with amyloid deposition in three dogs: an ultrastructural and immunoelectron microscopic study. *Ultrastruct. Pathol.*, **22** (5), 393–400.

36 Kupanoff, P.A., Popovitch, C.A., Goldschmidt, M.H. (2006) Colorectal plasmacytomas: a retrospective study of nine dogs. *J. Am. Anim. Hosp. Assoc.*, **42** (1), 37–43.

37 Trevor, P.B., Saunders, G.K., Waldron, D.R., *et al.* (1993) Metastatic extramedullary plasmacytoma of the colon and rectum in a dog. *J. Am. Vet. Med. Assoc.*, **203** (3), 406–409.

38 Rissetto, K., Villamil, J.A., Selting, K.A., *et al.* (2011) Recent trends in feline intestinal neoplasia: an epidemiologic study of 1,129 cases in the veterinary medical database from 1964 to 2004. *J. Am. Anim. Hosp. Assoc.*, **47** (1), 28–36.

39 Laurenson, M.P., Skorupski, K.A., Moore, P.F., *et al.* (2011) Ultrasonography of intestinal mast cell tumors in the cat. *Vet. Radiol. Ultrasound*, **52** (3), 330–334.

40 Sabattini, S., Giantin, M., Barbanera, A., *et al.* (2016) Feline intestinal mast cell tumours: clinicopathological characterization and KIT mutation analysis. *J. Feline Med. Surg.*, **18** (4), 280–289.

41 Henry, C., Herrera, C. (2013) Mast cell tumors in cats: clinical update and possible new treatment avenues. *J. Feline Med. Surg.*, **15** (1), 41–47.

42 Barrett, L.E., Skorupski, K., Brown, D.C., *et al.* (2018) Outcome following treatment of feline gastrointestinal mast cell tumours. *Vet. Comp. Oncol.*, **16** (2), 188–193.

43 Adamovich-Rippe, K.N., Mayhew, P.D., Marks, S.L., *et al.* (2017) Colonoscopic and histologic features of rectal masses in dogs: 82 cases (1995-2012). *J. Am. Vet. Med. Assoc.*, **250** (4), 424–430.

44 MacDonald, J.M., Mullen, H.S., Moroff, S.D. (1993) Adenomatous polyps of the duodenum in cats: 18 cases (1985-1990). *J. Am. Vet. Med. Assoc.*, **202** (4), 647–651.

45 Valerius, K.D., Powers, B.E., McPherron, M.A., *et al.* (1997) Adenomatous polyps and carcinoma in situ of the canine colon and rectum: 34 cases (1982–1994). *J. Am. Anim. Hosp. Assoc.*, **33** (2), 156–160.

46 Seiler, R.J. (1979) Colorectal polyps of the dog: a clinicopathologic study of 17 cases. *J. Am. Vet. Med. Assoc.*, **174** (1), 72–75.

47 Green, M.L., Smith, J.D., Kass, P.H. (2011) Surgical versus non-surgical treatment of feline small intestinal adenocarcinoma and the influence of metastasis on long-term survival in 18 cats (2000–2007). *Can. Vet. J.*, **52** (10), 1101–1105.

48 Patnaik, A.K., Hurvitz, A.I., Johnson, G.F. (1980) Canine intestinal adenocarcinoma and carcinoid. *Vet. Pathol.*, **17** (2), 149–163.

49 Czajkowski, P.S., Parry, N.M., Wood, C.A., *et al.* (2022) Outcome and prognostic factors in cats undergoing resection of intestinal adenocarcinomas: 58 cases (2008-2020). *Front. Vet. Sci.*, **9**, 911666. doi: 10.3389/fvets.2022.911666. Last accessed October 15, 2023.

50 Smith, A.A., Frimberger, A.E., Moore, A.S. (2019) Retrospective study of survival time and prognostic factors for dogs with small intestinal adenocarcinoma treated by tumor excision with or without adjuvant chemotherapy. *J. Am. Vet. Med. Assoc.*, **254** (2), 243–250.

51 Sako, T., Uchida, E., Okamoto, M., *et al.* (2003) Immunohistochemical evaluation of a malignant intestinal carcinoid in a dog. *Vet. Pathol.*, **40** (2), 212–215.

52 Nabeta, R., Kanaya, A., Ikeda, N., *et al.* (2019) A case of feline primary duodenal carcinoid with intestinal hemorrhage. *J. Vet. Med. Sci.*, **81** (8), 1086–1089.

53 Spugnini, E.P., Gargiulo, M., Assin, R., *et al.* (2008) Adjuvant carboplatin for the treatment of intestinal carcinoid in a dog. *In Vivo*, **22** (6), 759–761.

54 Sykes, G.P., Cooper, B.J. (1982) Canine intestinal carcinoids. *Vet. Pathol.*, **19** (2), 120–131.

55 Frost, D., Lasota, J., Miettinen, M. (2003) Gastrointestinal stromal tumors and leiomyomas in the dog: a histopathologic, immunohistochemical, and molecular genetic study of 50 cases. *Vet. Pathol.*, **40** (1), 42–54.

56 Russell, K.N., Mehler, S.J., Skorupski, K.A., *et al.* (2007) Clinical and immunohistochemical differentiation of gastrointestinal stromal tumors from leiomyosarcomas in dogs: 42 cases (1990–2003). *J. Am. Vet. Med. Assoc.*, **230** (9), 1329–1333.

57 Suwa, A., Shimoda, T. (2017) Intestinal gastrointestinal stromal tumor in a cat. *J. Vet. Med. Sci.*, **79** (3), 562–566.

58 Serpa, P.B.S., Santos, A.P. (2022) Incidental diagnosis of a spindle cell type gastrointestinal stromal tumor in a dog with ethylene glycol intoxication. *Vet. Clin. Pathol.*, **50** (Suppl 1), 70–75.

59 Gidcumb, E.M., Bolton, T.A., Trusiano, B., *et al.* (2023) Probable paraneoplastic leukocytosis in a dog with a gastrointestinal stromal tumor. *Vet. Clin. Pathol.*, **52** (1), 38–43.

60 Treggiari, E., Giantin, M., Ferro, S., *et al.* (2023) Canine gastrointestinal stromal tumours treated with surgery and imatinib mesylate: three cases (2018-2020). *J. Small Anim. Pract.*, **64** (3), 161–167.

61 Irie, M., Tomiyasu, H., Tsujimoto, H., *et al.* (2021) Prognostic factors for dogs with surgically resected gastrointestinal stromal tumors. *J. Vet. Med. Sci.*, **83** (9), 1481–1484.

62 Avallone, G., Pellegrino, V., Muscatello, L.V., *et al.* (2022) Canine smooth muscle tumors: a clinicopathological study. *Vet. Pathol.*, **59** (2), 244–255.

63 Henker, L.C., Dal Pont, T.P., Dos Santos, I.R., *et al.* (2022) Duodenal leiomyosarcoma in a cat: cytologic, pathologic, and immunohistochemical findings. *Vet. Clin. Pathol.*, **51** (4), 507–510.

64 Kapatkin, A.S., Mullen, H.S., Matthiesen, D.T., *et al.* (1992) Leiomyosarcoma in dogs: 44 cases (1983–1988). *J. Am. Vet. Med. Assoc.*, **201** (7), 1077–1079.

65 Cohen, M., Post, G.S., Wright, J.C. (2003) Gastrointestinal leiomyosarcoma in 14 dogs. *J. Vet. Intern. Med.*, **17** (1), 107–110.

66 Craig, L.E., Hardam, E.E., Hertzke, D.M., *et al.* (2009) Feline gastrointestinal eosinophilic sclerosing fibroplasia. *Vet. Pathol.*, **46** (1), 63–70.

67 Linton, M., Nimmo, J.S., Norris, J.M., *et al.* (2015) Feline gastrointestinal eosinophilic sclerosing fibroplasia: 13 cases and review of an emerging clinical entity. *J. Feline Med. Surg.*, **17** (5), 392–404.

68 Munday, J.S., Martinez, A.W., Soo, M. (2014) A case of feline gastrointestinal eosinophilic sclerosing fibroplasia mimicking metastatic neoplasia. *N. Z. Vet. J.*, **62** (6), 356–360.

69 Weissman, A., Penninck, D., Webster, C., *et al.* (2013) Ultrasonographic and clinicopathological features of feline gastrointestinal eosinophilic sclerosing fibroplasia in four cats. *J. Feline Med. Surg.*, **15** (2), 148–154.

70 Kambe, N., Okabe, R., Osada, H., *et al.* (2020) A case of feline gastrointestinal eosinophilic sclerosing fibroplasia limited to the mesentery. *J. Small Anim. Pract.*, **61** (1), 64–67.

71 Sivho, H.K., Simola, O.T., Vainionpää, M.H., *et al.* (2011) Pathology in practice. Severe chronic multifocal intramural fibrosing and eosinophilic enteritis, with occasional intralesional bacteria, consistent with feline gastrointestinal eosinophilic sclerosing fibroplasia. *J. Am. Vet. Med. Assoc.*, **238** (5), 585–587.

72 Broussard, J.D. (2003) Optimal fecal assessment. *Clin. Tech. Small Anim. Pract.*, **18** (4), 218–230.

73 Frezoulis, P.S., Angelidou, E., Diakou, A., *et al.* (2017) Optimization of fecal cytology in the dog: comparison of three sampling methods. *J. Vet. Diagn. Investig.*, **29** (5), 767–771.

74 Minamoto, Y., Otoni, C.C., Steelman, S.M., *et al.* (2015) Alteration of the fecal microbiota and serum metabolite profiles in dogs with idiopathic inflammatory bowel disease. *Gut Microbes*, **6** (1), 33–47.

75 Epe, C. (2009) Intestinal nematodes: biology and control. *Vet. Clin. North Am. Small Anim. Pract.*, **39** (6), 1091–1107.

76 Little, S.E., Johnson, E.M., Lewis, D., *et al.* (2009) Prevalence of intestinal parasites in pet dogs in the United States. *Vet. Parasitol.*, **166** (1–2), 144–152.

77 Nagamori, Y., Payton, M.E., Looper, E., *et al.* (2020) Retrospective survey of endoparasitism identified in feces of client-owned dogs in North America from 2007 to 2018. *Vet. Parasitol.*, **282**, 109137. doi: 10.1016/j.vetpar.2020.109137.

78 Gates, M.C., Nolan, T.J. (2014) Declines in canine endoparasite prevalence associated with the introduction of commercial heartworm and flea preventatives from 1984 to 2007. *Vet. Parasitol.*, **204** (3–4), 265–268.

79 Conboy, G. (2009) Cestodes of dogs and cats in North America. *Vet. Clin. North Am. Small Anim. Pract.*, **39** (6), 1075–1090.

80 Barta, J.R., Schrenzel, M.D., Carreno, R., *et al.* (2005) The genus Atoxoplasma (Garnham 1950) as a junior objective synonym of the genus Isospora (Schneider 1881) species infecting birds and resurrection of Cystoisospora (Frenkel 1977) as the correct genus for Isospora species infecting mammals. *J. Parasitol.*, **91** (3), 726–727.

81 Litster, A.L., Nichols, J., Hall, K., *et al.* (2014) Use of ponazuril paste to treat coccidiosis in shelter-housed cats and dogs. *Vet. Parasitol.*, **202** (3–4), 319–325.

82 Hecht, S., Penninck, D.G., Keating, J.H. (2007) Imaging findings in pancreatic neoplasia and nodular hyperplasia in 19 cats. *Vet. Radiol. Ultrasound*, **48** (1), 45–50.

83 Törner, K., Staudacher, M., Tress, U., *et al.* (2020) Histopathology and feline pancreatic lipase immunoreactivity in inflammatory, hyperplastic and neoplastic pancreatic diseases in cats. *J. Comp. Pathol.*, **174**, 63–72.

84 Seaman, R.L. Exocrine pancreatic neoplasia in the cat: a case series. *J. Am. Anim. Hosp. Assoc.*, **40** (3), 238–245.

85 Lin, F., Staerkel, G. (2003) Cytologic criteria for well differentiated adenocarcinoma of the pancreas in fine-needle aspiration biopsy specimens. *Cancer*, **99** (1), 44–50.

86 Cordner, A.P., Sharkey, L.C., Armstrong, P.J., *et al.* (2015) Cytologic findings and diagnostic yield in 92 dogs undergoing fine-needle aspiration of the pancreas. *J. Vet. Diagn. Investig.*, **27** (2), 236–240.

87 Bennett, P.F., Hahn, K.A., Toal, R.L., *et al.* (2001) Ultrasonographic and cytopathological diagnosis of exocrine pancreatic carcinoma in the dog and cat. *J. Am. Anim. Hosp. Assoc.*, **37** (5), 466–473.

88 Aupperle-Lellbach, H., Törner, K., Staudacher, M., *et al.* (2019) Characterization of 22 canine pancreatic carcinomas and review of the literature. *J. Comp. Pathol.*, **173**, 71–82.

89 Cony, F.G., Slaviero, M., Santos, I.R., *et al.* (2023) Pathological and immunohistochemical characterization of pancreatic carcinoma in cats. *J. Comp. Pathol.*, **201**, 123–129.

90 Pinard, C.J., Hocker, S.E., Weishaar, K.M. (2021) Clinical outcome in 23 dogs with exocrine pancreatic carcinoma. *Vet. Comp. Oncol.*, **19** (1), 109–114.

91 Veytsman, S., Amsellem, P., Husbands, B.D., *et al.* (2023) Retrospective study of 20 cats surgically treated for insulinoma. *Vet. Surg.*, **52** (1), 42–50.

92 Siliart, B., Stambouli, F. (1996) Laboratory diagnosis of insulinoma in the dog: a retrospective study and a new diagnostic procedure. *J. Small Anim. Pract.*, **37** (8), 367–370.

93 Goutal, C.M., Brugmann, B.L., Ryan, K.A. (2012) Insulinoma in dogs: a review. *J. Am. Anim. Hosp. Assoc.*, **48** (3), 151–163.

94 Ryan, D., Pérez-Accino, J., Gonçalves, R., *et al.* (2021) Clinical findings, neurological manifestations and survival of dogs with insulinoma: 116 case (2009-2020). *J. Small Anim. Pract.*, **62** (7), 531–539.

95 Polton, G.A., White, R.N., Brearley, M.J., *et al.* (2007) Improved survival in a retrospective cohort of 28 dogs with insulinoma. *J. Small Anim. Pract.*, **48** (3), 151–156.

96 Cleland, N.T., Morton, J., Delisser, P.J. (2021) Outcome after surgical management of canine insulinoma in 49 cases. *Vet. Comp. Oncol.*, **19** (3), 428–441.

97 Hoenerhoff, M., Kiupel, M. (2014) Concurrent gastrinoma and somatostatinoma in a 10-year-old Portuguese water dog. *J. Comp. Pathol.*, **130** (4), 313–318.

98 Struthers, J.D., Robl, N., Wong, V.M., *et al.* (2018) Gastrinoma and Zollinger-Ellison syndrome in canids: a literature review and a case in a Mexican gray wolf. *J. Vet. Diagn. Investig.*, **30** (4), 584–588.

99 Gal, A., Ridgway, M.D., Fredrickson, R.L. (2011) An unusual clinical presentation of a dog with gastrinoma. *Can. Vet. J.*, **52** (6), 641–644.

100 Myers-Nodes, J., Mazepa, A.S.W. (2022) Combined surgical and medical management of a cat with gastrinoma. *J. Small Anim. Pract.*, **63** (8), 632–634.

101 Lamb, C.R., Simpson, K.W., Boswood, A., *et al.* (1995) Ultrasonography of pancreatic neoplasia in the dog: a retrospective review of 16 cases. *Vet. Rec.*, **137** (3), 65–68.

102 Hayden, D.W., Waters, D.J., Burke, B.A., *et al.* (1993) Disseminated malignant histiocytosis in a golden retriever: clinicopathologic, ultrastructural, and immunohistochemical findings. *Vet. Pathol.*, **30** (3), 256–264.

103 Thompson, L.J., Seshadri, R., Raffe, M.R. (2009) Characteristics and outcomes in surgical management of severe acute pancreatitis: 37 dogs (2001-2007). *J. Vet. Emerg. Crit. Care*, **19** (2), 165–173.

104 Nemoto, Y., Haraguchi, T., Shimokawa Miyama, T., *et al.* (2017) Pancreatic abscess in a cat due to *Staphylococcus aureus* infection. *J. Vet. Med. Sci.*, **79** (7), 1146–1150.

105 Salisbury, S.K., Lantz, G.C., Nelson, R.W., *et al.* (1988) Pancreatic abscess in dogs: six cases (1978-1986). *J. Am. Vet. Med. Assoc.*, **193** (9), 1104–1008.

106 Talbot, C.T., Cheung, R., Holmes, E.J., *et al.* (2022) Medical and surgical management of pancreatic fluid accumulation in dogs: a retrospective study of 15 cases. *J. Vet. Intern. Med.*, **36** (3), 919–926.

107 Anderson, J.R., Cornell, K.K., Parnell, N.K., *et al.* (2008) Pancreatic abscess in 36 dogs: a retrospective analysis of prognostic indicators. *J. Am. Anim. Hosp. Assoc.*, **44** (4), 171–179.

108 Johnson, M.D., Mann, F.A. (2006) Treatment for pancreatic abscesses via omentalization with abdominal closure versus open peritoneal drainage in dogs: 15 cases (1994–2004). *J. Am. Vet. Med. Assoc.*, **228** (3), 397–402.

109 Son, T.T., Thompson, L., Serrano, S., *et al.* (2010) Surgical intervention in the management of severe acute pancreatitis in cats: 8 cases (2003–2007). *J. Vet. Emerg. Crit. Care*, **20** (4), 426–435.

110 VanEnkevort, B.A., O'Brien, R.T., Young, K.M. (1999) Pancreatic pseudocysts in 4 dogs and 2 cats: ultrasonographic and clinicopathologic findings. *J. Vet. Intern. Med.*, **13** (4), 309–313.

111 Healy, D.M., Cassidy, J.P., Martin, S.A. (2022) A true congenital pancreatic cyst in a dog. *BMC Vet. Res.*, **18** (1), 304.

10

Urinary

10.1 Kidney

10.1.1 Normal

10.1.1.1 Cytologic Appearance
Normal renal epithelial cells are round and may exfoliate individually or in small cohesive sheets. They have abundant clear to pale-blue cytoplasm and may contain coarse clear lipid vacuoles, particularly in cats (Figure 10.1). Glomerular tufts of capillaries may also be sampled (Figure 10.2).

10.1.2 Pyelonephritis

10.1.2.1 Cytologic Appearance
Generally characterized by a marked inflammatory infiltrate. Degenerative neutrophils containing intracellular bacteria are most common. Granulomatous inflammation is associated with fungal and *Mycobacterium* infections. Sheets of renal epithelial cells also may be seen (Figure 10.3).

10.1.2.2 Clinical Considerations
- Usually secondary to ascending infection.
- Clinical signs = acute pyelonephritis associated with anorexia, lethargy, abdominal pain, pyrexia, renomegaly, vomiting, polyuria/polydipsia. Chronic disease may not be associated with clinical signs [1, 2].
- Predisposing factors may include obstructive disease (uroliths and neoplasia), incontinence, chronic urinary tract infection, chronic kidney disease, and immunosuppressive therapies [2, 3].
- May cause acute kidney injury and lead to systemic infection and sepsis [4–6].
- Common bacterial isolates in dogs include *Escherichia coli, Pseudomonas aeruginosa*, and *Klebsiella pneumoniae* [3, 5–7].

10.1.2.3 Prognosis
Variable based on severity, any underlying kidney damage or concurrent disease. Mortality rates can be high, especially with systemic disease and multiple affected organs [2, 5, 6]. Dogs with urosepsis secondary to pyelonephritis can have good survival rates [5].

10.1.3 Renal Carcinomas

10.1.3.1 Cytologic Appearance
Renal carcinomas often exfoliate well in cohesive sheets with variably prominent intercellular borders. Nuclei are round to polygonal with a medium-blue cytoplasm that may contain small clear vacuoles. Nuclei are ovoid with finely granular chromatin and prominent, often multiple nucleoli. Anisocytosis/anisokaryosis vary from mild to moderate in well-differentiated tumors to marked in anaplastic neoplasms. Renal carcinoma (Figure 10.4), adenocarcinomas (tubular and papillary) (Figures 10.5 and 10.6), and transitional cell carcinoma (Figure 10.7), among others, are reported.

10.1.3.2 Clinical Considerations
- Most common primary tumor of the kidney in dogs [8].
- Unilateral > bilateral [9].
- Highly locally invasive (may invade vena cava) and high metastatic rate.
- Clinical signs = hematuria, polyuria/polydipsia, abdominal pain, lethargy. May be associated with azotemia and erythrocytosis [8, 9].
- *Note*: Metastatic disease of kidneys is more common than primary renal neoplasia [8, 10].
- May be associated with hypercalcemia of malignancy [11].

10.1.3.3 Prognosis
Guarded. All carcinoma types have similar clinical behavior. Nephrectomy for unilateral tumors with no evidence of metastatic disease may achieve moderate survival times [9].

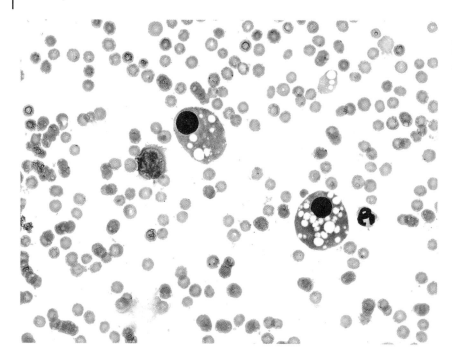

Figure 10.1 Normal renal tubular epithelial cells, cat, 50× objective. Note the coarse, clear lipid vacuoles in the cytoplasm.

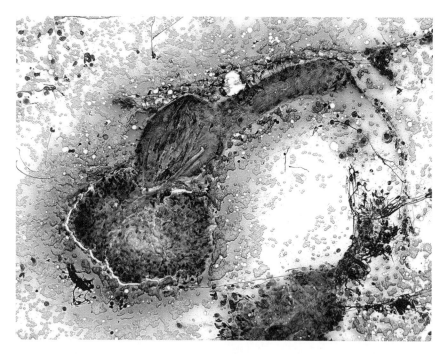

Figure 10.2 Glomerular tuft, cat, 10× objective. Note the linear renal tubule extending from the glomerular tuft.

Poor prognosis if surgery not performed/not possible. High mitotic counts within the tumor are associated with significantly shorter survival times [12].

10.1.4 Nephroblastoma

10.1.4.1 Cytologic Appearance

The epithelial component of nephroblastomas often exfoliates well as variably cohesive sheets of ovoid cells with a moderate volume of pale-blue cytoplasm. Bright-pink basement membrane-like material may be present (Figure 10.8). Nuclei are ovoid with finely clumped chromatin and small or inapparent nucleoli. Mitotic figures may be seen (Figure 10.9). Anisocytosis/anisokaryosis typically are mild to moderate (compared to renal carcinomas). Evaluation for areas of cohesion can be important to differentiate between loosely cohesive nephroblastomas and renal lymphoma (compare Figures 10.9 and 10.10).

Figure 10.3 Pyelonephritis, dog, 50× objective.

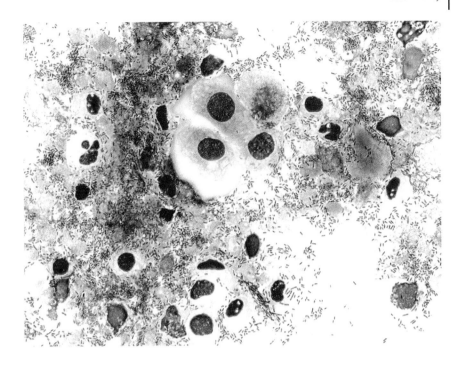

Figure 10.4 Renal carcinoma, dog, 50× objective.

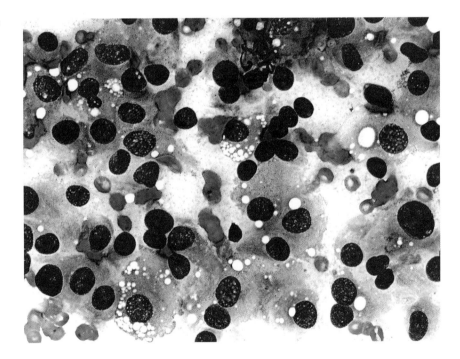

10.1.4.2 Clinical Considerations

- Rare tumors of embryonal metanephric blastema with epithelial and mesenchymal components.
- Dogs > cats
- Patients often younger than those with renal carcinoma or sarcomas and can be seen in dogs and cats <1 year of age [13–15].

- Solitary, unilateral tumors [9].
- May also be seen in the spinal cord (see Chapter 14).

10.1.4.3 Prognosis

Guarded to poor. Metastatic disease occurs early and widely, and survival times are short, even with surgery [9].

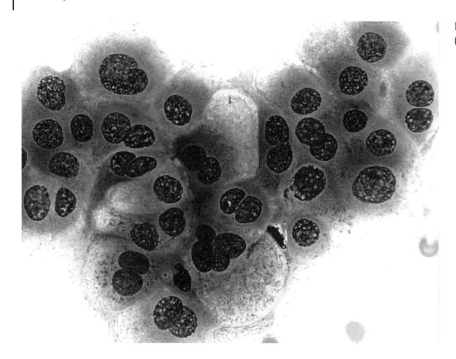

Figure 10.5 Renal adenocarcinoma (tubular), dog, 50× objective.

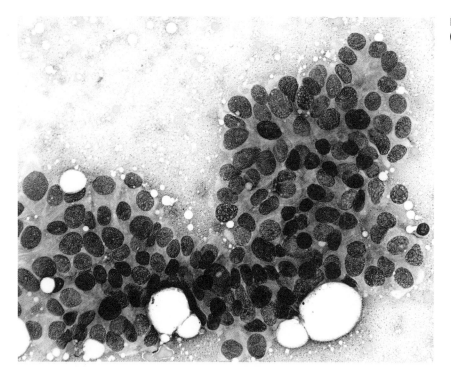

Figure 10.6 Renal adenocarcinoma (papillary), dog, 50× objective.

Nephrectomy in the absence of metastatic disease may lead to prolonged survival [15].

10.1.5 Lymphoma

10.1.5.1 Cytologic Appearance
Renal lymphomas often exfoliate in large numbers, comprising individualized cells with nuclei about twofold to threefold the size of red blood cells in diameter, and finely

stippled chromatin. The cells have a moderate volume of medium- to deep-blue cytoplasm that frequently contains fine clear vacuoles (Figure 10.10).

10.1.5.2 Clinical Considerations
- Bilateral > unilateral [16, 17].
- May be primary (more common in cats) or part of multicentric disease [18].

Figure 10.7 Renal transitional cell carcinoma, dog, 50× objective. Note the round, pink secretory material in the cytoplasm of some cells (arrows).

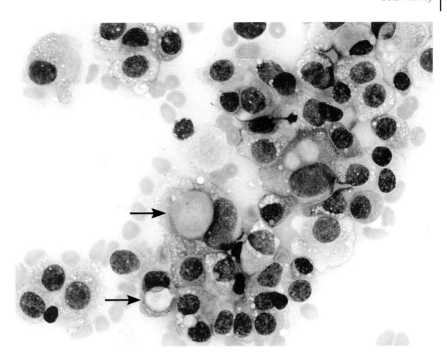

Figure 10.8 Nephroblastoma, dog, 50× objective. Note the bright-pink basement membrane between cells.

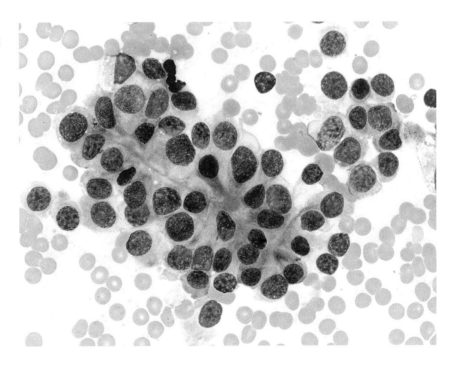

- Clinical findings = renomegaly, inappetence, weight loss, polyuria/polydipsia, azotemia, and erythrocytosis [16, 19].
- Cytology highly sensitive and specific for the diagnosis of renal lymphoma [20].
- Neoplastic cells may rarely exfoliate into urine [21].

10.1.5.3 Prognosis
Poor. Remission and survival times are short in both dogs and cats [17–19, 22, 23].

10.1.6 Renal Sarcomas

10.1.6.1 Cytologic Appearance
Sarcomas of the kidney exfoliate variably well, with cells seen individually or in aggregates. They have a small to moderate volume of cytoplasm forming bipolar tapering ends, and ovoid to elongated nuclei with granular chromatin and prominent nucleoli. Anisocytosis/anisokaryosis usually are moderate to marked and N/C ratios often are high (Figures 10.11 and 10.12).

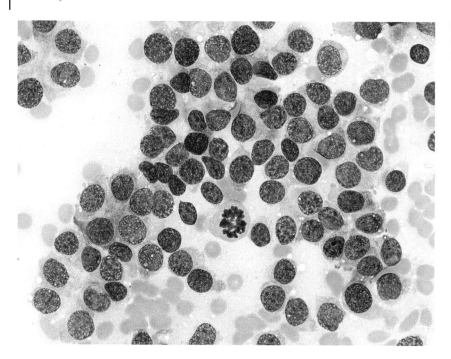

Figure 10.9 Nephroblastoma, dog, 50× objective. Cells are variably cohesive and mitotic figures are common (middle).

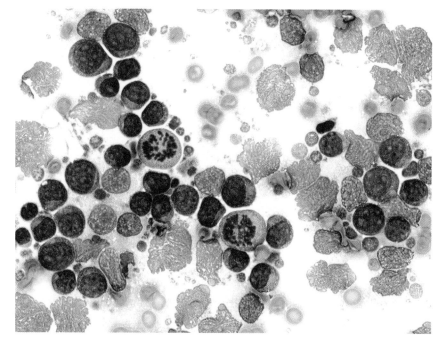

Figure 10.10 Renal lymphoma, dog, 50× objective.

10.1.6.2 Clinical Considerations
- Unilateral [9].
- Dogs > cats [9, 24].
- Hemangiosarcoma and renal sarcoma most common [9, 25].

10.1.6.3 Prognosis
Guarded to poor. High rates of metastasis and short survival times reported [9].

10.1.7 Renal Cysts

10.1.7.1 Cytologic Appearance
Renal cysts have a thick proteinaceous background that may be pink, blue, or purple. Cholesterol crystals and inflammatory cells – particularly reactive macrophages – often are present (Figure 10.13). Renal epithelial cells are variably present.

Figure 10.11 Renal sarcoma, dog, 50× objective.

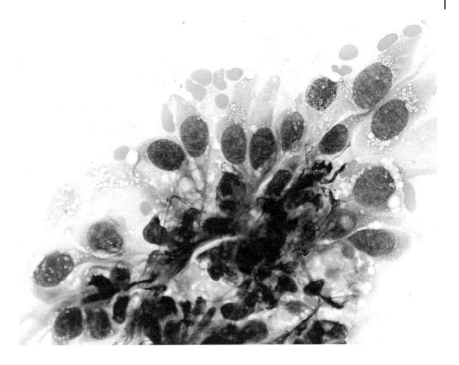

Figure 10.12 Renal hemangiosarcoma, dog, 50× objective.

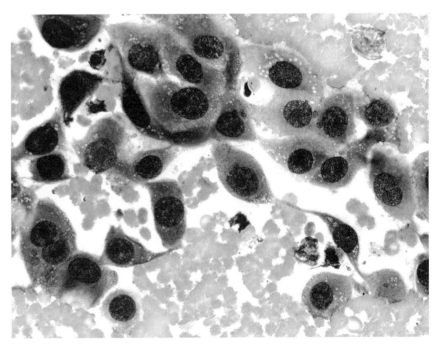

10.1.7.2 Clinical Considerations
- May be unilateral or bilateral.
- DDx = simple renal cysts, polycystic kidney disease, renal dysplasia, perinephric pseudocysts [26, 27].

10.1.7.3 Prognosis
Variable based on the underlying cause. Simple renal cysts often are incidental; perinephric pseudocysts carry a good prognosis [26, 27].

10.2 Bladder

10.2.1 Hyperplastic Epithelium

10.2.1.1 Cytologic Appearance
Hyperplastic transitional epithelium can be highly pleomorphic and may mimic neoplasia (compare Figures 10.14 and 10.16). It is normally seen secondary to inflammation (septic or sterile) or trauma/irritation (e.g., due to

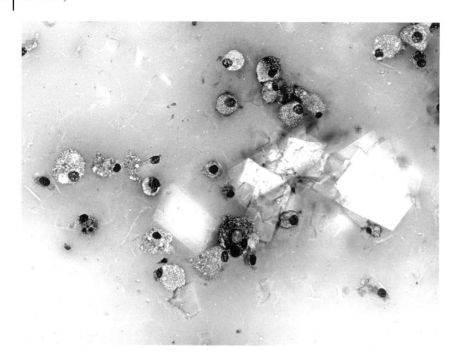

Figure 10.13 Renal cyst, cat, 20× objective. Note the large, rectangular, clear cholesterol crystals, and reactive macrophages.

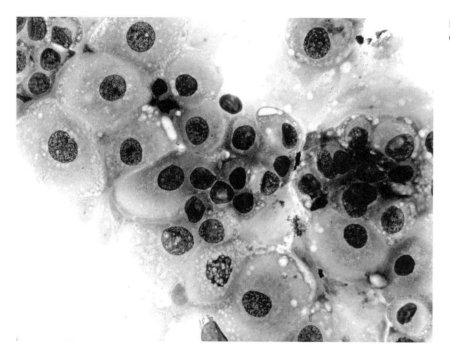

Figure 10.14 Bladder, transitional epithelial hyperplasia, dog, 50× objective.

urolithiasis), and evidence of inflammation, infectious organisms, or crystalluria frequently is present.

10.2.1.2 Clinical Considerations
- False-positive diagnoses of neoplasia may be made [28]. Always correlate with clinical/imaging findings, and histopathology may be required.

10.2.1.3 Prognosis
Excellent with treatment of the underlying inflammation/ infection.

10.2.2 Papilloma/Polyp

10.2.2.1 Cytologic Appearance
Papillomas and polyps exfoliate as cohesive sheets of monomorphic cells, in contrast to the gradient of pleomorphism seen with hyperplastic epithelium (compare Figures 10.15 and 10.14). Cells are round to polygonal and have a moderate volume of pale-blue cytoplasm. Nuclei are ovoid, with finely granular chromatin and small or inapparent nucleoli. Anisocytosis/anisokaryosis are mild and N/C ratios are moderate to low.

Figure 10.15 Bladder, polyp, dog, 50× objective.

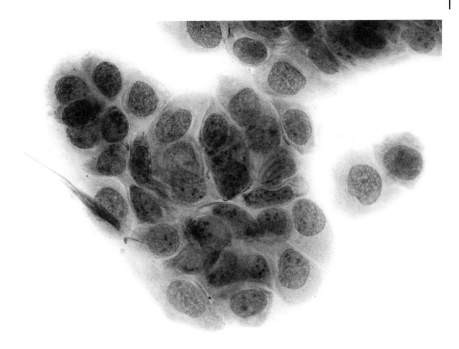

Figure 10.16 Bladder, transitional (urothelial) cell carcinoma, dog, 50× objective. Note the pink globular material within the cytoplasm of many cells (arrowheads) and the mitotic figure (arrow).

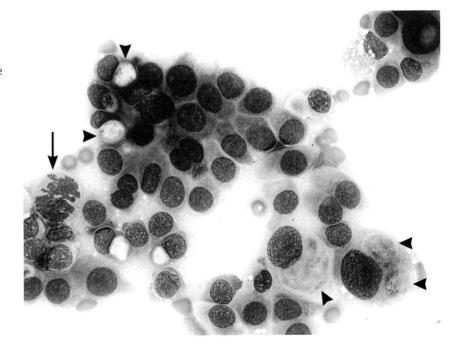

10.2.2.2 Clinical Considerations

- Much less common than malignant tumors [29].
- May represent benign neoplasia or nonneoplastic hyperplasia (e.g., polypoid cystitis) [30, 31].
- Unknown if papillomas/polyps represent a preneoplastic lesion [31].

10.2.2.3 Prognosis

Excellent.

10.2.3 Transitional Cell Carcinoma

10.2.3.1 Cytologic Appearance

Transitional cell carcinomas (TCCs) exfoliate as sheets of epithelial cells that are round to polygonal. They have a variable volume of cytoplasm that frequently contains bright-pink, spherical inclusions of secretory material, sometimes called *Melamed-Wolinska bodies* (Figure 10.16). Nuclei are ovoid, with granular chromatin and often multiple, prominent nucleoli. Multinucleation is common. Anisocytosis/anisokaryosis are marked and N/C ratios are variable.

10.2.3.2 Clinical Considerations
- Also known as *urothelial carcinoma.*
- Dogs >> cats. The most common bladder tumor in both species [32–34].
- Most often located in the trigone region in dogs. Location appears more variable in cats [35–37].
- Predisposing factors = females, neutered animals, breeds = Scottish Terrier, Shetland Sheepdog, Beagle, Wire-haired Fox Terrier, West Highland White Terrier [35].

10.2.3.3 Prognosis
Guarded to poor [35, 36, 38], though prolonged survival times are possible with therapy [37, 39]. Increased tumor size and the presence of metastatic disease significantly decrease survival times [35].

10.2.4 Lymphoma

10.2.4.1 Cytologic Appearance
Lymphoma of the bladder is characterized by large cells, with nuclei approximately twofold the size of RBCs in diameter, with stippled chromatin and often prominent nucleoli. The cells have a small rim of pale-blue cytoplasm that may contain punctate clear vacuoles (Figure 10.17).

10.2.4.2 Clinical Considerations
- Rarely reported in dogs and cats.
- Often localized to the bladder but may involve other organs [40–42].
- May cause wall thickening or mural masses and are indistinguishable on imaging from other bladder tumors [41, 43].
- Neoplastic cells may exfoliate into urine [40].

10.2.4.3 Prognosis
Guarded. Some reported cases have short survival times, while one patient experienced long-term remission with radiation and chemotherapy [40, 44].

10.2.5 Other Neoplasms

Other neoplasms that rarely affect the bladder include SCC (see Chapter 4), rhabdomyoma/sarcoma, leiomyoma/sarcoma (see Chapter 7), and hemangiosarcoma (see Section 10.1.6).

10.3 Urine

10.3.1 Normal/Hyperplastic Epithelium

10.3.1.1 Cytologic Appearance
Normal transitional epithelial cells are monomorphic, with minimal pleomorphism and low N/C ratios (Figure 10.18).

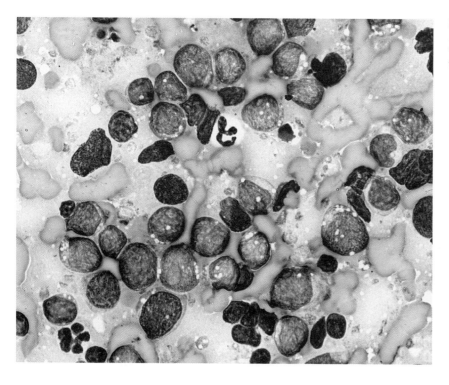

Figure 10.17 Bladder, lymphoma, cat, 50× objective. Note the punctate vacuoles in the cytoplasm of many of the cells.

Figure 10.18 Urine, normal transitional epithelium, dog, 50× objective.

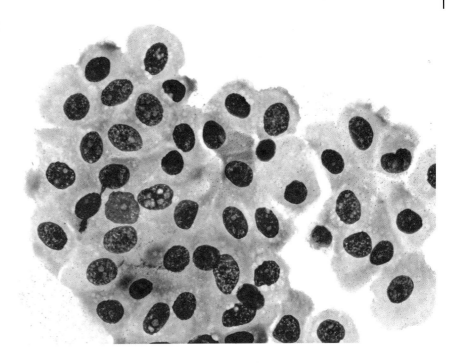

Figure 10.19 Urine, transitional epithelial hyperplasia, dog, 50× objective.

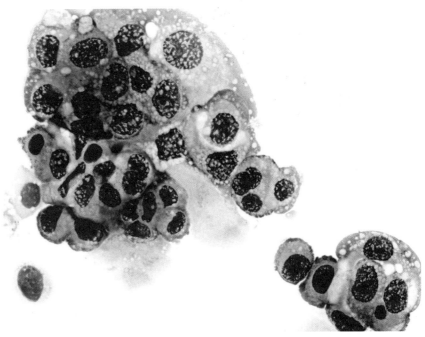

Hyperplastic transitional epithelial cells can exfoliate into urine and have increased pleomorphism that may mimic neoplasia (Figure 10.19). As described in Section 10.2.1, they often are accompanied by evidence of inflammation, infectious organisms, or crystals.

10.3.1.2 Clinical Considerations

- False-positive diagnoses of neoplasia may be made [28]. Always correlate with clinical/imaging findings, and histopathology may be required.

10.3.1.3 Prognosis

Excellent with treatment of the underlying inflammation/infection.

10.3.2 Neoplastic Epithelium

10.3.2.1 Cytologic Appearance

Exfoliation of neoplastic cells into urine is uncommon, and differentiation from epithelial hyperplasia can be difficult. Neoplastic cells should have marked criteria of malignancy, including marked anisocytosis/anisokaryosis, and prominent nucleoli ± mitotic figures (Figures 10.20 and 10.21).

10.3.2.2 Clinical Considerations

- Atypical epithelial cells should be correlated with clinical and diagnostic imaging findings.
- Traumatic catheterization or direct aspiration of any masses is more reliable for diagnosis.

10.3.2.3 Prognosis

Poor.

10.3.3 Inflammation/Infection

10.3.3.1 Cytologic Appearance

Leukocytes should be seen in low numbers in normal urine (<3 per 40× objective field in a wet preparation). Neutrophils are most frequently seen and may be

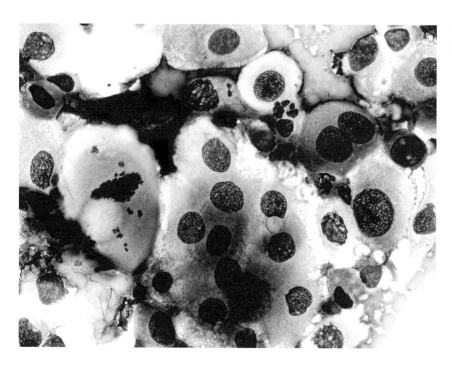

Figure 10.20 Urine, transitional cell carcinoma, dog, 50× objective. Note the bizarre mitotic figure on the left.

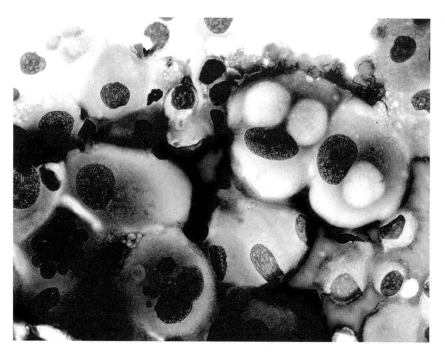

Figure 10.21 Urine, transitional cell carcinoma, dog, 50× objective. Note the multinucleated cells in the lower left.

associated with infectious organisms such as bacteria (Figure 10.22) or fungal agents (Figure 10.23).

10.3.3.2 Clinical Considerations
- Stained slides are recommended to most accurately evaluate infectious organisms [45, 46].

- Microbial culture and susceptibility testing is recommended even if bacteria are not seen.

10.3.3.3 Prognosis
Generally excellent, but variable with underlying cause of inflammation.

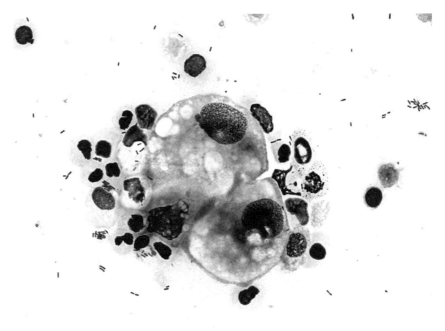

Figure 10.22 Urine, septic inflammation (bacterial), dog, 50× objective. Note bacteria within neutrophils and in the background.

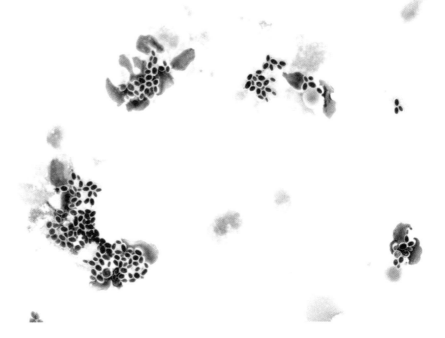

Figure 10.23 Urine, septic inflammation (fungal; *Candida* spp.), dog, 50× objective.

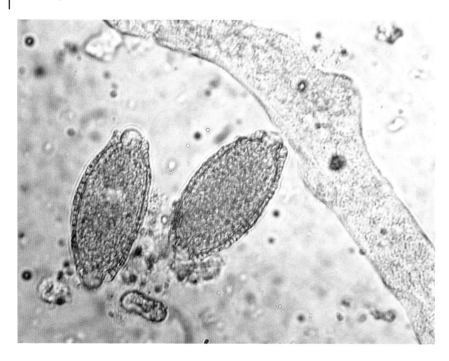

Figure 10.24 Urine, *Capillaria plica* ova, cat, 40× objective.

10.3.4 *Capillaria plica*

10.3.4.1 Cytologic Appearance
Eggs from *C. plica* (syn. *Pearsonema plica*) may be detected in urine samples. The eggs are lemon-shaped, with bipolar tilted terminal plugs (Figure 10.24).

10.3.4.2 Clinical Considerations
- Dogs and cats.
- Mostly incidental finding.
- Clinical signs (if present) = polyuria, pollakiuria, periuria, incontinence, dysuria, and urinary blockage [47, 48].

10.3.4.3 Prognosis
Generally excellent.

10.4 Urinary Crystals

The shape of crystals (habit) often provides a strong indication of composition. However, this is not always the case, and mixed crystals are possible. The following section provides classic examples of common crystal shapes seen in the urine of cats and dogs.

10.4.1 Struvite

10.4.1.1 Cytologic Appearance
Struvite crystals are colorless, mostly rectangular, and often have a characteristic 'coffin-lid' appearance (Figure 10.25). Struvite crystals may also appear as linear, needle-shaped crystals.

10.4.1.2 Clinical Considerations
- pH = alkaline urine.
- Common crystals in dogs and cats [49, 50].
- May be an incidental finding and may form *in vitro* in refrigerated or stored samples [51].
- Variably associated with struvite urolithiasis. Uroliths are radio-opaque.
- Uroliths amenable to medical dissolution [52].
- May be associated with sepsis due to urease-producing bacteria (e.g., *Staphylococcus*, *Enterococcus*, and *Proteus* spp.), especially in dogs [53].
- Mostly seen in small or toy-breed dogs; females > males [54].

10.4.2 Calcium Oxalate Dihydrate

10.4.2.1 Cytologic Appearance
Calcium oxalate dihydrate crystals are colorless, square, and have a characteristic cross pattern (Figure 10.26).

10.4.2.2 Clinical Considerations
- pH = mostly acidic urine.
- Common crystals in dogs and cats [49, 50].
- May form *in vitro* in refrigerated or stored samples [51].
- Often an incidental finding in clinically healthy patients.

Figure 10.25 Urine, struvite crystals, dog, 100× objective.

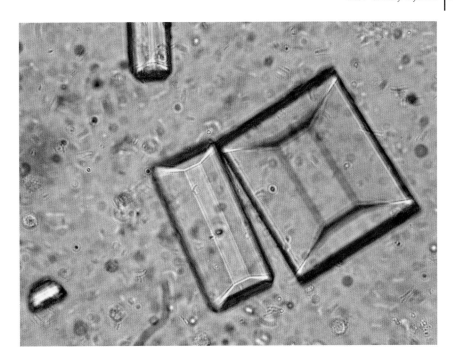

Figure 10.26 Urine, calcium oxalate dihydrate crystals, cat, 40× objective.

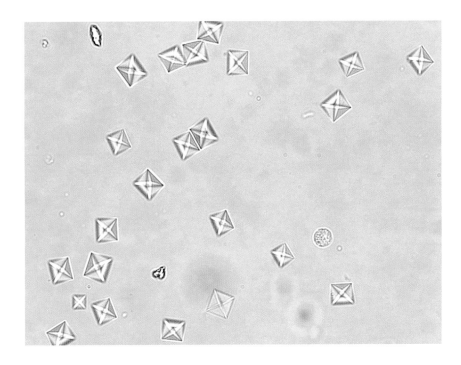

- Breed predisposition = long-haired cats (e.g., Persian and Himalayan) and small breed dogs (e.g., Miniature Schnauzer, Shih Tzu, and Yorkshire Terrier) [53].
- Uroliths not amenable to medical dissolution.
- High recurrence rate in dogs and cats [55, 56].

10.4.3 Calcium Oxalate Monohydrate

10.4.3.1 Cytologic Appearance

These crystals are variably shaped. Elongated crystals reminiscent of fence-posts often are associated with cases of ethylene glycol toxicity and may be accompanied by

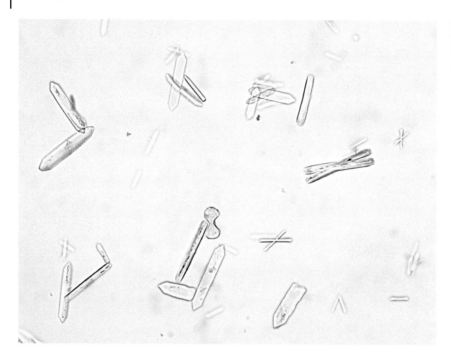

Figure 10.27 Urine, calcium oxalate monohydrate crystals, dog, 50× objective. Case of ethylene glycol toxicity. Slide courtesy of Dr. Reema Patel.

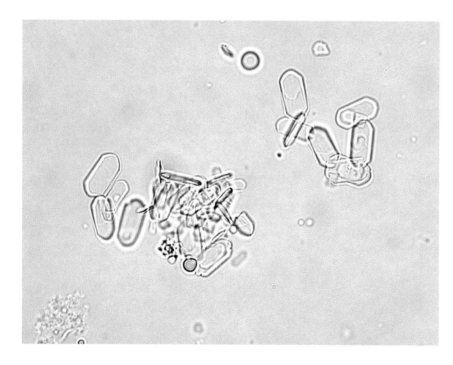

Figure 10.28 Urine, calcium oxalate monohydrate crystals, dog, 100× objective. Case of hypercalciuria. Note the small size and short nature of the crystals relative to those in Figure 10.27.

dumbbell and cross shapes (Figure 10.27). Crystals may also be associated with hypercalciuric or hyperoxaluric conditions and generally are smaller, shorter, and broader (Figure 10.28).

10.4.3.2 Clinical Considerations
- pH = acidic > neutral or alkaline urine.
- In large numbers, suggests hypercalciuric or hyperoxaluric conditions.

- The elongated form is most commonly seen in ethylene glycol toxicity, forming 3–9 hours post exposure, and may persist for up to 18 hours [57].

10.4.4 Ammonium Urate

10.4.4.1 Cytologic Appearance
Yellow/brown or amber crystals that are round to amorphous, with irregular spiny projections (Figure 10.29).

Figure 10.29   Urine, ammonium urate, dog, 50× objective.

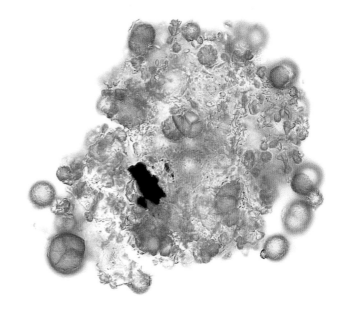

Figure 10.30   Urine, uric acid crystals, dog, 20× objective. Slide courtesy of Dr. Reema Patel.

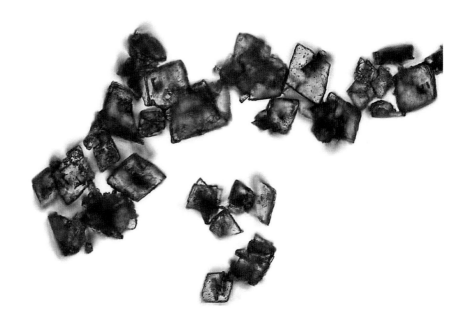

10.4.4.2   Clinical Considerations

- pH = mostly acidic urine
- Dogs > cats.
- Commonly associated with liver disease (e.g., portosystemic shunts) [58].
- Breed predisposition = Dalmatians and English Bulldogs [59].
- Medical dissolution possible (though not normally successful with untreated liver disease).

10.4.5   Uric Acid

10.4.5.1   Cytologic Appearance

Clear to yellow/brown, flat crystals that are diamond-shaped to six-sided (Figure 10.30). They may be seen individually or in aggregates. The crystals are birefringent under polarized light (Figure 10.31)

10.4.5.2   Clinical Considerations

- Similar to ammonium urate (see Section 10.4.4).

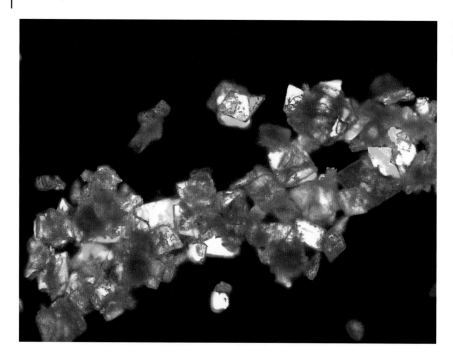

Figure 10.31 Urine, uric acid crystals under polarized light, dog, 20× objective. Slide courtesy of Dr. Reema Patel.

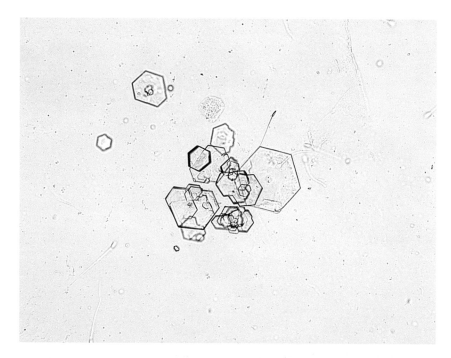

Figure 10.32 Urine, cystine crystals, dog, 20× objective. Note the spermatozoa in the background.

10.4.6 Cystine

10.4.6.1 Cytologic Appearance

Cystine crystals are colorless, flat, hexagonal crystals that may be seen individually but frequently stack in aggregates (Figure 10.32).

10.4.6.2 Clinical Considerations

- pH = acidic urine.
- Dogs > > cats.
- Due to proximal tubular defect in amino acid absorption (cystine, lysine, and arginine) [60].

Figure 10.33 Urine, bilirubin crystals, dog, 100× objective.

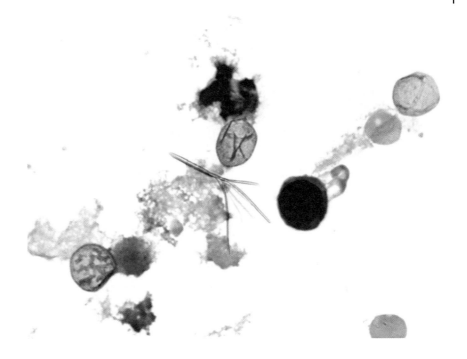

- Breed predisposition = Dachshunds, Basset Hounds, English Bulldogs, and Irish Terriers [59, 60].
- Uroliths frequently present and are amenable to medical dissolution.

10.4.7 Bilirubin

10.4.7.1 Cytologic Appearance
Needle-like crystals that are orange/amber, often seen in bundles and may be pinched in the middle (Figure 10.33).

10.4.7.2 Clinical Considerations
- pH = any
- May be seen in low numbers in concentrated urine from healthy male dogs.
- Indicate hemolytic or hepatobiliary disease.

10.5 Urinary Casts

10.5.1 Hyaline

10.5.1.1 Cytologic Appearance
Translucent and colorless, with parallel sides and rounded edges (Figure 10.34).

10.5.1.2 Clinical Considerations
- Comprised purely of mucoproteins (Tamm–Horsfall proteins) [61].
- Low numbers seen in normal/healthy patients (e.g., up to 2 per 10× objective field).

- Increased numbers may be seen secondary to fever, extreme exercise, renal disease, or diuresis.
- Increased contrast often required to visualize (either lower microscope condenser or close iris diaphragm).

10.5.1.3 Prognosis
Generally good – correlate with any possible underlying cause.

10.5.2 Granular

10.5.2.1 Cytologic Appearance
Granular casts are tubular and have a variably coarse, grainy appearance (Figures 10.34 and 10.35).

10.5.2.2 Clinical Considerations
- Thought to represent degenerated epithelial casts [59].
- Low numbers of granular casts are considered normal, especially in concentrated urine (e.g., 1–2 per 10× objective field).
- Similar rule-outs as epithelial casts.

10.5.2.3 Prognosis
Variable, based on the severity of the underlying disease.

10.5.3 Waxy

10.5.3.1 Cytologic Appearance
Waxy casts may appear similar to hyaline casts, but generally are wider, have blunt squared ends, are more opaque, and often have fissures (Figure 10.36).

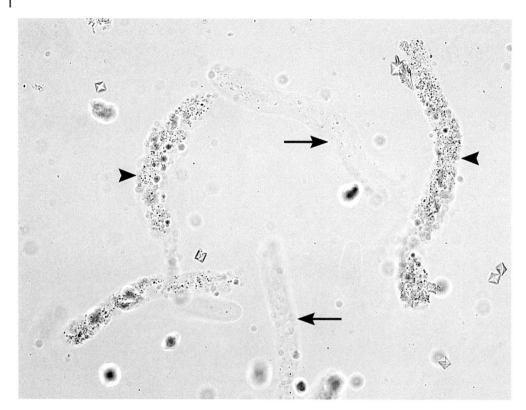

Figure 10.34 Urine, renal tubular casts, dog, 20× objective. Hyaline casts (arrows) are translucent and difficult to see. Note also the granular casts (arrowheads).

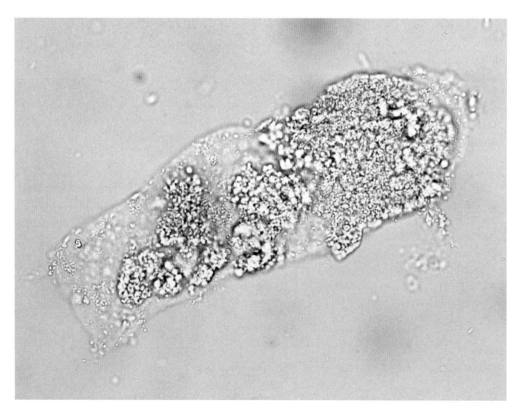

Figure 10.35 Urine, coarse granular cast, cat, 50× objective.

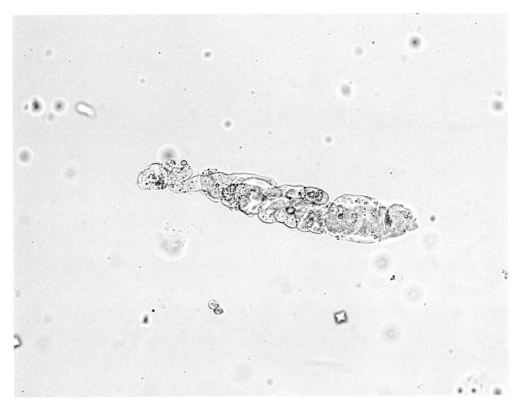

Figure 10.36 Urine, renal tubular cast (waxy), dog, 20× objective.

10.5.3.2 Clinical Considerations
- Considered the final stage of cast degeneration.
- Always considered pathologic and suggestive of chronic or prior renal tubular damage.

10.5.3.3 Prognosis
Variable, based on the severity/extent of disease.

10.5.4 Cellular

10.5.4.1 Cytologic Appearance
Sloughed/dead epithelial cells may become entrapped in mucoproteins and form epithelial casts. They are tubular and contain numerous nuclei of epithelial cells arranged in palisading rows (Figures 10.37 and 10.38). Cellular casts may also include leukocytes and red blood cells, indicating inflammation and hemorrhage, respectively.

10.5.4.2 Clinical Considerations
- Always considered abnormal and seen secondary to renal tubular disease.
- Rule-outs may include renal ischemia/infarction or drug/toxin exposure.

- May be seen prior to changes in serum renal markers or altered renal concentrating ability [59, 62].

10.5.4.3 Prognosis
Variable, based on the severity of underlying disease.

10.5.5 Fatty

10.5.5.1 Cytologic Appearance
Fatty casts contain numerous, variably sized round, highly refractile lipid droplets (Figure 10.39).

10.5.5.2 Clinical Considerations
- May be an incidental finding in low numbers, especially in cats.
- Seen in disorders of lipid metabolism such as diabetes mellitus [59].

10.5.5.3 Prognosis
Generally good but should be correlated with any underlying disease.

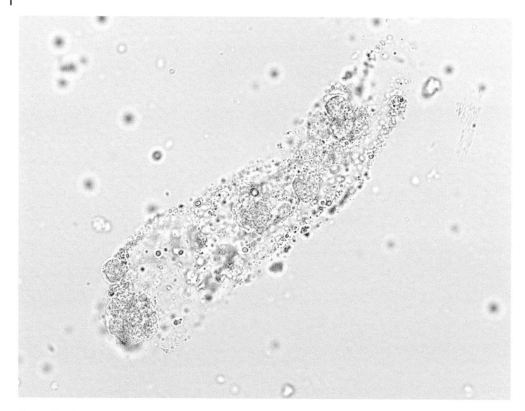

Figure 10.37 Urine, renal tubular cast (epithelial), cat, 20× objective. Note the epithelial cells trapped within the tubular cast.

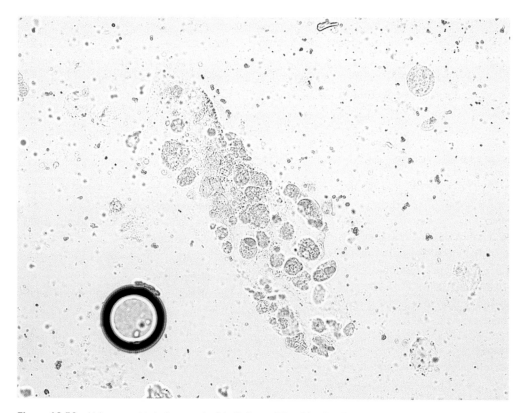

Figure 10.38 Urine, renal tubular cast (epithelial), cat, 20× objective. Renal tubular epithelial cells are seen in a tubular arrangement.

Figure 10.39 Urine, hyaline cast with entrapped lipid droplets, 40× objective. Courtesy of Dr. Annalisa Hernandez.

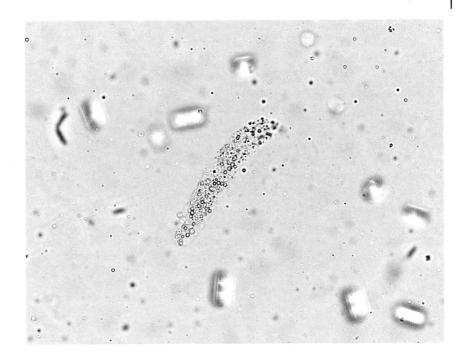

References

1 Dorsch, R., Teichmann-Knorrn, S., Sjetne Lund, H. (2019) Urinary tract infection and subclinical bacteriuria in cats: a clinical update. *J. Feline. Med. Surg.*, **21** (11), 1023–1038.

2 Bouillon, J., Snead, E., Caswell, J., *et al.* (2018) Pyelonephritis in dogs: retrospective study of 47 histologically diagnosed cases (2005-2015). *J. Vet. Intern. Med.*, **32** (1), 249–259.

3 Foster, J.D., Krishnan, H., Cole, S. (2018) Characterization of subclinical bacteriuria, bacterial cystitis, and pyelonephritis in dogs with chronic kidney disease. *J. Am. Vet. Med. Assoc.*, **252** (10), 1257–1262.

4 Chen, H., Dunaevich, A., Apfelbaum, N., *et al.* (2020) Acute on chronic kidney disease in cats: etiology, clinical and clinicopathologic findings, prognostic markers, and outcome. *J. Vet. Intern. Med.*, **34** (4), 1496–1506.

5 Perry, K.M., Lynch, A.M., Caudill, A., *et al.* (2022) Clinical features, outcome, and illness severity scoring in 32 dogs with urosepsis. *J. Vet. Emerg. Crit. Care*, **32** (2), 236–242.

6 Elbert, J.A., Rissi, D.R. (2022) Neuropathologic changes associated with systemic bacterial infection in 28 dogs. *J. Vet. Diagn. Investig.*, **34** (4), 752–756.

7 Wong, C., Epstein, S.E., Westropp, J.L. (2015) Antimicrobial susceptibility patterns in urinary tract infections in dogs (2010–2013). *J. Vet. Intern. Med.*, **29** (4), 1045–1052.

8 Burgess, K.E., DeRegis, C.J. (2019) Urologic oncology. *Vet. Clin. North Am. Small Anim. Pract.*, **49** (2), 311–323.

9 Bryan, J.N., Henry, C.J., Turnquist, S.E., *et al.* (2006) Primary renal neoplasia of dogs. *J. Vet. Intern. Med.*, **20** (5), 1155–1160.

10 Rossi, F., Gianni, B., Marconato, L., *et al.* (2023) Comparison of sonographic and CT findings for the identification of renal nodules in dogs and cats. *Vet. Radiol. Ultrasound*, **64** (3), 439–447.

11 Merrick, C.H., Schleis, S.E., Smith, A.N., *et al.* (2013) Hypercalcemia of malignancy associated with renal cell carcinoma in a dog. *J. Am. Anim. Hosp. Assoc.*, **49** (6), 385–388.

12 Edmonson, E.F., Hess, A.M., Powers, B.E. (2015) Prognostic significance of histologic features in canine renal cell carcinomas: 70 nephrectomies. *Vet. Pathol.*, **52** (2), 260–268.

13 Michael, H.T., Sharkey, L.C., Kovi, R.C., *et al.* (2013) Pathology in practice. Renal nephroblastoma in a young dog. *J. Am. Vet. Med. Assoc.*, **242** (4), 471–473.

14 Montinaro, V., Boston, S.E., Stevens, B. (2013) Renal nephroblastoma in a 3-month-old Golden Retriever. *Can. Vet. J.*, **54** (7), 683–686.

15 Hergt, F., Mortier, F., Werres, C., *et al.* (2019) Renal nephroblastoma in a 17-month-old Jack Russell Terrier. *J. Am. Anim. Hosp. Assoc.*, **55** (5), e55503. doi: 10.5326/ JAAHA-MS-6664. Last accessed October 15, 2023.

16 Taylor, A.J., Lara-Garcia, A., Benigni, L. (2014) Ultrasonographic characteristics of canine renal lymphoma. *Vet. Radiol. Ultrasound*, **55** (4), 441–446.

17 Taylor, A., Finotello, R., Vilar-Saavedra, P., *et al.* (2019) Clinical characteristics and outcome of dogs with presumed primary renal lymphoma. *J. Small Anim. Pract.*, **60** (11), 663–670.

18 Williams, A.G., Hohenhaus, A.E., Lamb, K.E. (2021) Incidence and treatment of feline renal lymphoma: 27 cases. *J. Feline. Med. Surg.*, **23** (10), 936–944.

19 Taylor, S.S., Goodfellow, M.R., Browne, W.J., *et al.* (2009) Feline extranodal lymphoma: response to chemotherapy and survival in 110 cats. *J. Small Anim. Pract.*, **50** (11), 584–592.

20 McAloney, C.A., Sharkey, L.C., Feeney, D.A., *et al.* (2018) Evaluation of the diagnostic utility of cytologic examination of renal fine-needle aspirates from dogs and the use of ultrasonographic features to inform cytologic diagnosis. *J. Am. Vet. Med. Assoc.*, **252** (10), 1247–1256.

21 Witschen, P.M., Sharkey, L.C., Seelig, D.M., *et al.* (2020) Diagnosis of canine renal lymphoma by cytology and flow cytometry of the urine. *Vet. Clin. Pathol.*, **49** (1), 137–142.

22 Vail, D.M., Moore, A.S., Ogilvie, G.K., *et al.* (1998) Feline lymphoma (145 cases): proliferation indices, cluster of differentiation 3 immunoreactivity, and their association with prognosis in 90 cats. *J. Vet. Intern. Med.*, **12** (5), 349–354.

23 Snead, E.C. (2005) A case of bilateral renal lymphosarcoma with secondary polycythaemia and paraneoplastic syndromes of hypoglycaemia and uveitis in an English Springer Spaniel. *Vet. Comp. Oncol.*, **3** (3), 139–144.

24 Henry, C.J., Turnquist, S.E., Smith, A., *et al.* (1999) Primary renal tumours in cats: 19 cases (1992–1998). *J. Feline Med. Surg.*, **1** (3), 165–170.

25 Locke, J.E., Barber, L.G. (2006) Comparative aspects and clinical outcomes of canine renal hemangiosarcoma. *J. Vet. Intern. Med.*, **20** (4), 962–967.

26 Zatelli, A., Bonfanti, U., D'Ippolito, P. (2005) Obstructive renal cyst in a dog: ultrasonography-guided treatment using puncture aspiration and injection with 95% ethanol. *J. Vet. Intern. Med.*, **19** (2), 252–254.

27 Ochoa, V.B., DiBartola, S.P., Chew, D.J., *et al.* (1999) Perinephric pseudocysts in the cat: a retrospective study and review of the literature. *J. Vet. Intern. Med.*, **13** (1), 47–55.

28 Cannon, C.M., Allstadt, S.D. (2015) Lower urinary tract cancer. *Vet. Clin. North Am. Small Anim. Pract.*, **45** (4), 807–824.

29 Norris, A.M., Laing, E.J., Valli, V.E., *et al.* (1992) Canine bladder and urethral tumors: a retrospective study of 115 cases (1980–1985). *J. Vet. Intern. Med.*, **6** (3), 145–153.

30 Patrick, D.J., Fitzgerald, S.D., Sesterhenn, I.A., *et al.* (2006) Classification of canine urinary bladder urothelial tumours based on the World Health Organization/International Society of Urological Pathology consensus classification. *J. Comp. Pathol.*, **135** (4), 190–199.

31 Martinez, I., Mattoon, J.S., Eaton, K.A., *et al.* (2003) Polypoid cystitis in 17 dogs (1978–2001). *J. Vet. Intern. Med.*, **17** (4), 499–509.

32 Mutsaers, A.J., Widmer, W.R., Knapp, D.W. (2003) Canine transitional cell carcinoma. *J. Vet. Intern. Med.*, **17** (2), 136–144.

33 Walker, D.B., Cowell, R.L., Clinkenbeard, K.D., *et al.* (1993) Carcinoma in the urinary bladder of a cat: cytologic findings and a review of the literature. *Vet. Clin. Pathol.*, **22** (4), 103–108.

34 Schwarz, P.D., Greene, R.W., Patnaik, A.K. (1985) Urinary bladder tumors in the cat: a review of 27 cases. *J. Am. Anim. Hosp. Assoc.*, **21** (2), 237–245.

35 Knapp, D.W., Glickman, N.W., Denicola, D.B., *et al.* (2000) Naturally-occurring canine transitional cell carcinoma of the urinary bladder: a relevant model of human invasive bladder cancer. *Urol. Oncol.*, **5** (2), 47–59.

36 Wilson, H.M., Chun, R., Larson, V.S., *et al.* (2007) Clinical signs, treatments, and outcome in cats with transitional cell carcinoma of the urinary bladder: 20 cases (1990–2004). *J. Am. Vet. Med. Assoc.*, **231** (1), 101–106.

37 Griffin, M.A., Culp, W.T.N., Giuffrida, M.A., *et al.* (2020) Lower urinary tract transitional cell carcinoma in cats: Clinical findings, treatments, and outcomes in 118 cases. *J. Vet. Intern. Med.*, **34** (1), 274–282.

38 Rocha, T.A., Mauldin, G.N., Patnaik, A.K., *et al.* (2000) Prognostic factors in dogs with urinary bladder carcinoma. *J. Vet. Intern. Med.*, **14** (5), 486–490.

39 Fulkerson, C.M., Knapp, D.W. (2015) Management of transitional cell carcinoma of the urinary bladder in dogs: a review. *Vet. J.*, **205** (2), 217–225.

40 Jeffries, C., Moore, A.R., Schlemmer, S.N. (2021) Urinary bladder wall mass with neoplastic lymphoid cells in the urine: diagnosis of an IgG secretory B-cell lymphoma with Bence-Jones proteinuria in a dog. *Vet. Clin. Pathol.*, **51** (3), 426–431.

41 Benigni, L., Lamb, C.R., Corzo-Menendez, N., *et al.* (2006) Lymphoma affecting the urinary bladder in three dogs and a cat. *Vet. Radiol. Ultrasound*, **47** (6), 592–596.

42 Adachi, M., Igarashi, H., Okamoto, M., *et al.* (2022) Large granular lymphocyte lymphoma in the skin and urinary bladder of a dog. *J. Vet. Med. Sci.*, **84** (2), 296–301.

43 Maiolino, P., DeVico, G. (2000) Primary epitheliotropic T-cell lymphoma of the urinary bladder in a dog. *Vet. Pathol.*, **37** (2), 184–186.

44 Kessler, M., Kandel-Tschiederer, B., Pfleghaar, S., *et al.* (2008) Primary malignant lymphoma of the urinary bladder in a dog: longterm remission following treatment with radiation and chemotherapy. *Schweiz. Arch. Tierheilkd.*, **150** (11), 565–569.

45 Swenson, C.L., Boisvert, A.M., Gibbons-Burgener, S.N., *et al.* (2011) Evaluation of modified Wright-staining of dried urinary sediment as a method for accurate detection of bacteriuria in cats. *Vet. Clin. Pathol.*, **40** (2), 256–264.

46 Swenson, C.L., Boisvert, A.M., Kruger, J.M., *et al.* (2004) Evaluation of modified Wright-staining of urine sediment as a method for accurate detection of bacteriuria in dogs. *J. Am. Vet. Med. Assoc.*, **224** (8), 1282–1289.

47 Basso, W., Spänhauer, Z., Arnold, S., *et al.* (2014) *Capillaria plica* (syn. *Pearsonema plica*) infection in a dog with chronic pollakiuria: challenges in the diagnosis and treatment. *Parasitol. Int.*, **63** (1), 140–142.

48 Rossi, M., Messina, N., Ariti, G., *et al.* (2011) Symptomatic *Capillaria plica* infection in a young European cat. *J. Feline. Med. Surg.*, **13** (10), 793–795.

49 Kopecny, L., Palm, C.A., Segev, G., *et al.* (2021) Urolithiasis in dogs: Evaluation of trends in urolith composition and risk factors (2006-2018). *J. Vet. Intern. Med.*, **35** (3), 1406–1415.

50 Kopecny, L., Palm, C.A., Segev, G., *et al.* (2021) Urolithiasis in cats: evaluation of trends in urolith composition and risk factors (2005-2018). *J. Vet. Intern. Med.*, **35** (3), 1397–1405.

51 Albasan, H., Lulich, J.P., Osborne, C.A., *et al.* (2003) Effects of storage time and temperature on pH, specific gravity, and crystal formation in urine samples from dogs and cats. *J. Am. Vet. Med. Assoc.*, **222** (2), 176–179.

52 Wingert, A.M., Murray, O.A., Lulich, J.P., *et al.* (2021) Efficacy of medical dissolution for suspected struvite cystoliths in dogs. *J. Vet. Intern. Med.*, **35** (5), 2287–2295.

53 Bartges, J.W., Callens, A.J. (2015) Urolithiasis. *Vet. Clin. North Am. Small Anim. Pract.*, **45** (4), 747–768.

54 Okafor, C.C., Pearl, D.L., Lefebvre, S.L., *et al.* (2013) Risk factors associated with struvite urolithiasis in dogs evaluated at general care veterinary hospitals in the United States. *J. Am. Vet. Med. Assoc.*, **243** (12), 1737–1745.

55 Lulich, J.P., Osborne, C.A., Lekcharoensuk, C., *et al.* (2004) Effects of diet on urine composition of cats with calcium oxalate urolithiasis. *J. Am. Anim. Hosp. Assoc.*, **40** (3), 185–191.

56 Bartges, J.W., Kirk, C., Lane, I.F. (2004) Update: Management of calcium oxalate uroliths in dogs and cats. *Vet. Clin. North Am. Small Anim. Pract.*, **34** (4), 969–987.

57 Thrall, M.A., Dial, S.M., Winder, D.R. (1985) Identification of calcium oxalate monohydrate crystals by X-ray diffraction in urine of ethylene glycolintoxicated dogs. *Vet. Pathol.*, **22** (6), 625–628.

58 Caporali, E.H.G., Phillips, H., Underwood, L., *et al.* (2015) Risk factors for urolithiasis in dogs with congenital extrahepatic portosystemic shunts: 95 cases (1999–2013). *J. Am. Vet. Med. Assoc.*, **246** (5), 530–536.

59 Callens, A.J., Bartges, J.W. (2015) Urinalysis. *Vet. Clin. North Am. Small Anim. Pract.*, **45** (4), 621–637.

60 Hoppe, A., Denneberg, T. (2001) Cystinuria in the dog: clinical studies during 14 years of medical treatment. *J. Vet. Intern. Med.*, **15** (4), 361–367.

61 De Loor, J., Daminet, S., Smets, P., *et al.* (2013) Urinary biomarkers for acute kidney injury in dogs. *J. Vet. Intern. Med.*, **27** (5), 998–1010.

62 Schentag, J.J., Gengo, F.M., Plaut, M.E., *et al.* (1979) Urinary casts as an indicator of renal tubular damage in patients receiving aminoglycosides. *Antimicrob. Agents Chemother.*, **16** (4), 468–474.

11

Respiratory

11.1 Nasal Cavity

11.1.1 Inflammation (Septic)

11.1.1.1 Cytologic Appearance
Septic rhinitis is characterized by large numbers of inflammatory cells, with neutrophils normally predominating in bacterial rhinitis (Figure 11.1), and macrophages seen with fungal, protozoal, or algal infections, which may also be accompanied by eosinophils.

11.1.1.2 Clinical Considerations
- Primary rhinitis = fungal > bacterial [1].
- Fungal disease more common in young patients [2].
- Clinical signs = sneezing, nasal discharge (unilateral > bilateral), and epistaxis [3].
- Septic inflammation may be secondary to the underlying neoplasia or foreign body [4].
- See Chapter 3 for details on infectious agents.

11.1.1.3 Prognosis
Highly variable, based on the causative agent and whether septic inflammation is primary or secondary.

11.1.2 Inflammation: Lymphoplasmacytic Rhinitis

11.1.2.1 Cytologic Appearance
Lymphoplasmacytic rhinitis is the most common sterile inflammatory condition and is associated with increased numbers of small mature and reactive lymphocytes with plasma cells (Figure 11.2).

11.1.2.2 Clinical Considerations
- Most common in large-breed dogs.
- Associated with mucoid nasal discharge and bilateral stertor [5].
- Bilateral > > unilateral, though discharge often is only unilateral [6].
- May cause epistaxis [7].

11.1.2.3 Prognosis
Generally good, but a common cause of chronic nasal disease in dogs.

11.1.3 Extramedullary Plasmacytoma

11.1.3.1 Cytologic Appearance
Plasmacytomas comprise a discrete population of plasma cells, which are mostly well differentiated with an abundant volume of medium-blue cytoplasm that frequently has a prominent perinuclear clearing (Golgi zone) and may have a bright-pink coloration to the periphery (flame cells) or contain bright-blue, round inclusions (Russell bodies) (Figure 11.3). Nuclei are round, often eccentrically placed, and have finely granular chromatin with multiple small basophilic nucleoli. Multinucleation is a common finding, and mitotic figures may be seen. Anisocytosis/anisokaryosis are variable and N/C ratios are mostly low.

11.1.3.2 Clinical Considerations
- Reported rarely in older dogs and cats [8–10].
- May present with a solitary mass or infiltrative disease [8–10].
- Important to rule out underlying multiple myeloma or myeloma-like disease.

11.1.3.3 Prognosis
Guarded. Prognosis is poor for reported feline cases, though the disease was often extensive and in geriatric patients [9, 10]. Prognosis appears better for solitary lesions in dogs [8].

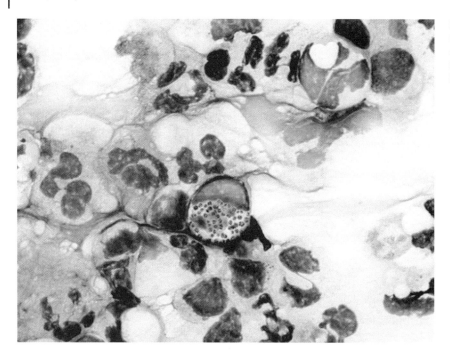

Figure 11.1 Bacterial rhinitis, dog, 100× objective. Note intracellular bacterial cocci within a degenerative neutrophil and smooth pink mucin in the background.

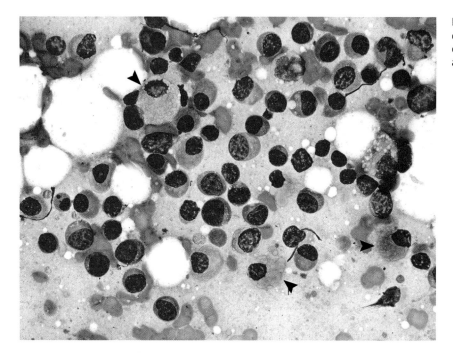

Figure 11.2 Lymphoplasmacytic rhinitis, dog, 50× objective. Lymphocytes, plasma cells, and even Mott cells (arrowheads) are seen.

11.1.4 Normal/Hyperplastic Epithelium

11.1.4.1 Cytologic Appearance

Both squamous and pseudostratified columnar epithelial cells are present in the nasal cavity. Hyperplasia may be seen secondary to inflammation, infection, chronic irritation, or adjacent neoplasia. Typically, these cells have a slightly decreased volume (higher N/C ratios) of more deeply basophilic cytoplasm and may lack cilia (Figure 11.4).

Anisocytosis/anisokaryosis generally are still mild and few criteria of malignancy are seen.

11.1.5 Nasal Adenocarcinoma

11.1.5.1 Cytologic Appearance

Adenocarcinomas exfoliate in variably cohesive sheets. Well-differentiated tumors have prominent intercellular borders, while anaplastic tumors may be poorly cohesive,

Figure 11.3 Extramedullary plasmacytoma, dog, 50× objective. Note the bright-blue globular inclusions in some cells (Russell bodies) and the bright-pink coloration to the periphery of many cells (flame cells).

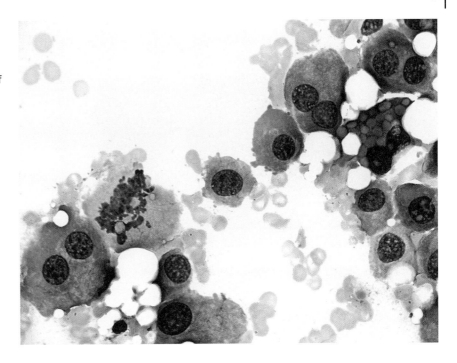

Figure 11.4 Hyperplastic nasal epithelium, dog, 50× objective.

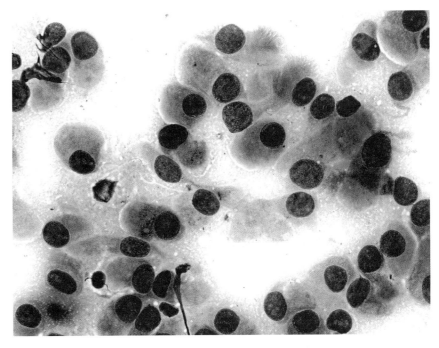

often mimicking lymphoma, particularly in cats [11]. Cells mostly are round, with a moderate volume of medium- to deep-blue cytoplasm, and round nuclei with stippled chromatin and prominent nucleoli. Anisocytosis/anisokaryosis mostly are moderate to marked and N/C ratios are high (Figure 11.5).

11.1.5.2 Clinical Considerations
- Dogs > cats. Most common nasal tumor in dogs [12].

- Mostly older patients, but reported in young dogs [4, 12, 13].
- Unilateral > bilateral [14].
- Clinical signs = nasal discharge (often unilateral progressing to bilateral), epistaxis, sneezing, and facial deformity.

11.1.5.3 Prognosis
Poor. Survival times are short both with and without therapy [15, 16]. Metastatic disease confers a grave prognosis [17].

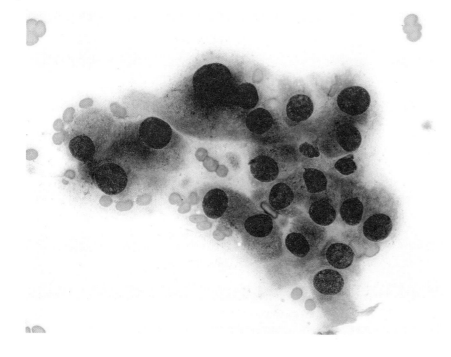

Figure 11.5 Nasal adenocarcinoma, cat, 50× objective.

11.1.6 Nasal Lymphoma

11.1.6.1 Cytologic Appearance

Nasal lymphoma often exfoliates well and comprises individualized cells with round nuclei, stippled chromatin, and variably prominent nucleoli. The cells have a small to moderate volume of medium- to deep-blue cytoplasm (Figure 11.6).

11.1.6.2 Clinical Considerations

- Cats > dogs. Most common nasal tumor in cats [3, 18].
- FeLV infection may predispose to the development of nasal lymphoma in cats [19].
- Clinical signs = nasal discharge (unilateral or bilateral), sneezing, decreased appetite, and increased upper respiratory noise [18].

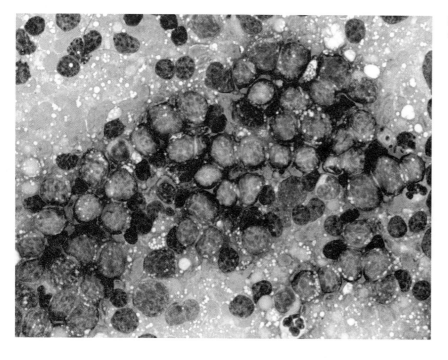

Figure 11.6 Nasal lymphoma, cat, 50× objective.

11.1.6.3 Prognosis

Guarded. Survival times generally short, even with therapy, though can be prolonged in some cats and dogs [4, 19–22]. Anemia may be a negative prognostic factor in cats [21].

11.1.7 Squamous Cell Carcinoma

11.1.7.1 Cytologic Appearance

Squamous cell carcinomas are characterized by variably cohesive sheets of cells ranging from polygonal to round. The cells frequently have keratinized, bright-blue cytoplasm (Figure 11.7). Perinuclear vacuolation also is a common finding. Anisocytosis/anisokaryosis are marked. Tumors frequently are accompanied by neutrophilic inflammation.

11.1.7.2 Clinical Considerations

- Dogs and cats [4, 15].
- Clinical signs = nasal discharge, epistaxis, sneezing, facial deformity, and exophthalmos.
- Low metastatic rates [23].

11.1.7.3 Prognosis

Guarded. Survival times are often short, even with therapy, which generally is palliative [15, 23, 24].

11.1.8 Chondrosarcoma

11.1.8.1 Cytologic Appearance

Chondrosarcomas are characterized by dense, metachromatic extracellular chondroid in which cells may be embedded, forming lacunae. Cells mostly are round but can be spindloid and have a pale-blue cytoplasm that contains pink granules (Figure 11.8). Nuclei are centrally placed, with finely stippled chromatin and multiple basophilic nucleoli.

11.1.8.2 Clinical Considerations

- Common cause of non-epithelial nasosinal tumor.
- Unilateral ≈ bilateral [25].
- Malignant transformation from nasal polyps reported [26].
- Metastasis rare, generally to lungs, but to other organs reported [27, 28].

11.1.8.3 Prognosis

Guarded. Prolonged survival times possible with appropriate therapy [29].

11.1.9 Fibrosarcoma

11.1.9.1 Cytologic Appearance

Fibrosarcomas exfoliate as spindloid cells seen individually or in aggregates, often associated with bright-pink

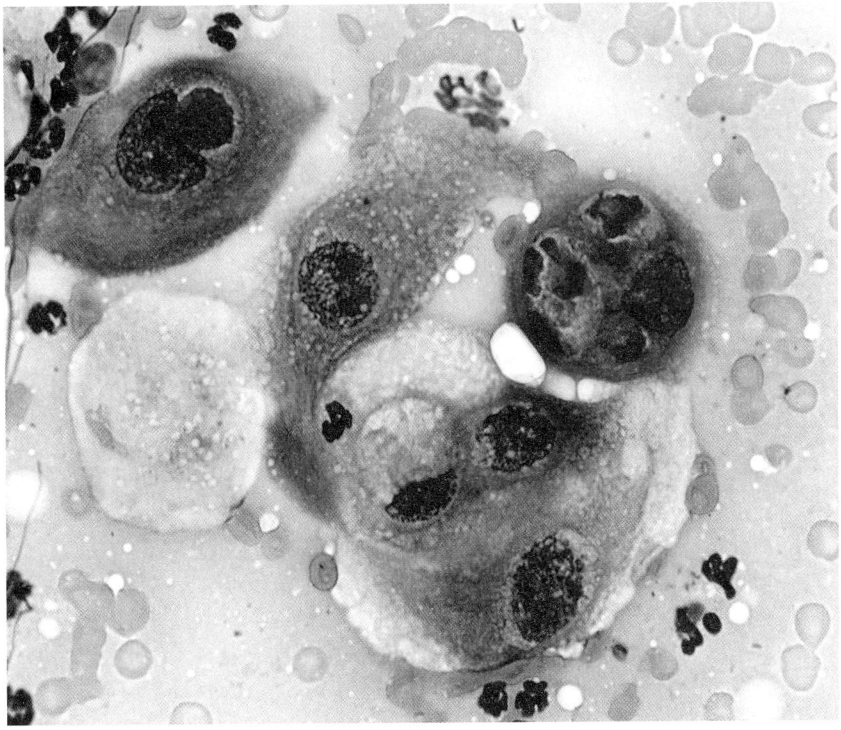

Figure 11.7 Nasal squamous cell carcinoma, cat, 50× objective.

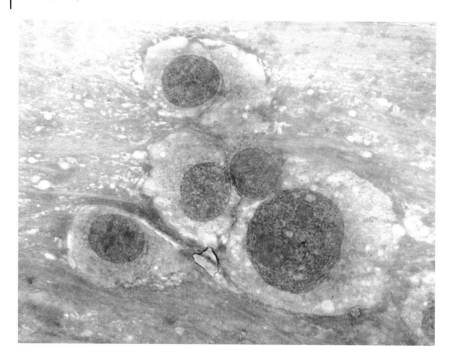

Figure 11.8 Nasal chondrosarcoma, dog, 100× objective.

extracellular matrix. The cells have a variable volume of cytoplasm forming tendrils and wisps and may contain fine pink granules or vacuoles (Figure 11.9). Nuclei are ovoid to elongated, with finely granular chromatin and prominent nucleoli. Anisocytosis/anisokaryosis often are marked and N/C ratios generally are high.

11.1.9.2 Clinical Considerations
- Dogs > cats.
- Middle-aged to older patients.
- Paraneoplastic erythrocytosis reported in a dog [30].

11.1.9.3 Prognosis
Guarded. Moderate survival times possible with appropriate therapy [29].

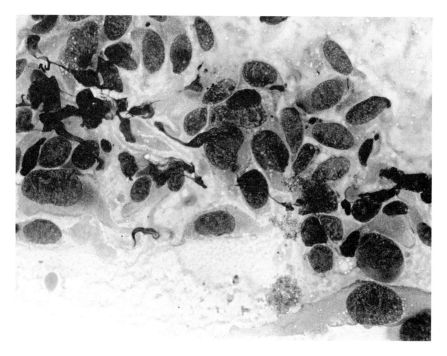

Figure 11.9 Nasal fibrosarcoma, dog, 50× objective.

11.1.10 Other Neoplasms

Numerous other neoplasms may rarely be seen in the nasal cavity, some of which include osteosarcoma (see Chapter 7), mast cell tumor (see Chapter 4), melanoma (see Chapter 4), and transmissible venereal tumors (see Chapter 4).

11.2 Lung

11.2.1 Hyperplastic Epithelium

11.2.1.1 Cytologic Appearance

Hyperplastic epithelium may be seen secondary to underlying inflammation, infection, hemorrhage, or neoplasia. Cells are variably pleomorphic, and criteria of malignancy such as high N/C ratios and increased anisocytosis/anisokaryosis may be seen (Figure 11.10). Care must be taken to distinguish between hyperplasia and neoplasia, which is not always possible, especially in the presence of inflammation.

11.2.2 Carcinoma (Bronchoalveolar and Adenocarcinoma)

11.2.2.1 Cytologic Appearance

Pulmonary carcinomas exfoliate as cohesive sheets of cuboidal to round cells, often seen in tubular or acinar-like arrangements. Degree of atypia is highly variable, ranging from well-differentiated (Figure 11.11) to pleomorphic (Figure 11.12). The cells often contain fine clear vacuoles in their cytoplasm (Figure 11.13). These tumors frequently are associated with a marked paraneoplastic inflammatory response. Note that metastatic carcinomas may appear cytologically similar.

11.2.2.2 Clinical Considerations

- Most common cause of primary pulmonary neoplasia in dogs [31].
- Bronchoalveolar, adenocarcinoma, anaplastic, papillary, solid, and adenosquamous reported [32].
- Most common = bronchoalveolar (dogs) and adenocarcinoma (cats) [33, 34].
- Mostly a solitary, well-defined nodule, but multiple nodules can be seen, and concurrent metastatic lesions may be present [32, 35].
- Most common in caudal lung lobes [36, 37].
- Clinical signs frequently not present at the time of diagnosis [38].

11.2.2.3 Prognosis

Guarded to poor. High metastatic rates reported in cats [32]. Poor prognostic factors include clinical signs present, metastatic disease, presence of pleural effusion, large tumor size, older age, and higher canine lung carcinoma stage classification [31, 37–41].

11.2.3 Squamous Cell Carcinoma

11.2.3.1 Cytologic Appearance

Squamous cell carcinomas are characterized by variably cohesive sheets of cells ranging from polygonal to round.

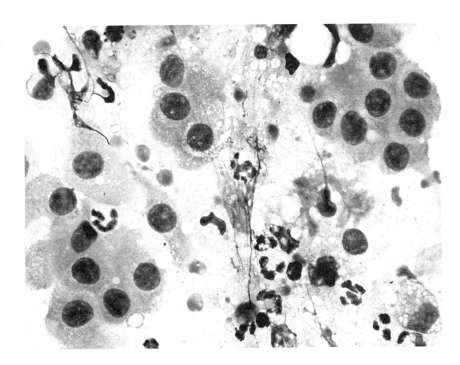

Figure 11.10 Lung, hyperplastic epithelium, dog, 50× objective. Note the concurrent inflammation.

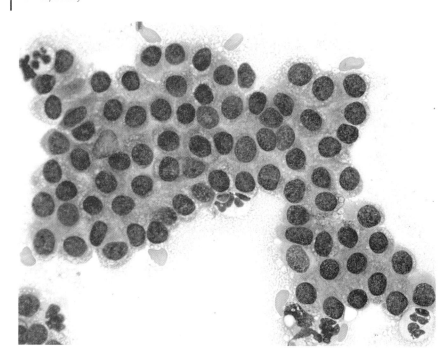

Figure 11.11 Lung, carcinoma (well differentiated), dog, 50× objective. Large sheets of cuboidal cells are arranged in tubular arrangements.

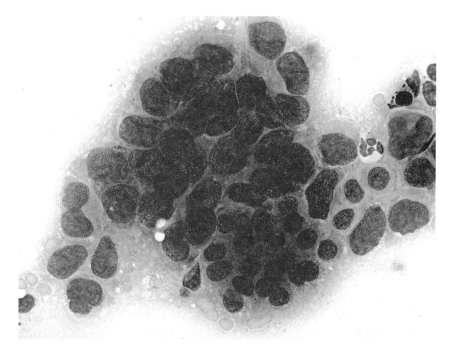

Figure 11.12 Lung, carcinoma (pleomorphic), dog, 50× objective.

The cells frequently have keratinized, bright-blue cytoplasm (Figure 11.14). Perinuclear vacuolation also is a common finding. Anisocytosis/anisokaryosis often are marked. Tumors frequently are accompanied by concurrent inflammation.

11.2.3.2 Clinical Considerations
Mostly a solitary, well-defined nodule [36].

11.2.3.3 Prognosis
Poor. High metastatic rates and short survival times reported [37, 42, 43].

11.2.4 Histiocytic Sarcoma

11.2.4.1 Cytologic Appearance
Histiocytic sarcoma is characterized by individualized cells with many criteria of malignancy, including marked

Figure 11.13 Lung, carcinoma (pleomorphic), dog, 50× objective. Note the prominent vacuolation in many of the cells.

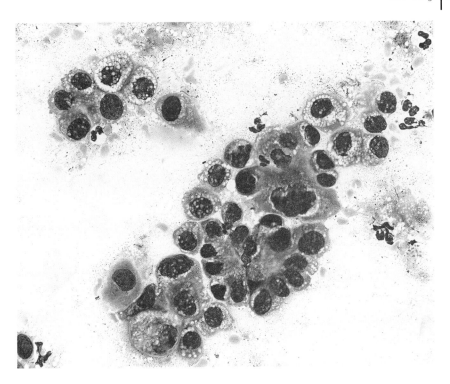

Figure 11.14 Lung, squamous cell carcinoma, dog, 50× objective. Note the bright-blue, hyalinized appearance of the cytoplasm, consistent with keratinization.

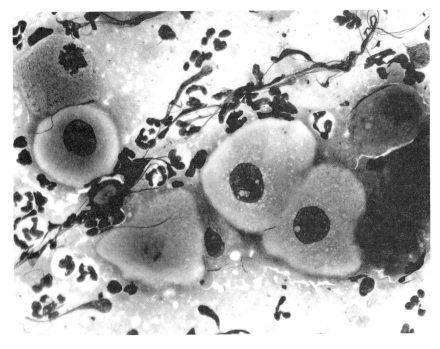

anisocytosis and anisokaryosis, with karyomegaly a common finding. Multinucleation, nuclear fragmentation, and hyperchromasia also are common (Figure 11.15). The cytoplasm is variably vacuolated.

11.2.4.2 Clinical Considerations
- Most common sarcoma in dog lungs [36, 44]. May reflect primary or disseminated disease [45].

- Significantly larger than other primary pulmonary tumors [36].
- Most commonly found in the left cranial and right middle lung lobes [36].

11.2.4.3 Prognosis
Poor. Survival times in dogs are significantly shorter compared to pulmonary carcinomas [31], and metastatic disease

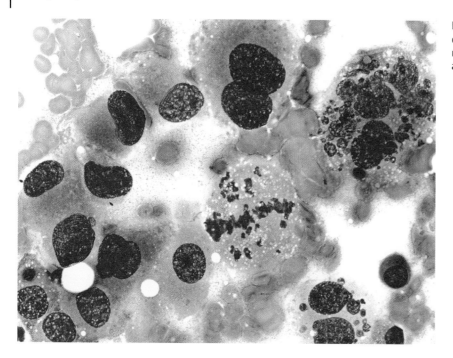

Figure 11.15 Lung, histiocytic sarcoma, dog, 50× objective. Note prominent multinucleation/nuclear fragmentation and the bizarre mitotic figure (center).

is a poor prognostic indicator [46]. Survival times may increase with appropriate therapy of localized tumors [46, 47].

11.2.5 Inflammation/Infection

11.2.5.1 Cytologic Appearance
Inflammatory lesions in the lung frequently exfoliate well and contain large numbers of leukocytes that may indicate the underlying disease process. Neutrophils often are associated with bacterial agents, macrophages are most common with fungal or protozoal agents (Figure 11.16), and eosinophils may be seen with fungal, protozoal, or algal organisms (see Chapter 3 for details).

11.2.5.2 Clinical Considerations
Paraneoplastic inflammation is common with many neoplasms, especially pulmonary carcinomas and squamous cell carcinomas (see Sections 11.2.2 and 11.2.3).

11.2.5.3 Prognosis
Variable, based on the underlying cause.

11.3 Bronchoalveolar Lavage/ Transtracheal Wash

11.3.1 Normal/Hyperplastic Airway Epithelium

11.3.1.1 Cytologic Appearance
The airways are lined by pseudostratified, columnar, ciliated, respiratory epithelium with goblet cells (Figure 11.17). Hyperplastic epithelial cells are cytologically similar to

normal cells but appear in greater numbers. Hyperplastic cells may have decreased N/C ratios, increased cytoplasmic basophilia, and may not be ciliated.

11.3.1.2 Clinical Considerations
- Low numbers seen normally in bronchoalveolar lavage (BAL)/transtracheal wash (TTW) samples.
- Epithelial hyperplasia (especially goblet cell hyperplasia) often associated with chronic inflammation or airway irritation (Figure 11.18).

11.3.2 Oropharyngeal Contamination

11.3.2.1 Cytologic Appearance
Well-differentiated, polygonal squamous epithelial cells with pyknotic or absent nuclei are considered contaminants from the oropharynx. These may be accompanied by normal oral bacterial flora such as *Simonsiella*-like spp. that have a characteristic appearance (Figures 11.19 and 3.50). They are rod-shaped bacteria and form striated stacks of bacteria.

11.3.2.2 Clinical Considerations
- Oropharyngeal flora may be present in cases of aspiration pneumonia [48].
- Careful interpretation of microbial culture results is warranted.

11.3.3 Mucus and Curschmann's Spirals

11.3.3.1 Cytologic Appearance
Mucus is seen in BAL/TTW samples as pools and streaming strands of material ranging from blue to pink. Curschmann's

Figure 11.16 Lung, *Toxoplasma gondii*, dog, 100× objective. Protozoal organisms are accompanied by mixed inflammatory cells.

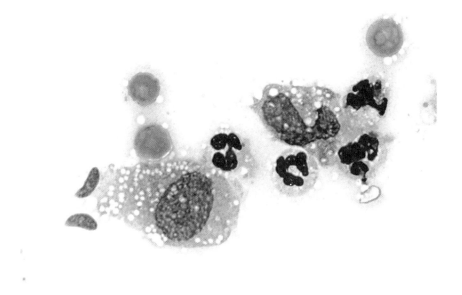

Figure 11.17 BAL, normal respiratory epithelium, dog, 50× objective. Note the purple granules of mucin in the cytoplasm of some cells.

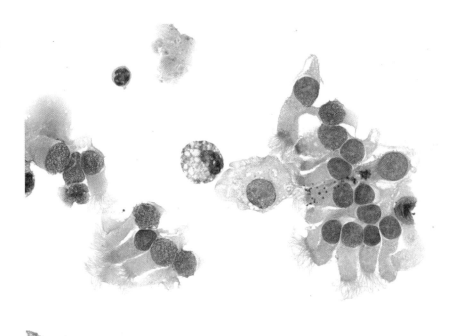

spirals are bright-pink/purple, serpiginous spirals of mucus (Figure 11.20).

11.3.3.2 Clinical Considerations

- A small amount of mucus is normal. Increased mucus may be seen secondary to inflammation, irritation, or chronic airway disease.
- Curschmann's spirals represent mucous casts of bronchioles, associated with chronic or obstructive disease of the small airways.

11.3.4 Inflammation (Neutrophilic)

11.3.4.1 Cytologic Appearance

Neutrophils may appear similar to those in the blood (non-degenerative) or may be degenerative, suggestive of infectious organisms (see Figure 11.21).

11.3.4.2 Clinical Considerations

- Normal neutrophil % = ~5% in dogs and cats [49, 50].
- DDx = infectious disease (especially bacterial), aspiration pneumonia, chronic bronchitis, obstructive/dynamic

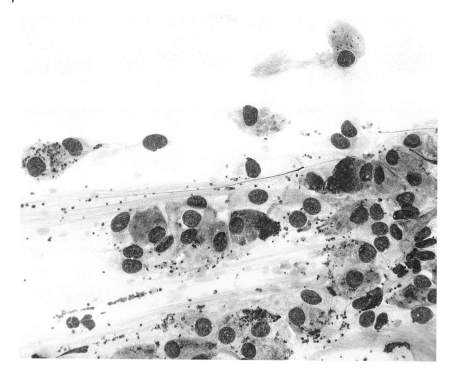

Figure 11.18 BAL, epithelial hyperplasia, dog, 50× objective. Note the increased goblet cells with abundant magenta mucin granules in their cytoplasm.

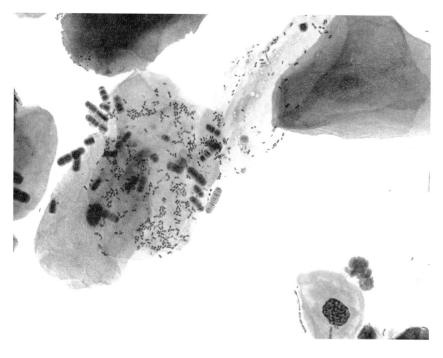

Figure 11.19 BAL, oropharyngeal contamination, dog, 50× objective. Squamous epithelial cells with adherent bacteria (*Simonsiella*-like spp. and coccobacilli).

airway disease, trauma, neoplasia, and foreign body reaction [51].

- May be seen in acute and chronic inflammation.
- Repeat BAL procedures may cause an increase in neutrophil % [48].

11.3.4.3 Prognosis

Variable, based on the underlying/predisposing causes.

11.3.5 Infectious Agents

11.3.5.1 Cytologic Appearance

Many infectious organisms may affect the lungs. Common agents include bacteria (e.g., *Bordetella bronchiseptica* and *Mycobacteria*), fungi (e.g., *Cryptococcus*, *Blastomyces*, *Coccidioides*, and *Pneumocystis*), parasites (*Aelurostrongylus abstrusus* and *Filaroides hirthi*), and protozoal agents (e.g., *Toxoplasma gondii*) (see Chapter 3 for details).

Figure 11.20 BAL, Curschmann's spiral, dog, 50× objective.

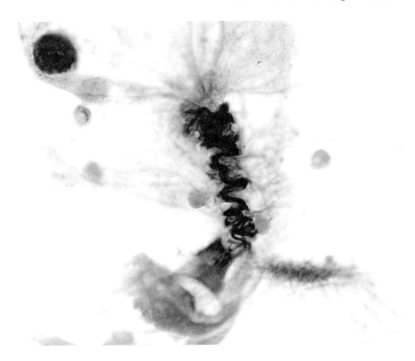

Figure 11.21 BAL, bacterial sepsis, dog, 100× objective.

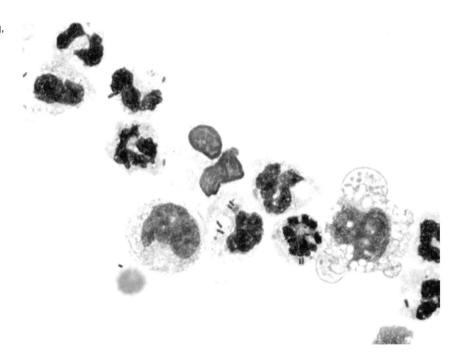

11.3.5.2 Clinical Considerations

- Presence of inflammation warrants close examination for infectious organisms. Figure 11.22 shows fungal hyphae in a BAL (*Conidiobolus* spp.) with mixed inflammation, while Figure 11.23 shows *B. bronchiseptica* adhered to respiratory epithelial cilia (see Chapter 3 for details).
- Airway cytology is extremely useful in the diagnosis of infectious agents in BAL and TTW samples [52, 53].

11.3.5.3 Prognosis

Variable, based on the infectious agent present and extent of disease.

11.3.6 Inflammation (Eosinophilic)

11.3.6.1 Cytologic Appearance

Eosinophil granules vary greatly in color in BAL/TTW samples from bright-pink (Figure 11.24) to brick-red or

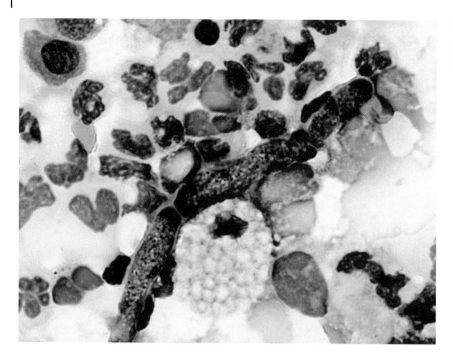

Figure 11.22 BAL, fungal sepsis, dog, 100× objective. Hyphae of *Conodiobolus* spp. are accompanied by a mixed inflammatory response.

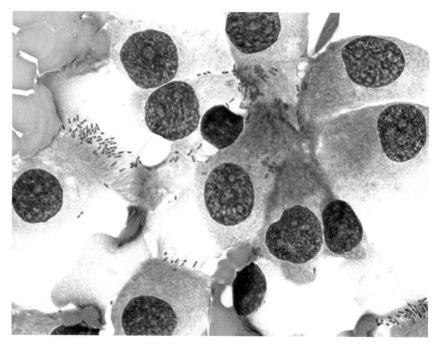

Figure 11.23 BAL, *Bordetella bronchiseptica*, dog, 100× objective. Note the ciliotropic coccobacilli.

even brown. Eosinophil granules are rod-shaped in cats and round in dogs but may coalesce to form large amorphous inclusions. Eosinophilic inflammation often is associated with increased mucus production.

11.3.6.2 Clinical Considerations
- Normal eosinophil % = ~4% in dogs and ~16% in cats (though normal counts up to 25% are reported in healthy cats) [49, 50, 54].

- DDx = allergic/hypersensitivity disease, infectious organisms (e.g., fungal, protozoal, *Mycoplasma*, or parasites such as lungworm), and idiopathic [55].
- Eosinophilic inflammatory airway disease more common in young cats [51].

11.3.6.3 Prognosis
Variable, based on the underlying cause.

Figure 11.24 BAL, eosinophilic inflammation, dog, 50× objective.

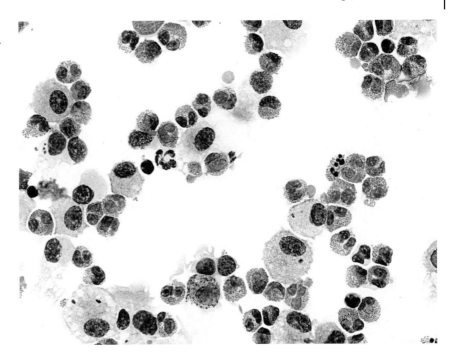

11.3.7 Inflammation (Mononuclear)

11.3.7.1 Cytologic Appearance

Macrophages normally predominate in BAL/TTW samples. Increased numbers and/or % indicate mononuclear inflammation. Multinucleation or reactive changes (e.g., highly vacuolated or basophilic cytoplasm) also suggest inflammation (Figure 11.25).

11.3.7.2 Clinical Considerations

- Normal macrophage % = ~78% in dogs and ~71% in cats [49].
- DDx = chronic inflammation, irritation, or hemorrhage, infectious agents (e.g., fungi, *Mycobacteria*), and foreign body/material reaction.

Figure 11.25 BAL, mononuclear inflammation, dog, 50× objective.

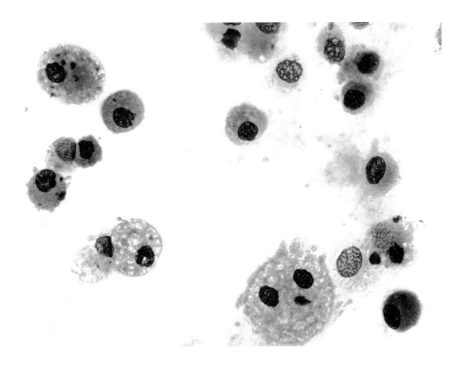

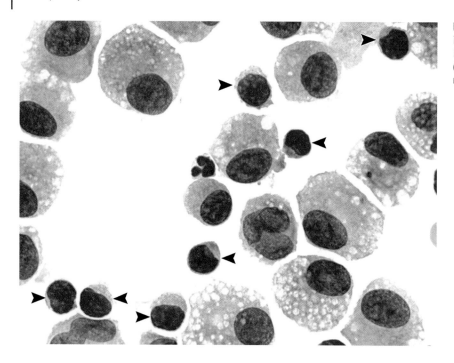

Figure 11.26 BAL, lymphocytic inflammation, dog, 100× objective. Increased small mature lymphocytes (arrowheads) are admixed with reactive macrophages and a single neutrophil.

11.3.7.3 Prognosis
Variable, based on the underlying/predisposing cause.

11.3.8 Inflammation (Lymphocytic)

11.3.8.1 Cytologic Appearance
Lymphocytic inflammation is characterized by a mixed population of lymphocytes, mostly dominated by small mature cells and plasma cells (Figure 11.26).

11.3.8.2 Clinical Considerations
- Normal lymphocyte % = ~7% of cells in dogs and ~5% in cats [49].
- DDx = chronic inflammation/antigenic stimulation, infectious disease [56]. Frequently accompany other inflammatory processes [57].
- Associated with airway collapse in dogs [57].

11.3.8.3 Prognosis
Variable, based on the underlying/predisposing causes.

11.3.9 Hemorrhage

11.3.9.1 Cytologic Appearance
Blood should not be present in BAL/TTW samples. Erythrocytes may represent acute hemorrhage, and chronic hemorrhage is confirmed by the presence of macrophages that are erythrophagocytic or contain heme-breakdown pigment (hemosiderophages) (Figure 11.27).

11.3.9.2 Clinical Considerations
- More common in BAL samples from cats than dogs [58].
- DDx = neoplasia, cardiac failure, rhinitis, asthma, bleeding diatheses, trauma, or inhaled irritants [58, 59].

11.3.9.3 Prognosis
Variable, based on the underlying/predisposing cause.

11.3.10 Foreign Material

11.3.10.1 Cytologic Appearance
Aspirated foreign material incites an inflammatory response, generally dominated by macrophages that ingest the material. Crystalline material (barium) is seen phagocytosed by macrophages in Figure 11.28.

11.3.10.2 Clinical Considerations
- Barium and sucralfate reported [60, 61].
- May be accompanied by evidence of hemorrhage or Curschmann's spirals.

11.3.10.3 Prognosis
Generally good, but dependent on the type of material and extent of disease.

Figure 11.27 BAL, hemorrhage, dog, 50× objective. Note erythrophagia (arrowhead) and hemosiderin pigment (arrow) within macrophages.

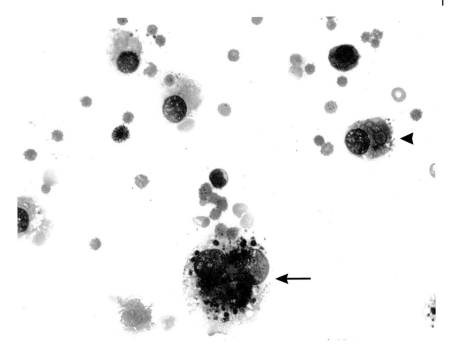

Figure 11.28 BAL, foreign material (barium), dog, 100× objective. Crystalline barium material is phagocytosed by a macrophage (arrow).

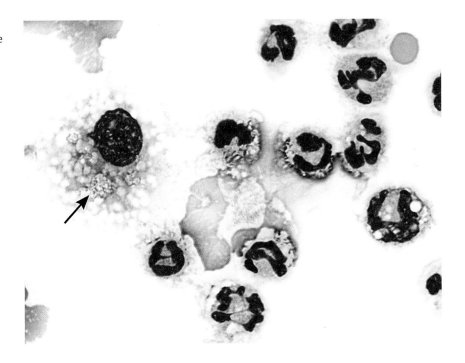

11.3.11 Neoplasia

11.3.11.1 Cytologic Appearance
Neoplastic cells from the lungs or airways may rarely be seen in BAL/TTW fluid samples and appear similar to the underlying neoplasm. Carcinoma cells are most commonly seen, with marked criteria of malignancy including anisocytosis/anisokaryosis (Figure 11.29).

11.3.11.2 Clinical Considerations
- Carcinomas must be distinguished from hyperplastic epithelium.
- Lymphoma is also occasionally seen in BAL samples [62].

11.3.11.3 Prognosis
Poor.

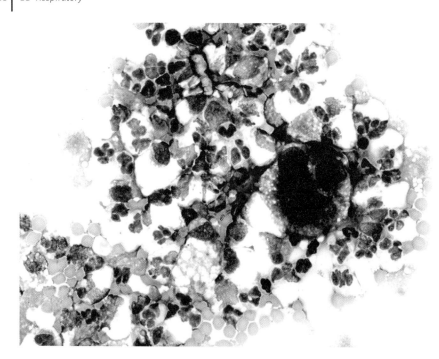

Figure 11.29 BAL, carcinoma, dog, 50× objective. A large, multinucleated carcinoma cell is accompanied by mixed inflammation.

References

1 Meler, E., Dunn, M., Lecuyer, M. (2008) A retrospective study of canine persistent nasal disease: 80 cases (1998–2003). *Can. Vet. J.*, **49** (1), 71–76.

2 Plickert, H.D., Tichy, A., Hirt, R.A. (2014) Characteristics of canine nasal discharge related to intranasal diseases: a retrospective study of 105 cases. *J. Small Anim. Pract.*, **55** (3), 145–152.

3 Ferguson, S., Smith, K.C., Welsh, C.E., *et al.* (2020) A retrospective study of more than 400 feline nasal biopsy samples in the UK (2006–2013). *J. Feline. Med. Surg.*, **22** (8), 736–743.

4 Henderson, S.M., Bradley, K., Day, M.J., *et al.* (2004) Investigation of nasal disease in the cat – a retrospective study of 77 cases. *J. Feline Med. Surg.*, **6** (4), 245–257.

5 Lobetti, R. (2014) Idiopathic lymphoplasmacytic rhinitis in 33 dogs. *J. South Afr. Vet. Assoc.*, **85** (1), 1151.

6 Windsor, R.C., Johnson, L.R., Herrgesell, E.J., *et al.* (2004) Idiopathic lymphoplasmacytic rhinitis in dogs: 37 cases (1997–2002). *J. Am. Vet. Med. Assoc.*, **224** (12), 1952–1957.

7 Bissett, S.A., Drobatz, K.J., McKnight, A., *et al.* (2007) Prevalence, clinical features, and causes of epistaxis in dogs: 176 cases (1996–2001). *J. Am. Vet. Med. Assoc.*, **231** (12), 1843–1850.

8 Elliott, J., Looper, J., Keyerleber, M., *et al.* (2020) Response and outcome following radiation therapy of macroscopic canine plasma cell tumours. *Vet. Comp. Oncol.*, **18** (4), 718–726.

9 Sykes, S.E., Byfield, V., Sullivan, L., *et al.* (2017) Feline respiratory extramedullary plasmacytoma with lymph node metastasis and intrahistiocytic amyloid. *J. Comp. Pathol.*, **156** (2–3), 173–177.

10 Schöniger, S., Bridger, N., Allenpasch, K., *et al.* (2007) Sinonasal plasmacytoma in a cat. *J. Vet. Diagn. Investig.*, **19** (5), 573–577.

11 Nagata, K., Lamb, M., Goldschmidt, M.H., *et al.* (2014) The usefulness of immunohistochemistry to differentiate between nasal carcinoma and lymphoma in cats: 140 cases (1986–2000). *Vet. Comp. Oncol.*, **12** (1), 52–57.

12 Avner, A., Dobson, J.M., Sales, J.I., *et al.* (2008) Retrospective review of 50 canine nasal tumours evaluated by low-field magnetic resonance imaging. *J. Small Anim. Pract.*, **49** (5), 233–239.

13 Lefebvre, J., Kuehn, N.F., Wortinger, A. (2005) Computed tomography as an aid in the diagnosis of chronic nasal disease in dogs. *J. Small Anim. Pract.*, **46** (6), 280–285.

14 Bouyssou, S., Hammond, G.J., Eivers, C. (2021) Comparison of CT features of 79 cats with intranasal mass lesions. *J. Feline. Med. Surg.*, **23** (10), 987–995.

15 Woodruff, M.J., Heading, K.L., Bennett, P. (2019) Canine intranasal tumours treated with alternating carboplatin and doxorubicin in conjunction with oral piroxicam: 29 cases. *Vet. Comp. Oncol.*, **17** (1), 42–48.

16 Rassnick, K.M., Goldkamp, C.E., Erb, H.N., *et al.* (2006) Evaluation of factors associated with survival in dogs with untreated nasal carcinomas: 139 cases (1993–2003). *J. Am. Vet. Med. Assoc.*, **229** (3), 401–406.

17 Henry, C.J., Brewer, W.G., Jr, Tyler, J.W., *et al.* (1998) Survival in dogs with nasal adenocarcinoma: 64 cases (1981–1995). *J. Vet. Intern. Med.*, **12** (6), 436–439.

18 Little, L., Patel, R., Goldschmidt, M. (2007) Nasal and nasopharyngeal lymphoma in cats: 50 cases (1989–2005). *Vet. Pathol.*, **44** (6), 885–892.

19 Santagostino, S.F., Mortellaro, C.M., Boracchi, P., *et al.* (2015) Feline upper respiratory tract lymphoma: site, cytohistology, phenotype, FeLV expression, and prognosis. *Vet. Pathol.*, **52** (2), 250–259.

20 Reczynska, A.I., LaRue, S.M., Boss, M.K., *et al.* (2022) Outcome of sterotactic body radiation for treatment of nasal and nasopharyngeal lymphoma in 32 cats. *J. Vet. Intern. Med.*, **36** (2), 733–742.

21 Haney, S.M., Beaver, L., Turrel, J., *et al.* (2009) Survival analysis of 97 cats with nasal lymphoma: a multi-institutional retrospective study (1986–2006). *J. Vet. Intern. Med.*, **23** (2), 287–294.

22 George, R., Smith, A., Schleis, S., *et al.* (2016) Outcome of dogs with intranasal lymphoma treated with various radiation and chemotherapy protocols: 24 cases. *Vet. Radiol. Ultrasound*, **57** (3), 306–312.

23 Rogers, K.S., Walker, M.A., Helman, R.G. (1996) Squamous cell carcinoma of the canine nasal cavity and frontal sinus: eight cases. *J. Am. Anim. Hosp. Assoc.*, **32** (2), 103–110.

24 Gieger, T., Rassnick, K., Siegel, S., *et al.* (2008) Palliation of clinical signs in 48 dogs with nasal carcinomas treated with coarse-fraction radiation therapy. *J. Am. Anim. Hosp. Assoc.*, **44** (3), 116–123.

25 Patnaik, A.K., Lieberman, P.H., Erlandson, R.A., *et al.* (1984) Canine sinonasal skeletal neoplasms: chondrosarcomas and osteosarcomas. *Vet. Pathol.*, **21** (5), 475–482.

26 Sumner, J.A., Witham, A.I., Stent, A.W., *et al.* (2018) Emergence of nasal chondrosarcoma in a dog with nasal polyposis. *Clin. Case. Rep.*, **6** (5), 821–826.

27 Durham, A.C., Popovitch, C.A., Goldschmidt, M.H. (2008) Feline chondrosarcoma: a retrospective study of 67 cats (1987-2005). *J. Am. Anim. Hosp. Assoc.*, **44** (3), 124–130.

28 Hahn, K.A., McGavin, M.D., Adams, W.H. (1997) Bilateral renal metastases of nasal chondrosarcoma in a dog. *Vet. Pathol.*, **34** (4), 352–355.

29 Sones, E., Smith, A., Schleis, S., *et al.* (2013) Survival times for canine intranasal sarcomas treated with radiation therapy: 86 cases (1996–2011). *Vet. Radiol. Ultrasound*, **54** (2), 194–201.

30 Couto, C.G., Boudrieau, R.J., Zanjani, E.D. (1989) Tumor-associated erythrocytosis in a dog with nasal fibrosarcoma. *J. Vet. Intern. Med.*, **3** (3), 183–185.

31 McPhetridge, J.B., Scharf, V.F., Regier, P.J., *et al.* (2021) Distribution of histopathologic types of primary pulmonary neoplasia in dogs and outcome of affected dogs: 340 cases (2010-2019). *J. Am. Vet. Med. Assoc.*, **260** (2), 234–243.

32 Santos, I.R., Raiter, J., Lamego, E.C., *et al.* (2023) Feline pulmonary carcinoma: gross, histological, metastatic, and immunohistochemical aspects. *Vet. Pathol.*, **60** (1), 8–20.

33 Griffey, S.M., Kraegel, S.A., Madewell, B.R. (1998) Rapid detection of K-ras gene mutations in canine lung cancer using single-strand conformational polymorphism analysis. *Carcinogenesis*, **19** (6), 959–963.

34 D'Costa, S., Yoon, B.I., Kim, D.Y., *et al.* (2012) Morphologic and molecular analysis of 39 spontaneous feline pulmonary carcinomas. *Vet. Pathol.*, **49** (6), 971–978.

35 Marolf, A.J., Gibbons, D.S., Podell, B.K., *et al.* (2011) Computed tomographic appearance of primary lung tumors in dogs. *Vet. Radiol. Ultrasound*, **52** (2), 168–172.

36 Barrett, L.E., Pollard, R.E., Zwingenberger, A., *et al.* (2014) Radiographic characterization of primary lung tumors in 74 dogs. *Vet. Radiol. Ultrasound*, **55** (5), 480–487.

37 Maritato, K.C., Schertel, E.R., Kennedy, S.C. (2014) Outcome and prognostic indicators in 20 cats with surgically treated primary lung tumors. *J. Feline Med. Surg.*, **16** (12), 979–984.

38 McNiel, E.A., Ogilvie, G.K., Powers, B.E., *et al.* (1997) Evaluation of prognostic factors for dogs with primary lung tumors: 67 cases (1985–1992). *J. Am. Vet. Med. Assoc.*, **211** (11), 1422–1427.

39 Mehlhaff, C.J., Leifer, C.E., Patnaik, A.K., *et al.* (1984) Surgical treatment of primary pulmonary neoplasia in 15 dogs. *J. Am. Anim. Hosp. Assoc.*, **20** (5), 799–803.

40 Polton, G.A., Brearley, M.J., Powell, S.M., *et al.* (2008) Impact of primary tumour stage on survival in dogs with solitary lung tumours. *J. Small Anim. Pract.*, **49** (2), 66–71.

41 Ichimata, M., Kagawa, Y., Namiki, K., *et al.* (2023) Prognosis of primary pulmonary adenocarcinoma after surgical resection in small-breed dogs: 52 cases (2005-2021). *J. Vet. Intern. Med.*, **37** (4) 1466–1474.

42 Morey-Matamalas, A., de Stefani, A., Corbetta, D., *et al.* (2018) Pulmonary basaloid squamous cell carcinoma in a dog. *J. Comp. Pathol.*, **159**, 11–15.

43 Moulton, J.E., von Tscharner, C., Schneider, R. (1981) Classification of lung carcinomas in the dog and cat. *Vet. Pathol.*, **18** (4), 513–528.

44 Bleakley, S., Duncan, C.G., Monnet, E. (2015) Thoracoscopic lung lobectomy for primary lung tumors in 13 dogs. *Vet. Surg.*, **44** (8), 1029–1035.

45 Purzycka, K., Peters, L.M., Elliott, J., *et al.* (2020) Histiocytic sarcoma in Miniature Schnauzers: 30 cases. *J. Small Anim. Pract.*, **61** (6), 338–345.

46 Marlowe, K.W., Robat, C.S., Clarke, D.M., *et al.* (2018) Primary pulmonary histiocytic sarcoma in dogs: a retrospective analysis of 37 cases (2000-2015). *Vet. Comp. Oncol.*, **16** (4), 658–663.

47 Murray, C.A., Wilcox, J.L., De Mello Souza, C.H., *et al.* (2022) Outcome in dogs with curative-intent treatment of localized primary pulmonary histiocytic sarcoma. *Vet. Comp. Oncol.*, **20** (2), 458–464.

48 Andreasen, C.B. (2003) Bronchoalveolar lavage. *Vet. Clin. North Am. Small Anim. Pract.*, **33** (1), 69–88.

49 Hawkins, E.C., DeNicola, D.B., Kuehn, N.F. (1990) Bronchoalveolar lavage in the evaluation of pulmonary disease in the dog and cat. State of the art. *J. Vet. Intern. Med.*, **4** (5), 267–274.

50 Rebar, A.H., DeNicola, D.B., Muggenburg, B.A. (1980) Bronchopulmonary lavage cytology in the dog: normal findings. *Vet. Pathol.*, **17** (3), 294–304.

51 Lee, E.A., Johnson, L.R., Johnson, E.G., *et al.* (2020) Clinical features and radiographic findings in cats with eosinophilic, neutrophilic, and mixed airway inflammation (2011–2018). *J. Vet. Intern. Med.*, **34** (3), 1291–1299.

52 Howard, J., Reinero, C.R., Almond, G., *et al.* (2021) Bacterial infection in dogs with aspiration pneumonia at 2 tertiary referral practices. *J. Vet. Intern. Med.*, **35** (6), 2763–2771.

53 Osathanon, R., Lamb, C.R., Church, D.B. (2022) Associations between respiratory signs, thoracic CT findings and results of tracheobronchoscopy and bronchoalveolar lavage in dogs. *Vet. Rec.*, **191** (4), e1385. doi: 10.1002/vetr.1385. Last accessed October 15, 2023.

54 Padrid, P.A., Feldman, B.F., Funk, K., *et al.* (1991) Cytologic, microbiologic, and biochemical analysis of bronchoalveolar lavage fluid obtained from 24 healthy cats. *Am. J. Vet. Res.*, **52** (8), 1300–1307.

55 Casamian-Sorrosal, D., Silvestrini, P., Blake, R., *et al.* (2020) Clinical features and long-term follow-up of 70 cases of canine idiopathic eosinophilic lung disease. *Vet. Rec.*, **187** (8), e65. doi: 10.1136/vr.105193. Last accessed October 15, 2023.

56 Crisi, P.E., Johnson, L.R., Di Cesare, A., *et al.* (2019) Evaluation of bronchoscopy and bronchoalveolar lavage findings in cats with Aelurostrongylus abstrusus in comparison to cats with feline bronchial disease. *Front. Vet. Sci.*, **6**, 337. doi: 10.3389/fvets.2019.0033. Last accessed October 15, 2023

57 Johnson, L.R., Vernau, W. (2019) Bronchoalveolar lavage fluid lymphocytosis in 104 dogs (2006–2016). *J. Vet. Intern. Med.*, **33** (3), 1315–1321.

58 Hooi, K.S., Defarges, A.M., Jelovcic, S.V., *et al.* (2019) Bronchoalveolar lavage hemosiderosis in dogs and cats with respiratory disease. *Vet. Clin. Pathol.*, **48** (1), 42–49.

59 DeHeer, H.L., McManus, P. (2005) Frequency and severity of tracheal wash hemosiderosis and association with underlying disease in 96 cats: 2002–2003. *Vet. Clin. Pathol.*, **34** (1), 17–22.

60 Colledge, S.L., Messick, J.B., Huang, A. (2013) What is your diagnosis? Transtracheal wash fluid from a dog. *Vet. Clin. Pathol.*, **42** (2), 238–239.

61 Nunez-Ochoa, L., Desnoyers, M., Lecuyer, M. (1993) What is your diagnosis? Transtracheal wash from a 2-year-old dog. *Vet. Clin. Pathol.*, **22** (4), 122.

62 Hawkins, E.C., Morrison, W.B., DeNicola, D.B., *et al.* (1993) Cytologic analysis of bronchoalveolar lavage fluid from 47 dogs with multicentric malignant lymphoma. *J. Am. Vet. Med. Assoc.*, **203** (10), 1418–1425.

12

Endocrine

12.1 Thyroid

12.1.1 Thyroid Adenoma

12.1.1.1 Cytologic Features

Thyroid adenomas comprise sheets of uniform, cuboidal to columnar epithelial cells, frequently arranged in palisading rows and acinar arrangements (Figure 12.1). Bright-pink colloid may be seen in the background, and bare nuclei are a common finding. The cells often lack prominent intercellular borders. They have a moderate volume of cytoplasm that may contain green/black pigment (tyrosine). Nuclei are centrally or eccentrically placed and have stippled chromatin with small basophilic nucleoli. Anisocytosis/anisokaryosis are mild and N/C ratios are low. Note that adenomatous hyperplasia appears cytologically similar.

12.1.1.2 Clinical Considerations

Cats
- Very common, and responsible for 97–99% of cases of hyperthyroidism [1].
- Rare in patients <8 years of age.
- 71–85% of cases of adenoma/adenomatous hyperplasia are bilateral [1, 2].

Dogs
- Less common than cats, usually small, clinically silent, and an incidental finding [3].

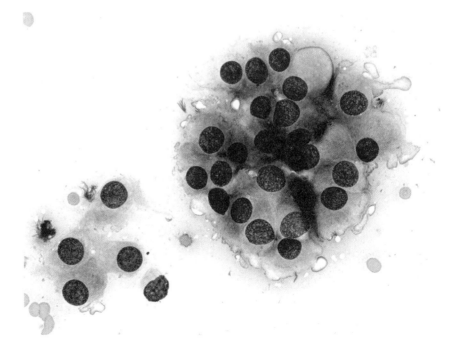

Figure 12.1 Thyroid adenoma, cat, 50× objective. Note the acinar arrangement of the cells and the subtle pink colloid around the periphery of the cytoplasm.

Clinical Atlas of Small Animal Cytology and Hematology, Second Edition. Andrew G. Burton.
© 2024 John Wiley & Sons, Inc. Published 2024 by John Wiley & Sons, Inc.

12.1.1.3 Prognosis
Excellent.

12.1.2 Thyroid Adenocarcinoma

12.1.2.1 Cytologic Features
Cytologic appearance of thyroid carcinomas is highly variable, ranging from well-differentiated (making them difficult to distinguish from adenomas; compare Figures 12.1 and 12.2) to markedly pleomorphic (see Figures 12.3–12.5). They frequently have a densely bloody background, as carcinomas are more vascular than benign tumors [4]. The cells often form palisading rows or acinar arrangements, and bright-pink, smooth colloid may be seen in the background (Figure 12.3). Green/black tyrosine granules may be present in the cytoplasm (Figure 12.6)

12.1.2.2 Clinical Considerations
Dogs
- The majority of clinically detectable tumors are carcinomas [3].
- Most are nonfunctional.

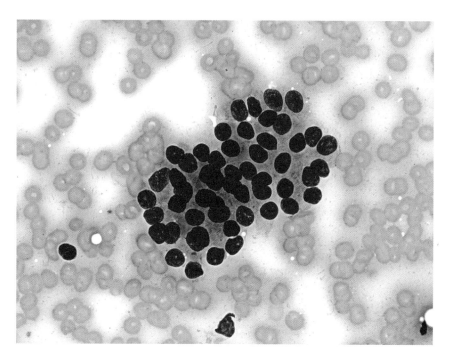

Figure 12.2 Thyroid adenocarcinoma (well-differentiated), dog 50× objective. The cells have mild criteria of malignancy, but note the high N/C ratios and cellular crowding.

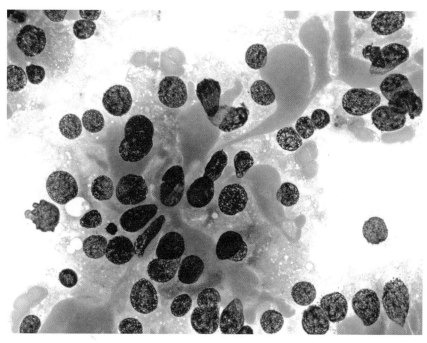

Figure 12.3 Thyroid adenocarcinoma, dog, 50× objective. There is an abundant bright-pink colloid. Cells have indistinct intercellular borders and are disorganized.

Figure 12.4 Thyroid adenocarcinoma, cat, 50× objective. Note the marked anisocytosis, anisokaryosis, and large basophilic nucleoli.

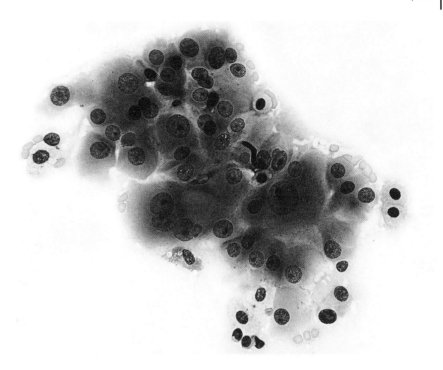

Figure 12.5 Thyroid carcinoma, dog, 50× objective. Neoplastic cells are poorly cohesive and have marked anisokaryosis.

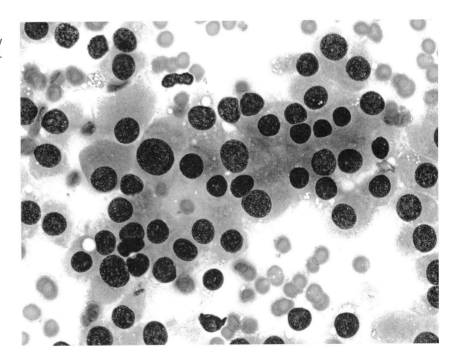

- Seen mostly in older dogs. Boxers, Golden Retrievers, Beagles, and Siberian Huskies are predisposed [3, 5, 6].
- Good correlation between results of cytology and histopathology [7].
- Metastatic potential has been linked to tumor size and was 14% for tumors $\leq$20 cm^3, 74% for tumors 21–100 cm^3, and 100% in tumors >100 cm^3 in one study [6].
- Local lymph nodes and lungs are the most common locations for metastases [5, 6, 8].

- Metastatic disease is common at the time of diagnosis and is 16-fold more likely for bilateral tumors than unilateral tumors [6, 8].

Cats
- Uncommon. Seen in 1–3% of hyperthyroid cats [1], and nonfunctional carcinomas are rare.
- Metastatic disease to local lymph nodes and lungs is common [9].

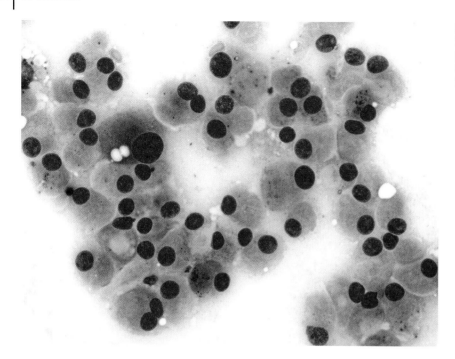

Figure 12.6 Thyroid carcinoma, dog, 50× objective. The cells are arranged in palisading rows and have marked anisocytosis/anisokaryosis. Green/blue tyrosine granules are seen in many cells.

12.1.2.3 Prognosis

Variable. Dogs and cats treated with thyroidectomy can have prolonged survival times; however, undifferentiated carcinomas carry a poor prognosis in dogs [5, 9, 10]. Impact of metastatic disease at the time of diagnosis is variable and may not reduce survival time, but it may increase tumor-related fatality [5, 10]. Invasive tumors may result in shorter survival times, even in the absence of metastatic disease at the time of diagnosis [11].

12.1.3 Thyroid C Cell (Medullary) Carcinoma

12.1.3.1 Cytologic Features

Thyroid C cell carcinomas often have a distinctive 'plasmacytoid' appearance, similar to those described in humans [12]. The cells are ovoid, with a moderate volume of pink granular cytoplasm (which may represent cytoplasmic calcitonin) and eccentrically placed nuclei that have finely stippled chromatin and single basophilic nucleoli (Figure 12.7). Anisokaryosis is moderate. The

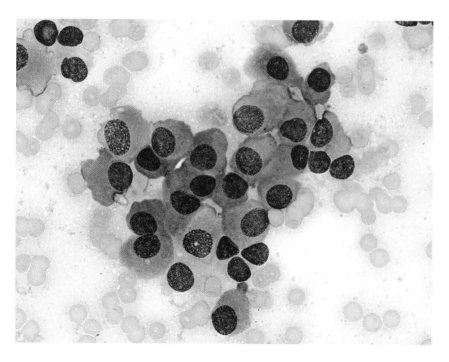

Figure 12.7 Thyroid C cell (medullary) carcinoma, dog, 50× objective. Note the faint pink granular appearance of the cytoplasm.

pink cytoplasm can make differentiating these tumors from carotid body tumors difficult (compare to Figure 12.10); however, the cytoplasm of carotid body tumors mostly has a more coarse granular appearance.

12.1.3.2 Clinical Considerations
- Derived from C cells of the thyroid.
- May account for up to 30% of thyroid tumors in dogs [5]. Not reported in cats.
- Elevated calcitonin is used as a tumor marker in humans but is not reported in dogs [13]. Hypocalcemia is an inconsistent finding [14, 15].

12.1.3.3 Prognosis
Less malignant potential than thyroid adenocarcinomas, a finding mirrored in human patients [13, 14]. In one study, 30% of surgically resected cases had at least one-year survival [14]; however, others have found a higher risk of tumor-related death than follicular thyroid carcinomas [5].

12.2 Parathyroid

12.2.1 Parathyroid Adenoma

12.2.1.1 Cytologic Features
Parathyroid adenomas comprise sheets of uniform cuboidal to columnar cells in palisading rows and acinar arrangements. They have a moderate volume of cytoplasm, which may contain eosinophilic material (Figure 12.8) that has also been reported in parathyroid carcinomas [16].

Nuclei are round with granular chromatin and inapparent nucleoli. Tumors of parathyroid origin may appear similar to those of the thyroid and can be difficult to distinguish without histopathology.

12.2.1.2 Clinical Considerations
- Derived from parathyroid chief cells.
- Rare tumors in dogs and cats.
- Adenomas are more common than carcinomas [17–20].
- Frequently functional and associated with hypercalcemia [17, 20, 21].

12.2.1.3 Prognosis
Excellent.

12.2.2 Parathyroid Carcinoma

12.2.2.1 Cytologic Features
Parathyroid carcinomas can appear similar to adenomas. Increased anisokaryosis/anisocytosis and high N/C ratios generally are seen as well as cellular crowding (compare Figures 12.9 and 12.8).

12.2.2.2 Clinical Considerations
- Usually larger than adenomas and may be palpable in cats, though rarely palpable in dogs [18, 22].
- Frequently functional and associated with hypercalcemia [23].
- Bilateral tumors are rare, though multiple nodules may be present [23].

Figure 12.8 Parathyroid adenoma, dog, 50× objective. Cells are arranged in palisading rows. Note the smooth pink material in the cytoplasm of many cells.

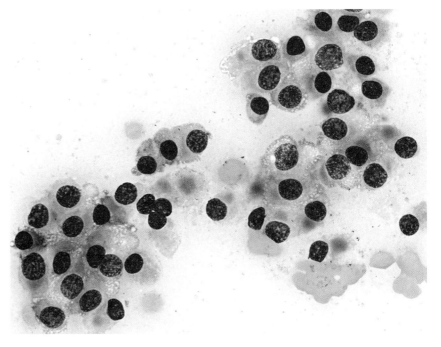

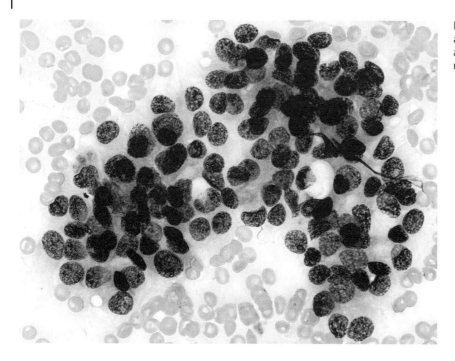

Figure 12.9 Parathyroid adenocarcinoma, dog, 50× objective. Cells are crowded, piled and have high N/C ratios and moderate anisokaryosis.

- Clinical signs = often associated with hypercalcemia and polyuria/polydipsia, hindlimb paresis, hyporexia, weight loss, and vomiting [23].
- Metastatic disease or recurrence after surgery is rare [23, 24].

12.2.2.3 Prognosis
Good, with long-term survival and resolution of hypercalcemia reported after surgical excision [23, 24].

12.3 Chemoreceptor Tumors

12.3.1 Chemodectomas

12.3.1.1 Cytologic Features
Chemodectomas often are highly cellular and have a moderate amount of pale-blue cytoplasm that frequently contains abundant, diffuse, pink granules that are helpful to distinguish them from thyroid/parathyroid tumors (Figures 12.10 and 12.11). Some tumors may lack pink

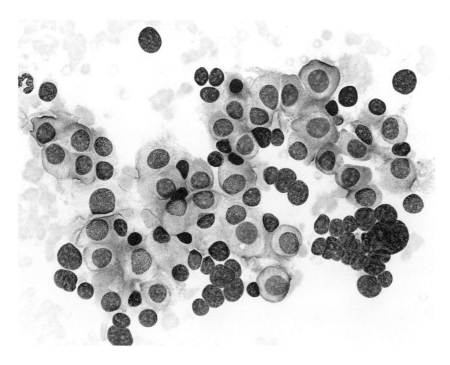

Figure 12.10 Carotid body tumor, dog, 50× objective. Note the variably cohesive sheets of cells with many bare nuclei. Many cells have pink granules diffusely through their cytoplasm.

Figure 12.11 Carotid body tumor, dog, 100× objective. The cytoplasm contains many fine pink granules.

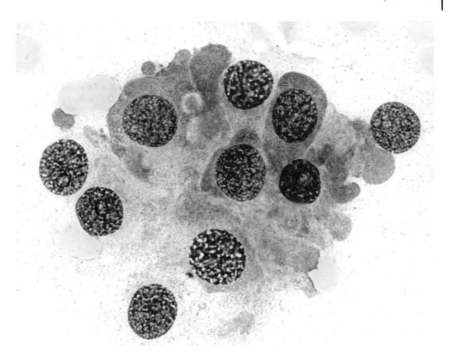

granules (Figure 12.12), and special stains may be required for further assessment (Figure 12.13). Nuclei are round, with finely stippled chromatin and small basophilic nucleoli. Anisocytosis/anisokaryosis generally are mild.

12.3.1.2 Clinical Considerations
- Chemodectomas include aortic body tumors (more common) and carotid body tumors [25].
- Dogs >> cats. Rare tumors in both species [25, 26].

- Usually affect middle-aged to older patients but reported in young dogs [25].
- There is an increased incidence of aortic body tumors in brachycephalic breeds [27].

12.3.1.3 Prognosis
Carotid body tumors frequently are locally invasive and have a propensity to metastasize widely [28]. Aortic body tumors often are benign with a low incidence of metastatic

Figure 12.12 Carotid body tumor, dog, 50× objective. Cells are seen in loosely cohesive sheets and lack the pink granulation seen in Figures 12.10 and 12.11.

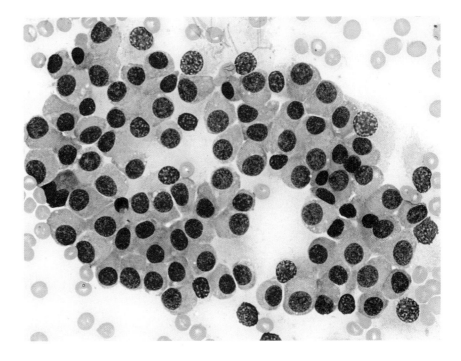

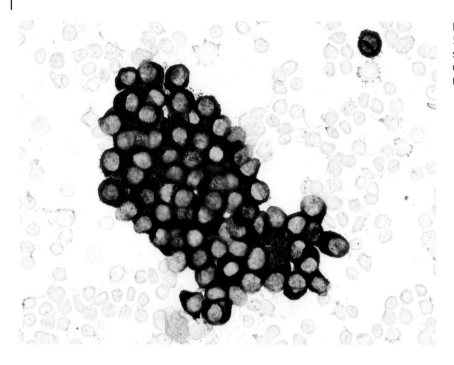

Figure 12.13 Carotid body tumor, dog, 50× objective. Cell cytoplasm is staining strongly positive for synaptophysin, confirming a neuroendocrine origin (same case as Figure 12.12).

disease, but are associated with pericardial effusion, cardiac tamponade, or heart failure. Dogs treated with pericardectomy had significantly longer survival times [29].

12.4 Adrenal Gland

12.4.1 Adrenocortical Adenoma

12.4.1.1 Cytologic Features
Adrenocortical adenomas often exfoliate as individualized, ovoid cells but may also be seen in small sheets associated with capillaries (Figure 12.14). The cells have abundant pale-blue/gray cytoplasm that contains numerous small, coarse, clear vacuoles. Nuclei are round, centrally located, and have reticulated chromatin with small, prominent, single nucleoli. Anisocytosis/anisokaryosis are mild and N/C ratios are low (Figure 12.15). Hyperplastic nodules appear cytologically similar and require histopathology for differentiation.

12.4.1.2 Clinical Considerations
- May be functional or nonfunctional.
- Often an incidental finding [30].

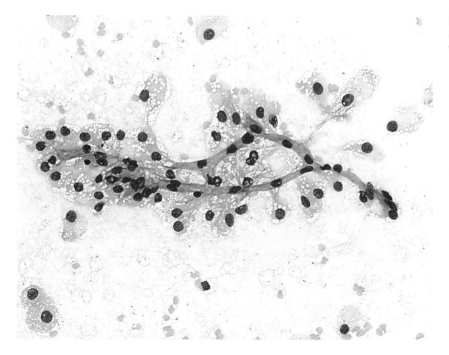

Figure 12.14 Adrenocortical adenoma, dog, 20× objective. Cells are emanating from linear capillaries.

Figure 12.15 Adrenocortical adenoma, dog, 50× objective. The cells are uniform and have an abundant vacuolated cytoplasm.

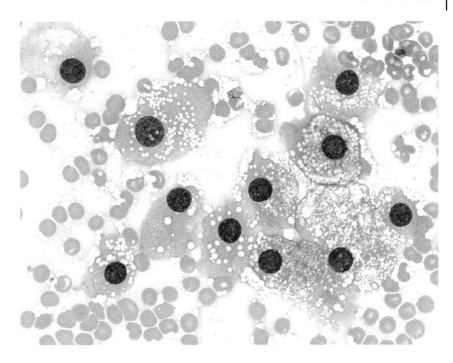

- Adrenocortical adenomas were nearly fourfold more common than carcinomas in dogs in one study [31], while the incidence appears similar in cats [32].
- Extramedullary hematopoiesis can be seen in adrenal tumors (Figure 12.16) and is more likely to be present in adenomas than carcinomas [33].

12.4.1.3 Prognosis

Variable. Many tumors are incidental findings. Dogs surviving surgery for functional adrenocortical adenomas have an excellent prognosis [34]. Cats surviving adrenalectomy also have good long-term survival [32].

12.4.2 Adrenocortical Carcinoma

12.4.2.1 Cytologic Features

Variably cohesive tumors comprising round to polygonal cells with variably vacuolated cytoplasm. The nuclei are round, centrally located with reticulated chromatin, and often with multiple, basophilic nucleoli. Relative to adenomas, adrenocortical carcinomas have higher N/C ratios,

Figure 12.16 Adrenocortical adenoma, dog, 50× objective. Note the erythroid precursors at the right of the photo confirming extramedullary hematopoiesis.

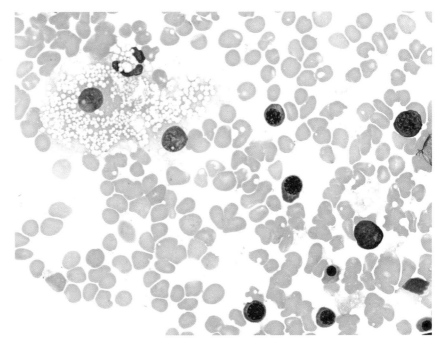

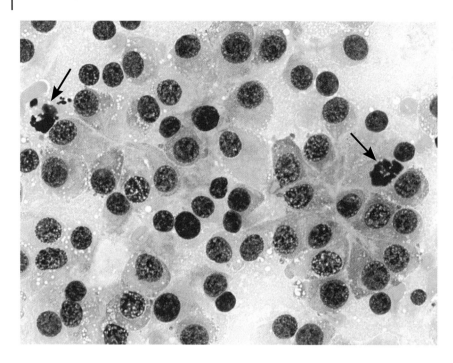

Figure 12.17 Adrenocortical adenocarcinoma, dog, 50× objective. The cells have high N/C ratios and are poorly vacuolated. Note the mitotic figures (arrows).

often contain fewer vacuoles, have a more basophilic cytoplasm, and have greater nuclear atypia (compare Figures 12.17 and 12.15).

12.4.2.2 Clinical Considerations
- May be functional or nonfunctional (functional tumors are more common) [32].
- Typically larger than adenomas, with tumors >2 cm more likely to be carcinomas [33].
- Metastatic disease is seen in approximately 50% of cases [33].

12.4.2.3 Prognosis
Variable. Prolonged survival times are reported in both dogs and cats surviving surgery [32, 35]. Survival times are significantly decreased in the presence of metastatic disease [35].

12.4.3 Pheochromocytoma

12.4.3.1 Cytologic Features
Pheochromocytomas frequently exfoliate well, as papillary sheets of polygonal cells that often lack prominent intercellular borders. The cells have a variable volume of cytoplasm, which might have a distinctive eosinophilic granular appearance (Figure 12.18). The nuclei are ovoid, with coarsely granular chromatin and small basophilic nucleoli. Anisokaryosis often is marked.

12.4.3.2 Clinical Considerations
- Arise from chromaffin cells of the adrenal medulla.
- Uncommon in dogs and rare in cats. Typically occur in middle-aged to older patients [32, 36].
- Often incidental findings. A high frequency of concurrent neoplasia, including other endocrine origin, is reported [37].
- Clinical signs such as polyuria/polydipsia, weakness, and hypertension associated with catecholamine release [36].
- Metastatic disease is seen in up to 36% of canine cases, in local lymph nodes, or widely disseminated [37, 38].

12.4.3.3 Prognosis
Highly variable based on tumor size, local invasion, or presence of metastatic disease. Patients without metastatic disease that survive surgical removal have a good prognosis [32].

12.5 Pituitary Gland

12.5.1 Pituitary Carcinoma

12.5.1.1 Cytologic Features
Cells from pituitary carcinomas exfoliate individually and in variably cohesive sheets. The cells are round, with a moderate volume of medium-blue cytoplasm that frequently contains fine clear vacuoles. Nuclei mostly are ovoid, but often are amoeboid or cleaved, and have very finely stippled, immature chromatin with multiple basophilic nucleoli. Anisocytosis/anisokaryosis are moderate to marked and

Figure 12.18 Pheochromocytoma, dog, 50× objective. The cells have a characteristic faint pink cytoplasm and prominent anisokaryosis.

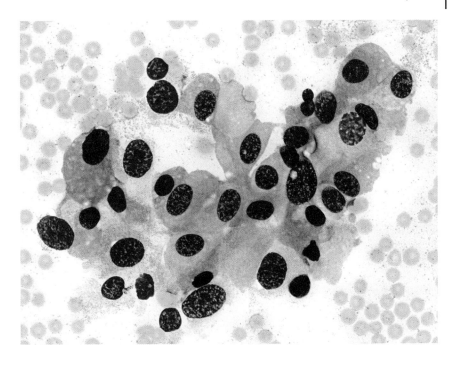

N/C ratios are moderate to high. These tumors frequently have a very high mitotic rate (Figure 12.19).

12.5.1.2 Clinical Considerations
- Rare tumors in dogs and cats [39, 40].
- Typically older patients, but reported in a dog <1-year old [41].

- Less common than adenomas [39, 42, 43].
- Variable hormone production, but often secrete ACTH [41, 44].

12.5.1.3 Prognosis
Poor [40, 41].

Figure 12.19 Pituitary carcinoma, dog, 50× objective.

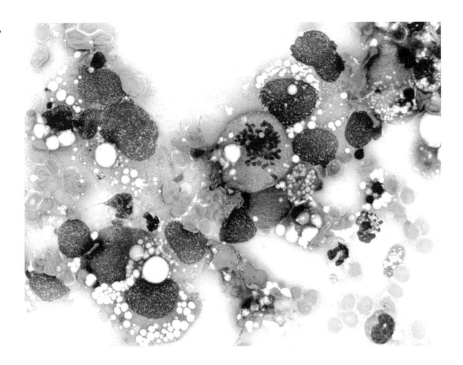

References

1 Naan, E.C., Kirpensteijn, J., Kooistra, H.S., *et al.* (2006) Results of thyroidectomy in 101 cats with hyperthyroidism. *Vet. Surg.*, **35** (3), 287–293.

2 Peterson, M.E., Kintzer, P.P., Cavanagh, P.G., *et al.* (1983) Feline hyperthyroidism: pretreatment clinical and laboratory evaluation of 131 cases. *J. Am. Vet. Med. Assoc.*, **183** (1), 103–110.

3 Wucherer, K.L., Wilke, V. (2010) Thyroid cancer in dogs: an update based on 638 cases (1995–2005). *J. Am. Anim. Hosp. Assoc.*, **46** (4), 249–254.

4 Kent, M.S., Griffey, S.M., Verstraete, F.J., *et al.* (2002) Computer-assisted image analysis of neovascularization in thyroid neoplasms from dogs. *Am. J. Vet. Res.*, **63** (3), 363–369.

5 Enache, D., Ferro, L., Morello, E.M., *et al.* (2023) Thyroidectomy in dogs with thyroid tumors: survival analysis in 144 cases (1994-2018). *J. Vet. Intern. Med.*, **37** (2), 635–647.

6 Leav, I., Schiller, A.L., Rijnberk, A., *et al.* (1976) Adenomas and carcinomas of the canine and feline thyroid. *Am. J. Pathol.*, **83** (1), 61–122.

7 Thompson, E.J., Stirtzinger, T., Lumsden, J.H., *et al.* (1980) Fine needle aspiration cytology in the diagnosis of canine thyroid carcinoma. *Can. Vet. J.*, **21** (6), 186–188.

8 Skinner, O.T., Souza, C.H.M., Kim, D.Y. (2021) Metastasis to ipsilateral medial retropharyngeal and deep cervical lymph nodes in 22 dogs with thyroid carcinoma. *Vet. Surg.*, **50** (1), 150–157.

9 Oramas, A., Boston, S., Wavreille, V. (2020) The outcome for feline non-hypersecretory thyroid carcinoma after thyroidectomy. *Can. Vet. J.*, **61** (7), 719–723.

10 Giannasi, C., Rushton, S., Rook, A., *et al.* (2021) Canine thyroid carcinoma prognosis following the utilisation of computed tomography assisted staging. *Vet. Rec.*, **189** (1), e55.

11 Klein, M.K., Powers, B.E., Withrow, S.J., *et al.* (1995) Treatment of thyroid carcinoma in dogs by surgical resection alone: 20 cases (1981–1989). *J. Am. Vet. Med. Assoc.*, **206** (7), 1007–1009.

12 Mehdi, G., Maheshwari, V., Ansari, H.A., *et al.* (2010) FNAC diagnosis of medullary carcinoma thyroid: a report of three cases with review of literature. *J. Cytol.*, **27** (2), 66–68.

13 Melvin, K.E., Miller, H.H., Tashjian, A.H., Jr. (1971) Early diagnosis of medullary carcinoma of the thyroid gland by means of calcitonin assay. *N. Engl. J. Med.*, **285** (20), 1115–1120.

14 Carver, J.R., Kapatkin, A., Patnaik, A.K. (1995) A comparison of medullary thyroid carcinoma and thyroid adenocarcinoma in dogs: a retrospective study of 38 cases. *Vet. Surg.*, **24** (4), 315–319.

15 Patnaik, A.K., Lieberman, P.H., Erlandson, R.A., *et al.* (1978) Canine medullary carcinoma of the thyroid. *Vet. Pathol.*, **15** (5), 590–599.

16 Ramaiah, S.K., Alleman, A.R., Hanel, R., *et al.* (2001) A mass in the ventral neck of a hypercalcemic dog. *Vet. Clin. Pathol.*, **30** (4), 177–179.

17 Young, K.M., Degner, D.A. (2023) Surgical description and outcome of ultrasound-guided minimally invasive parathyroidectomy in 50 dogs with primary hyperparathyroidism. *Vet. Surg.*, **52** (1), 18–25.

18 Kallet, A.J., Richter, K.P., Feldman, E.C., *et al.* (1991) Primary hyperparathyroidism in cats: seven cases (1984–1989). *J. Am. Vet. Med. Assoc.*, **199** (12), 1767–1771.

19 Berger, B., Feldman, E.C. (1987) Primary hyperparathyroidism in dogs: 21 cases (1976–1986). *J. Am. Vet. Med. Assoc.*, **191** (3), 350–356.

20 Singh, A., Giuffrida, M.A., Thomson, C.B., *et al.* (2019) Perioperative characteristics, histological diagnosis, and outcome in cats undergoing surgical treatment of primary hyperparathyroidism. *Vet. Surg.*, **48** (3), 367–374.

21 DeRouen, A.E. (2023) Concurrent parathyroid adenoma and thyroid carcinoma in a domestic shorthaired feline. *J. Am. Anim. Hosp. Assoc.*, **59** (1), 32–35.

22 Secrest, S., Grimes, J. (2019) Ultrasonographic size of the canine parathyroid gland may not correlate with histopathology. *Vet. Radiol. Ultrasound*, **60** (6), 729–733.

23 Erickson, A.K., Regier, P.J., Watt, M.M., *et al.* (2021) Incidence, survival time, and surgical treatment of parathyroid carcinomas in dogs: 100 cases (2010-2019). *J. Am. Vet. Med. Assoc.*, **259** (11), 1309–1317.

24 Sawyer, E.S., Northrup, N.C., Schmiedt, C.W., *et al.* (2012) Outcome of 19 dogs with parathyroid carcinoma after surgical excision. *Vet. Comp. Oncol.*, **10** (1), 57–64.

25 Teh, A.P., Pratakpiriya, W., Hidaka, Y., *et al.* (2017) An atypical case of recurrent carotid body carcinoma in a young adult dog: histopathological, immunohistochemical and electron microscopic study. *J. Vet. Med. Sci.*, **79** (4), 714–718.

26 Hansen, S.C., Smith, A.N., Kuo, K.W., *et al.* (2016) Metastatic neuroendocrine carcinoma of aortic body origin in a cat. *Vet. Clin. Pathol.*, **45** (3), 490–494.

27 Hayes, H.M. (1975) An hypothesis for the aetiology of canine chemoreceptor neoplasms, based upon an epidemiological study of 73 cases among hospital patients. *J. Small Anim. Pract.*, **16** (5), 337–343.

28 Obradovich, J.E., Withrow, S.J., Powers, B.E., *et al.* (1992) Carotid body tumors in the dog. Eleven cases (1978-1988). *J. Vet. Intern. Med.*, **6** (2), 96–101.

29 Ehrhart, N., Ehrhart, E.J., Willis, J., *et al.* (2002) Analysis of factors affecting survival in dogs with aortic body tumors. *Vet. Surg.*, **31** (1), 44–48.

30 Baum, J.I., Boston, S.E., Case, J.B. (2016) Prevalence of adrenal gland masses as incidental findings during abdominal computed tomography in dogs: 270 cases (2013-2014). *J. Am. Vet. Med. Assoc.*, **249** (10), 1165–1169.

31 Labelle, P., De Cock, H.E. (2005) Metastatic tumors to the adrenal glands in domestic animals. *Vet. Pathol.*, **42** (1), 52–58.

32 Daniel, G., Mahony, O.M., Markovich, J.E., *et al.* (2016) Clinical findings, diagnostics and outcome in 33 cats with adrenal neoplasia (2002-2013). *J. Feline. Med. Surg.*, **18** (2), 77–84.

33 Labelle, P., Kyles, A.E., Farver, T.B. (2004) Indicators of malignancy of canine adrenocortical tumors: histopathology and proliferation index. *Vet. Pathol.*, **41** (5), 490–497.

34 Schwartz, P., Kovak, J.R., Koprowski, A., *et al.* (2008) Evaluation of prognostic factors in the surgical treatment of adrenal gland tumors in dogs: 41 cases (1999–2005). *J. Am. Vet. Med. Assoc.*, **232** (1), 77–84.

35 Massari, F., Nicoli, S., Romanelli, G., *et al.* (2011) Adrenalectomy in dogs with adrenal gland tumors: 52 cases (2002–2008). *J. Am. Vet. Med. Assoc.*, **239** (2), 216–221.

36 Prego, M.T., Dias, M.J., Ferreira, R.L., *et al.* (2023) Plasma and urinary metanephrine and normetanephrine concentrations using liquid chromatography with tandem mass spectrometry in healthy cats an in a cat with pheochromocytoma. *J. Vet. Intern. Med.*, **37** (3), 910–914.

37 Barthez, P.Y., Marks, S.L., Woo, J., *et al.* (1997) Pheochromocytoma in dogs: 61 cases (1984–1995). *J. Vet. Intern. Med.*, **11** (5), 272–278.

38 Gilson, S.D., Withrow, S.J., Wheeler, S.L., *et al.* (1994) Pheochromocytoma in 50 dogs. *J. Vet. Intern. Med.*, **8** (3), 228–232.

39 Rissi, D.R. (2015) A retrospective study of skull base neoplasia in 42 dogs. *J. Vet. Diagn. Investig.*, **27** (6), 743–748.

40 Kimitsuki, K., Boonsriroj, H., Kojima, D., *et al.* (2014) A case report of feline pituitary carcinoma with hypercortisolism. *J. Vet. Med. Sci.*, **76** (1), 133–138.

41 Gestier, S., Cook, R.W., Agnew, W., *et al.* (2012) Silent pituitary corticotroph carcinoma in a young dog. *J. Comp. Pathol.*, **146** (4), 327–331.

42 Miller, M.A., Piotrowski, S.L., Donovan, T.A., *et al.* (2021) Feline pituitary adenomas: correlation of histologic and immunohistochemical characteristics with clinical findings and case outcome. *Vet. Pathol.*, **58** (2), 266–275.

43 Hyde, B.R., Martin, L.G., Chen, A.V., *et al.* (2023) Clinical characteristics and outcome in 15 dogs treated with transsphenoidal hypophysectomy for nonfunctional sellar masses. *Vet. Surg.*, **52** (1), 69–80.

44 Nakaichi, M., Iseri, T., Horikirizono, H., *et al.* (2020) Clinical features and their course of pituitary carcinoma with distant metastasis in a dog. *J. Vet. Med. Sci.*, **82** (11), 1671–1675.

13

Reproductive

Male

13.1 Testes

13.1.1 Normal Testicle

13.1.1.1 Cytologic Appearance

An appreciation of normal testicular cytology is important when interpreting pathologic changes. Readers are referred to the review in Ref. 1 for an excellent and comprehensive summary of normal testicular cytology. Cells from testicle aspirates can be grouped into three major categories: Sertoli cells, Leydig cells, and spermatogenic cells. Sertoli cells have large ovoid nuclei with finely stippled chromatin and single, prominent nucleoli (Figure 13.1). Leydig cells are seen rarely and have abundant cytoplasm with numerous punctate, clear vacuoles (Figure 13.2). Spermatogenic cells include (from most immature to mature): spermatogonia, spermatocytes, early spermatids, late spermatids, and spermatozoa (Figures 13.1, 13.3, and 13.4). Spermatogonia are rare and have characteristic parachromatin condensation that causes a crescent shape. Spermatocytes have a characteristic cord-like chromatin pattern (Figure 13.1). Spermatids are the most common. Early spermatids have a small to moderate volume of pale cytoplasm that contains small, clear vacuoles. Multinucleation is common. Late spermatids have progressively elongated nuclei with condensed chromatin and scant to absent cytoplasm (Figure 13.4).

13.1.2 Seminoma

13.1.2.1 Cytologic Appearance

Seminomas exfoliate well, comprising many large, individualized, discrete cells with a moderate volume of encircling, pale-blue cytoplasm. Nuclei are round, with very finely granular, immature chromatin, and multiple prominent basophilic nucleoli. Binucleation, multinucleation, and mitotic figures often are present. Small mature lymphocytes may be seen (Figure 13.5) [2, 3].

13.1.2.2 Clinical Considerations

- Derived from germinal epithelium of the seminiferous tubules.
- Dogs >> cats.
- Gross appearance = variably sized, soft, bulging, and cream-colored on the cut surface [4].
- Increased risk in cryptorchid testes [3, 5].
- Can be bilateral and associated with other testicular tumors of different origin [6].
- Feminization syndrome is rare [7].

13.1.2.3 Prognosis

Generally good. In the absence of metastatic disease, orchiectomy may be curative. Metastatic disease is uncommon for testicular tumors in general and, if present, seminomas tend to metastasize to inguinal or sublumbar lymph nodes, with wide dissemination reported rarely [4].

13.1.3 Sertoli Cell Tumor

13.1.3.1 Cytologic Appearance

These tumors exfoliate variably well and comprise round cells distributed individually and in loose aggregates, often with a palisading arrangement. The cells have a moderate volume of medium-blue cytoplasm that frequently contains characteristic coarse, clear vacuoles, which can be helpful in differentiating these tumors from seminomas (compare Figures 13.6 and 13.5). The nuclei are round, with coarsely granular chromatin, and prominent, single nucleoli. Anisocytosis/anisokaryosis generally are mild to moderate. Cells may be seen in rosettes surrounding pink basement membrane material (Call-Exner bodies) [8].

Clinical Atlas of Small Animal Cytology and Hematology, Second Edition. Andrew G. Burton.
© 2024 John Wiley & Sons, Inc. Published 2024 by John Wiley & Sons, Inc.

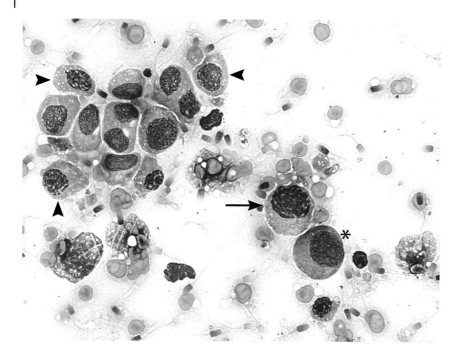

Figure 13.1 Normal testicle, cat, 50× objective. Sertoli cell (asterisk), spermatocyte (arrow), early spermatids (arrowheads), and spermatozoa in the background.

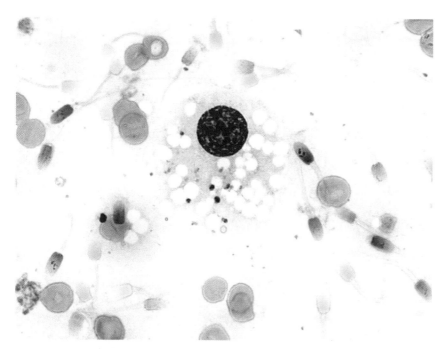

Figure 13.2 Normal testicle, cat, 100× objective. Leydig cell with cytoplasmic vacuoles and numerous spermatozoa in the background.

13.1.3.2 Clinical Considerations
- Derived from sustentacular cells of the seminiferous tubules.
- Dogs >> cats.
- Gross appearance = variably sized, firm, lobulated, and white/gray [4].
- Increased risk in cryptorchid testes [5, 9].
- Less common than seminomas and interstitial cell tumors in descended testicles, but more common in cryptorchid testicles [5, 6, 10].

- May produce estrogen and may be associated with feminizing syndrome. Clinical signs = bilaterally symmetrical alopecia, hyperpigmentation, gynecomastia, and bone marrow suppression [11].

13.1.3.3 Prognosis
Variable, based on the presence of metastatic disease, bone marrow suppression, and feminizing syndrome [11]. Pancytopenia often resolves with the removal of the tumor and prolonged survival is possible [11]. Signs of

Figure 13.3 Normal testicle, cat, 50× objective. Early (arrows) and late (arrowheads) spermatids with many mature spermatozoa in the background.

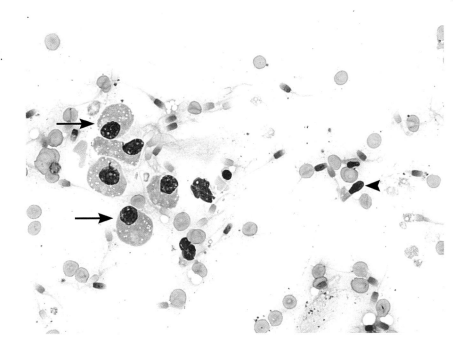

Figure 13.4 Normal testicle, cat, 100× objective. Stages of spermiogenesis: early spermatids (arrowheads), Golgi phase (asterisk), cap phase (open arrow), maturation phase (long arrow), and mature spermatozoa (short arrows).

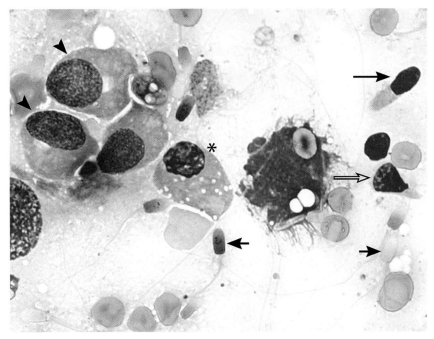

feminization also frequently resolve with the removal of the tumor [12]. Metastatic rates typically are low, and if absent, orchiectomy may be curative.

13.1.4 Interstitial Cell Tumor (Leydig Cell Tumor)

13.1.4.1 Cytologic Appearance
Neoplastic cells are elongated, and may even appear spindloid, and often exfoliate centered around capillaries (Figure 13.7). They have a moderate volume of pale-blue cytoplasm that frequently contains numerous fine, clear vacuoles (Figure 13.8) compared to the coarse clear vacuoles in Sertoli cell tumors (see Figure 13.6). Nuclei often are eccentrically placed and have finely granular chromatin with small basophilic nucleoli. Anisocytosis/anisokaryosis generally are mild to moderate.

13.1.4.2 Clinical Considerations
- Derived from Leydig cells between seminiferous tubules.
- Dogs >> cats.

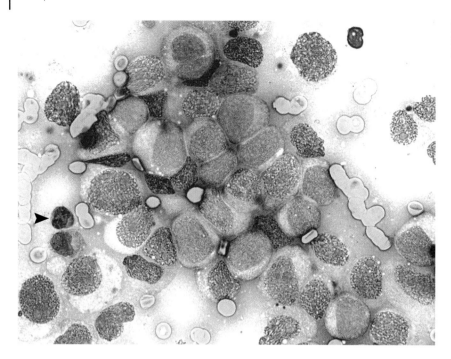

Figure 13.5 Seminoma, dog, 50× objective. Note the small mature lymphocyte (arrowhead).

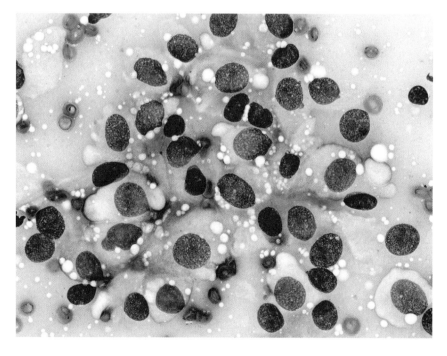

Figure 13.6 Sertoli cell tumor, dog, 50× objective. Note the coarse, clear vacuoles in the cytoplasm.

- Gross appearance = generally small, soft, bulging, and yellow/orange on the cut surface. Often contain cysts [4].
- Cryptorchidism is not a risk factor for development [5].
- Produce testosterone and are associated with an increased risk of perianal gland tumors and prostatic disease [4].

13.1.4.3 Prognosis

Typically good. Most tumors are benign with low metastatic rates, and orchiectomy is curative for these tumors.

Rare malignant variants have been reported which have a guarded prognosis [13].

13.1.5 Orchitis

13.1.5.1 Cytologic Appearance

Orchitis is characterized by an inflammatory infiltrate, interspersed with variable numbers of spermatogenic precursor cells (Figure 13.9). Neutrophilic inflammation is common with infectious agents. Infectious agents such as

Figure 13.7 Interstitial (Leydig) cell tumor, dog, 50× objective. Neoplastic cells radiate from a central linear capillary.

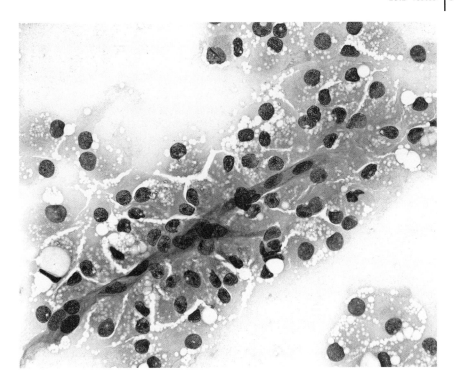

Figure 13.8 Interstitial (Leydig) cell tumor, dog, 50× objective. Note the punctate clear vacuoles in the cytoplasm.

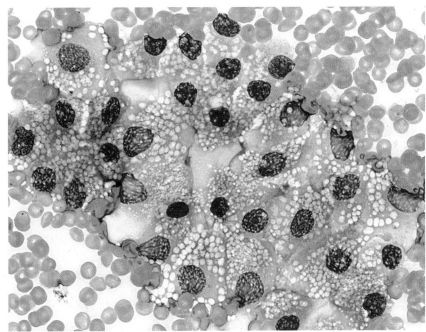

bacteria, fungi, or protozoa may be seen. Lymphocytes and plasma cells are common with chronic inflammation and immune-mediated disease.

13.1.5.2 Clinical Considerations
- *Brucella canis* is a common cause. *B. canis* has zoonotic potential.
- Other bacteria, *Blastomyces dermatitidis* and *Leishmania infantum* reported in dogs [14–16], as well as fibrinous

and necrotic orchitis secondary to feline infectious peritonitis in a cat [17].
- May be seen secondary to trauma, including bite wounds [18].
- Immune-mediated orchitis is reported [19].

13.1.5.3 Prognosis
The prognosis for maintaining fertility is guarded in cases of acute orchitis and poor for chronic orchitis.

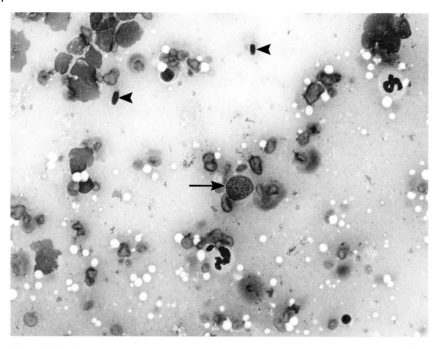

Figure 13.9 Orchitis, dog, 50× objective. Neutrophils are seen with scattered normal spermatogenic cells including spermatozoa heads (arrowheads) and an early spermatid (arrow).

13.2 Semen Analysis

Section 13.2.1 describes the morphologic characteristics of spermatozoa. Readers are referred to other excellent resources for a full description of semen analysis [20, 21].

13.2.1 Sperm Morphology

13.2.1.1 Cytologic Appearance
Spermatozoa morphology is shown in Figure 13.10.

Normal spermatozoa have a single, ovoid head, attached to a single, straight tail.

Primary morphologic changes occur during spermatogenesis and are considered more serious than secondary changes [22]. These changes include double tail, tightly coiled tail, deformed head (including bent head or abnormal shape), proximal droplet, and double head.

Secondary morphologic changes occur during maturation or collection of samples and include detached head, bent tail, distal coiled tail, and distal droplet.

Normal semen should have <10% primary and <20% secondary abnormalities [22].

The samples should also be assessed for any evidence of inflammation (Figure 13.11).

13.2.1.2 Clinical Considerations
- Slides are best prepared using similar spreading techniques as when making a blood smear [20]. Diff-Quik stains are adequate for analysis [23].

- At least 200 spermatozoa should be assessed on two separate slides. Assess spermatozoa in the middle third of the slides for optimal morphology.
- Semen quality may vary significantly between collections, and repeat evaluation is often required [18].
- Aspiration of the testicle, if required, is a safe procedure, with no significant adverse side effects or effects on testicular function [24].

13.2.1.3 Prognosis
Fertility in dogs appears to be most adversely affected when the percentage of normal spermatozoa morphology drops below 60% [25]. *Note*: The morphologic assessment of spermatozoa is only one facet of assessing fertility, with other factors being sperm concentration and motility, and the physical and hormonal characteristics of the patient.

13.3 Prostate

13.3.1 Prostatic Hyperplasia

13.3.1.1 Cytologic Features
Prostatic hyperplasia (PH) is characterized by sheets of uniform cells, with minimal anisocytosis and anisokaryosis. Cells have prominent intercellular borders and are cuboidal to polygonal, giving them a characteristic "honeycomb" appearance (Figure 13.12). Nuclei have clumped, mature chromatin and mostly inapparent nucleoli.

(A)

(B)

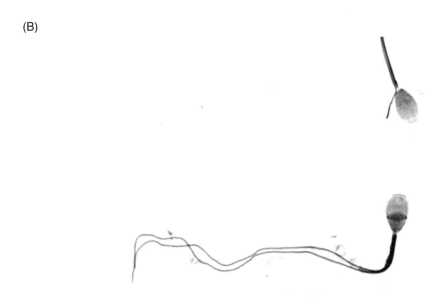

Figure 13.10 Sperm morphology, (A) normal spermatozoon, (B) double tail.

(C)

(D)

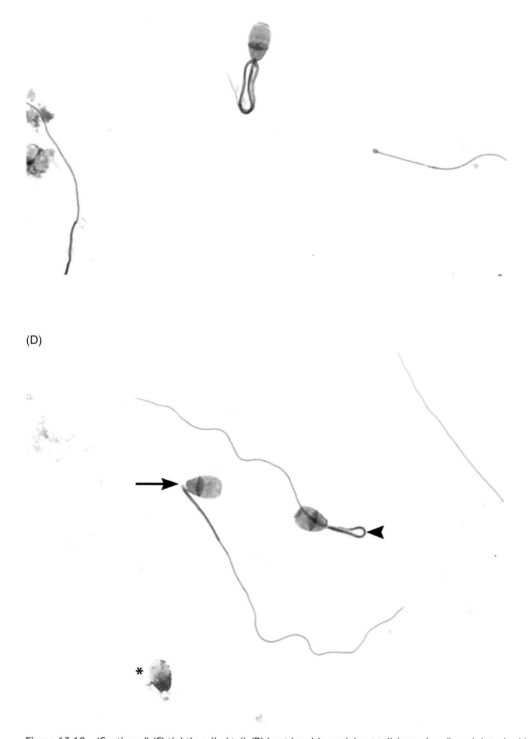

Figure 13.10 (Continued) (C) tightly coiled tail, (D) bent head (arrow), bent tail (arrowhead), and detached head (asterisk).

(E)

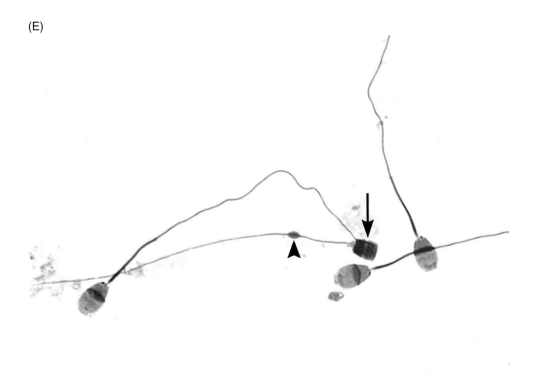

(F)

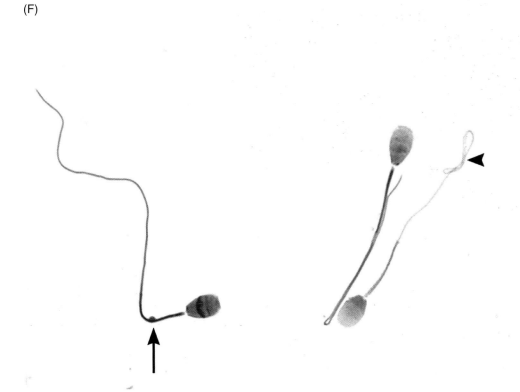

Figure 13.10 (Continued) (E) abnormally shaped head (arrow) and a proximal droplet (arrowhead), and (F) a spermatozoon is seen (arrowhead) with a distal coil. The two other spermatozoa have bent tails, and a proximal droplet is present (arrow).

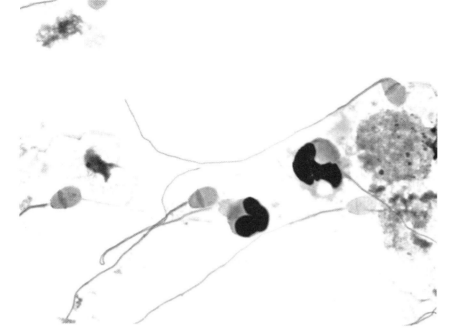

Figure 13.11 Neutrophilic inflammation, semen, dog, 100× objective.

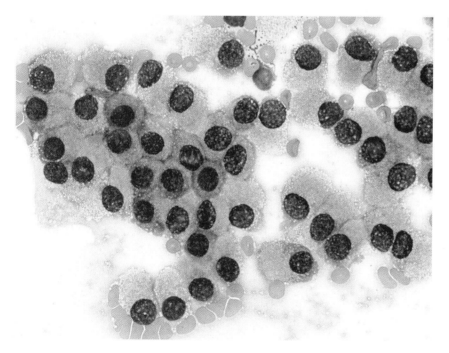

Figure 13.12 Prostatic hyperplasia, dog, 50× objective.

13.3.1.2 Clinical Considerations

- Previously termed *benign prostatic hyperplasia* (BPH). PH is now the current recommendation in veterinary medicine [26].
- Androgen-dependent condition, common in older, intact dogs [27].
- Reported prevalence in intact dogs of 80% ≥6 years and 95% ≥9 years old [28].
- Clinical signs: urinary incontinence, dysuria, hematuria, and/or difficult/painful defecation. Many dogs are asymptomatic. Severity of clinical signs not linked to prostate size [29].
- Prostate usually symmetrical, smooth, and non-painful [29].
- May be primary or secondary to underlying inflammation [29].
- Not a risk factor for subsequent development of carcinoma [26, 30].

13.3.1.3 Prognosis
Excellent.

13.3.2 Prostatic Adenocarcinoma

13.3.2.1 Cytologic Features
Prostatic adenocarcinomas exfoliate as sheets of cohesive cells but differ from PH in that the cells become more round/ovoid and have a variable amount of cytoplasm. Cell sheets also become more crowded and less uniform than those seen in PH. Anisokaryosis is increased, nuclei have more open chromatin, and nucleoli become more prominent and numerous (compare Figures 13.13 and 13.12).

13.3.2.2 Clinical Considerations
- Dogs >> cats
- Castrated dogs may be at increased risk relative to intact dogs [31].
- Frequently associated with mineralization, necrosis, and inflammation (see Figures 2.2 and 2.7), which may constitute the majority of the sample [32–34].
- Prostate often asymmetrically and irregularly enlarged.
- High metastatic rates (70–80% of cases), commonly to regional lymph nodes, lung, liver, urethra, bladder, spleen, and kidney [35].

13.3.2.3 Prognosis
Grave. Tumors are locally aggressive with high metastatic rates, and short survival times are reported even with medical and surgical therapy [36, 37]. Metastatic disease and intact signalment are poor prognostic indicators [36].

13.3.3 Prostatic Urothelial Carcinoma

13.3.3.1 Cytologic Features
Prostatic urothelial carcinomas can be difficult to differentiate from prostatic adenocarcinomas cytologically, and even histologically, and mixed urothelial and glandular phenotypes exist [35, 38]. Urothelial carcinomas frequently contain bright-pink secretory material within the cytoplasm, sometimes called *Melamed-Wolinska bodies*, (Figure 13.14), though these are not pathognomonic for this tumor type. Criteria of malignancy frequently are marked, similar to those described for prostatic carcinoma.

13.3.3.2 Clinical Considerations
- Arise from urothelial cells of the prostatic urethra or periurethral ducts.
- Castrated dogs may be at increased risk relative to intact dogs [31].

13.3.3.3 Prognosis
Grave. High metastatic rates and short survival times reported [33, 39].

13.3.4 Prostate: Squamous Metaplasia

13.3.4.1 Cytologic Features
Prostatic epithelial cells assume a more squamous appearance and are large, angular, and flattened, with abundant pale-/sky-blue cytoplasm consistent with keratinization.

Figure 13.13 Prostatic carcinoma, dog, 50× objective.

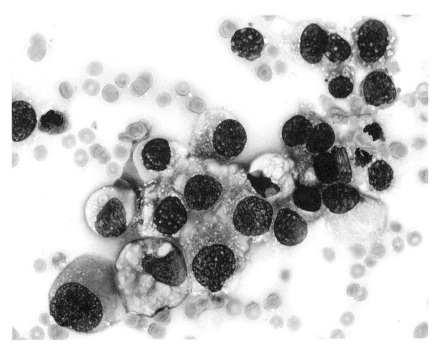

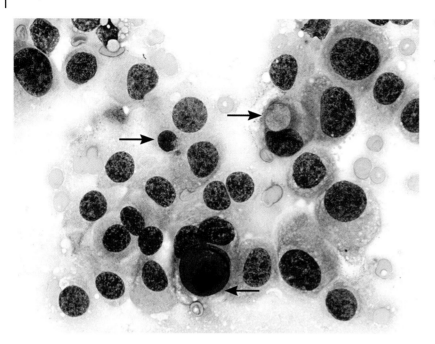

Figure 13.14 Transitional cell carcinoma, prostatic urethra, dog, 50× objective. Bright-pink secretory material (Melamed-Wolinska bodies) is seen within the cytoplasm of many cells (arrows).

Nuclei are single, centrally located, and have stippled to variably clumped chromatin. Hyperplastic epithelium also may be seen (Figure 13.15).

13.3.4.2 Clinical Considerations

- Most commonly associated with increased concentration of estrogen or testosterone, including Sertoli cell tumors in dogs and interstitial cell tumors in cats [40, 41].
- Also may be seen secondary to chronic inflammation/irritation.
- Squamous metaplasia is not considered a pre-neoplastic change [35].

13.3.4.3 Prognosis

Excellent. Changes reversible with the removal of the source of estrogen/irritation [35].

13.3.5 Prostatic Cyst

13.3.5.1 Cytologic Appearance

Cysts generally have a pink-stippled, proteinaceous background with a minimal amount of blood. Nucleated cells are seen in low numbers and may include rare quiescent macrophages, non-degenerative neutrophils, and small mature lymphocytes. Mineralized material may be present (Figure 13.16) [42].

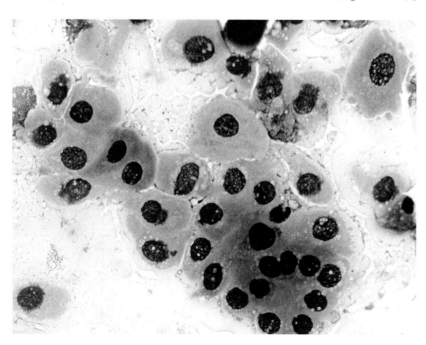

Figure 13.15 Squamous metaplasia, prostate, dog, 50× objective. Note the sky-blue appearance of the cytoplasm consistent with keratinization.

Figure 13.16 Prostatic cyst, dog, 50× objective. Note the aggregates of refractile mineralized material, and a single macrophage (far left).

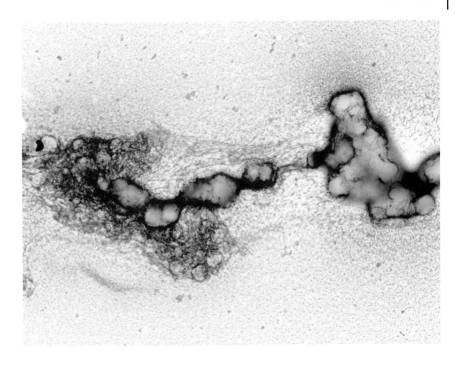

13.3.5.2 Clinical Considerations
- Dogs >> cats [43, 44].
- Often associated with PH and may be septic [43, 45].
- May form within prostatic parenchyma (retention cysts) or outside the prostate gland (paraprostatic cysts).

13.3.5.3 Prognosis
Good with appropriate therapy.

13.3.6 Septic Prostatitis

13.3.6.1 Cytologic Appearance
Septic prostatitis appears similar to septic inflammation elsewhere, with degenerative neutrophils predominating, often containing intracellular bacteria. Hyperplastic prostatic epithelium may be present and confirms the prostate as the source of the septic inflammation (Figure 13.17).

Figure 13.17 Septic prostatitis, dog, 50× objective. Neutrophils that frequently contain rod-shaped bacteria (arrows) are intimately associated with hyperplastic prostatic epithelium.

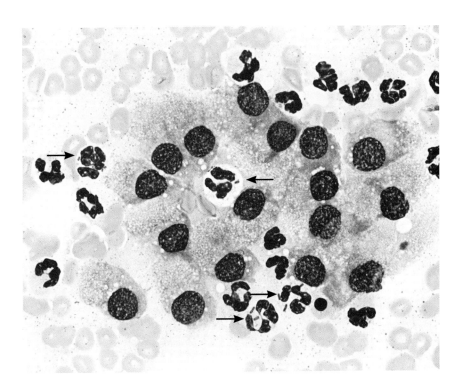

13.3.6.2 Clinical Considerations

- Intact >> castrated dogs [35].
- Ascending infection from bladder > hematogenous spread [43].
- Predisposing factors = PH and prostatic cysts [46].
- Mostly aerobic bacteria, with *Escherichia coli* being the most common isolate in both dogs and cats [47, 48]. Other common isolates include *Staphylococcus* spp., *Streptococcus* spp., *Pseudomonas* spp., *Klebsiella* spp., *Enterobacter* spp., and *Pasteurella* spp. [35].
- Clinical signs = fever, anorexia, lethargy, straining to urinate or defecate, hematuria, and edema of the scrotum or hindlimbs [35].

13.3.6.3 Prognosis

Generally good with appropriate therapy. Prolonged antibiotic therapy and castration often required [46].

13.4 Penis

The most frequent neoplasms affecting the penis include squamous cell carcinoma (SCC), transmissible venereal tumor (TVT), and tumors of the skin (prepuce). See Chapter 4 for details.

Female

13.5 Ovary

13.5.1 Dysgerminoma

13.5.1.1 Cytologic Appearance

Dysgerminomas are highly exfoliative, composed of discrete, large, round cells with a small to moderate volume of pale-blue/purple cytoplasm. Nuclei are ovoid to occasionally amoeboid and have finely granular, immature chromatin with multiple basophilic nucleoli. Multinucleation and satellite nuclei are frequent, and many mitotic figures are present (Figure 13.18). Anisocytosis/anisokaryosis are moderate to marked. Small mature lymphocytes may be present [49].

13.5.1.2 Clinical Considerations

- Mostly older dogs and cats (>10 years), but have been reported in patients as young as 2 years [50, 51].
- Usually unilateral, frequently affecting the right ovary [50].
- Clinical signs mostly attributable to a space-occupying abdominal mass.
- Metastatic disease present in 10–33% of cases, involving regional lymph nodes and widely disseminated [52, 53].

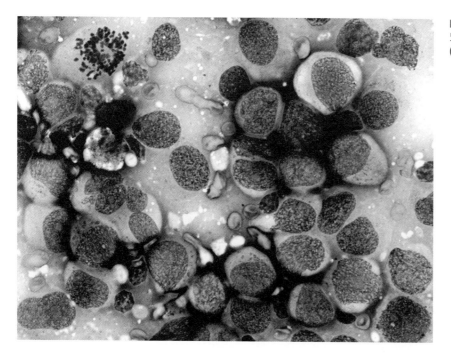

Figure 13.18 Dysgerminoma, dog, 50× objective. Note the mitotic figure (top left).

13.5.1.3 Prognosis

Good with surgical excision if no metastatic disease is present; however, prognosis is variable in the presence of metastases [50, 54].

13.5.2 Granulosa Cell Tumor

13.5.2.1 Cytologic Appearance

Highly cellular, arranged in loose aggregates and often associated with streaming or pooling eosinophilic extracellular mucinous material (Figure 13.19). Cells are round to polyhedral, with a large amount of pale-blue cytoplasm that contains many punctate clear vacuoles. Nuclei are round, eccentrically placed, and have finely stippled chromatin, with single, basophilic nucleoli. Anisocytosis/anisokaryosis are moderate to rarely marked, and N/C ratios are low. Cells may be seen in rosettes surrounding pink basement membrane material (Call-Exner bodies) [49].

13.5.2.2 Clinical Considerations

- Sex cord-stromal tumors.
- Constitute approximately 50% of ovarian tumors in dogs and cats [4, 54].
- May develop in female spayed dogs with ovarian remnants or ectopic ovarian tissue [55, 56].
- Most are functional and produce estrogen or progesterone, causing persistent estrus, vulvar swelling, pyometra, mammary gland hyperplasia, and/or myelotoxicity [57].
- Approximately 20% of tumors are malignant in dogs, 50% are malignant in cats, and the tumors metastasize widely [4, 53].

13.5.2.3 Prognosis

Surgical excision may be curative, but the prognosis is guarded with evidence of metastatic disease, which is common [4, 53–55].

13.5.3 Ovarian Adenoma

13.5.3.1 Cytologic Appearance

Ovarian adenomas comprise cohesive sheets of round epithelial cells that have a moderate to abundant amount of pale-blue cytoplasm. Nuclei are round, centrally located, and have coarsely granular chromatin with small nucleoli. Anisocytosis/anisokaryosis are mild, and N/C ratios are low (Figure 13.20).

13.5.3.2 Clinical Considerations

- Dogs > cats.
- Occur unilaterally.
- Often associated with cystic endometrial hyperplasia [58].

13.5.3.3 Prognosis

Excellent. Ovarian adenomas do not metastasize, and ovariohysterectomy is curative [58].

13.5.4 Ovarian Adenocarcinoma

13.5.4.1 Cytologic Appearance

Ovarian adenocarcinomas also exfoliate as cohesive sheets. Relative to adenomas the cells often are crowded or piled and have high N/C ratios. Chromatin is more "ropey," and hyperchromasia of nuclei is often more prominent (compare Figures 13.21 and 13.20).

Figure 13.19 Granulosa cell tumor, dog, 50× objective.

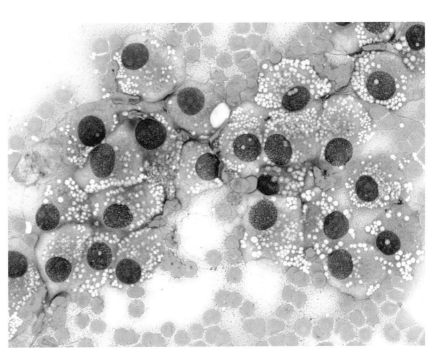

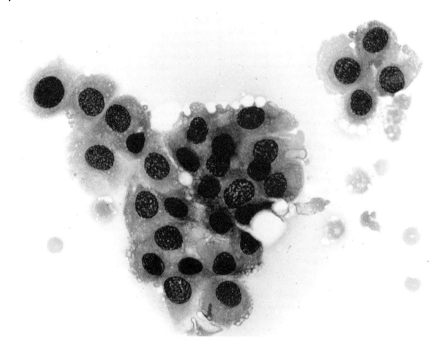

Figure 13.20 Ovarian adenoma, dog, 50× objective.

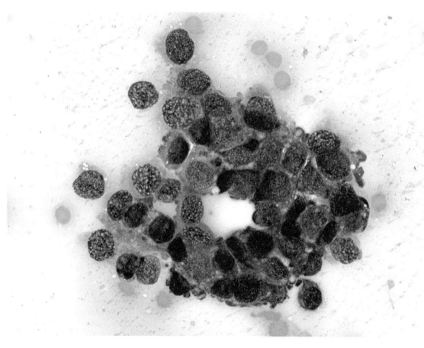

Figure 13.21 Ovarian papillary adenocarcinoma, dog, 50× objective. Note the cell crowding, disorganization, and higher N/C ratios compared to the adenoma in Figure 13.20.

13.5.4.2 Clinical Considerations
- Dogs > cats.
- Frequently the most common ovarian tumor in dogs [58, 59].
- Papillary, tubular, and undifferentiated variants.
- Unilateral involvement most common.

13.5.4.3 Prognosis
Guarded. Approximately 50% will metastasize, generally within the peritoneal cavity, and is often associated with a neoplastic effusion, though prolonged survival is possible with surgical and medical therapy [60]. A larger tumor size is linked to malignancy [58].

13.5.5 Teratoma

13.5.5.1 Cytologic Appearance
Teratomas arise from more than one germ cell layer (ectoderm, mesoderm, and/or endoderm), and as such their appearance is highly variable. Epithelial-origin cells

Figure 13.22 Teratoma, cat, 20× objective.

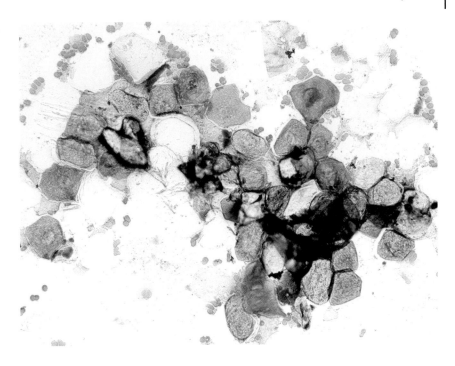

are the most common, varying from poorly differentiated to well-differentiated (see squamous epithelial cells in Figure 13.22) [49]. Hair shafts, cartilage/bone, muscle, and nervous tissue may all be seen. These tumors often are cystic.

13.5.5.2 Clinical Considerations
- Rare in dogs and cats.
- Mostly young animals, but may be seen in older patients [61].
- Most commonly affect the left ovary. Extragonadal sites are rare [50].
- May be benign or malignant.

13.5.5.3 Prognosis
Good for benign tumors, but poor if metastatic disease is present [50, 62].

13.6 Mammary Glands

13.6.1 Benign Mammary Tumors

13.6.1.1 Cytologic Appearance
Epithelial origin: Hyperplastic lesions of ducts and adenomas appear cytologically similar and comprise variably sized sheets of uniform, cuboidal to round epithelial cells. Cell clusters frequently have a tubular (Figure 13.23) or papillary arrangement (Figures 13.24 and 13.25). Anisocytosis/anisokaryosis generally are mild; however, small clusters with increased atypia can be seen. N/C ratios are low to moderate. *Note*: Well-differentiated carcinomas can

mimic benign lesions, and histopathology is required for definitive characterization of biologic behavior (compare to Figure 13.26).

Mesenchymal origin: Benign mesenchymal neoplasms are rare and usually seen in conjunction with an epithelial component (e.g., fibroadenoma).

13.6.1.2 Clinical Considerations
- Dogs > cats – malignant tumors more common in cats (see Section 13.6.2).
- Mammary tumors are rare in male dogs and cats (intact or neutered) and most appear to be benign epithelial tumors in dogs and carcinomas in cats [63, 64].
- Usually small, well-encapsulated, firm.
- May be single or multiple, and other concurrent masses may not share biologic behavior [65, 66].

13.6.1.3 Prognosis
Good to excellent, with surgical excision generally curative.

13.6.2 Malignant Mammary Tumors

13.6.2.1 Cytologic Appearance
Epithelial origin: Mammary gland carcinomas often are highly pleomorphic, but can be well-differentiated (Figure 13.26). The cells often exfoliate in sheets that have a papillary or acinar arrangement. Nuclei range from round to amoeboid and often have prominent basophilic nucleoli. Mitotic figures are common. Anisocytosis/anisokaryosis are marked and N/C ratios are variable. Many variants are

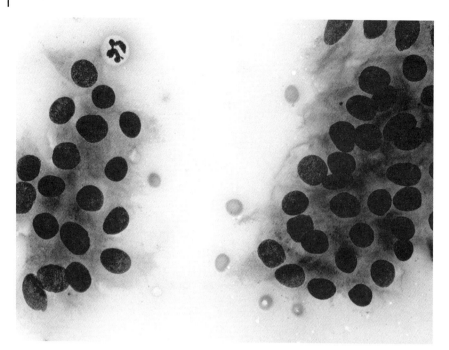

Figure 13.23 Tubular mammary adenoma, dog, 50× objective.

Figure 13.24 Papillary mammary adenoma, dog, 50× objective.

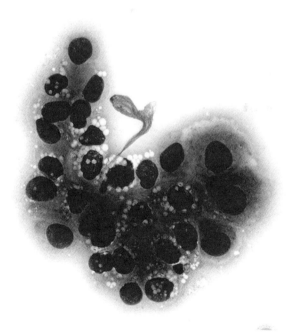

described that require histopathology for differentiation. Some of these include ductal (Figure 13.27), simple tubular (Figure 13.28), adenocarcinoma (Figure 13.29), and anaplastic (Figure 13.30) [67].

Mesenchymal origin: Cytologic appearance reflects the cell of origin. Osteosarcoma is the most common (Figure 13.31), while chondrosarcoma, fibrosarcoma, and hemangiosarcoma are also possible.

13.6.2.2 Clinical Considerations
Dogs
- Middle-aged to older, increased risk over time.
- Ovariohysterectomy is protective. The risk of tumor development increases from 0.5% to 26% in dogs with no estrous cycle, to the third estrous cycle [68].
- Up to 70% of intact females have more than one tumor at diagnosis (benign or malignant) [65, 68].

Figure 13.25 Papillary mammary adenoma, dog, 50× objective.

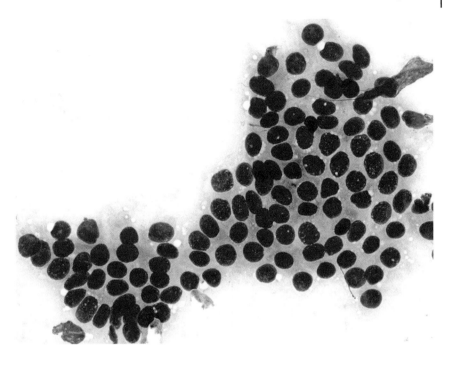

Figure 13.26 Mammary carcinoma (well differentiated), cat, 50× objective.

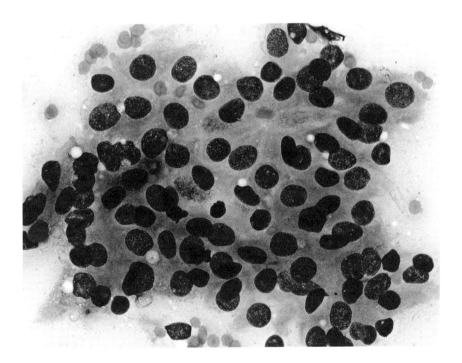

Cats

- Middle-aged to older, increased risk over time.
- Siamese breed overrepresented [66].
- Sevenfold higher risk in intact cats as compared to spayed cats [69].
- Rare in male cats and have similar biologic behavior to females [64].

- Multiple tumors may be present at the time of diagnosis (benign or malignant) [66].

13.6.2.3 Prognosis

Variable. Low rates of lymphatic invasion and distant metastatic disease in dogs, but high in cats. Surgical excision of localized tumors may be curative. Important prognostic

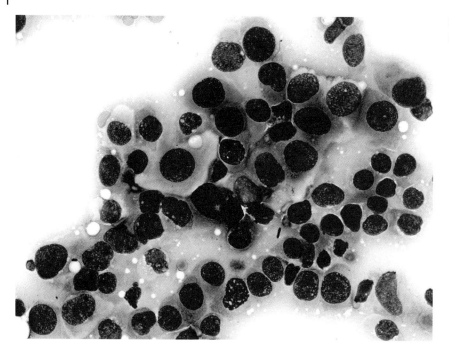

Figure 13.27 Mammary carcinoma (ductal), cat, 50× objective.

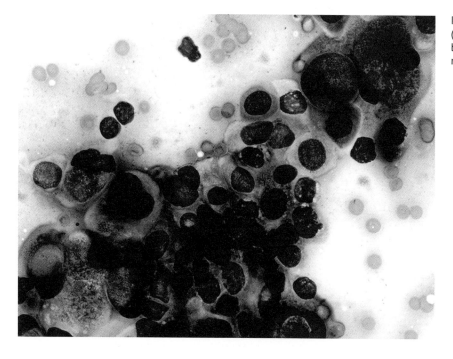

Figure 13.28 Mammary carcinoma (tubular), cat, 50× objective. Note the bright-pink secretory material within many cells.

factors in both dogs and cats include (i) tumor type (ductal carcinomas are more aggressive), (ii) tumor size (tumors <3 cm in diameter have been associated with longer survival and tumors >3 cm have been associated with poor prognosis in cats), and (iii) lymph node involvement (poor prognosis if present) [64, 70–72].

13.6.3 Complex/Mixed Mammary Gland Tumors

13.6.3.1 Cytologic Appearance

Complex tumors contain an epithelial and a mesenchymal component (Figure 13.32), while mixed tumors involve an epithelial population with the proliferation of cartilage ± bone ± adipose tissue (Figure 13.33).

Figure 13.29 Mammary carcinoma (adenocarcinoma), dog, 50× objective. Note the vacuolated cytoplasm and multiple prominent nucleoli.

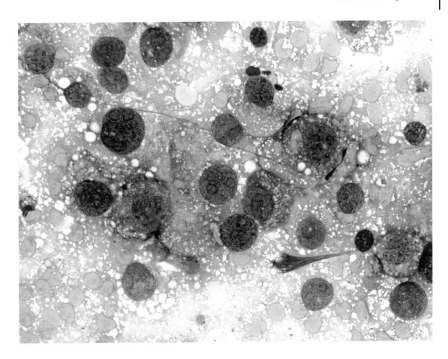

Figure 13.30 Mammary carcinoma (anaplastic), dog, 50× objective.

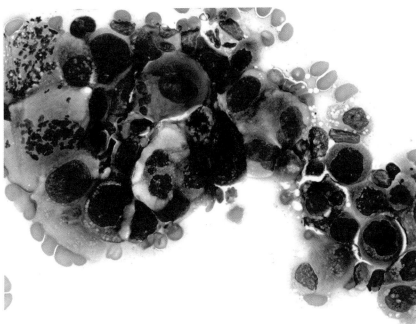

13.6.3.2 Prognosis

Variable, based on tumor types involved. Carcinosarcomas (malignant epithelial and mesenchymal components) metastasize widely and carry a poor prognosis [69].

13.6.4 Mastitis

13.6.4.1 Cytologic Appearance

Samples frequently contain large numbers of inflammatory cells. Degenerative neutrophils containing intracellular bacteria are the most common (Figure 13.34), with lesser numbers of macrophages and lymphocytes.

13.6.4.2 Clinical Considerations

- Mostly seen postpartum or in pseudopregnancy.
- Clinical signs = swollen, painful, warm glands ± discoloration of skin.
- *E. coli*, *Staphylococcus* spp., and *Streptococcus* spp. are the most common bacterial isolates [73].
- Other infectious organisms (*Mycobacterium*, fungal agents, and protozoa) rarely noted [74–76].

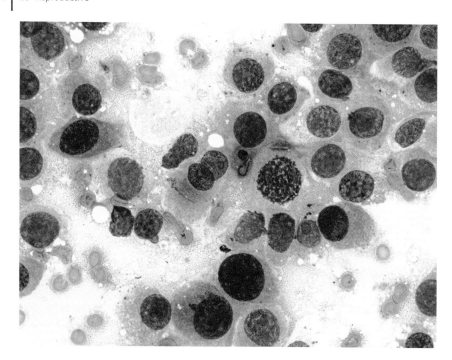

Figure 13.31 Mammary gland osteosarcoma, dog, 50× objective.

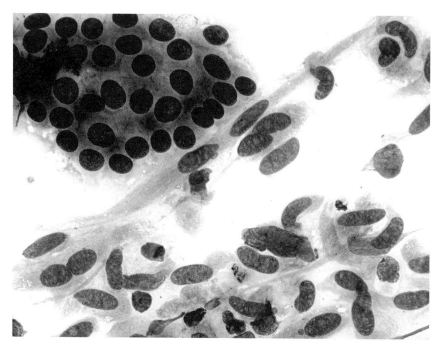

Figure 13.32 Benign complex mammary gland tumor, dog, 50× objective. Note the epithelial cells (top left) and mesenchymal cells.

13.6.4.3 Prognosis

Mostly good with appropriate therapy. Abscessation or gangrenous mastitis may carry a more guarded prognosis.

13.7 Vaginal Cytology

The cells that need to be identified on vaginal cytology include basal cells, parabasal cells, intermediate cells, and superficial cells (Figure 13.35).

1) Basal cells = These cells are small, round, and have very high N/C ratios. They have a deep epithelial location and are not routinely seen in vaginal cytology samples.
2) Parabasal cells = These cells are small and round, with high N/C ratios, and large nuclei with stippled chromatin.
3) Intermediate cells = These cells are ovoid with a more abundant volume of pale-blue cytoplasm. They have nuclei similar to parabasal cells, which are round with stippled chromatin.

Figure 13.33 Mixed mammary gland tumor, dog, 50× objective. Note the sheet of epithelial cells adjacent to an island of deep metachromatic chondroid that contains embedded chondrocytes.

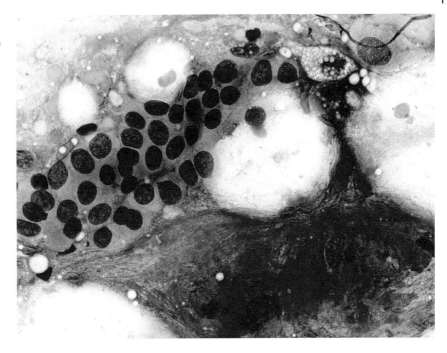

Figure 13.34 Mastitis, dog, 50× objective. Hyperplastic epithelial cells are accompanied by many variably degenerative neutrophils that contain intracellular bacteria (arrow).

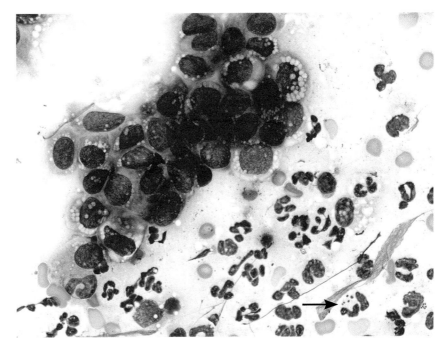

4) Superficial cells = These cells are polygonal with abundant pale-blue cytoplasm. They can be anucleated or have small, pyknotic, round nuclei with condensed chromatin.

13.7.1 Anestrus

13.7.1.1 Cytologic Appearance

Anestrus in dogs is dominated by parabasal cells, admixed with occasional intermediate cells (Figure 13.36). Superficial cells and red blood cells are absent during anestrus.

Rare neutrophils and extracellular bacteria may be present but are most often absent. In cats, nucleated superficial cells may be seen [77].

13.7.1.2 Clinical Considerations
- Anestrus varies from 1 to 6 months [78].
- Associated with uterine involution and endometrial repair.
- Females not attractive to, or receptive to, males.
- No discharge, and the vulva is small.

(A)

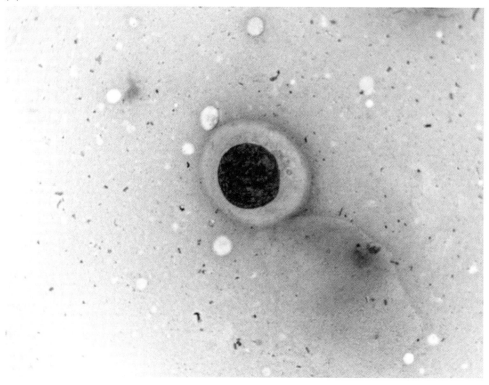

(B)

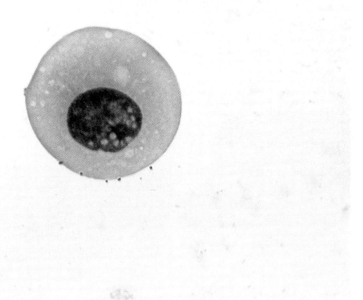

Figure 13.35 Normal vaginal epithelial cells, (A) basal cell, (B) parabasal cell.

(C)

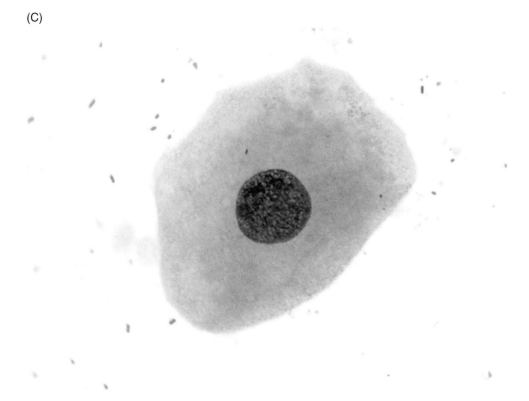

(D)

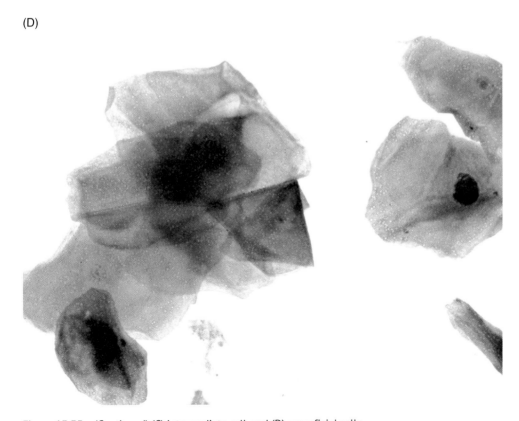

Figure 13.35 (Continued) (C) intermediate cell, and (D) superficial cells.

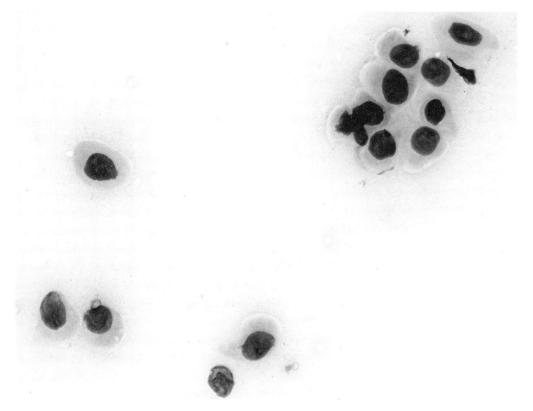

Figure 13.36 Vaginal cytology, anestrus, cat, 50× objective. Only parabasal cells are seen.

- During late anestrus, progesterone concentrations are at their nadir ($<1\,ng\,ml^{-1}$) and estrogen is at basal levels ($\sim2-10\,pg\,ml^{-1}$) [78–80].

13.7.2 Proestrus

13.7.2.1 Cytologic Appearance

Increasing concentrations of estrogen lead to progressive cornification of the vaginal epithelium. As such, in addition to intermediate and parabasal cells, proestrus is characterized by the presence of superficial cells, which constitute <50% of cells in early proestrus (Figure 13.37) and >50% of cells in late proestrus (Figure 13.38). An increasing estrogen concentration also results in capillary fragility, and erythrocytes generally are present in large numbers, accompanied by nondegenerative neutrophils ± extracellular bacteria [81].

13.7.2.2 Clinical Considerations

- Proestrus length is highly variable, ranging from 3 days to 3 weeks (mean = 9 days) [78].

- Females become attractive to males, but usually are not receptive.
- Vulva mildly enlarged ± serosanguinous or hemorrhagic discharge (dogs).
- Estrogen levels peak during late proestrus ($\sim50-100\,pg\,ml^{-1}$) and progesterone concentration is low, but increases with the luteinizing hormone (LH) surge (typically $>2\,ng\,ml^{-1}$) [78–80].

13.7.3 Estrus

13.7.3.1 Cytologic Appearance

In dogs, estrus is characterized by an almost exclusive population (>90%) of superficial cells (Figure 13.39). Neutrophils are absent, but extracellular bacteria may be present (Figure 13.40). In cats, anucleated superficial cells constitute 40–60% of the cells [82].

13.7.3.2 Clinical Considerations

- Females are receptive and passive toward males. *Note*: Both estrus behavior and cornification of epithelial cells

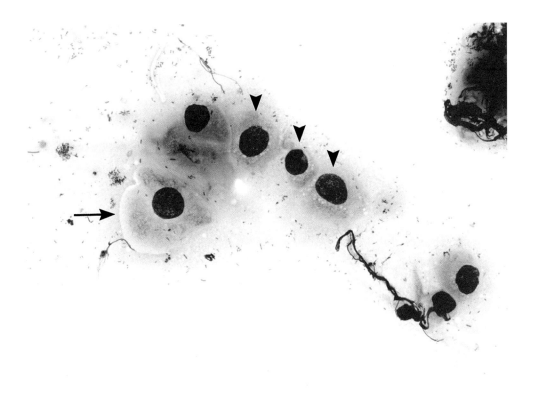

Figure 13.37 Vaginal cytology, early proestrus, dog, 50× objective. Parabasal cells (arrowheads) and a small superficial cell (arrow) are seen. Many extracellular bacteria are present.

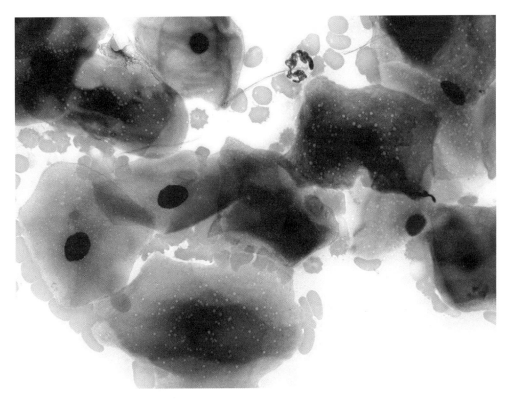

Figure 13.38 Vaginal cytology, late proestrus, dog, 50× objective. Large superficial cells predominate, accompanied by many red blood cells and a neutrophil.

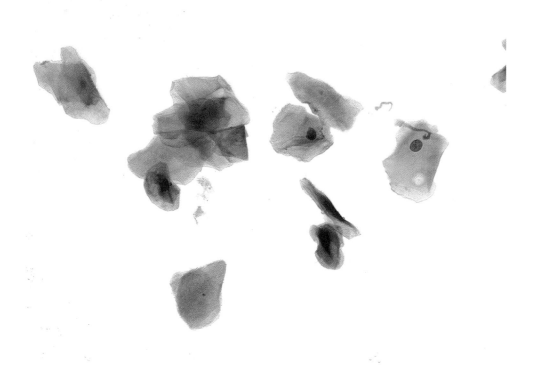

Figure 13.39 Vaginal cytology, estrus, dog, 20× objective.

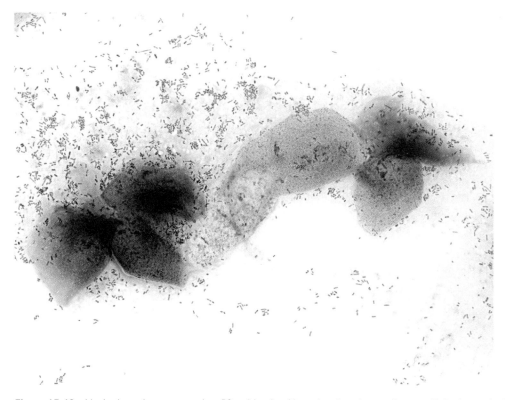

Figure 13.40 Vaginal cytology, estrus, dog, 50× objective. Note the abundance of extracellular bacteria, but the absence of any neutrophils.

may precede or follow the LH surge and do not always correlate with the fertile estrus period.

- Estrus lasts 3 days to 3 weeks (mean = 9 days) [78].
- Vulvar enlargement is maximal (dogs).
- The serosanguinous/hemorrhagic discharge seen in proestrus tends to diminish.
- Estrogen levels drop precipitously after the LH surge, while progesterone increases (usually 4–$10\,ng\,ml^{-1}$ at ovulation) [78–80].

13.7.4 Diestrus

13.7.4.1 Cytologic Appearance

During diestrus, there is a dramatic decrease in the percentage of superficial cells and a return of intermediate and parabasal cells. Within 24 hours, superficial cells decrease from approximately 100% to 20–40% of the population. Neutrophils often return during diestrus, and intracellular bacteria may be noted (Figure 13.41).

13.7.4.2 Clinical Considerations

- Females become refractory to breeding. Vulvar swelling and any residual discharge decrease.
- Breedings after the onset of diestrus rarely are fertile.
- Onset of diestrus is an accurate determinant of the time of ovulation and hence can be used to estimate gestation length. In dogs, ovulation occurs 5–7 days prior to the onset of diestrus. Gestation time is therefore 57 days ± 1 day from the onset of diestrus [78].
- Progesterone levels rise to a peak (15–$80\,ng\,ml^{-1}$), before progressively declining in late diestrus [78–80].

- Diestrus typically lasts 2–3 months in the absence of pregnancy.

13.7.5 Vaginitis/Metritis

13.7.5.1 Cytologic Appearance

Large numbers of neutrophils typically are seen that may be degenerative and contain intracellular bacteria (Figure 13.42). Squamous epithelial cells (anucleated or with pyknotic nuclei) may be seen.

13.7.5.2 Clinical Considerations

- Intracellular bacteria may be seen during diestrus normally – correlate with epithelial cell populations and clinical signs.
- Common aerobic bacterial isolates include *E. coli*, beta-hemolytic *Streptococcus,* and *Staphylococcus intermedius*, though microbial culture and susceptibility testing are recommended [83].

13.7.5.3 Prognosis

Generally excellent with appropriate antimicrobial therapy and treatment of any underlying predisposing causes. Prognosis for cases of pyometra is more guarded [84].

13.7.6 Neoplasia

Common neoplasms that affect the vagina include leiomyoma/leiomyosarcoma (see Chapter 7) and TVT (see Chapter 4).

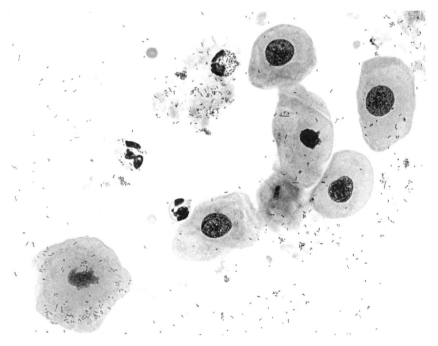

Figure 13.41 Vaginal cytology, diestrus, dog, 50× objective. Intermediate cells predominate, admixed with increased neutrophils and bacteria (both intracellular and extracellular).

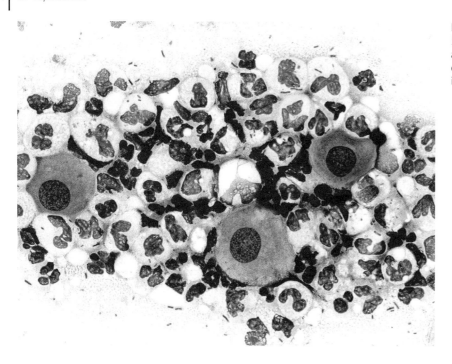

Figure 13.42 Vaginitis, dog, 50× objective. Vaginal epithelial cells are surrounded by abundant degenerative neutrophils that contain intracellular bacteria.

13.7.7 Clitoral Adenocarcinoma

13.7.7.1 Cytologic Appearance

Cells are seen in dense cohesive clusters that often lack prominent intercellular borders, and frequently form palisading rows or vague acinar arrangements that may be associated with pink extracellular matrix. Nuclei are round, centrally located, and have finely stippled chromatin with small nucleoli. Anisocytosis/anisokaryosis are mild and N/C ratios are moderate. Bare nuclei may be seen in the background, and low numbers of macrophages are often present [85]. The morphologic appearance is similar to that seen in anal sac apocrine gland adenocarcinomas (see Figure 13.43).

13.7.7.2 Clinical Considerations

- Rare tumors, most frequently reported in older female spayed dogs [85].
- Masses typically firm, nodular, and hyperemic [85, 86].

Figure 13.43 Clitoral adenocarcinoma, dog, 50× objective. Note the lack of prominent intercellular borders and palisading arrangement of the cells.

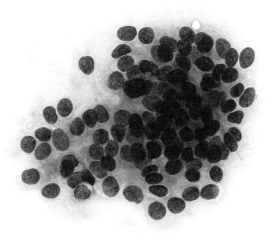

- Clinical signs: polyuria/polydipsia, licking vulva, and hemorrhagic vulvar discharge.
- Metastatic disease common to inguinal and/or iliac lymph nodes [85–87].
- Hypercalcemia may be present [85, 87].

13.7.7.3 Prognosis

Guarded. Tumors often have aggressive, infiltrative regional growth with a high incidence of metastasis. Long-term outcomes are mostly poor; however, cases amenable to surgical excision and free of metastases may have a better prognosis [85].

References

1 Santos, M., Marcos, R., Caniatti, M. (2010) Cytologic study of normal canine testis. *Theriogenology*, **73** (2), 208–214.

2 Masserdotti, C., Bonfanti, U., De Lorenzi, D., *et al.* (2005) Cytologic features of testicular tumours in dog. *J. Vet. Med. A Physiol. Pathol. Clin. Med.*, **52** (7), 339–346.

3 Scott, T.N., Swenson, C.L., Stein, L., *et al.* (2022) What is your diagnosis? Abdominal mass from a dog. *Vet. Clin. Pathol.*, **51** (4), 591–594.

4 McEntee, M.C. (2002) Reproductive oncology. *Clin. Tech. Small Anim. Pract.*, **17** (3), 133–149.

5 Liao, A.T., Chu, P.Y., Yeh, L.S., *et al.* (2009) A 12-year retrospective study of canine testicular tumors. *J. Vet. Med. Sci.*, **71** (7), 919–923.

6 Grieco, V., Riccardi, E., Greppi, G.F., *et al.* (2008) Canine testicular tumours: a study on 232 dogs. *J. Comp. Pathol.*, **138** (2–3), 86–89.

7 Lipowitz, A.J., Schwartz, A., Wilson, G.P., *et al.* (1973) Testicular neoplasms and concomitant clinical changes in the dog. *J. Am. Vet. Med. Assoc.*, **163** (12), 1364–1368.

8 Masserdotti, C., De Lorenzi, D., Gasparotto, L. (2008) Cytologic detection of Call-Exner bodies in Sertoli cell tumors from 2 dogs. *Vet. Clin. Pathol.*, **37** (1), 112–114.

9 Dill, J.A., Janosco, M.E., Miller, D.M. (2018) Pathology in practice. *J. Am. Vet. Med. Assoc.*, **253** (9), 1129–1131.

10 Moreau, A.M., Scruggs, J.L. (2018) What is your diagnosis? Inguinal mass in a dog. *Vet. Clin. Pathol.*, **47** (1), 155–156.

11 Salyer, S.A., Lapsley, J.M., Palm, C.A., *et al.* (2022) Outcome of dogs with bone marrow suppression secondary to Sertoli cell tumour. *Vet. Comp. Oncol.*, **20** (2), 484–490.

12 Withers, S.S., Lawson, C.M., Burton, A.G., *et al.* (2016) Management of an invasive and metastatic Sertoli cell tumor with associated myelotoxicosis in a dog. *Can. Vet. J.*, **57** (3), 299–304.

13 Kudo, T., Kamiie, J., Aihara, N., *et al.* (2019) Malignant Leydig cell tumor in dogs: two cases and a review of the literature. *J. Vet. Diagn. Investig.*, **31** (4), 557–561.

14 Wanke, M.M. (2004) Canine brucellosis. *Anim. Reprod. Sci.*, **82–83**, 195–207.

15 Diniz, S.A., Melo, M.S., Borges, A.M., *et al.* (2005) Genital lesions associated with visceral leishmaniasis and shedding of *Leishmania* sp. in the semen of naturally infected dogs. *Vet. Pathol.*, **42** (5), 650–658.

16 Ober, C.P., Spaulding, K., Breitschwerdt, E.B., *et al.* (2004) Orchitis in two dogs with Rocky Mountain spotted fever. *Vet. Radiol. Ultrasound*, **45** (5), 458–465.

17 Foster, R.A., Caswell, J.L., Rinkardt, N. (1996) Chronic fibrinous and necrotic orchitis in a cat. *Can. Vet. J.*, **37** (11), 681–682.

18 Prochowska, S., Niżański, W. (2022) Infertility in toms: clinical approach, experiences and challenges. *J. Feline. Med. Surg.*, **24** (9), 837–846.

19 Davidson, A.P., von Dehn, B.J., Schlafer, D.H. (2015) Adult-onset lymphoplasmacytic orchitis in a Labrador retriever stud dog. *Top. Companion Anim. Med.*, **30** (1), 31–34.

20 Root Kustritz, M.V. (2007) The value of canine semen evaluation for practitioners. *Theriogenology*, **68** (3), 329–337.

21 Zambelli, D., Cunto, M. (2006) Semen collection in cats: techniques and analysis. *Theriogenology*, **66** (2), 159–165.

22 Freshman, J.L. (2002) Semen collection and evaluation. *Clin. Tech. Small Anim. Pract.*, **17** (3), 104–107.

23 Root Kustritz, M.V., Olson, P.N., Johnston, S.D., *et al.* (1998) The effects of stains and investigators on assessment of the morphology of canine spermatozoa. *J. Am. Anim. Hosp. Assoc.*, **34** (4), 348–352.

24 Gouletsou, P.G., Galatos, A.D., Leontides, L.S., *et al.* (2010) Impact of fine or large needle aspiration on the dog's testis: in vitro ultrasonographic, bacteriological, gross anatomy and histological assessment. *Theriogenology*, **74** (9), 1604–1614.

25 Oettle, E.E. (1993) Sperm morphology and fertility in the dog. *J. Reprod. Fertil. Suppl.*, **47**, 257–260.

26 Palmieri, C., Foster, R.A., Grieco, V., *et al.* (2019) Histopathologic terminology standards for the reporting of prostatic epithelial lesions in dogs. *J. Comp. Pathol.*, **171**, 30–37.

27 Holst, B.S., Nilsson, S. (2023) Age, weight and circulating concentrations of total testosterone are associated with the relative prostatic size in adult intact male dogs. *Theriogenology*, **198**, 356–360.

28 Berry, S.J., Strandberg, J.D., Saunders, W.J., *et al.* (1986) Development of canine benign prostatic hyperplasia with age. *Prostate*, **9** (4), 363–373.

29 Ruetten, H., Wehber, M., Murphy, M., *et al.* (2021) A retrospective review of canine benign prostatic hyperplasia with and without prostatitis. *Clin. Theriogenol.*, **13** (4), 360–366.

30 LeRoy, B.E., Northrup, N. (2009) Prostate cancer in dogs: comparative and clinical aspects. *Vet. J.*, **180** (2), 149–162.

31 Bryan, J.N., Keeler, M.R., Henry, C.J., *et al.* (2007) A population study of neutering status as a risk factor for canine prostate cancer. *Prostate*, **67** (11), 1174–1181.

32 Bradbury, C.A., Westropp, J.L., Pollard, R.E. (2009) Relationship between prostatomegaly, prostatic mineralization, and cytologic diagnosis. *Vet. Radiol. Ultrasound*, **50** (2), 167–171.

33 Yang, N.S., Johnson, E.G., Palm, C.A., *et al.* (2023) MRI characteristics of canine prostatic neoplasia. *Vet. Radiol. Ultrasound*, **64** (1), 105–112.

34 de Brot, S., Lothion-Roy, J., Grau-Roma, L., *et al.* (2022) Histological and immunohistochemical investigation of canine prostate carcinoma with identification of common intraductal carcinoma component. *Vet. Comp. Oncol.*, **20** (1), 38–49.

35 Palmieri, C., Fonseca-Alves, C.E., Laufer-Amorim, R. (2022) A review on canine and feline prostate pathology. *Front. Vet. Sci.*, **9**, 881232. doi: 10.3389/fvets.2022.881232. Last accessed June 11, 2023.

36 Ravicini, S., Baines, S.J., Taylor, A., *et al.* (2018) Outcome and prognostic factors in medically treated canine prostatic carcinomas: a multi-institutional study. *Vet. Comp. Oncol.*, **16** (4), 450–458.

37 Bennett, T.C., Matz, B.M., Henderson, R.A., *et al.* (2018) Total prostatectomy as a treatment for prostatic carcinoma in 25 dogs. *Vet. Surg.*, **47** (3), 367–377.

38 LeRoy, B.E., Nadella, M.V.P., Toribio, R.E., *et al.* (2004) Canine prostate carcinomas express markers of urothelial and prostatic differentiation. *Vet. Pathol.*, **41** (2), 131–140.

39 Allstadt, S.D., Rodriguez, C.O., Jr., Boostrom, B., *et al.* (2015) Randomized phase III trial of piroxicam in combination with mitoxantrone or carboplatin for first-line treatment of urogenital tract transitional cell carcinoma in dogs. *J. Vet. Intern. Med.*, **29** (1), 261–267.

40 Powe, J.R., Canfield, P.J., Martin, P.A. (2004) Evaluation of the cytologic diagnosis of canine prostatic disorders. *Vet. Clin. Pathol.*, **33** (3), 150–154.

41 Tucker, A.R., Smith, J.R. (2008) Prostatic squamous metaplasia in a cat with interstitial cell neoplasia in a retained testis. *Vet. Pathol.*, **45** (6), 905–909.

42 Renfrew, H., Barrett, E.L., Bradley, K.J., *et al.* (2008) Radiographic and ultrasonographic features of canine paraprostatic cysts. *Vet. Radiol. Ultrasound*, **49** (5), 444–448.

43 Smith, J. (2008) Canine prostatic disease: a review of anatomy, pathology, diagnosis, and treatment. *Theriogenology*, **70** (3), 375–383.

44 Newell, S.M., Mahaffey, M.B., Binhazim, A., *et al.* (1992) Paraprostatic cyst in a cat. *J. Small Anim. Pract.*, **33** (8), 399–401.

45 Black, G.M., Ling, G.V., Nyland, T.G., *et al.* (1998) Prevalence of prostatic cysts in adult, large-breed dogs. *J. Am. Anim. Hosp. Assoc.*, **34** (2), 177–180.

46 Niżański, W., Levy, X., Ochota, M., *et al.* (2014) Pharmacological treatment for common prostatic conditions in dogs – benign prostatic hyperplasia and prostatitis: an update. *Reprod. Domest. Anim.*, **49** (Suppl. 2), 8–15.

47 Krawiec, D.R., Heflin, D. (1992) Study of prostatic disease in dogs: 177 cases (1981–1986). *J. Am. Vet. Med. Assoc.*, **200** (8), 1119–1122.

48 Mordecai, A., Liptak, J.M., Hofstede, T., *et al.* (2008) Prostatic abscess in a neutered cat. *J. Am. Anim. Hosp. Assoc.*, **44** (2), 90–94.

49 Bertazzolo, W., Dell'Orco, M., Bonfanti, U., *et al.* (2004) Cytological features of canine ovarian tumours: a retrospective study of 19 cases. *J. Small Anim. Pract.*, **45** (11), 539–545.

50 Greenlee, P.G., Patnaik, A.K. (1985) Canine ovarian tumors of germ cell origin. *Vet. Pathol.*, **22** (2), 117–122.

51 Fernandez, T., Diez-Bru, N., Rios, A., *et al.* (2001) Intracranial metastases from an ovarian dysgerminoma in a 2-year-old dog. *J. Am. Anim. Hosp. Assoc.*, **37** (6), 553–556.

52 Herron, M.A. (1983) Tumors of the canine genital system. *J. Am. Anim. Hosp. Assoc.*, **19**, 981–994.

53 Stein, B.S. (1981) Tumors of the feline genital tract. *J. Am. Anim. Hosp. Assoc.*, **17**, 1022–1025.

54 Goto, S., Iwasaki, R., Sakai, H., *et al.* (2021) A retrospective analysis on the outcome of 18 dogs with malignant ovarian tumours. *Vet. Comp. Oncol.*, **19** (3), 442–450.

55 Spoor, M.S., Flesner, B.K., Trzil, J.E., *et al.* (2014) What is your diagnosis? Intra-abdominal mass in a female spayed dog. *Vet. Clin. Pathol.*, **43** (1), 109–110.

56 Ball, R.L., Birchard, S.J., May, L.R., *et al.* (2010) Ovarian remnant syndrome in dogs and cats: 21 cases (2000-2007). *J. Am. Vet. Med. Assoc.*, **236** (5), 548–553.

57 McCandlish, I.A., Munro, C.D., Breeze, R.G., *et al.* (1979) Hormone-producing ovarian tumours in the dog. *Vet. Rec.*, **105** (1), 9–11.

58 Patnaik, A.K., Greenlee, P.G. (1987) Canine ovarian neoplasms: a clinicopathologic study of 71 cases, including histology of 12 granulosa cell tumors. *Vet. Pathol.*, **24** (6), 509–514.

59 Banco, B., Antuofermo, E., Borzacchiello, G., *et al.* (2011) Canine ovarian tumors: an immunohistochemical study with HBME-1 antibody. *J. Vet. Diagn. Investig.*, **23** (5), 977–981.

60 Itoh, T., Kojimoto, A., Uchida, K., *et al.* (2021) Long-term treatment results for ovarian tumors with malignant effusion in seven dogs. *J. Am. Anim. Hosp. Assoc.*, **57** (3), 106–113.

61 Yamaguchi, Y., Sato, T., Shibuya, H., *et al.* (2004) Ovarian teratoma with a formed lens and nonsuppurative inflammation in an old dog. *J. Vet. Med. Sci.*, **66** (7), 861–864.

62 Coggeshall, J.D., Franks, J.N., Wilson, D.U., *et al.* (2012) Primary ovarian teratoma and GCT with intra-abdominal metastasis in a dog. *J. Am. Anim. Hosp. Assoc.*, **48** (6), 424–428.

63 Saba, C.F., Rogers, K.S., Newman, S.J., *et al.* (2007) Mammary gland tumors in male dogs. *J. Vet. Intern. Med.*, **21** (5), 1056–1059.

64 Skorupski, K.A., Overley, B., Shofer, F.S., *et al.* (2005) Clinical characteristics of mammary carcinoma in male cats. *J. Vet. Intern. Med.*, **19** (1), 52–55.

65 Sorenmo, K.U., Kristiansen, V.M., Cofone, M.A., *et al.* (2009) Canine mammary gland tumours: a histological continuum from benign to malignant: clinical and histopathological evidence. *Vet. Comp. Oncol.*, **7** (3), 162–172.

66 Hayes, H.M., Jr, Milne, K.L., Mandell, C.P. (1981) Epidemiological features of feline mammary carcinoma. *Vet. Rec.*, **108** (22), 476–479.

67 Goldschmidt, M., Pena, L., Rasotto, R., *et al.* (2011) Classification and grading of canine mammary tumors. *Vet. Pathol.*, **48** (1), 117–131.

68 Schneider, R., Dorn, C.R., Taylor, D.O. (1969) Factors influencing canine mammary cancer development and postsurgical survival. *J. Natl. Cancer Inst.*, **43** (6), 1249–1261.

69 Dorn, C.R., Taylor, D.O., Schneider, R., *et al.* (1968) Survey of animal neoplasms in Alameda and Contra Costa Counties, California. II. Cancer morbidity in dogs and cats from Alameda County. *J. Natl. Cancer Inst.*, **40** (2), 307–318.

70 Benjamin, S.A., Lee, A.C., Saunders, W.J. (1999) Classification and behavior of canine mammary epithelial neoplasms based on life-span observations in beagles. *Vet. Pathol.*, **36** (5), 423–436.

71 Chang, S.C., Chang, C.C., Chang, T.J., *et al.* (2005) Prognostic factors associated with survival two years after surgery in dogs with malignant mammary tumors: 79 cases (1998–2002). *J. Am. Vet. Med. Assoc.*, **227** (10), 1625–1629.

72 MacEwen, E.G., Hayes, A.A., Harvey, H.J., *et al.* (1984) Prognostic factors for feline mammary tumors. *J. Am. Vet. Med. Assoc.*, **185** (2), 201–204.

73 Biddle, D., Macintire, D.K. (2000) Obstetrical emergencies. *Clin. Tech. Small Anim. Pract.*, **15** (2), 88–93.

74 Murai, A., Maruyama, S., Nagata, M., *et al.* (2013) Mastitis caused by *Mycobacterium kansasii* infection in a dog. *Vet. Clin. Pathol.*, **42** (3), 377–381.

75 Ditmyer, H., Craig, L. (2011) Mycotic mastitis in three dogs due to *Blastomyces dermatitidis*. *J. Am. Anim. Hosp. Assoc.*, **47** (5), 356–358.

76 Park, C.H., Ikadai, H., Yoshida, E., *et al.* (2007) Cutaneous toxoplasmosis in a female Japanese cat. *Vet. Pathol.*, **44** (5), 683–687.

77 Mills, J.N., Valli, V.E., Lumsden, J.H. (1979) Cyclical changes of vaginal cytology in the cat. *Can. Vet. J.*, **20** (4), 95–101.

78 Olson, P.N., Husted, P.W., Allen, T.A., *et al.* (1984) Reproductive endocrinology and physiology of the bitch and queen. *Vet. Clin. North Am. Small Anim. Pract.*, **14** (4), 927–946.

79 Root Kustritz, M.V. (2012) Managing the reproductive cycle in the bitch. *Vet. Clin. North Am. Small Anim. Pract.*, **42** (3), 423–437.

80 Hollinshead, F.K., Hanlon, D.W. (2019) Normal progesterone profiles during estrus in the bitch: a prospective analysis of 1420 estrous cycles. *Theriogenology*, **125**, 37–42.

81 Groppetti, D., Pecile, A., Barbero, C., *et al.* (2012) Vaginal bacterial flora and cytology in proestrous bitches: role on fertility. *Theriogenology*, **77** (8), 1549–1556.

82 Shille, V.M., Lundstrom, K.E., Stabenfeldt, G.H. (1979) Follicular function in the domestic cat as determined by estradiol-17 beta concentrations in plasma: relation to estrous behavior and cornification of the exfoliated vaginal epithelium. *Biol. Reprod.*, **21** (4), 953–963.

83 Bjurstrom, L. (1993) Aerobic bacteria occurring in the vagina of bitches with reproductive disorders. *Acta Vet. Scand.*, **34** (1), 29–34.

84 Jitpean, S., Strom-Holst, B., Emanuelson, U., *et al.* (2014) Outcome of pyometra in female dogs and predictors of peritonitis and prolonged postoperative hospitalization in surgically treated cases. *BMC Vet. Res.*, **10**, 6. doi: 10.1186/1746-6148-10-6. Last accessed May 1, 2017.

85 Verin, R., Cian, F., Stewart, J., *et al.* (2018) Canine clitoral carcinoma: a clinical, cytologic, histopathologic, immunohistochemical, and ultrastructural study. *Vet. Pathol.*, **55** (4), 501–509.

86 Rout, E.D., Hoon-Hanks, L.L., Gustafson, T.L., *et al.* (2016) What is your diagnosis? Clitoral mass in a dog. *Vet. Clin. Pathol.*, **45** (1), 197–198.

87 Neihaus, S.A., Winter, J.E., Goring, R.L., *et al.* (2010) Primary clitoral adenocarcinoma with secondary hypercalcemia of malignancy in a dog. *J. Am. Anim. Hosp. Assoc.*, **46** (3), 193–196.

14

Neurologic

14.1 Brain

14.1.1 Meningioma

14.1.1.1 Cytologic Appearance

Meningiomas exfoliate in variably tight aggregates that may be associated with pink extracellular matrix and may be seen in whorls. Cells mostly are fusiform to stellate, but can be ovoid, and have a moderate volume of pale-blue cytoplasm (Figures 14.1 and 14.2). Nuclei are ovoid with finely granular chromatin and multiple prominent nucleoli. Round, prominent structures may be seen in the nucleus (nuclear pseudoinclusions) that represent projection of the cytoplasm into nuclear grooves (Figure 14.3) [1–3]. Anisocytosis/anisokaryosis usually are moderate and N/C ratios are variable.

14.1.1.2 Clinical Considerations

- The most common brain tumor of dogs and cats [4–6].
- Affects older patients.
- Many subtypes in dogs, including psammomatous meningiomas that are associated with mineralized "psammoma bodies" (Figure 14.4) [7].
- Mostly benign tumors, but metastatic disease does occur [4, 8].

14.1.1.3 Prognosis

Variable, based on treatment methods, but long-term survival is possible [8].

14.1.2 Astrocytoma

14.1.2.1 Cytologic Appearance

The cytologic appearance of astrocytomas varies with the degree of differentiation of the neoplastic cells. Differentiated tumors comprise spindloid cells with scant cytoplasm forming long bipolar cytoplasmic processes, and elongated nuclei that have finely granular chromatin and small basophilic nucleoli (Figures 14.5 and 14.6) [1]. Anisocytosis/anisokaryosis are mild to moderate and N/C ratios are high. Anaplastic variants comprise round cells that may be difficult to differentiate from oligodendrogliomas.

14.1.2.2 Clinical Considerations

- Dogs > cats.
- Typically older patients, but reported in a young dog [9].
- Brachycephalic dog breeds appear overrepresented [4].
- Clinical signs = mentation change, seizures, vestibular syndrome, and vision loss [4, 5].

14.1.2.3 Prognosis

Limited data are available. Prognosis without treatment is poor [10, 11].

14.1.3 Oligodendroglioma

14.1.3.1 Cytologic Appearance

Oligodendrogliomas often are associated with abundant coursing capillaries (Figure 14.7) [1]. Neoplastic cells are fragile, and many bare nuclei may be present. Cells are seen individually, and are ovoid, with a moderate volume of medium-blue cytoplasm. Nuclei are ovoid, eccentrically placed, and have coarsely granular chromatin with prominent nucleoli (Figure 14.8). The chromatin pattern and the amount of cytoplasm are most useful in differentiating from lymphoma (compare to Figure 14.9).

14.1.3.2 Clinical Considerations

- Dogs > cats [4, 12].
- Typically solitary masses in the forebrain white matter [13].
- Brachycephalic dog breeds appear overrepresented [4, 13].

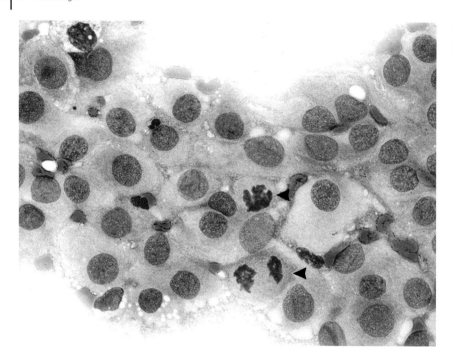

Figure 14.1 Meningioma, dog, 50× objective. Note the increased number of mitotic figures (arrowheads).

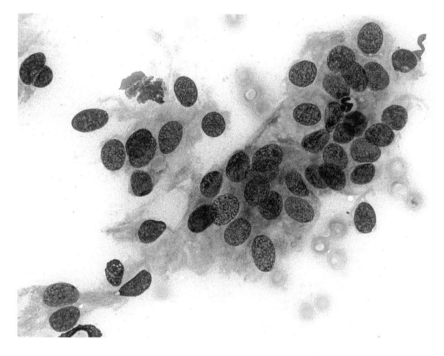

Figure 14.2 Meningioma, dog, 50× objective.

- Clinical signs = seizures and mentation changes most common [4, 5].
- Neoplastic cells may be seen in cerebrospinal fluid (CSF) [12].

14.1.3.3 Prognosis
Limited data are available. Prognosis without therapy is poor, but long-term survival is reported with therapy [10, 14].

14.1.4 Lymphoma

14.1.4.1 Cytologic Appearance
Lymphoma of the central nervous system (CNS) appears similar to that in other organs, with an expanded population of discrete, round cells with round to indented nuclei approximately twofold to threefold the size of red blood cells in diameter, and finely stippled, immature chromatin (Figure 14.9). Mitotic figures may be seen [1].

Figure 14.3 Meningioma, dog, 100× objective. Note the prominent nuclear pseudoinclusion (arrow) that should not be mistaken for a nucleolus.

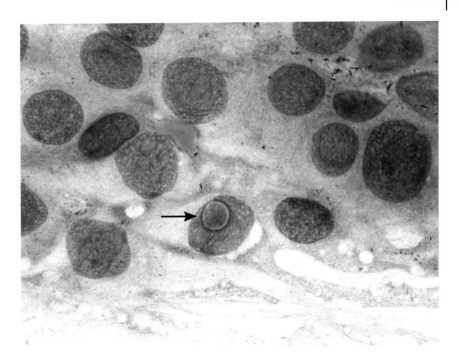

Figure 14.4 Psammoma body, psammomatous meningioma, dog, 20× objective. The psammoma body is refractile and mineralized, surrounded by neoplastic cells.

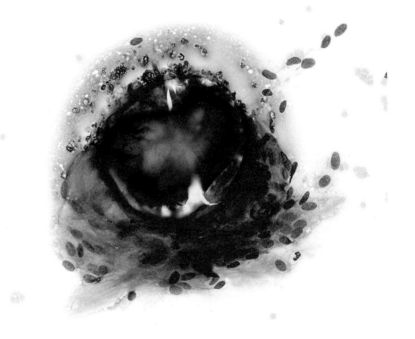

14.1.4.2 Clinical Considerations

- Cats > dogs. Second most common brain neoplasm in cats [5].
- May be primary or an extension of multicentric lymphoma [15, 16].
- Focal and multifocal lesions are possible [6].

14.1.4.3 Prognosis

Generally poor. Response rates to therapy are moderate to low, and survival times are short [5, 17, 18].

14.1.5 Primitive Neuroectodermal Tumors

14.1.5.1 Cytologic Appearance

Primitive neuroectodermal tumors (PNETs) mostly exfoliate in loosely cohesive sheets, and cells often are seen individually such that they may be difficult to differentiate from lymphoma. Compared to lymphoma, the cells often aggregate and tend to form vague palisading and acinar-like arrangements (compare Figures 14.10 and 14.9). They have

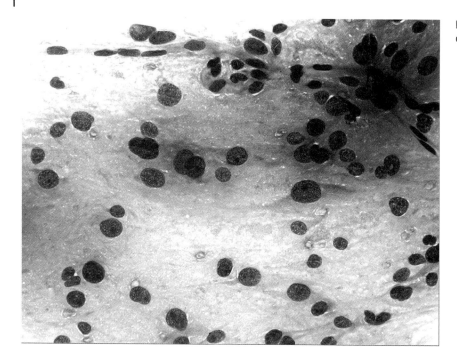

Figure 14.5 Astrocytoma, dog, 20× objective. Photo courtesy of Dr. Bill Vernau.

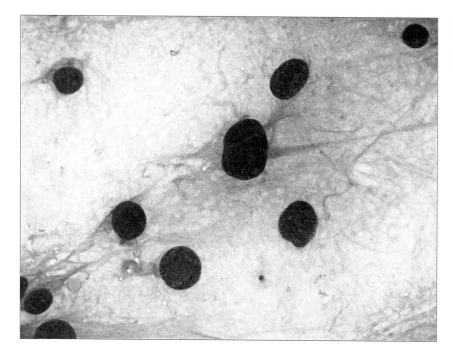

Figure 14.6 Astrocytoma, dog, 50× objective. Note the fine, delicate tendrils of the cytoplasm. Photo courtesy of Dr. Bill Vernau.

ovoid nuclei with stippled chromatin and variably prominent nucleoli. Anisocytosis/anisokaryosis are mild to moderate, N/C ratios are high, and many mitotic figures usually are present [19].

14.1.5.2 Clinical Considerations
- Medulloblastomas and neuroblastomas are the most common PNETs [20, 21].

- Medulloblastomas most common in the cerebellum [20].
- Dogs > cats. Rare in both.
- Typically affect younger patients [21].

14.1.5.3 Prognosis
Limited data are available, but prognosis generally is guarded to poor [19–21].

Figure 14.7 Oligodendroglioma, dog, 20× objective. There are numerous capillaries coursing across the sample.

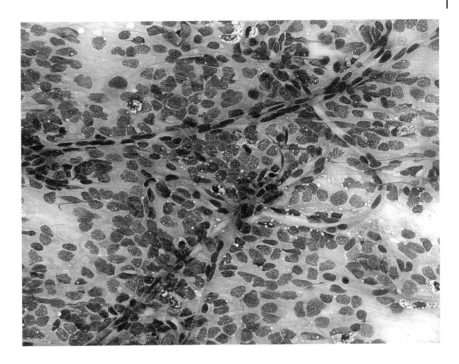

Figure 14.8 Oligodendroglioma, dog, 50× objective. Many cells are lysed. Intact cells are round and discrete.

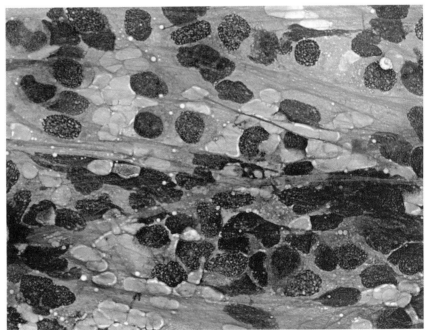

14.1.6 Histiocytic Sarcoma

14.1.6.1 Cytologic Appearance

Histiocytic sarcoma is characterized by a population of large, atypical discrete cells. These cells are round, with a variable volume of medium-blue cytoplasm that often is vacuolated. Nuclei are ovoid to amoeboid and have finely stippled chromatin with multiple prominent nucleoli (Figure 14.11). Anisocytosis/ anisokaryosis are marked and N/C ratios are variable.

14.1.6.2 Clinical Considerations

- May be primary or an extension of disseminated disease [22, 23].
- Primary lesions most frequently affect the cerebrum [6].
- Predisposed breeds = Bernese Mountain Dogs, Labrador Retrievers, Golden Retrievers, Rottweilers, and Pembroke Welsh Corgis [22].

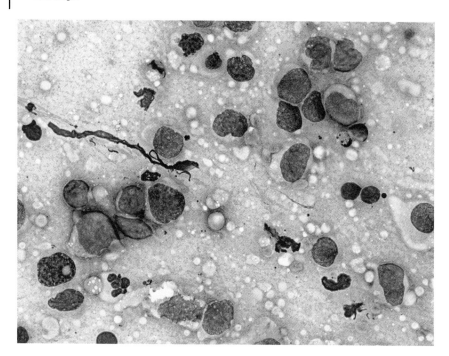

Figure 14.9 Lymphoma, dog, 50× objective.

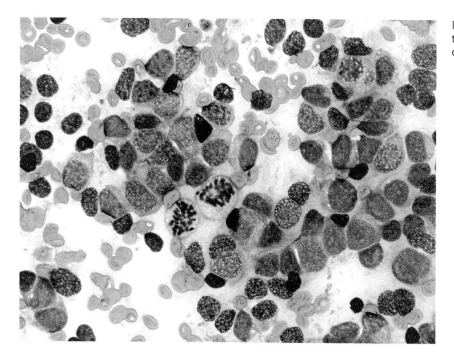

Figure 14.10 Primitive neuroectodermal tumor (neuroblastoma), dog, 50× objective.

14.1.6.3 Prognosis
Grave [22].

14.1.7 Choroid Plexus Papilloma

14.1.7.1 Cytologic Appearance
Choroid plexus papillomas comprise cohesive sheets of round cells with moderate-to-abundant amounts of mid-blue cytoplasm that contains a variable number of fine, pink granules

(Figure 14.12). Nuclei are round to ovoid, eccentrically placed, and have small or inapparent nucleoli. Anisocytosis/anisokaryosis are mild and N/C ratios are moderate to low.

14.1.7.2 Clinical Considerations
- Median age of 5 years in dogs [24].
- Clinical signs = mentation change, central vestibular disease, and neck pain [4].
- Rarely locally invasive.

Figure 14.11 Histiocytic sarcoma, dog, 50× objective.

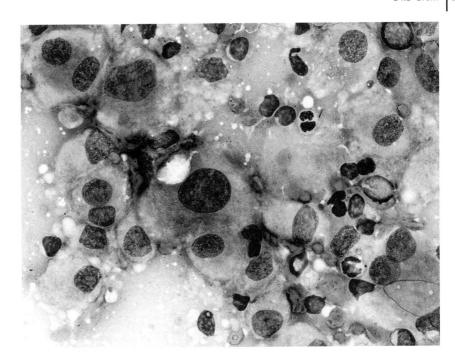

Figure 14.12 Choroid plexus papilloma, dog, 50× objective.

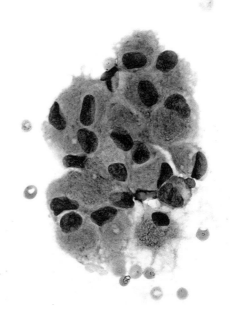

14.1.7.3 Prognosis

Limited data are available, but prognosis appears guarded to poor. Most patients have short survival times [10, 25]. Long-term survival is rarely reported [26].

14.1.8 Choroid Plexus Carcinoma

14.1.8.1 Cytologic Appearance

Choroid plexus carcinomas also exfoliate in sheets, often in palisading rows (Figure 14.13). The cells have a small to moderate volume of mid-blue cytoplasm and round nuclei

with coarsely granular chromatin and variably prominent nucleoli. Anisocytosis/anisokaryosis are mild to moderate, and N/C ratios are high.

14.1.8.2 Clinical Considerations

- Median age of 7 years in dogs [24].
- Clinical signs = mentation change, central vestibular disease, and neck pain [4].
- Locally invasive tumors, which may metastasize within the brain, or less commonly to the spinal cord [24, 27, 28].

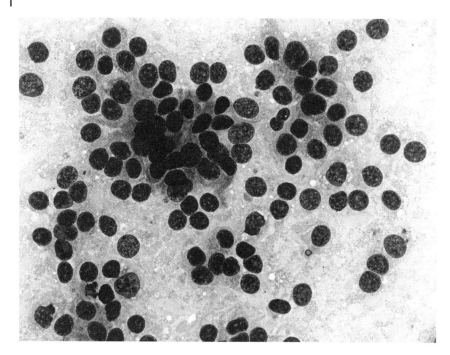

Figure 14.13 Choroid plexus carcinoma, dog, 50× objective.

14.1.8.3 Prognosis

Limited data are available, but prognosis generally is poor [10, 25, 27].

14.1.9 Ependymoma

14.1.9.1 Cytologic Appearance

Ependymomas exfoliate as tightly cohesive clusters, often in acinar-like arrangements (Figure 14.14). Cells have a moderate volume of medium-blue cytoplasm that may contain clear vacuoles. Nuclei are round, eccentrically placed, and have granular chromatin and single nucleoli. Anisocytosis/anisokaryosis are mild to moderate.

14.1.9.2 Clinical Considerations

- Rare in dogs and cats.
- May affect the brain or spinal cord. Most common in the lateral ventricle [29].
- Locally invasive and may metastasize via the CSF [30].

14.1.9.3 Prognosis

Limited data are available. Prognosis generally is poor for intracranial masses, but better for spinal lesions [30–32].

14.1.10 Encephalitis

14.1.10.1 Cytologic Appearance

Inflammatory lesions in the CNS are characterized by variable numbers of inflammatory cells (Figure 14.15). The type of cells may indicate the underlying cause, such as neutrophils in cases of bacterial disease, lymphoplasmacytic inflammation in sterile/immune-mediated inflammatory lesions or secondary to viral disease, and eosinophils secondary to parasitic, fungal, or protozoal agents.

14.1.10.2 Clinical Considerations

- Inflammatory mass lesions less common than neoplasia [33, 34].
- May be sterile or due to infectious agents.

14.1.10.3 Prognosis

Variable, based on the underlying cause.

14.2 Cerebrospinal Fluid

14.2.1 Normal CSF

14.2.1.1 Cytologic Appearance

Normal CSF has low cell and protein concentrations. Nucleated cell counts should be <5 cells μl^{-1} [35]. Protein concentration is <25 mg dl^{-1} for cisternal samples, and <35 mg dl^{-1} for lumbar samples [35]. Nucleated cells are seen in low numbers, and are dominated by quiescent macrophages, with low numbers of small, mature lymphocytes (Figure 14.16). Neutrophils and eosinophils should be absent, or seen rarely if blood is present in the samples.

14.2.1.2 Clinical Considerations

- Grossly clear and colorless.

Figure 14.14 Ependymoma, dog, 100× objective.

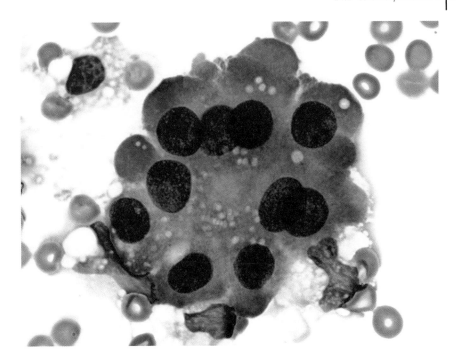

Figure 14.15 Encephalitis, dog, 50× objective. Note the foamy, pink white matter in the background, and numerous small, mature lymphocytes, a plasma cell, and a neutrophil.

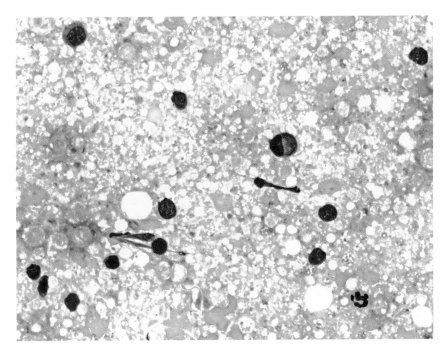

• Lack of cytologic abnormalities does not exclude pathology in the CNS, nor future involvement of CSF in disease.

14.2.2 Intervertebral Disc Material

14.2.2.1 Cytologic Appearance
Intervertebral disc material appears as variably sized, amorphous, smooth to fibrillar, deep-magenta extracellular material (Figure 14.17).

14.2.2.2 Clinical Considerations
• May be inadvertently sampled during CSF collection or indicate underlying intervertebral disc disease if present in large amounts.

14.2.2.3 Prognosis
The presence of disc material does not affect prognosis – correlate with the severity of underlying disease.

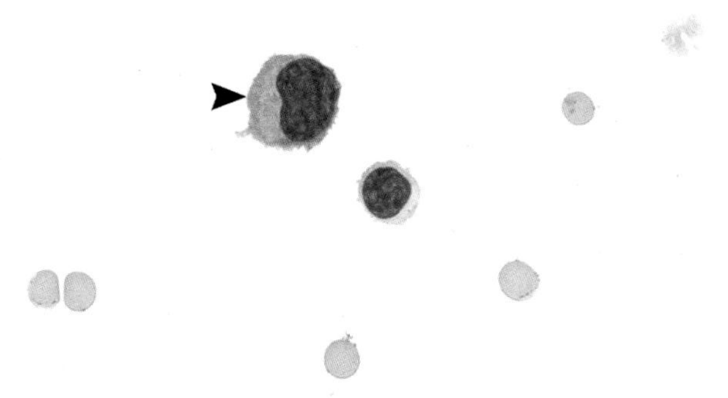

Figure 14.16 Normal CSF, dog, 50× objective. Low numbers of cells are seen on a clear background with a small amount of blood. A quiescent macrophage is seen (arrowhead) next to a small, mature lymphocyte.

Figure 14.17 Intervertebral disc material, CSF, dog, 50× objective. Note the quiescent macrophage.

14.2.3 Myelin-like Material

14.2.3.1 Cytologic Appearance
Myelin-like material may be sampled during CSF collection. It appears as variably sized aggregates of pale-pink, foamy material, often with internal circular structures giving a "honeycomb" appearance (Figure 14.18).

14.2.3.2 Clinical Considerations
- Mostly an incidental finding in CSF samples.

- Larger amounts associated with intervertebral disc disease [36].
- No association with disease outcome.
- More likely to be seen in lumbar (than cerebromedullary) samples, and in small dogs (<10 kg) [36].

14.2.3.3 Prognosis
Mostly excellent. May rarely be associated with myelomalacia, which carries a poor prognosis [37].

Figure 14.18 Myelin-like material, CSF, dog, 50× objective.

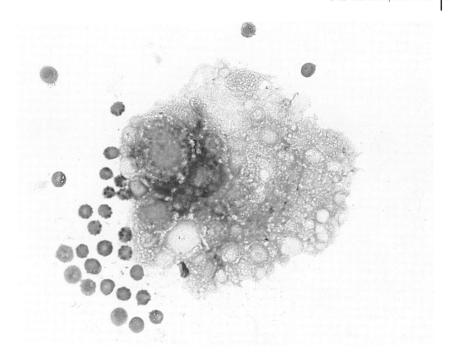

14.2.4 Surface Epithelial Cells

14.2.4.1 Cytologic Appearance

Surface epithelial cells may include ependymal, meningeal, and choroid plexus cells, which are seen individually or in small cohesive sheets. These cells may be round, with a moderate volume of pink granular cytoplasm and eccentric nuclei (ependymal or choroid plexus origin; Figure 14.19), or more polygonal/spindloid with pale-blue cytoplasm and round/ovoid nuclei (meningeal origin; Figure 14.20). Anisocytosis/anisokaryosis are mild.

14.2.4.2 Clinical Considerations

• Uncommon, mostly an incidental finding [38].

14.2.4.3 Prognosis

Excellent.

Figure 14.19 Surface epithelial cells, ependymal/choroid plexus origin, CSF, dog, 50× objective.

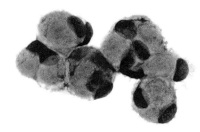

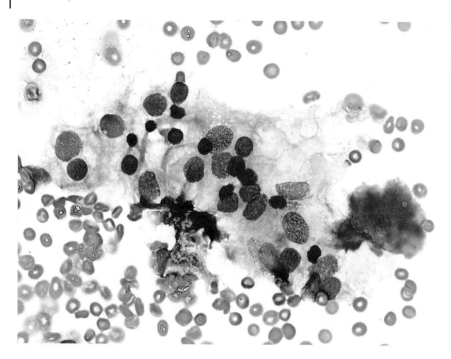

Figure 14.20 Surface epithelial cells, meningeal origin, CSF, dog, 50× objective. Note the small aggregate of intervertebral disc material on the right.

14.2.5 Neutrophilic Inflammation

14.2.5.1 Cytologic Appearance
Neutrophils should be absent in CSF. Low numbers may be seen if blood contamination is present. A predominance of neutrophils confirms neutrophilic inflammation. Neutrophils may be non-degenerative in sterile processes (Figure 14.21), or degenerative with infectious etiologies (Figure 14.22).

14.2.5.2 Clinical Considerations
DDx = infectious meningitis, steroid-responsive meningitis-arteritis (acute), neoplasia, fibrocartilaginous emboli, trauma, and necrosis [22, 39–41].

14.2.5.3 Prognosis
Variable, based on the underlying cause.

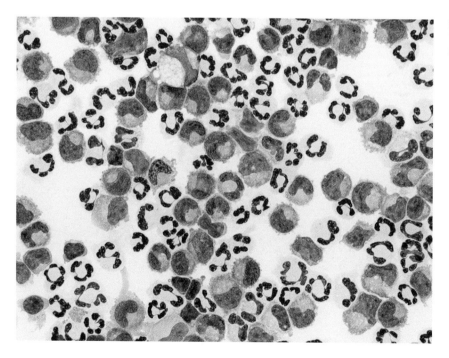

Figure 14.21 Neutrophilic inflammation (sterile), CSF, dog, 50× objective.

Figure 14.22 Neutrophilic inflammation (septic), CSF, dog, 100× objective. Note the variably sized/shaped bacterial rods in the phagolysosomes of degenerative neutrophils.

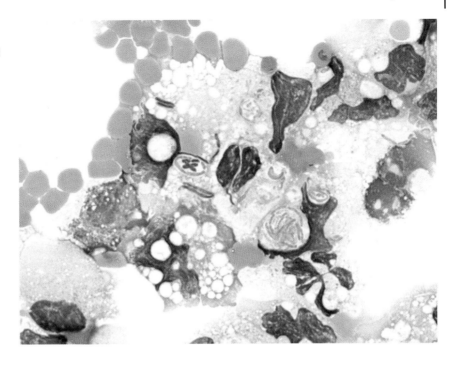

14.2.6 Eosinophilic Inflammation

14.2.6.1 Cytologic Appearance

Eosinophils should be absent in CSF. Mildly increased numbers of eosinophils may be seen in many inflammatory conditions. Eosinophils >10–20% are supportive of eosinophilic meningitis (Figure 14.23) [42, 43].

14.2.6.2 Clinical Considerations

- DDx = infectious agents (especially protozoa, fungal agents, algae, and migrating parasites), intervertebral disc extrusions, and idiopathic eosinophilic meningoencephalomyelitis [43, 44].

Figure 14.23 Eosinophilic inflammation (idiopathic eosinophilic meningoencephalomyelitis), CSF, dog, 50× objective.

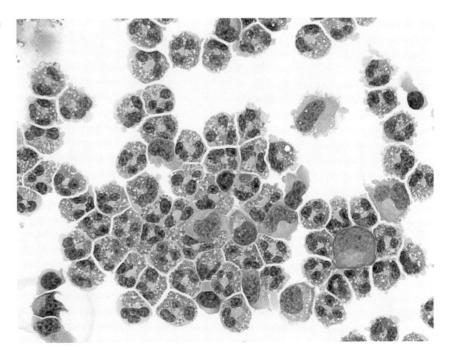

14.2.6.3 Prognosis

Variable, based on the underlying cause – infectious agents generally confer a poor prognosis [43, 45].

14.2.7 Lymphocytic Inflammation

14.2.7.1 Cytologic Appearance

Lymphocytes are present in low numbers in normal CSF. Lymphocytic inflammation is characterized by an increased number of heterogeneous lymphocytes, usually dominated by small, mature cells, with lesser numbers of intermediate cells, reactive variants, or plasma cells (Figure 14.24).

14.2.7.2 Clinical Considerations

- DDx = intervertebral disc disease (especially chronic), granulomatous/necrotizing meningoencephalitis, and infectious agents (especially viral) [46–49].

14.2.7.3 Prognosis

Variable, based on the underlying cause.

14.2.8 Mononuclear Inflammation

14.2.8.1 Cytologic Appearance

Macrophages predominate in normal CSF; however, increased numbers may be seen in cases of mononuclear inflammation, frequently accompanied by reactive changes such as an increased volume of vacuolated cytoplasm (Figure 14.25).

14.2.8.2 Clinical Considerations

- DDx = steroid responsive meningitis-arteritis (chronic), meningoencephalitis of unknown etiology (MUE), granulomatous meningoencephalitis (GME), infectious agents (e.g., fungal and feline infectious peritonitis), and storage diseases [40, 50].

14.2.8.3 Prognosis

Variable, based on the underlying cause.

14.2.9 Mononuclear Reactivity

14.2.9.1 Cytologic Appearance

Macrophages predominate in normal CSF. In cases of mononuclear reactivity, these cells are present in normal numbers, but have reactive changes including an increased volume of vacuolated cytoplasm (most common) or increased cytoplasmic basophilia (Figure 14.26).

14.2.9.2 Clinical Considerations

- Reactive macrophages are not associated with blood contamination of samples and are useful indicators of pathology [51].
- A nonspecific but important marker of underlying disease. Can be seen secondary to inflammation, seizure activity, non-exfoliating neoplasia, vascular disease, necrosis, etc.

14.2.9.3 Prognosis

Variable, based on the underlying cause.

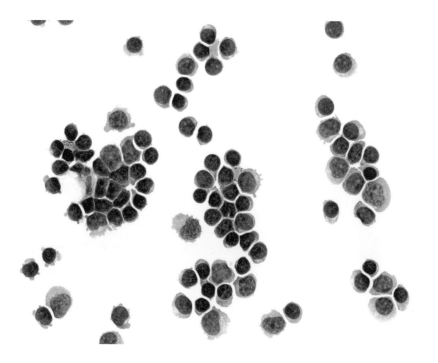

Figure 14.24 Lymphocytic inflammation, CSF, dog, 50× objective.

Figure 14.25 Mononuclear inflammation, CSF, cat, 50× objective.

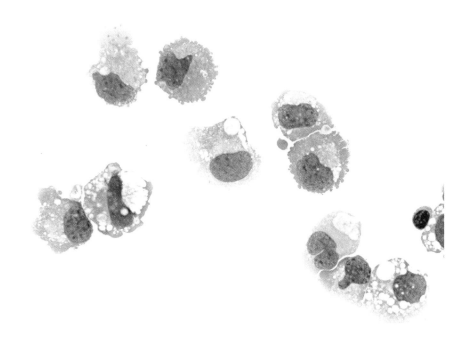

Figure 14.26 Mononuclear reactivity, CSF, dog, 50× objective. Macrophages are reactive, but seen in low/normal numbers.

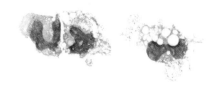

14.2.10 Mixed Inflammation

14.2.10.1 Cytologic Appearance

Frequently, a mixture of inflammatory cells is present, without any obvious predominance of type (Figure 14.27). Combinations of increased lymphocytes, neutrophils, macrophages, and eosinophils are seen. Cell and protein concentrations usually are also increased.

14.2.10.2 Clinical Considerations

- DDx = MUE, GME, steroid-responsive meningitis-arteritis, trauma, intervertebral disc disease, ischemia, and non-exfoliating neoplasia [52].

14.2.10.3 Prognosis

Variable, based on the underlying cause.

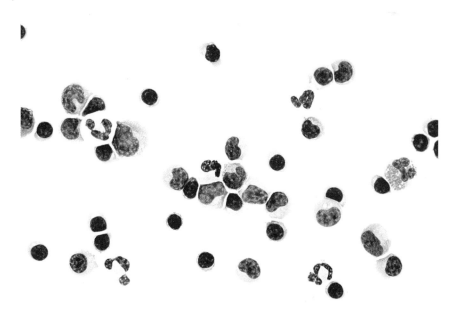

Figure 14.27 Mixed inflammation, CSF, dog, 50× objective. Note the mixture of inflammatory cells including macrophages, small, mature lymphocytes, neutrophils, and an eosinophil.

14.2.11 Hemorrhage

14.2.11.1 Cytologic Appearance

Erythrocytes should not be present in normal CSF. Pathologic hemorrhage may be acute or chronic. Chronic hemorrhage is confirmed with the presence of either erythrophagia or heme-breakdown pigments (e.g., hemosiderin) in macrophages (Figure 14.28). Acute hemorrhage may be pathologic or iatrogenic at the time of sampling and it is difficult to differentiate via cytology. Reactive changes in macrophages and lymphocytes are not associated with blood contamination and may be helpful markers [51].

14.2.11.2 Clinical Considerations

- CSF grossly may appear yellow (xanthochromic) with mild chronic hemorrhage, or red with acute hemorrhage.
- DDx = trauma (including intervertebral disc disease), degenerative conditions, inflammation, bleeding

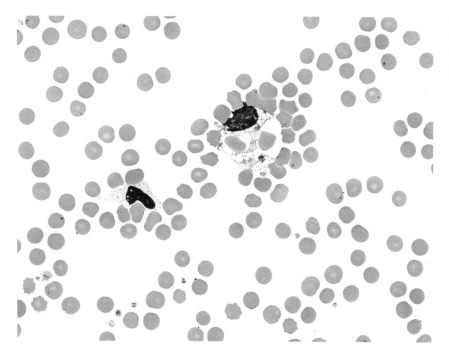

Figure 14.28 Hemorrhage, CSF, dog, 50× objective. Phagocytosed red blood cells are seen within a reactive macrophage. Note the neutrophil to the lower left.

diatheses, infectious disease, neoplasia, and vascular lesions [52–54].

- Blood contamination results in increased percentages of neutrophils and eosinophils, and an increased protein concentration [51]. Platelets are also commonly present.

14.2.11.3 Prognosis
Variable, based on the underlying cause.

SPECIFIC DISEASES ASSOCIATED WITH CSF

14.2.12 Granulomatous Meningoencephalitis

14.2.12.1 Cytologic Appearance
GME is characterized by a variably mixed population of leukocytes, but most often is dominated by lymphocytes. Small, mature lymphocytes are admixed with lesser numbers of intermediate-sized or reactive lymphocytes, and a variable number of non-degenerative neutrophils, macrophages, and even rare eosinophils (Figure 14.29).

14.2.12.2 Clinical Considerations
- Most common in toy and terrier breed dogs [47].
- Any age may be affected (2 months to 15 years in one study) [55].
- Clinical signs = cranial nerve deficits, visual disturbances, seizures, and ataxia [56].
- DDx = necrotizing meningoencephalitis and necrotizing encephalitis [55].

14.2.12.3 Prognosis
Guarded to poor [47].

14.2.13 Feline Infectious Peritonitis

14.2.13.1 Cytologic Appearance
Feline infectious peritonitis (FIP) often manifests with changes in CSF. The fluid frequently has a very high protein concentration, associated with a medium to thick purple background. Reactive macrophages usually predominate; however, neutrophils may also predominate, and small, mature lymphocytes often are present (Figure 14.30).

14.2.13.2 Clinical Considerations
- Common cause of neurologic signs in young cats [57].
- Normal CSF analysis does not rule out underlying FIP [58]; however, most cases are associated with a marked increase in cell and protein concentrations [59].

14.2.13.3 Prognosis
Guarded. Grave prognosis if untreated [59]. New treatment options show promise for long-term survival [60].

14.2.14 Septic Meningitis

14.2.14.1 Cytologic Appearance
Septic meningitis is associated with large numbers of inflammatory cells, the type of which often suggests the underlying organism. Bacterial meningitis is associated

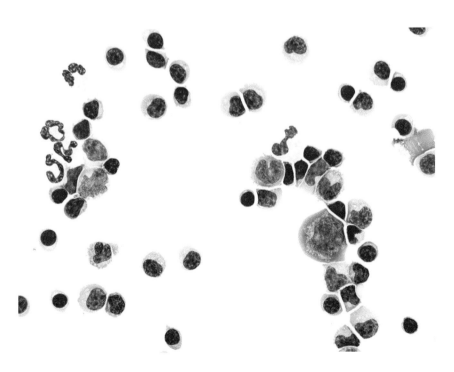

Figure 14.29 Granulomatous meningoencephalitis, CSF, dog, 50× objective.

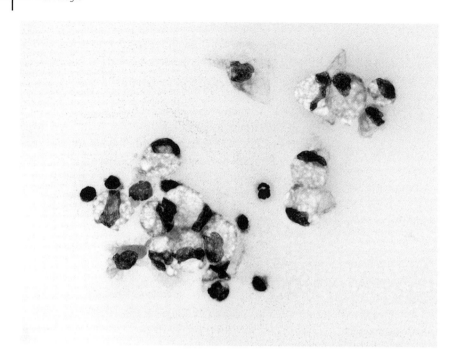

Figure 14.30 Feline infectious peritonitis (FIP), CSF, cat, 50× objective. Note the thick proteinaceous background; the protein concentration was 3212 mg dl^{-1}.

with neutrophilic inflammation, and bacteria often are present within degenerative neutrophils (see Figure 14.22). Fungal, protozoal, and algal infections are mostly associated with eosinophilic inflammation (Figure 14.31).

14.2.14.2 Clinical Considerations

- Clinical signs = pyrexia, cranial nerve deficits, mentation changes, ataxia, head tilt, conscious proprioception deficits, and seizures [39, 61].
- May result from hematogenous spread, extension from the middle/inner ear, or direct inoculation [55, 61].

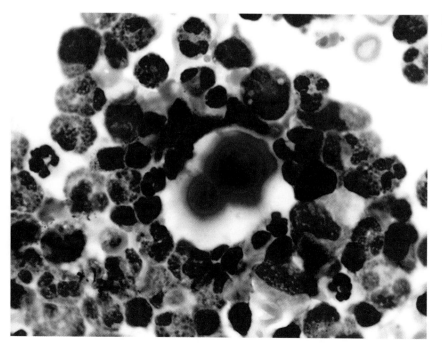

Figure 14.31 Septic meningitis (*Cryptococcus* spp.), CSF, dog, 100× objective.

- Neutrophilic inflammation invariably present with bacterial meningitis, with intracellular bacteria confirming sepsis [61].
- Bacteria may be more commonly seen in CSF samples than identified with microbial culture [61].

14.2.14.3 Prognosis

Variable, based on the stage and severity of disease, as well as the etiological agent. Bacterial meningitis is often associated with favorable outcomes, while fungal and protozoal agents tend to confer a worse prognosis, though this is highly dependent on the specific organism [39, 44, 61–63].

NEOPLASIA AND THE CSF

14.2.15 Lymphoma

14.2.15.1 Cytologic Appearance

Lymphoma in the CSF exfoliates as discrete, round cells that are large, with nuclei approximately twofold to threefold the size of red blood cells in diameter. The nuclei may be round, indented, or have irregular borders. Chromatin is finely granular, nucleoli are prominent, and mitotic figures are common (Figure 14.32).

14.2.15.2 Clinical Considerations

- Dogs and cats.
- May be restricted to the CNS or extension of generalized disease.

- Clinical signs: gait abnormalities, reduced conscious proprioception, head tilt, and cranial nerve deficits [52].
- Neoplastic cells do not always exfoliate into CSF, and absence does not rule out lymphoma [5].

14.2.15.3 Prognosis

Generally poor. Response rates to therapy are moderate to low, and survival times are short [5, 17, 18].

14.2.16 Histiocytic Sarcoma

14.2.16.1 Cytologic Appearance

Similar to other locations, histiocytic sarcoma cells are large and have marked atypia. Nuclei vary from ovoid to amoeboid, and multinucleation is common, as are mitotic figures. Anisocytosis/anisokaryosis are marked and N/C ratios are variable. Importantly, histiocytic sarcoma frequently is accompanied by a mixed inflammatory response (Figure 14.33). Immunocytochemical stains may be required for definitive diagnosis (Figure 14.34).

14.2.16.2 Clinical Considerations

- Dogs >> cats.
- Often associated with concurrent inflammation, and neoplastic cells may not be seen [22, 23].
- Marked inflammation more common with primary than disseminated disease [23].

Figure 14.32 Lymphoma, CSF, dog, 50× objective.

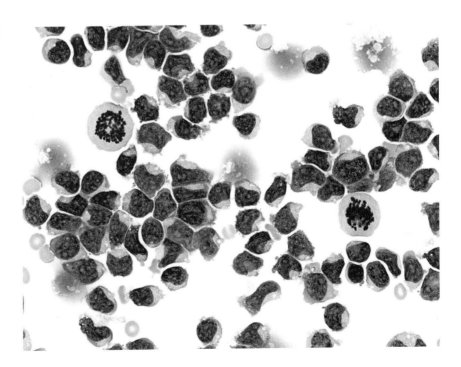

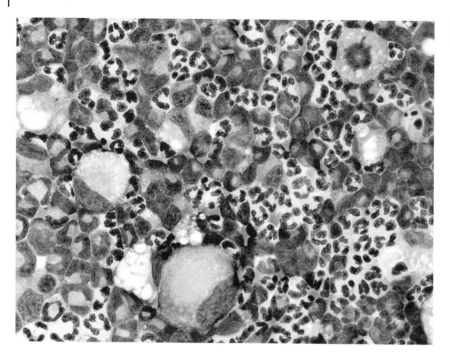

Figure 14.33 Histiocytic sarcoma, CSF, dog, 50× objective.

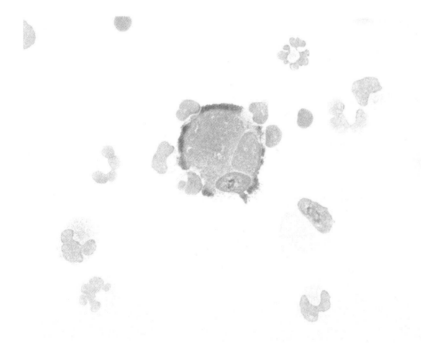

Figure 14.34 Histiocytic sarcoma, CSF, dog, CD1c stain, 50× objective. Same case as Figure 14.33.

14.2.16.3 Prognosis
Grave [22, 23].

14.2.17 Choroid Plexus Carcinoma

14.2.17.1 Cytologic Appearance
Choroid plexus carcinomas may be seen in CSF as cohesive sheets (often in palisading rows) (Figure 14.35), or as individualized cells that are round, with a moderate volume of mid-blue cytoplasm, and round, eccentrically placed nuclei with granular chromatin and prominent nucleoli (Figure 14.36).

14.2.17.2 Clinical Considerations
Choroid plexus carcinomas have higher CSF protein concentrations than papillomas. In one study, only carcinomas had protein >80 mg dl^{-1} [24].

Figure 14.35 Choroid plexus carcinoma, dog, 50× objective.

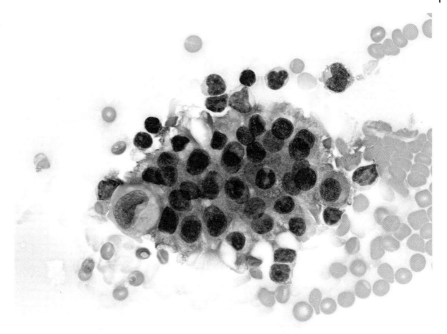

Figure 14.36 Choroid plexus carcinoma, dog, 100× objective.

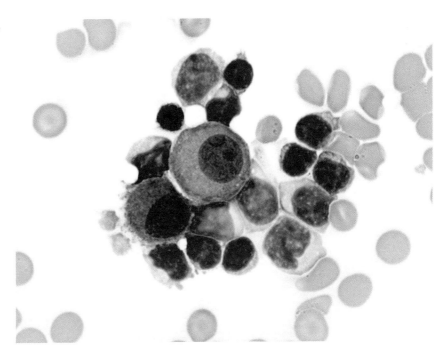

14.2.17.3 Prognosis

Limited data are available, but the prognosis generally is poor [10, 25].

14.2.18 Mast Cell Neoplasia

14.2.18.1 Cytologic Appearance

Mast cells may rarely be seen in the CSF. Neoplastic mast cells often appear atypical, with variable granulation and vacuolation, and have finely stippled, immature chromatin with prominent nucleoli (Figure 14.37). Anisocytosis/anisokaryosis are moderate and N/C ratios are variable. Eosinophilic inflammation is reported with mast cell neoplasia in the CSF [64].

14.2.18.2 Clinical Considerations

- Rare tumor of CNS.
- Spinal cord > brain [64, 65].
- May be associated with primary mast cell neoplasia of the CNS or metastatic disease [64–68].

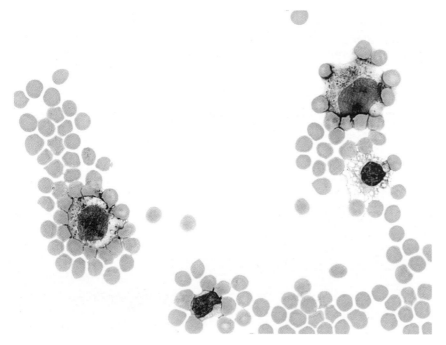

Figure 14.37 Mast cell neoplasia, CSF, dog, 50× objective.

14.2.18.3 Prognosis

Limited data available. Metastatic disease to CNS appears to confer a poor prognosis, as do primary mast cell tumors of the brain [64, 65]. Primary, well-differentiated spinal mast cell tumors may have a good prognosis with appropriate therapy [65, 68].

14.3 Spinal Cord

14.3.1 Spinal Cord Nephroblastoma

14.3.1.1 Cytologic Description

Similar to those in the kidney (see Chapter 10), spinal cord nephroblastomas exfoliate well, often as individualized cells, and rarely in sheets (Figure 14.38). The cells are round, with ovoid to amoeboid nuclei and finely stippled chromatin. Nucleoli, when visible, are single. Many mitotic figures are seen. The cells have a small volume of pale-blue cytoplasm. These tumors can be difficult to differentiate from lymphoma (compare to Figures 14.9 and 14.32).

14.3.1.2 Clinical Considerations

- Rare tumors of young dogs (typically aged <4 years, but may be as young as 5 months) [69].
- Breed predilection = Labrador Retrievers, Golden Retrievers, and German Shepherds [69, 70].
- Progressive gait abnormalities the most common clinical signs.

- Most common in the distal thoracic to early lumbar segments [69, 70].
- Metastatic disease is uncommon [71].

14.3.1.3 Prognosis

Grave. Short survival times generally, even in patients undergoing surgery ± radiation therapy [70, 71].

14.3.2 Nerve-sheath Tumor

14.3.2.1 Cytologic Appearance

These tumors are variably exfoliative, with cells seen individually and in aggregates that may be associated with a bright-pink extracellular matrix. The cells are spindloid and plump, with a moderate volume of medium-blue cytoplasm that forms tendrils and wisps and may contain clear vacuoles (Figure 14.39). Nuclei are ovoid, with coarsely granular chromatin and prominent nucleoli. Anisocytosis/anisokaryosis are mild to moderate and N/C ratios are moderate to high. These tumors can be difficult to differentiate from meningiomas; however, the presence of long, delicate cytoplasmic wisps is more suggestive of nerve-sheath tumors (compare to Figures 14.1 and 14.2).

14.3.2.2 Clinical Considerations

- This category includes Schwannomas, neurofibromas, and neurofibrosarcomas [72].
- May be benign or malignant – histopathology required to assess malignancy.

Figure 14.38 Nephroblastoma, spinal cord, dog, 50× objective.

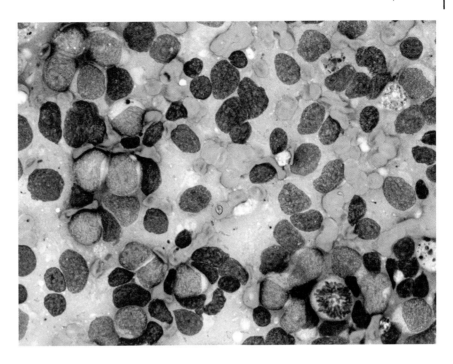

Figure 14.39 Nerve-sheath tumor, spinal cord, dog, 50× objective.

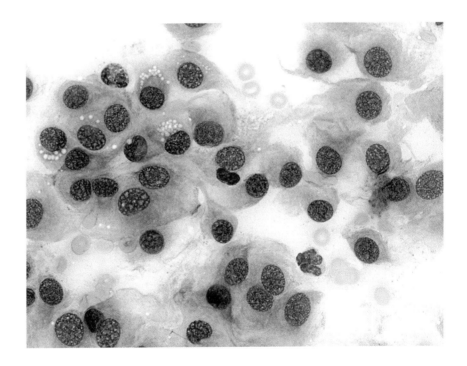

14.3.2.3 Prognosis

Guarded to poor. Dogs with tumors close to the nerve root have short survival times [72].

14.3.3 Other Neoplasms

Other neoplasms that can affect the spinal cord include meningioma, ependymoma, and lymphoma, which are described earlier in this chapter.

References

1 Vernau, K.M., Higgins, R.J., Bollen, A.W., *et al.* (2001) Primary canine and feline nervous system tumors: intraoperative diagnosis using the smear technique. *Vet. Pathol.*, **38** (1), 47–57.

2 Gould, A., Naskou, M.C., Brinker, E. (2023) What is your diagnosis? Impression smear from a dog with an intracranial mass. *Vet. Clin. Pathol.*, **52** (Suppl. 2), 122–126.

3 Harms, N.J., Dickinson, R.M., Nibblett, B.M., *et al.* (2009) What is your diagnosis: Intracranial mass in a dog. *Vet. Clin. Pathol.*, **38** (4), 537–540.

4 Snyder, J.M., Shofer, F.S., Van Winkle, T.J., *et al.* (2006) Canine intracranial primary neoplasia: 173 cases (1986–2003). *J. Vet. Intern. Med.*, **20** (3), 669–675.

5 Troxel, M.T., Vite, C.H., Van Winkle, T.J., *et al.* (2003) Feline intracranial neoplasia: retrospective review of 160 cases (1985–2001). *J. Vet. Intern. Med.*, **17** (6), 850–859.

6 Kishimoto, T.E., Uchida, K., Chambers, J.K., *et al.* (2020) A retrospective study on canine intracranial tumors between 2007 and 2017. *J. Vet. Med. Sci.*, **82** (1), 77–83.

7 Montoliu, P., Añor, S., Vidal, E., *et al.* (2006) Histological and immunohistochemical study of 30 cases of canine meningioma. *J. Comp. Pathol.*, **135** (4), 200–207.

8 Motta, L., Mandara, M.T., Skerritt, G.C. (2012) Canine and feline intracranial meningiomas: an updated review. *Vet. J.*, **192** (2), 153–165.

9 Petrukovich, B.N., Kilburn, G.A. (2015) What is your neurologic diagnosis? Astrocytoma affecting the pontine region of the brainstem. *J. Am. Vet. Med. Assoc.*, **247** (9), 1015–1017.

10 Heidner, G.L., Kornegay, J.N., Page, R.L., *et al.* (1991) Analysis of survival in a retrospective study of 86 dogs with brain tumors. *J. Vet. Intern. Med.*, **5** (4), 219–226.

11 Kube, S.A., Bruyette, D.S., Hanson, S.M. (2003) Astrocytomas in young dogs. *J. Am. Anim. Hosp. Assoc.*, **39** (3), 288–293.

12 Dickinson, P.J., Keel, M.K., Higgins, R.J., *et al.* (2000) Clinical and pathologic features of oligodendrogliomas in two cats. *Vet. Pathol.*, **37** (2), 160–167.

13 Rissi, D.R., Levine, J.M., Eden, K.B., *et al.* (2015) Cerebral oligodendroglioma mimicking intraventricular neoplasia in three dogs. *J. Vet. Diagn. Investig.*, **27** (3), 396–400.

14 Tamura, M., Hasegawa, D., Uchida, K., *et al.* (2013) Feline anaplastic oligodendroglioma: long-term remission through radiation therapy and chemotherapy. *J. Feline Med. Surg.*, **15** (12), 1137–1140.

15 Degl'Innocenti, S., Camera, N.D., Falzone, C., *et al.* (2019) Canine cerebral intravascular lymphoma: neuropathological and immunohistochemical findings. *Vet. Pathol.*, **56** (2), 239–243.

16 Brunati, G., Pintore, L., Avallone, G., *et al.* (2023) A case of spermatic cord B-cell lymphoma relapsing to the brain in a dog. *Can. Vet. J.*, **64** (6), 529–533.

17 Taylor, S.S., Goodfellow, M.R., Browne, W.J., *et al.* (2009) Feline extranodal lymphoma: response to chemotherapy and survival in 110 cats. *J. Small Anim. Pract.*, **50** (11), 584–592.

18 Couto, C.G., Cullen, J., Pedroia, V., *et al.* (1984) Central nervous system lymphosarcoma in the dog. *J. Am. Vet. Med. Assoc.*, **184** (7), 809–813.

19 Thompson, C.A., Russell, K.E., Levine, J.M., *et al.* (2003) Cerebrospinal fluid from a dog with neurologic collapse. *Vet. Clin. Pathol.*, **32** (3), 143–146.

20 Steinberg, H., Galbreath, E.J. (1998) Cerebellar medulloblastoma with multiple differentiation in a dog. *Vet. Pathol.*, **35** (6), 543–546.

21 Trudel, C., Culang, D., Atmane, M.I., *et al.* (2022) What is your diagnosis? Cerebellar tumor in a dog. *Vet. Clin. Pathol.*, **51** (2), 283–285.

22 Mariani, C.L., Jennings, M.K., Olby, N.J., *et al.* (2015) Histiocytic sarcoma with central nervous system involvement in dogs: 19 cases (2006–2012). *J. Vet. Intern. Med.*, **29** (2), 607–613.

23 Toyoda, I., Vernau, W., Sturges, B.K., *et al.* (2020) Clinicopathological characteristics of histiocytic sarcoma affecting the central nervous system in dogs. *J. Vet. Intern. Med.*, **34** (2), 828–837.

24 Westworth, D.R., Dickinson, P.J., Vernau, W., *et al.* (2008) Choroid plexus tumors in 56 dogs (1985–2007). *J. Vet. Intern. Med.*, **22** (5), 1157–1165.

25 Zaki, F.A., Nafe, L.A. (1980) Choroid plexus tumors in the dog. *J. Am. Vet. Med. Assoc.*, **176** (4), 328–330.

26 Itoh, T., Uchida, K., Nishi, A., *et al.* (2016) Choroid plexus papilloma in a dog surviving for 15 months after diagnosis with symptomatic therapy. *J. Vet. Med. Sci.*, **78** (1), 167–169.

27 Carisch, L., Golini, L., Schurna, L., *et al.* (2023) Hypertensive, nonobstructive hydrocephalus as main magnetic resonance imaging feature in a dog with disseminated choroid plexus carcinomatosis. *J. Vet. Intern. Med.*, **37** (4), 1493–1500.

28 Frezoulis, P.S., Urraca, C., Altuzarra, R., *et al.* (2023) Choroid plexus carcinoma with meningeal carcinomatosis in a dog. *J. Small Anim. Pract.*, **64** (9), 595. doi:10.1111/jsap.13603. Last accessed October 15, 2023.

29 Miller, A.D., Koehler, J.W., Donovan, T.A., *et al.* (2019) Canine ependymoma: diagnostic criteria and common pitfalls. *Vet. Pathol.*, **56** (6), 860–867.

30 Vural, S.A., Besalti, O., Ilhan, F., *et al.* (2006) Ventricular ependymoma in a German Shepherd dog. *Vet. J.*, **172** (1), 185–187.

31 Traslavina, R.P., Kent, M.S., Mohr, F.C., *et al.* (2013) Clear cell ependymoma in a dog. *J. Comp. Pathol.*, **149** (1), 53–56.

32 Ueno, H., Morimoto, M., Kobayashi, Y., *et al.* (2006) Surgical and radiotherapy treatment of a spinal cord ependymoma in a dog. *Aust. Vet. J.*, **84** (1–2), 36–39.

33 De Lorenzi, D., Mandara, M.T., Tranquillo, M., *et al.* (2006) Squash-prep cytology in the diagnosis of canine and feline nervous system lesions: a study of 42 cases. *Vet. Clin. Pathol.*, **35** (2), 208–214.

34 Koblik, P.D., LeCouteur, R.A., Higgins, R.J., *et al.* (1999) CT-guided brain biopsy using a modified Pelorus Mark III sterotactic system: experience with 50 dogs. *Vet. Radiol. Ultrasound*, **40** (5), 434–440.

35 Di Terlizzi, R., Platt, S. (2006) The function, composition and analysis of cerebrospinal fluid in companion animals: part I – function and composition. *Vet. J.*, **172** (3), 422–431.

36 Zabolotzky, S.M., Vernau, K.M., Kass, P.H., *et al.* (2010) Prevalence and significance of myelin-like material in canine cerebrospinal fluid. *Vet. Clin. Pathol.*, **39** (1), 90–95.

37 Fallin, C.W., Raskin, R.E., Harvey, J.W. (1996) Cytologic identification of neural tissue in the cerebrospinal fluid of two dogs. *Vet. Clin. Pathol.*, **25** (4), 127–129.

38 Wessmann, A., Volk, H.A., Chandler, K., *et al.* (2010) Significance of surface epithelial cells in canine cerebrospinal fluid and relationship to central nervous system disease. *Vet. Clin. Pathol.*, **39** (3), 358–364.

39 Radaelli, S.T., Platt, S.R. (2002) Bacterial meningoencephalomyelitis in dogs: a retrospective study of 23 cases (1990–1999). *J. Vet. Intern. Med.*, **16** (2), 159–163.

40 Lowrie, M., Penderis, J., McLaughlin, M., *et al.* (2009) Steroid responsive meningitis-arteritis: a prospective study of potential disease markers, prednisolone treatment, and long-term outcome in 20 dogs (2006–2008). *J. Vet. Intern. Med.*, **23** (4), 862–870.

41 De Risio, L., Adams, V., Dennis, R., *et al.* (2008) Association of clinical and magnetic resonance imaging findings with outcome in dogs suspected to have ischemic myelopathy: 50 cases (2000–2006). *J. Am. Vet. Med. Assoc.*, **233** (1), 129–135.

42 Kuberski, T. (1981) Eosinophils in cerebrospinal fluid: criteria for eosinophilic meningitis. *Hawaii Med. J.*, **40** (4), 97–98.

43 Windsor, R.C., Sturges, B.K., Vernau, K.M., *et al.* (2009) Cerebrospinal fluid eosinophilia in dogs. *J. Vet. Intern. Med.*, **23** (2), 275–281.

44 Jacobson, E., Morton, J.M., Woerde, D.J., *et al.* (2022) Clinical features, outcomes, and long-term survival times of cats and dogs with central nervous sytem cryptococcosis in Australia: 50 cases (2000-2020). *J. Am. Vet. Med. Assoc.*, **261** (2), 246–257.

45 Duncan, C., Stephen, C., Campbell, J. (2006) Clinical characteristics and predictors of mortality for *Cryptococcus gattii* infection in dogs and cats of southwestern British Columbia. *Can. Vet. J.*, **47** (10), 993–998.

46 Windsor, R.C., Vernau, K.M., Sturges, B.K., *et al.* (2008) Lumbar cerebrospinal fluid in dogs with type I intervertebral disc herniation. *J. Vet. Intern. Med.*, **22** (4), 954–960.

47 Granger, N., Smith, P.M., Jeffery, N.D. (2010) Clinical findings and treatment of non-infectious meningoencephalomyelitis in dogs: a systematic review of 457 published cases from 1962 to 2008. *Vet. J.*, **184** (3), 290–297.

48 Levine, J.M., Fosgate, G.T., Porter, B., *et al.* (2008) Epidemiology of necrotizing meningoencephalitis in Pug dogs. *J. Vet. Intern. Med.*, **22** (4), 961–968.

49 Amude, A.M., Alfieri, A.A., Alfieri, A.F. (2007) Clinicopathological findings in dogs with distemper encephalomyelitis presented without characteristic signs of disease. *Res. Vet. Sci.*, **82** (3), 416–422.

50 Johnsrude, J.D., Alleman, A.R., Schumacher, J., *et al.* (1996) Cytologic findings in cerebrospinal fluid from two animals with GM2-gangliosidosis. *Vet. Clin. Pathol.*, **25** (3), 80–83.

51 Doyle, C., Solano-Gallego, L. (2009) Cytologic interpretation of canine cerebrospinal fluid samples with low total nucleated cell concentration, with and without blood contamination. *Vet. Clin. Pathol.*, **38** (3), 392–396.

52 Singh, M., Foster, D.J., Child, G., *et al.* (2005) Inflammatory cerebrospinal fluid analysis in cats: clinical diagnosis and outcome. *J. Feline. Med. Surg.*, **7** (2), 77–93.

53 West, N., Butterfield, S., Rusbridge, C., *et al.* (2023) Non-traumatic hemorrhagic myelopathy in dogs. *J. Vet. Intern. Med.*, **37** (3), 1129–1138.

54 Williams, M.J., Baughman, B.S., Shores, A., *et al.* (2023) CSF from a puppy with a cerebral vascular hamartoma. *Vet. Clin. Pathol.*, **52** (1), 97–101.

55 Elbert, J.A., Yau, W., Rissi, D.R. (2022) Neuroinflammatory diseases of the central nervous system of dogs: a retrospective study of 207 cases (2008-2019). *Can. Vet. J.*, **63** (2), 178–186.

56 Adamo, P.F., Adams, W.M., Steinberg, H. (2007) Granulomatous meningoencephalomyelitis in dogs. *Compend. Contin. Educ. Vet.*, **29** (11), 678–690.

57 Bradshaw, J.M., Pearson, G.R., Gruffydd-Jones, T.J. (2004) A retrospective study of 286 cases of neurological disorders of the cat. *J. Comp. Pathol.*, **131** (2–3), 112–120.

58 Boettcher, I.C., Steinberg, T., Matiasek, K., *et al.* (2007) Use of anti-coronavirus antibody testing of cerebrospinal fluid for diagnosis of feline infectious peritonitis involving the central nervous system in cats. *J. Am. Vet. Med. Assoc.*, **230** (2), 199–205.

59 Crawford, A.H., Stoll, A.L., Sanchez-Masian, D., *et al.* (2017) Clinicopathologic features and magnetic resonance imaging findings in 24 cats with histopathologically confirmed neurologic feline infectious peritonitis. *J. Vet. Intern. Med.*, **31** (5), 1477–1486.

60 Dickinson, P.J., Bannasch, M., Thomasy, S.M., *et al.* (2020) Antiviral treatment using the adenosine nucleoside analogue GS-441524 in cats with clinically diagnosed neurological feline infectious peritonitis. *J. Vet. Intern. Med.*, **34** (4), 1587–1593.

61 Rawson, F., Foreman, M., Mignan, T., *et al.* (2023) Clinical presentation, treatment, and outcome of 24 dogs with bacterial meningitis or meningoencephalitis without empyema (2010-2020). *J. Vet. Intern. Med.*, **37** (1), 223–229.

62 Griffin, J.F., Levine, J.M., Levine, G.J., *et al.* (2008) Meningomyelitis in dogs: a retrospective review of 28 cases (1999–2007). *J. Small Anim. Pract.*, **49** (10), 509–517.

63 Kelley, A.J., Stainback, L.B., Knowles, K.E., *et al.* (2021) Clinical characteristics, magnetic resonance imaging features, treatment, and outcome for presumed intracranial coccidioidomycosis in 45 dogs (2009-2019). *J. Vet. Intern. Med.*, **35** (5), 2222–2231.

64 Yang, N.S., Griffin, L.R., Frank, C.B., *et al.* (2022) What is your diagnosis? *J. Am. Vet. Med. Assoc.*, **259** (S1), 1–4.

65 Moore, T.W., Bentley, T., Moore, S.A., *et al.* (2017) Spinal mast cell tumors in dogs: imaging features and clinical outcome of four cases. *Vet. Radiol. Ultrasound*, **58** (1), 44–52.

66 Cooper, M.A., Bennett, P.F., Laverty, P.H. (2009) Metastatic mast cell tumour in a dog presenting with spinal pain. *Aust. Vet. J.*, **87** (4), 157–159.

67 Tyrrell, D., Davis, R.M. (2001) Progressive neurologic signs associated with systemic mastocytosis in a dog. *Aust. Vet. J.*, **79** (2), 106–108.

68 Guevar, J., Shihab, N., English, K., *et al.* (2013) What is your neurologic diagnosis? Mast cell tumor. *J. Am. Vet. Med. Assoc.*, **242** (5), 619–621.

69 Brewer, D.M., Cerda-Gonzalez, S., Dewey, C.W., *et al.* (2011) Spinal cord nephroblastoma in dogs: 11 cases (1985–2007). *J. Am. Vet. Med. Assoc.*, **238** (5), 618–624.

70 Liebel, F.X., Rossmeisl, J.H., Jr, Lanz, O.I., *et al.* (2011) Canine spinal nephroblastoma: long-term outcomes associated with treatment of 10 cases (1996–2009). *Vet. Surg.*, **40** (2), 244–252.

71 De New, K.M., Coates, J.R., Millman, Z., *et al.* (2023) What is your diagnosis? Spinal mass in a young dog. *Vet. Clin. Pathol.*, **52** (Suppl. 2), 97–99.

72 Brehm, D.M., Vite, C.H., Steinberg, H.S., *et al.* (1995) A retrospective evaluation of 51 cases of peripheral nerve sheath tumors in the dog. *J. Am. Anim. Hosp. Assoc.*, **31** (4), 349–359.

15

Ocular and Special Senses

15.1 Eyes: Cornea

15.1.1 Normal Epithelium

Normal corneal epithelium from scrapings of the cornea comprises mostly intermediate squamous epithelial cells. These cells are polygonal, with abundant pale-blue cytoplasm that may contain a small amount of melanin pigment. The nuclei are round, centrally located, and have clumped chromatin with small or inapparent nucleoli. Anisocytosis/anisokaryosis are mild and N/C ratios are low (Figure 15.1). Lesser numbers of basal squamous epithelial cells may be seen with deep scrapings.

15.1.2 Epithelial Hyperplasia/Dysplasia

15.1.2.1 Cytologic Appearance
Relative to the normal corneal epithelium, hyperplastic or dysplastic epithelial cells generally have higher N/C ratios and deeper-blue cytoplasm. The nuclei often are larger and have stippled chromatin and more prominent nucleoli. Anisocytosis/anisokaryosis ranges from mild to moderate (Figure 15.2).

15.1.2.2 Clinical Considerations
- Frequently accompany cases of chronic irritation/inflammation.

15.1.2.3 Prognosis
Good – hyperplastic changes will resolve with treatment of the underlying cause.

15.1.3 Squamous Cell Carcinoma

15.1.3.1 Cytologic Appearance
Squamous cell carcinomas of the cornea and conjunctiva mostly have marked criteria of malignancy. Cells have a variable volume of cytoplasm that frequently has a bright, sky-blue, hyalinized appearance consistent with keratinization. This is accompanied by large, immature nuclei that have prominent nucleoli (nuclear to cytoplasmic dissociation) (Figure 15.3). Anisocytosis/anisokaryosis are marked and N/C ratios are variable. These features can overlap with dysplastic changes (see Section 15.1.2), and histopathology is often required for definitive diagnosis.

15.1.3.2 Clinical Considerations
- Rare on the cornea, more commonly arise from the conjunctiva.
- Often associated with chronic or pigmentary keratitis [1].
- Brachycephalic dogs predisposed [2].

15.1.3.3 Prognosis
Good with appropriate therapy. Metastatic potential is low [1, 2].

15.1.4 Bacterial Keratitis

15.1.4.1 Cytologic Appearance
Bacterial keratitis generally is characterized by a neutrophilic infiltrate of variably degenerative neutrophils, with intracellular bacteria confirming bacterial sepsis (Figure 15.4). Bacteria may be present in the background only or may be absent in cytologic samples. Often accompanied by epithelial hyperplasia.

15.1.4.2 Clinical Considerations
- Dogs > cats [3, 4].
- Usually associated with concurrent ulceration (ulcerative keratitis).
- Common bacteria = *Staphylococcus*, *Streptococcus*, and *Pseudomonas* spp. [4, 5]
- Microbial culture and susceptibility testing is recommended to increase successful diagnosis [6].

Clinical Atlas of Small Animal Cytology and Hematology, Second Edition. Andrew G. Burton.
© 2024 John Wiley & Sons, Inc. Published 2024 by John Wiley & Sons, Inc.

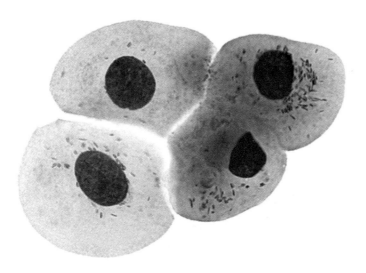

Figure 15.1 Normal corneal epithelium, dog, 100× objective. These cells contain a fine dusting of melanin pigment granules.

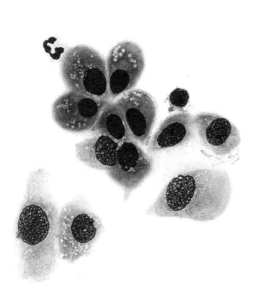

Figure 15.2 Corneal epithelial hyperplasia, dog, 50× objective. The cells have higher N/C ratios and more basophilic cytoplasm. Note the neutrophils in the background.

15.1.4.3 Prognosis

Generally good with appropriate, early therapy, but variable based on severity of the disease.

15.1.5 Fungal Keratitis

15.1.5.1 Cytologic Appearance

Fungal hyphae often are seen in dense mats, and close investigation of thick areas of corneal scrapes is warranted.

Fungal hyphae have parallel sides, internal structures, and may be septated or branching (Figure 15.5). Inflammatory cells and epithelial hyperplasia are variably present.

15.1.5.2 Clinical Considerations

- *Aspergillus* spp. are most common. *Candida* and *Fusarium* spp. are also common [7].
- Predisposing factors = corneal trauma, prolonged use of antibiotics or corticosteroids, endocrinopathies [8].

Figure 15.3 Corneal squamous cell carcinoma, dog, 50× objective. The cells have sky-blue, keratinized cytoplasm with immature nuclei. Criteria of malignancy are marked.

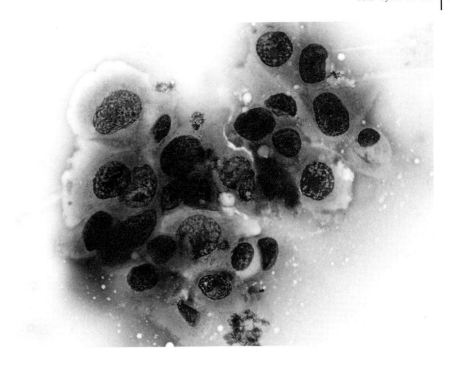

Figure 15.4 Bacterial keratitis, dog, 100× objective. Note the degenerative neutrophils that contain intracellular rod-shaped bacteria (arrow).

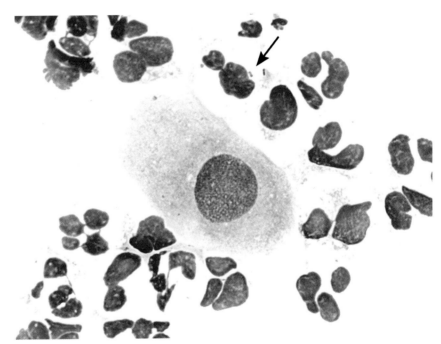

15.1.5.3 Prognosis
Variable, based on the severity of disease and the underlying cause. Enucleation is sometimes necessary [8].

15.1.6 Eosinophilic Keratitis

15.1.6.1 Cytologic Appearance
Eosinophilic keratitis or keratoconjunctivitis is characterized by increased eosinophils, and numerous eosinophil granules may be present in the background (Figure 15.6). Low numbers of other inflammatory cells, especially small mature lymphocytes, may be present, as well as mast cells, non-degenerative neutrophils, and globule leukocytes [9].

15.1.6.2 Clinical Considerations
- Cats.
- Unilateral > bilateral [10].

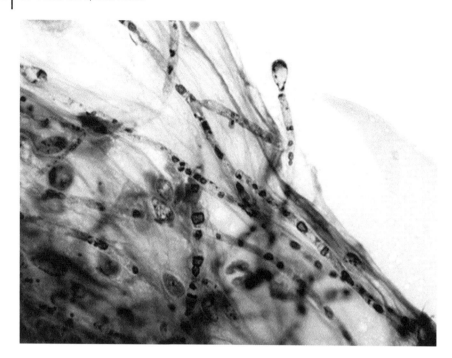

Figure 15.5 Fungal keratitis, dog, 100× objective. Fungal hyphae are seen in a large mat.

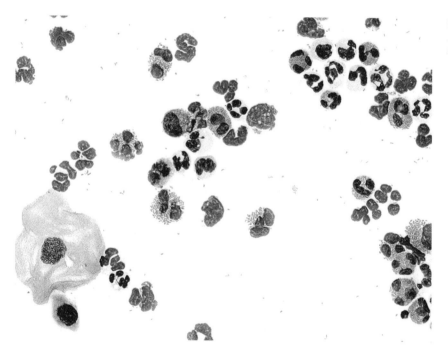

Figure 15.6 Eosinophilic keratitis, cat, 50× objective. A corneal epithelial cell is seen at the lower left.

- Grossly = pink/white plaques with gritty, yellow material and most commonly affects the superotemporal quadrant [10–12].
- Often associated with Feline Herpes Virus 1 [10, 11].

15.1.6.3 Prognosis
Good with appropriate therapy, but recurrence is common [12, 13].

15.1.7 Chronic Superficial Keratitis

15.1.7.1 Cytologic Appearance
Characterized by an infiltrate of mixed lymphocytes, dominated by small mature cells, and plasma cells may also be present (Figure 15.7). Well-differentiated corneal epithelial cells may be present, which may contain abundant melanin pigment.

Figure 15.7 Chronic superficial keratitis, dog, 50× objective. Numerous small mature lymphocytes are present, accompanied by well-differentiated, pigmented corneal epithelial cells.

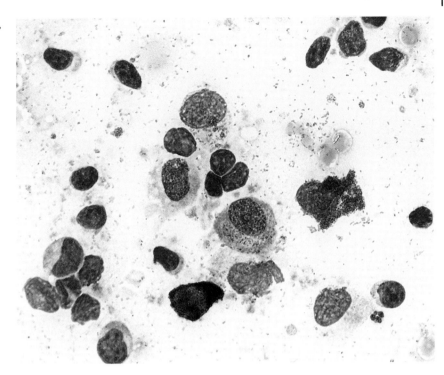

15.1.7.2 Clinical Considerations

- Also known as *pannus*.
- Usually bilateral.
- Immune-mediated etiology [14, 15].
- Most common in German Shepherds. Other predisposed breeds include Greyhounds, Belgian Tervurens, Border Collies, and Australian Shepherds [14, 16–18].
- Clinical signs = raised, red/brown/gray corneal pigmentation with corneal vascularization and edema. Lesions often arise from the ventrotemporal or temporal limbus [18].

15.1.7.3 Prognosis

Good with appropriate therapy [19].

15.1.8 Pigmentary Keratitis

15.1.8.1 Cytologic Appearance

In pigmentary keratitis, excessive melanin pigment accumulates within corneal epithelial cells. The melanin pigment is green/black and varies from fine elongated granules to coarse clumps (Figure 15.8).

15.1.8.2 Clinical Considerations

- Most common secondary to irritating stimuli (e.g., entropion, distichiasis, keratoconjunctivitis sicca, or chronic inflammation) [20].
- Bilateral >> unilateral [21].

- Common in Pugs, with or without predisposing stimuli [20–22].

15.1.8.3 Prognosis

Typically good, but variable based on the underlying cause and ability to control the underlying disease [23, 24].

15.2 Eyes: Conjunctiva

15.2.1 Inflammation

15.2.1.1 Cytologic Appearance

Conjunctivitis is most commonly neutrophilic in dogs and cats, but other inflammatory cells may be seen. Bacteria may be identified within neutrophils or associated with epithelial cells such as *Chlamydia* (Figure 15.9) or *Mycoplasma* (Figure 15.10).

15.2.1.2 Clinical Considerations

- May be primary or secondary and sterile or infectious.
- DDx: (dogs) = viral (*Distemper*), bacterial, keratoconjunctivitis sicca, neoplasia, immune-mediated; (cats) = Viral (herpesvirus), bacterial (*Mycoplasma*, *Chlamydia*), and neoplasia [25, 26].

15.2.1.3 Prognosis

Generally good, but variable based on the underlying cause.

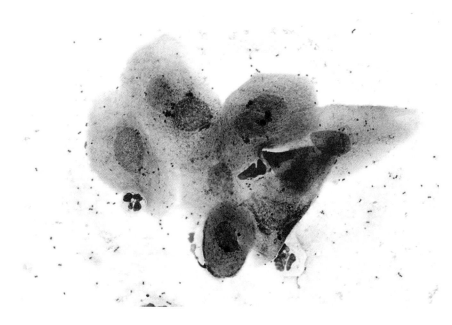

Figure 15.8 Pigmentary keratitis, dog, 50× objective. Abundant melanin pigment is noted, often in aggregates, associated with corneal epithelial cells. Three neutrophils are seen, and many coccoid bacteria are noted in the background.

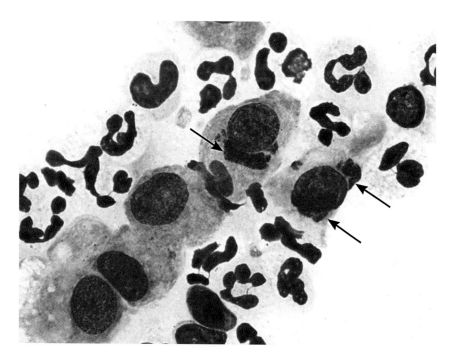

Figure 15.9 *Chlamydia felis* elementary bodies, conjunctiva, cat, 100× objective. Note the basophilic, perinuclear inclusions (arrows). Courtesy of Dr. Bill Vernau.

15.2.2 Mastocytic conjunctivitis

15.2.2.1 Cytologic Appearance

Mastocytic conjunctivitis is characterized by a predominance of well-granulated mast cells, though other inflammatory cells may be present, including eosinophils and neutrophils. The mast cells may be intimately associated with the conjunctival epithelium, and numerous extracellular granules may be present, which may be difficult to distinguish from bacteria (Figure 15.11).

15.2.2.2 Clinical Considerations

- Most commonly associated with allergic/hypersensitivity disease.
- Feline epitheliotropic mastocytic conjunctivitis is an uncommon, benign condition thought to have an allergic etiology [27]. It may be unilateral or bilateral.
- Mast cell neoplasia can affect conjunctiva in dogs and is a differential for a predominance of mast cells [28].

Figure 15.10 *Mycoplasma felis*, conjunctiva, cat, 100× objective. Fine, basophilic organisms are scattered over the surface of a squamous epithelial cell (arrow). Compare them to the melanin pigment in the cells on the right (arrowhead).

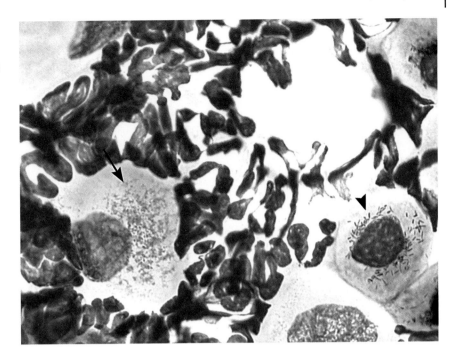

Figure 15.11 Mastocytic conjunctivitis, cat, 50× objective. Many well-granulated mast cells (arrows) are intimately associated with well-differentiated epithelial cells. Note the abundant extracellular granules.

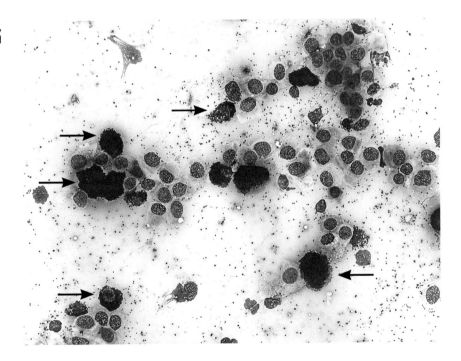

15.2.2.3 Prognosis

Good with treatment of the underlying cause. Patients with feline epitheliotropic mastocytic conjunctivitis typically respond well to therapy [27].

15.2.3 Neoplasia

Numerous neoplasms affect the conjunctiva, including squamous cell carcinoma (see Section 15.1.3), melanoma, mast cell tumor, papilloma, and lymphoma, which is specifically discussed in the following section.

15.2.4 Conjunctival Lymphoma

15.2.4.1 Cytologic Appearance

Lymphoma of the conjunctiva may present with variably sized lymphocytes, though they are typically large, with nuclei approximately 2-fold to 3-fold the size of RBCs in

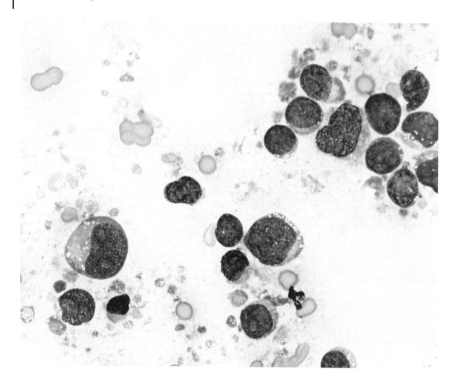

Figure 15.12 Conjunctival lymphoma, cat, 50× objective. The cells have large nuclei with immature chromatin and prominent nucleoli. Note the clear vacuoles in the cytoplasm.

diameter, with finely stippled chromatin and prominent nucleoli (Figure 15.12). They have a small volume of medium-blue cytoplasm which may contain punctate clear vacuoles.

15.2.4.2 Clinical Considerations
- May be localized (primary disease) or a part of systemic/metastatic disease [29, 30].
- Present with a diffuse thickening of the conjunctiva ± discrete masses [29, 31].
- T-cell phenotype more common in dogs and B-cell phenotype more common in cats [31, 32].

15.2.4.3 Prognosis
Prognosis is better for conjunctival lymphoma than intraocular lymphoma. Prolonged survival times with therapy have been reported, but prognosis is still guarded [29, 32].

15.3 Ears

15.3.1 Ceruminous Gland Adenoma

15.3.1.1 Cytologic Features
Ceruminous adenomas exfoliate in cohesive sheets of relatively uniform ovoid cells with a pale-blue cytoplasm that may contain clear secretory material. Nuclei are round, with granular chromatin and small basophilic nucleoli.

Anisocytosis/anisokaryosis are mild and N/C ratios are low (Figure 15.13). Cytologically similar to ceruminous cystic hyperplasia. Extracellular blue/black granular secretory material may be present [33].

15.3.1.2 Clinical Considerations
- Typically exophytic, smooth, pedunculated masses that rarely ulcerate.
- Seen in older dogs (9 years) but also in cats typically younger than those with adenocarcinomas [34].
- Cocker Spaniels and Poodles appear predisposed [34].
- Otitis externa is a common concurrent finding [35].

15.3.1.3 Prognosis
Excellent. Surgical excision is typically curative [35].

15.3.2 Ceruminous Gland Adenocarcinoma

15.3.2.1 Cytologic Features
These tumors comprise crowded sheets of ovoid to polygonal cells, often distributed in papillary or vague acinar arrangements. They have a variable volume of medium-blue cytoplasm that may be distended with clear secretory material. Nuclei are ovoid with finely stippled chromatin and prominent basophilic nucleoli. Anisocytosis/anisokaryosis are marked and N/C ratios are moderate to high (Figures 15.14 and 15.15).

Figure 15.13 Ceruminous gland adenoma, dog, 50× objective.

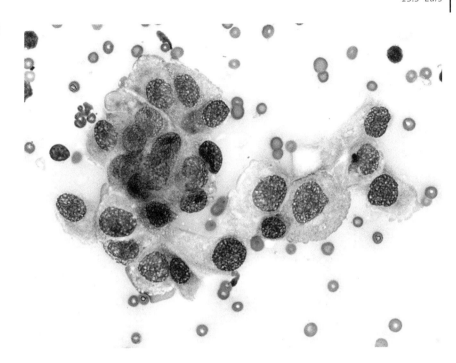

Figure 15.14 Ceruminous gland adenocarcinoma, dog, 50× objective.

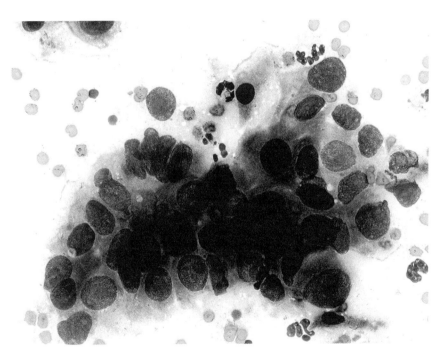

15.3.2.2 Clinical Considerations

- Most common malignant tumor of the ear canal in dogs and cats [34].
- Low metastatic rate, though the metastatic potential increases over time. Tumors are locally aggressive and invasive [36].

15.3.2.3 Prognosis

Variable. Long-term survival is possible with appropriate local therapy [37]. Metastatic disease confers a poor prognosis [34].

15.3.3 Otitis Externa (Bacterial)

15.3.3.1 Cytologic Features

Large numbers of bacteria are seen individually and as colonies in the background of the slide (Figures 15.16 and 15.17). Inflammatory cells are not always present, but sepsis is confirmed if intracellular bacteria are seen. *Note*: Low numbers of bacteria can be normal. Mean bacteria counts of <5 (dogs) and <4 (cats) per 40× objective field have been proposed as normal, while ≥25 (dogs) and ≥15

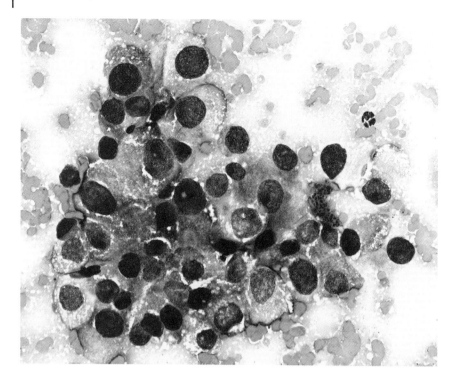

Figure 15.15 Ceruminous gland adenocarcinoma, dog, 50× objective. Note the marked anisokaryosis, cellular crowding and prominent basophilic nucleoli.

Figure 15.16 Bacterial otitis externa, dog, 100× objective. Colonies of bacterial cocci are noted, associated with squamous epithelial cells.

(cats) per 40× objective field have a high specificity for abnormal overgrowth or infection [38].

15.3.3.2 Clinical Considerations
- Dogs > cats.
- Bilateral > unilateral.
- Most common bacteria = *Staphylococcus pseudintermedius/ intermedius* and *Pseudomonas aeruginosa* [39]. Other common isolates include *Proteus, Enterococcus, Streptococcus,* and *Corynebacterium* spp. [40].
- Clinical signs = pruritus, head shaking, otic erythema/ discharge, malodor, and pain.
- Underlying predisposing factors (e.g., ear anatomy/breed and moisture) and primary causes (e.g., allergic dermatitis, parasites, and foreign bodies) should be investigated [41, 42].

Figure 15.17 Bacterial otitis externa, dog, 100× objective. Colonies of bacterial rods are noted, associated with squamous epithelial cells.

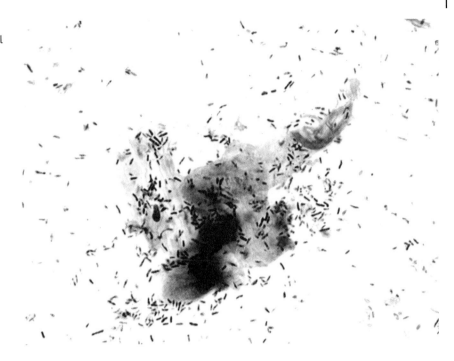

- Heat-fixing slides does not improve sample quality for cytologic analysis [43].

15.3.3.3 Prognosis
Generally excellent with appropriate therapy, but may be complicated by underlying predisposing causes, and recurrence is common [44, 45].

15.3.4 Otitis Externa (Fungal)

15.3.4.1 Cytologic Features
Otitis externa due to fungal agents (otomycosis) is most commonly associated with *Malassezia* spp. These are ovoid to bilobed organisms that stain intensely basophilic and may have a fine clear halo (Figure 15.18). *Note: Malassezia* may be seen normally in ears in low numbers, with ≤2 yeast organisms per 40× objective field considered normal [38]. Mean *Malassezia* counts of ≥5 (dogs) and ≥12 (cats) per 40× objective field have a high specificity for abnormal overgrowth or infection [38]. Inflammatory cells are seen rarely.

15.3.4.2 Clinical Considerations
- Dogs > cats.
- Bilateral > unilateral.
- Underlying predisposing factors (e.g., ear anatomy and moisture) and primary causes (e.g., allergic dermatitis, parasites, and foreign bodies) should be investigated [42].
- Most commonly due to *Malassezia pachydermatis*. Rarely associated with other fungal agents such as *Candida* and *Aspergillus* spp. [46].

- Associated with ceruminous discharge; rarely purulent [47].
- Concurrent otitis media occurs in approximately 20% of cases [48].
- Heat-fixing slides does not improve sample quality for cytologic analysis [43, 49].

15.3.4.3 Prognosis
Generally excellent with appropriate therapy, but may be complicated by underlying predisposing causes, and recurrence is common [44, 48, 50].

15.3.5 Otitis Externa (Parasitic)

15.3.5.1 Cytologic Appearance
Otodectes cynotis is the most common cause of parasitic otitis externa. They have two anterior and two posterior pairs of legs (see Figure 3.55). Sometimes only eggs of mites will be present, which are ovoid and ~200 μm long (Figure 15.19). *Demodex* spp. and other mites are less common (Figure 15.20).

15.3.5.2 Clinical Considerations
- Common primary causes of otitis externa [42].
- Often associated with black, granular discharge [51].
- Clinical signs = head shaking, ear scratching, and ear droop.
- May be accompanied by neutrophilic inflammation as well as secondary bacterial or yeast infection.

15.3.5.3 Prognosis
Excellent.

Figure 15.18 Mixed fungal and bacterial otitis externa, dog, 50× objective. Numerous bilobed *Malassezia* spp. organisms are seen, as well as bacteria.

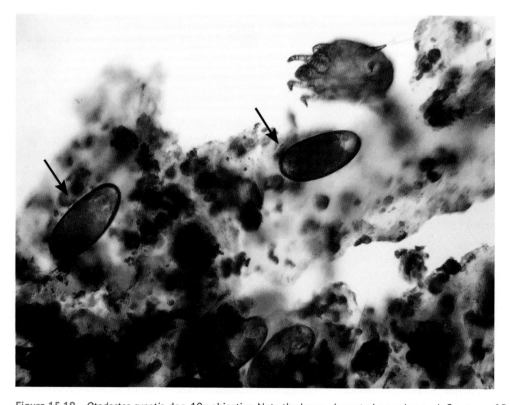

Figure 15.19 *Otodectes cynotis*, dog, 10× objective. Note the large, elongated eggs (arrows). Courtesy of Dr. Eric Franson.

Figure 15.20 *Demodex* nymph, dog, 20× objective.

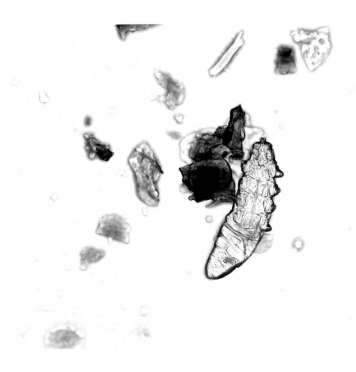

References

1 Takiyama, N., Terasaki, E., Uechi, M. (2010) Corneal squamous cell carecinoma in two dogs. *Vet. Ophthalmol.*, **13** (4), 266–269.

2 Dreyfus, J., Schobert, C.S., Dubielzig, R.R. (2011) Superficial corneal squamous cell carcinoma occurring in dogs with chronic keratitis. *Vet. Ophthalmol.*, **14** (3), 161–168.

3 Ollivier, F.J. (2003) Bacterial corneal diseases in dogs and cats. *Clin. Tech. Small Anim. Pract.*, **18** (3), 193–198.

4 Goldreich, J.E., Franklin-Guild, R.J., Ledbetter, E.C. (2020) Feline bacterial keratitis: clinical features, bacterial isolates, and in vitro antimicrobial susceptibility patterns. *Vet. Ophthalmol.*, **23** (1), 90–96.

5 McKeever, J.M., Ward, D.A., Hendrix, D.V.H. (2021) Comparison of antimicrobial resistance patterns in dogs with bacterial keratitis presented to a veterinary teaching hospital over two multi-year time periods (1993–2003 and 2013–2019) in the Southeastern United States. *Vet. Ophthalmol.*, **24** (6), 653–658.

6 Massa, K.L., Murphy, C.J., Hartmann, F.A., *et al.* (1999) Usefulness of aerobic microbial culture and cytologic evaluation of corneal specimens in the diagnosis of infectious ulcerative keratitis in animals. *J. Am. Vet. Med. Assoc.*, **215** (11), 1671–1674.

7 Andrew, S.E. (2003) Corneal fungal disease in small animals. *Clin. Tech. Small Anim. Pract.*, **18** (3), 186–192.

8 Scott, E.M., Carter, R.T. (2014) Canine keratomycosis in 11 dogs: a case series (2000–2011). *J. Am. Anim. Hosp. Assoc.*, **50** (2), 112–118.

9 Lucyshyn, D.R., Vernau, W., Maggs, D.J., *et al.* (2021) Correlations between clinical signs and corneal cytology in feline eosinophilic keratoconjunctivitis. *Vet. Ophthalmol.*, **24** (6), 620–626.

10 Dean, E., Meunier, V. (2013) Feline eosinophilic keratoconjunctivitis: a retrospective study of 45 cases (56 eyes). *J. Feline Med. Surg.*, **15** (8), 661–666.

11 Nasisse, M.P., Glover, T.L., Moore, C.P., *et al.* (1998) Detection of feline herpesvirus 1 DNA in corneas of cats with eosinophilic keratitis or corneal sequestration. *Am. J. Vet. Res.*, **59** (7), 856–858.

12 Morgan, R.V., Abrams, K.L., Kern, T.J. (1996) Feline eosinophilic keratitis: a retrospective study of 54 cases (1989–1994). *Vet. Comp. Ophthalmol.*, **6** (2), 131–134.

13 Labelle, A., Labelle, P. (2023) Eosinophilic keratoconjunctivitis in cats. *Vet. Clin. North Am. Small Anim. Pract.*, **53** (2), 353–365.

14 Barrientos, L.S., Zapata, G., Crespi, J.A., *et al.* (2013) A study of the association between chronic superficial keratitis and polymorphisms in the upstream regulatory regions of DLA-DRB$_1$, DLA-DQB$_1$ and DLA-DQA$_1$. *Vet. Immunol. Immunopathol.*, **156** (3–4), 205–210.

15 Jokinen, P., Rusanen, E.M., Kennedy, L.J., *et al.* (2011) MHC class II risk haplotype associated with canine chronic superficial keratitis in German Shepherd dogs. *Vet. Immunol. Immunopathol.*, **140** (1–2), 37–41.

16 Drahovska, Z., Balicki, I., Trbolova, A., *et al.* (2014) A retrospective study of the occurrence of chronic

superficial keratitis in 308 German Shepherd dogs: 1999-2010. *Pol. J. Vet. Sci.*, **17** (3), 543–546.

17 Cheng, S., Wigney, D., Haase, B., *et al.* (2016) Inheritence of chronic superficial keratitis in Australian Greyhounds. *Anim. Genet.*, **47** (5), 629.

18 Andrew, S.E. (2008) Immune-mediated canine and feline keratitis. *Vet. Clin. North Am. Small Anim. Pract.*, **38** (2), 269–290.

19 Nell, B., Walde, I., Billich, A., *et al.* (2005) The effect of topical pimecrolimus on keratoconjunctivitis sicca and chronic superficial keratitis in dogs: results from an exploratory study. *Vet. Ophathalmol.*, **8** (1), 39–46.

20 Labelle, A.L., Dresser, C.B., Hamor, R.E., *et al.* (2013) Characteristics of, prevalence of, and risk factors for corneal pigmentation (pigmentary keratopathy) in Pugs. *J. Am. Vet. Med. Assoc.*, **243** (5), 667–674.

21 Maini, S., Everson, R., Dawson, C., *et al.* (2019) Pigmentary keratitis in pugs in the United Kingdom: prevalence and associated features. *BMC Vet. Res.*, **15** (1), 384.

22 Vallone, L.V., Enders, A.M., Mohammed, H.O., *et al.* (2017) In vivo confocal microscopy of brachycephalic dogs with and without superficial corneal pigment. *Vet. Ophthalmol.*, **20** (4), 294–303.

23 Labelle, A., Labelle, P. (2023) Diagnosing corneal pigmentation in small animals. *Vet. Clin. North Am. Small Anim. Pract.*, **53** (2), 339–352.

24 Azoulay, T. (2014) Adjunctive cryotherapy for pigmentary keratitis in dogs: a study of 16 corneas. *Vet. Ophthalmol.*, **17** (4), 241–249.

25 Peña, M.A., Leiva, M. (2008) Canine conjunctivitis and blepharitis. *Vet. Clin. North Am. Small Anim. Pract.*, **38** (2), 233–249.

26 Tîrziu, A., Herman, V., Imre, K., *et al.* (2022) Occurrence of Chlamydia spp. in conjunctival samples of stray cats in Timişoara municipality, Western Romania. *Microorganisms*, **10** (11), 2187.

27 Beckwith-Cohen, B., Dubielzig, R.R., Maggs, D.J., *et al.* (2017) Feline epitheliotropic mastocytic conjunctivitis in 15 cats. *Vet. Pathol.*, **54** (1), 141–146.

28 Fife, M., Blocker, T., Fife, T., *et al.* (2011) Canine conjunctival mast cell tumors: a retrospective study. *Vet. Ophthalmol.*, **14** (3), 153–160.

29 Wiggins, K.T., Skorupski, K.A., Reilly, C.M., *et al.* (2014) Presumed solitary intraocular or conjunctival lymphoma in dogs and cats: 9 cases (1985–2013). *J. Am. Vet. Med. Assoc.*, **244** (4), 460–470.

30 Kang, S., Jeong, M., Seo, K. (2019) Corneoconjunctival manifestations of lymphoma in three dogs. *J. Vet. Sci.*, **20** (1), 98–101.

31 Radi, Z.A., Miller, D.L., Hines, M.E. 2nd (2004) B-cell conjunctival lymphoma in a cat. *Vet. Ophthalmol.*, **7** (6), 413–415.

32 McCowan, C., Malcolm, J., Hurn, S., *et al.* Conjunctival lymphoma: immunophenotype and outcome in five dogs and three cats. *Vet. Ophthalmol.*, **17** (5), 351–357.

33 De Lorenzi, D., Bonfanti, U., Masserdotti, C., *et al.* (2005) Fine-needle biopsy of external ear canal masses in the cat: cytologic results and histologic correlations in 27 cases. *Vet. Clin. Pathol.*, **34** (2), 100–105.

34 London, C.A., Dubilzeig, R.R., Vail, D.M., *et al.* (1996) Evaluation of dogs and cats with tumors of the ear canal: 145 cases (1978–1992). *J. Am. Vet. Med. Assoc.*, **208** (9), 1413–1418.

35 Pavletic, M.M. (2019) Partial vertical ear canal resection in two cats. *J. Am. Vet. Med. Assoc.*, **255** (12), 1365–1368.

36 Théon, A.P., Barthez, P.Y., Madewell, B.R., *et al.* (1994) Radiation therapy of ceruminous gland carcinomas in dogs and cats. *J. Am. Vet. Med. Assoc.*, **205** (4), 566–569.

37 Marino, D.J., MacDonald, J.M., Matthiesen, D.T., *et al.* (1994) Results of surgery in cats with ceruminous gland adenocarcinoma. *J. Am. Anim. Hosp. Assoc.*, **30** (1), 54–58.

38 Ginel, P.J., Lucena, R., Rodriguez, J.C., *et al.* (2002) A semiquantitative cytological evaluation of normal and pathological samples from the external ear canal of dogs and cats. *Vet. Dermatol.*, **13** (3), 151–156.

39 Oliveira, L.C., Leite, C.A., Brilhante, R.S., *et al.* (2008) Comparative study of the microbial profile from bilateral canine otitis externa. *Can. Vet. J.*, **49** (8), 785–788.

40 Bajwa, J. (2019) Canine otitis externa – treatment and complications. *Can. Vet. J.*, **60** (1), 97–99.

41 O'Neill, D.G., Volk, A.V., Soares, T., *et al.* (2021) Frequency and predisposing factors for canine otitis externa in the UK – a primary veterinary care epidemiological view. *Canine. Med. Genet.*, **8** (1), 7.

42 Rosser, E.J., Jr (2004) Causes of otitis externa. *Vet. Clin. North Am. Small Anim. Pract.*, **34** (2), 459–468.

43 Toma, S., Cornegliani, L., Persico, P., *et al.* (2006) Comparison of 4 fixation and staining methods for the cytologic evaluation of ear canals with clinical evidence of ceruminous otitis externa. *Vet. Clin. Pathol.*, **35** (2), 194–198.

44 Saridomichelakis, M.N., Farmaki, R., Leontides, L.S., *et al.* (2007) Aetiology of canine otitis externa: a retrospective study of 100 cases. *Vet. Dermatol.*, **18** (5), 341–347.

45 Logas, D., Maxwell, E.A. (2021) Collaborative care improves treatment outcome for dogs with chronic otitis externa: a collaborative care coalition study. *J. Am. Anim. Hosp. Assoc.*, **57** (5), 212–216.

46 Goodale, E.C., Outerbridge, C.A., White, S.D. (2016) *Aspergillus* otitis in small animals – a retrospective study of 17 cases. *Vet. Dermatol.*, **27** (1), 3–8.

47 Guillot, J., Bond, R. (2020) Malassezia yeasts in veterinary dermatology: an updated review. *Front. Cell. Infect.*

Microbiol., **10**, 79. doi: 10.3389/fcimb.2020.00079. Last accessed October 15, 2023.

48 Boone, J.M., Bond, R., Loeffler, A., *et al.* (2021) Malassezia otitis unresponsive to primary care: outcome in 59 dogs. *Vet. Dermatol.*, **32** (5), 441.

49 Griffin, J.S., Scott, D.W., Erb, H.N. (2007) *Malassezia* otitis externa in the dog: the effect of heat-fixing otic exudate for cytological analysis. *J. Vet. Med. A Physiol. Pathol. Clin. Med.*, **54** (8), 424–427.

50 Bond, R., Morris, D.O., Guillot, J., *et al.* (2020) Biology, diagnosis and treatment of Malassezia dermatitis in dogs and cats: clinical consensus guidelines of the World Association for Veterinary Dermatology. *Vet. Dermatol.*, **31** (1), 75. doi: 10.1111/vde.12834. Last accessed October 15, 2023.

51 Thomson, P., Carreño, N., Núñez, A. (2023) Main mites associated with dermatopathies present in dogs and other members of the Canidae family. *Open. Vet. J.*, **13** (2), 131–142.

16

Blood Smear Preparation and Evaluation

16.1 The Importance of Blood Smear Evaluation

Inspection of a blood smear is a critical component of complete hematology assessment. A thorough evaluation of a high-quality blood smear complements results from hematology analyzers and is ideally reviewed for all hematology samples, especially those from sick patients. Some of the parameters for which blood smear evaluation plays a critical role include, but are not limited to, identifying left shift and toxic changes in neutrophils, infectious agents, platelet clumping, presence and morphology of nucleated red blood cells, erythrocyte morphology, neoplastic cells, and background features.

In-clinic options for digital hematology have increased dramatically in recent years, further necessitating that clinics are able to make and stain high-quality blood smears. This chapter provides a detailed description of how to make, stain, and evaluate a high-quality blood smear. Subsequent chapters provide a detailed analysis to evaluate and interpret erythrocytes, leukocytes, platelets, and extracellular components of the blood smear.

16.2 Making a Blood Smear

Blood smears should be prepared using fresh EDTA anticoagulated blood within 2 hours of collection to avoid storage artifacts, which mostly affect erythrocyte morphology [1–3]. The blood tube should be at room temperature and should be mixed well by inverting the EDTA tube gently at least 10 times.

Supplies
- Latex or nitrile gloves.
- Glass microscope slides with a frosted edge.
- +/− Camelhair brush.
- A pencil.
- EDTA anticoagulated blood sample at room temperature.
- Plain microhematocrit tube.
- Cotton swabs
- +/− Hairdryer.

Procedure
1) Label the slides by writing patient details on the frosted edge of the slide with a pencil.
2) Use a camel hair brush to remove any debris or glass grit from the slides as needed.
3) Wear gloves when handling blood. The wooden end of a cotton swab can be used to stir the sample to evaluate for any gross clots.
4) Fill a plain microhematocrit tube with the blood sample and use this to place a small (1/4 cm diameter) drop of blood approximately 1 cm from the frosted edge of the slide. Do not tap the microhematocrit tube on the glass slide; instead, allow gravity to create the dot of blood. The use of a hematocrit tube (rather than a needle and syringe) is both safer and reduces shearing damage to cells. Alternatively, the wooden end of the cotton swabs used to stir the blood tube may be used to apply the drop of blood to the slide.
5) On a smooth, flat surface, hold the slide in place with a finger. Hold a second spreader slide in the dominant hand between the thumb and index finger at approximately a 45° angle to the lower slide in front of the drop of blood (Figure 16.1). *Note*: This angle may be altered based on the composition of the blood. For thin samples (e.g., from patients with moderate to marked anemia), this angle should be increased, while for thick samples (e.g., from patients with erythrocytosis), this angle should be decreased to ensure an appropriate monolayer.
6) Back the spreader slide into the drop of blood and allow blood to spread along the edge of the spreader slide (Figure 16.2). When the blood has nearly spread the

Clinical Atlas of Small Animal Cytology and Hematology, Second Edition. Andrew G. Burton.
© 2024 John Wiley & Sons, Inc. Published 2024 by John Wiley & Sons, Inc.

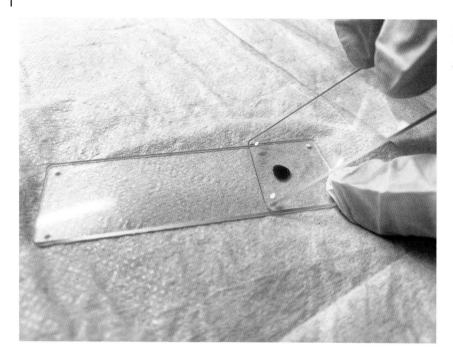

Figure 16.1 The slide is placed on a solid surface and stabilized with a finger. Note the size of the blood spot and the angle of the spreader slide.

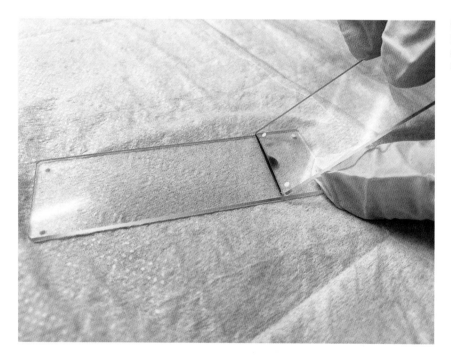

Figure 16.2 The spreader slide is backed into the blood spot, and blood is allowed to spread along the edge of the spreader slide.

entire length of the spreader slide edge, push it forward in a smooth, moderately paced motion along the entire length of the slide, using gentle, even pressure (Figure 16.3). Do not lift the slide at the end of this motion or stop spreading abruptly.

7) Dry the smear immediately by blowing gently on the slide or using the cool setting on a hair dryer [4]. This will prevent artifactual changes in erythrocytes, including crenation (Figure 16.4).

8) The smears should be fixed within the first hour of preparation to preserve cell morphology. Ensure that the slides are completely dry prior to fixation. They can be stained immediately after fixation, or at a later time. See Section 16.3 for details on staining blood smears.

A good quality blood smear has a bullet or thumbprint shape with three distinct regions for review: a feathered edge, a monolayer, and a body.

Figure 16.3 The spreader slide is pushed forward in a smooth, moderately paced motion along the entire length of the slide without lifting up at any time.

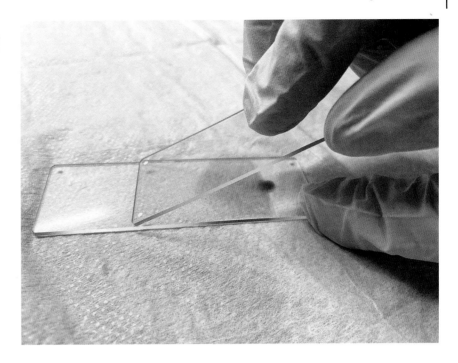

Figure 16.4 Blood smear, dog, 100× objective field. Crenation of erythrocytes. Note the regularly spaced, sharp spicules, and the decreased intensity of central pallor.

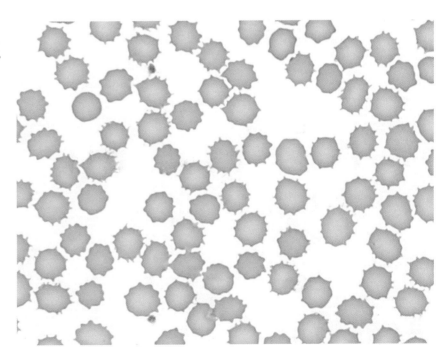

- Feathered edge: The feathered edge is the leading edge of the blood smear and should have a fine feathery appearance.
- Monolayer: The monolayer abuts the feathered edge and is the region of the slide where half of the red blood cells are touching each other, and half are not touching.

- Body: The body of the smear makes up the majority of the smear and should blend seamlessly into the monolayer.

Blood smears may lack some of the above regions or suffer from other artifacts of preparation (Figures 16.5 and 16.6). These artifacts, as well as potential underlying causes and fixes, are detailed in Table 16.1.

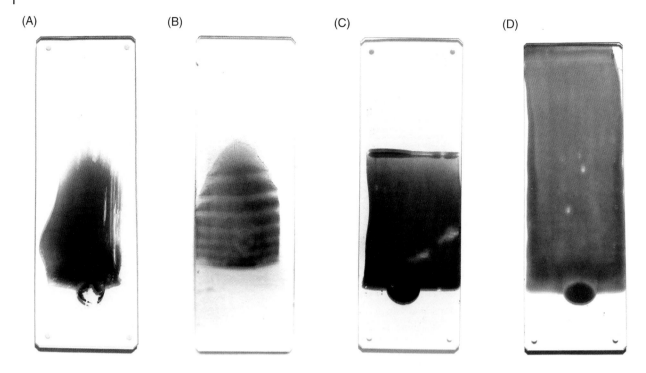

Figure 16.5 Blood smear preparation artifacts: (A) streaking (linear), (B) streaking (horizontal), (C) flat end, and (D) blood pushed off edge.

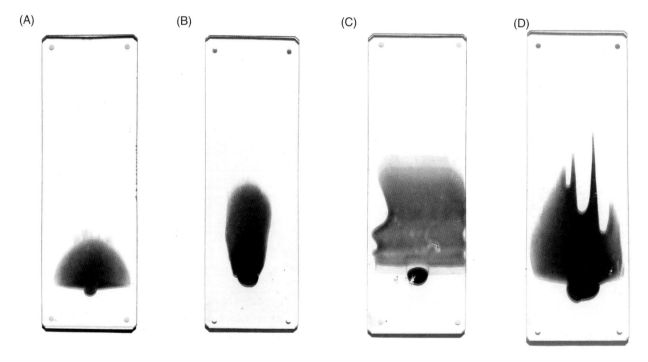

Figure 16.6 Blood smear preparation artifacts: (A) smear too short, (B) narrow smear, (C) irregular/wavy smear, and (D) irregular feathered edge.

Table 16.1 Common artifacts of blood smear preparation, with potential causes and solutions.

Problem	Potential cause	Potential fix	Figure
Streaking (linear)	• Debris on slide • Dried blood on spreader slide • Slow spreading	• Clean slide surface • Clean the end of the spreader slide if making multiple smears for the same patient • Spread blood in steady constant motion	Figure 16.5A
Streaking (horizontal)	• Hesitation or uneven pressure when spreading	• Push spreader slide with constant, even pressure	Figure 16.5B
Flat end of the smear	• Abrupt stop or lifting at the end of spreading motion • Slow spreading	• Push the spreader slide to the end of the smear without lifting or stopping motion • Spread blood in steady constant motion	Figure 16.5C
Blood pushed off the edge	• Drop of blood too big • Spreader slide angle too low	• Use smaller drops of blood • Increase the angle of the spreader slide	Figure 16.5D
Smear too short	• Drop of blood too small • Spreader slide angle too high	• Increase the size of blood drop • Decrease the angle of the spreader slide	Figure 16.6A
Narrow smear	• Drop of blood too small • Smear made before blood spread across the spreader slide	• Increase the size of blood drop • Allow blood to spread along the full edge of the spreader slide	Figure 16.6B
Irregular/wavy smear	• Excessive downward pressure • Wobbling spreader slide	• Do not place a finger on top of the spreader slide • Hold spreader slide with light but constant pressure	Figure 16.6C
Irregular feathered edge	• Wobbling spreader slide	• Hold spreader slide with light but constant pressure	Figure 16.6D

16.3 Blood Smear Staining and Handling

Blood smears are typically stained with Romanowsky-type stains for routine assessment. Examples of Romanowsky stains include Wright stain, Giemsa stain, May-Grünwald-Giemsa, and Leishman stain. These stains contain eosin that binds to basic components of the cells and stains them pink (e.g., hemoglobin in erythrocytes), and methylene blue that binds to the acidic components of cells and stains them blue (e.g., nuclei).

16.3.1 Rapid Romanowsky-type Stains

Rapid Romanowsky-type stains including Diff-Quik (Siemens, Munich, Germany) and Hema 3® (Fisher Scientific, Pittsburgh, PA) are available for in-clinic use. Methanol is used as fixative; however, the stains are aqueous-based.

16.3.1.1 Rapid Stain Procedure
The following steps detail how to maximize the stain quality of blood smears using rapid Romanowsky-type stains:

1) Gloves should be worn when staining slides, and forceps or a wooden peg can be used to hold the slide during staining.

2) Slides should be fixed within 1 hour of blood smear preparation. They cannot be over-fixed; however, under-fixation of slides greatly affects stain quality and may lead to cellular lysis or poor stain uptake. Increasing fixation time greatly increases the stain quality of the smear. Slides should be dipped in the fixative until evenly and completely covered and then allowed to sit in the fixative for 1–2 minutes. After this time, remove them and allow excess fixative to drain by holding the slide onto an absorbent pad.

3) Dip the slide into solution 1 (eosin) to completely and evenly cover it and then dip the slide a further 4–6 times for approximately 1 second per dip.

4) Allow excess stain to drain before repeating this step for solution 2 (methylene blue). *Note*: The number of dips and time spent in the eosin and methylene blue stains can and should be tailored to the needs of the sample and preference of the observer to increase or decrease stain intensity.

5) Rinse the slide thoroughly with water (ideally deionized) and stand it vertically with the feathered edge up to dry.

It is imperative that slides are completely dry prior to staining to avoid artifacts, especially those affecting erythrocytes such as refractile inclusions, which may also be

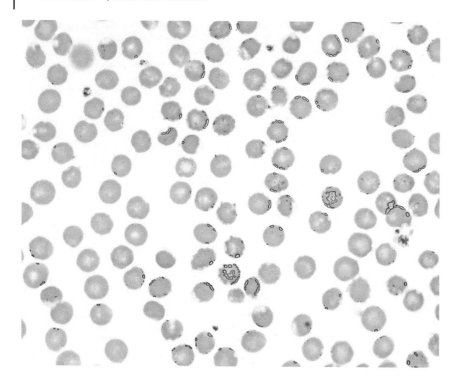

Figure 16.7 Blood smear, dog, 100× objective. Refractile artifact. Note the irregular, shiny refractile artifacts, often along the periphery of the erythrocytes.

seen if there is water contamination of the fixative solution (Figure 16.7). Slides should never be heat fixed (to avoid heat damage of cells); rather air-dried by blowing on the slide or using the cool setting on a hair dryer [4].

16.3.2 New Methylene Blue

New methylene blue (NMB) is a supravital stain that is helpful in evaluating Heinz bodies, as well as reticulocytes, especially in cats where punctate reticulocytes are prevalent and do not typically stain as blue/purple-tinged polychromatophils with routine hematology stains.

Methylene blue stains precipitate RNA, which is visible under the microscope as dark blue granules known as *reticulum* within immature anucleated red blood cells (reticulocytes) (see Figure 17.11). Increased numbers of reticulocytes in circulation indicate the release of immature red blood cells by the bone marrow, most frequently associated with a regenerative response to anemia. Such stains also stain aggregates of oxidized hemoglobin (Heinz bodies).

Supplies
- EDTA anticoagulated blood.
- NMB stain.
- Disposable pipettes.
- Glass or plastic test tubes.
- Timer.
- Microscope slides.

Procedure
1) Place 1 drop of well-mixed EDTA anticoagulated blood into a test tube.
2) Add 1 drop of reticulocyte stain to the test tube containing patient blood and mix thoroughly.
3) Set the timer for 10 minutes.
4) After 10 minutes, mix the contents of the test tube again.
5) Use a clean pipette to place 1 small drop of well-mixed sample onto a glass slide and prepare a blood smear (see Section 16.2).
6) Dry the slide quickly and allow it to sit for 5 minutes to dry completely.

Important considerations
- Optimal results obtained on fresh samples (refrigerated and <48 hours old).
- Gently mix NMB stain prior to use.
- Periodic filtering using Whatman Grade 4 filter paper may be required if increased precipitation is seen in stored NMB stain.

Interpretation
Mature erythrocytes have a homogeneous blue/green appearance. Immature anucleated erythrocytes contain aggregated RNA (reticulum) that appears as fine dots (punctate reticulocytes) or larger strings/clumps of coarse granules (aggregate reticulocytes) (see Chapter 17, Figure 17.11).

Figure 16.8 Blood smear, dog, 100× objective. Stain precipitation. Fine, variably clumped, purple granular material is seen across the background of the smear and overlaying red blood cells. This can mimic infectious organisms including *Mycoplasma* spp. (compare to Figure 17.49).

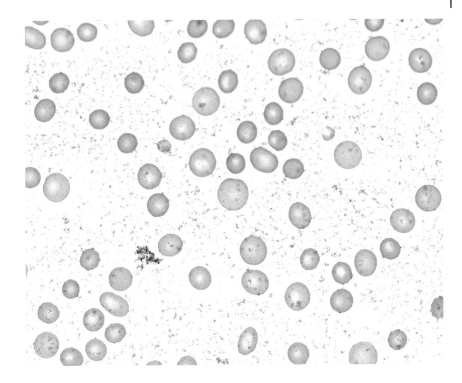

16.3.3 Stain Care and Quality Assurance

Careful maintenance of stains will dramatically affect stain quality. Ensure that fresh, clean stains are used to prevent excessive stain precipitation or contamination artifacts, which can mimic infectious organisms (Figure 16.8) [5]. Using separate Coplin jars for hematology, and cytology stains is preferable, as this reduces contamination artifacts on blood smears and increases the lifespan of the stains used for hematology. For further details on stain care, quality assurance, and the advantages and limitations of rapid Romanowsky-type stains, please refer to Chapter 1, Section 1.3.

16.3.4 Slide Handling

Stained hematology slides should be stored at room temperature, preferably in plastic slide containers to prevent breaking. Slides should not be stored in the refrigerator, or exposed to extreme temperatures. This is especially true for unstained slides, as hemoglobin crystal formation may occur, preventing evaluation of red blood cells and leukocytes that frequently rupture (Figure 16.9).

16.4 Blood Smear Evaluation

16.4.1 Approach to Blood Smear Evaluation

Four major categories should be evaluated on a blood smear:

1) Erythrocytes.
2) Leukocytes.
3) Platelets.
4) Background features and miscellaneous cells.

Each of these will be discussed in detail in the following chapters. Much like performing a physical exam, it is helpful to follow a routine when evaluating blood smears to ensure all these elements are evaluated and no findings are missed. While it can be tempting to focus only on abnormalities detected by hematology analyzers (e.g., low platelet concentration) or other diagnostic test results (e.g., altered PCV), it is important to still evaluate all components of the blood smear for a comprehensive analysis. This is especially important as many crucial pathologic findings may not be obvious or detected by automated instruments or other tests, and the ultimate cause of these changes may be separate from the cell line(s) affected. For example, Rickettsial organisms may be seen in leukocytes of a patient with thrombocytopenia.

While each category could be assessed prior to moving to the next (i.e., full evaluation of erythrocytes, then leukocytes, etc.), important findings for each require examination at both low- and high-power objectives, such that the author recommends starting at a low-power objective and evaluating relevant components of all four categories each time the objective is changed. This is an efficient way to constantly move forward with slide evaluation, without moving between objectives, which is time consuming and cumbersome, especially when using coverslips or oil.

Slide evaluation should start on a low-power objective such as 4× or 10× where the reviewer can comfortably and confidently evaluate relevant features. Think about the

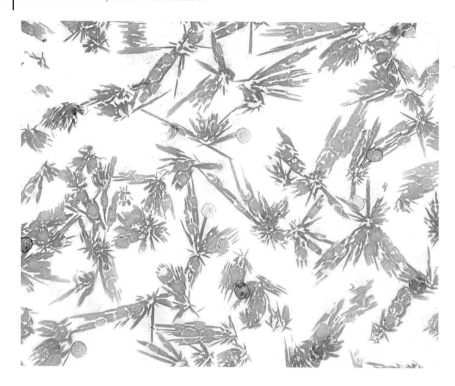

Figure 16.9 Blood smear, dog, 100× objective. Hemoglobin crystal formation secondary to exposure to cold temperatures (slide transported with ice packs). The blue round structures represent lysed nuclei of leukocytes.

four features to be evaluated, and which components are visible at that objective. Once erythrocytes, leukocytes, platelets, and background features have all been considered, move to the next higher objective, and repeat this process. In general, large objects and the distribution of cells are evaluated at lower power objectives, while small objects and cellular details are reviewed at higher power objectives. The remainder of this section will outline this approach to blood smear evaluation in more detail based on the important features to evaluate on each objective, and can be used as a helpful checklist when reviewing blood smears.

16.4.1.1 4× or 10× Objective
Erythrocytes
- Evaluate red blood cell density. The monolayer will be longer with anemia and shorter with erythrocytosis. This is an important quality control check for results from the erythrogram (HCT, Hb, and RBCC) and manual PCV.
- Evaluate red blood cell distribution, especially for any agglutination.

Leukocytes
- Evaluate leukocyte distribution. Subjectively estimate leukocytosis, leukopenia, or normal leukocyte concentration and check if the cells are distributed evenly across the slide or if they are clumped at the feathered edge. This will help the observer perform and interpret a manual differential.

- Evaluate for any large leukocytes such as mast cells or neoplastic cells that are often more obvious at lower objectives (and may be missed if present in low numbers and only higher objectives are evaluated). Such cells are often pushed to the feathered edge.

Platelets
- Assess for any large platelet clumps. These are often pushed to the feathered edge of the slide; however, the body of the smear should also be evaluated for platelet clumps at this objective.

Background features
- Evaluate for any large infectious agents, especially microfilaria.
- Evaluate the background for any color change or evidence of cryoglobulinemia.
- Look for any large or atypical cells, including megakaryocytes.

16.4.1.2 40× or 50× Objective
Erythrocytes
- Evaluate for any rouleaux formation.

Leukocytes
- The best objectives to perform a leukocyte differential.
- Often the best objectives to perform a quantitative leukocyte concentration estimate if required, though a lower objective (in cases of leukopenia) or higher

objective (in cases of leukocytosis) may be required (see Chapter 18, Section 18.1 for details).

- Evaluate for toxic changes within the neutrophil line.
- Examine carefully for infectious agents (e.g., *Hepatozoon* spp., Rickettsial morulae, etc.).

Platelets

- Examine any platelet aggregates that were noted on lower objectives to ensure platelets are present and they are not just fibrin clots.

Background features

- Evaluate overall stain quality, including even and adequate staining of red and white blood cells.
- Evaluate for medium-sized infectious agents including *Trypanosoma cruzi*, *Hepatozoon* spp., etc.
- Evaluate for atypical cells including apoptotic cells, mitotic figures, and plasma cells, as well as ruptured cells and cytoplasmic fragments.

16.4.1.3 100× Objective

Erythrocytes

- Evaluate red blood cell morphology, including shape changes (poikilocytosis) and color changes (e.g., polychromatophils and hypochromasia).
- Carefully examine the red blood cells for inclusions, which may include organisms (e.g., *Mycoplasma* spp. or *Babesia* spp.) as well as basophilic stippling, Howell Jolly bodies, Heinz bodies, etc.

Leukocytes

- Evaluate leukocyte morphology, especially slight toxic changes in neutrophils.
- Examine for leukocyte inclusions, including infectious agents, granules within lymphocytes, and granules/pigment within neutrophils.

Platelets

- Platelet estimates are performed at 100× objective.
- Also, evaluate platelet morphology (platelet activation, degranulation, vacuolation, infectious agents).

Background features

- Evaluate for small background features including stain precipitation and infectious agents such as bacteria, including *Mycoplasma* spp. that may detach from erythrocytes, especially in stored blood.

16.4.2 Important Considerations

It is important to evaluate cell morphology (including red blood cell shape and leukocyte identification) and to perform most cell analyses (including platelet estimates and leukocyte differentials) within the monolayer of the smear. The monolayer is a relatively short region that lies between the feathered edge and the body of the smear. Within this region, approximately half of the red blood cells are touching each other and half are not touching other erythrocytes (Figure 16.10). It is still important to evaluate other areas

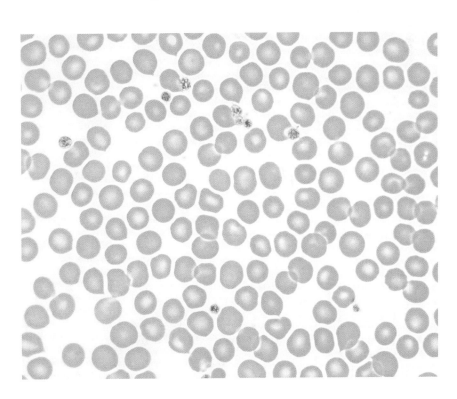

Figure 16.10 Blood smear, dog, 100× objective. Erythrocyte monolayer. Note that approximately half the cells are touching, and half are individualized.

of the slide, particularly the feathered edge, where larger cells or organisms may be pushed.

Note: 40× objectives are designed to be used with a coverslip! This objective will appear opaque or foggy if a coverslip is not used – regardless of the cleanliness of the objective lens. The coverslip can be placed on top of the dry slide, which allows easy removal and toggling to lower objectives if required. Alternatively, a small drop of oil can be placed on the slide to keep the coverslip in place and then removed to allow examination of the slide on oil objectives (50× or 100× objective lenses).

16.5 Hematology Procedures and Techniques

Some procedures discussed in the following hematology chapters are incredibly helpful to maximize the diagnostic potential of blood samples or increase the efficiency of diagnosis. Some of these procedures include a saline agglutination test (SAT) and buffy coat evaluation, which are described in Sections 16.5.1 and 16.5.2.

16.5.1 Saline Agglutination Test

Rouleaux formation (stacking of red blood cells in linear rows) and red blood cell agglutination (aggregation of erythrocytes) can be difficult to distinguish accurately by microscopic inspection of a peripheral blood smear. A SAT may be required to differentiate these erythrocyte distribution patterns.

Supplies
- EDTA anticoagulated blood.
- Phosphate buffered normal saline.
- Glass or plastic test tubes.
- Disposable pipettes (×3).
- Glass slides and coverslips.
- Microscope.

Procedure
1) Place 1 drop of well-mixed anticoagulated blood into the test tube using a clean pipette.
2) Use a new pipette and add 4 drops of saline into the test tube.
3) Gently mix the blood and saline mixture.
4) Use a new pipette to place 1 drop of the 1:5 dilution onto the glass slide and cover with a coverslip.
5) Examine the slides as a wet-mount preparation using the 10× and 40× objectives on the microscope.

Interpretation
Dispersion of red blood cells individually across the slide supports the presence of rouleaux, and the SAT is

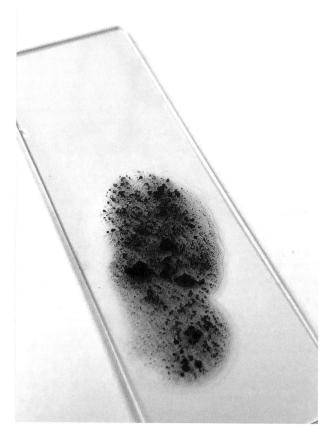

Figure 16.11 Saline agglutination test. Gross agglutination in a sample from a dog with immune-mediated hemolytic anemia.

considered negative. Clumping of red blood cells supports autoagglutination (and a positive SAT), especially if large or numerous clumps are present, which may be visible grossly on the slide (Figure 16.11). If only rare clumps are seen or the separation of red blood cells is unclear, a 1:10 dilution may be necessary and is often required in patients with marked hyperglobulinemia. If red blood cell clumping does not disperse after a 1:10 dilution, the sample is considered positive for autoagglutination (Figure 16.12). This procedure has high sensitivity, and specificity increases with increased dilution [6].

16.5.2 Buffy Coat

Centrifuged blood separates into three distinct visual layers (Figure 16.13). Erythrocytes are located at the bottom of a hematocrit tube as a prominent red layer. Plasma or serum is the top layer, and is clear in healthy dogs and cats, but may be discolored in disease (e.g., red with intravascular hemolysis or yellow with icterus). Located between the red cells and plasma/serum layers, is a variably thick (mostly thin) white layer, comprising leukocytes and platelets, known as the *buffy coat*. Buffy coat preparations examine this concentrated layer for efficient review of nucleated

Figure 16.12 Saline agglutination test. Positive microscopic agglutination in a dog with immune-mediated hemolytic anemia.

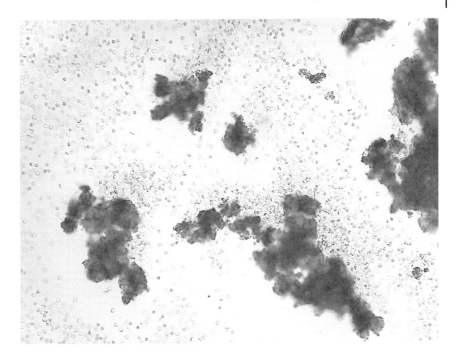

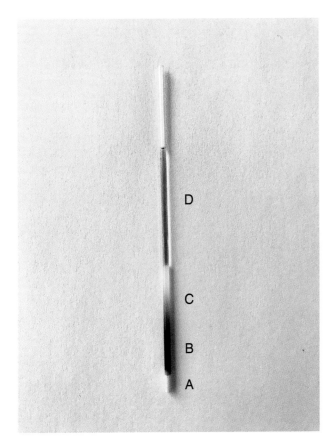

Figure 16.13 Microhematocrit tube of centrifuged blood from a dog with chronic lymphocytic leukemia (lymphocyte concentration of 1 200 000 cells μl⁻¹). A clay plug (A) is at the bottom of the tube. A column of red blood cells settles above this (B) and above that is the 'buffy coat' (C) of white blood cells and platelets, which is very wide in this case due to the marked lymphocytosis. The plasma column (D) is seen above the buffy coat and is clear.

cells. This may facilitate the identification of mast cells [7, 8], megakaryocytes, other atypical nucleated cells, or infectious agents within leukocytes such as Rickettsial bacteria and *Hepatozoon* spp. [9, 10]

Supplies
- Fresh (less than 24 hours old) EDTA anticoagulated whole blood.
- Microhematocrit tubes.
- Clay or tube sealing compound.
- Microhematocrit centrifuge.
- Glass slide or etcher.
- Glass slides.
- Personal protective equipment (latex or nitrile gloves and protective eyewear).

Procedure
1) A well-mixed sample is imperative. EDTA blood should be ideally mixed for 5 minutes on a rocker or inverted gently a minimum of 25 times.
2) Fill four microhematocrit tubes to 75% capacity.
3) Seal the end of the microhematocrit tube with clay or sealing compound.
4) Centrifuge the microhematocrit tubes at 10 000 RPM for 5 minutes.
5) Use an etcher or glass slide to score the tubes just below the white buffy coat layer.
6) Place gentle pressure at the score line to break the tube in the direction away from the face.
7) Tap the section of the microhematocrit tube with the buffy coat layer gently onto a clean glass slide, mixing cells, and a small amount of plasma.

8) Make a pull smear by placing a second clean glass slide on top of the slide with the white blood cell/plasma mixture, and gently pull the top spreader slide over the bottom slide to create a monolayer of cells.

9) Repeat steps 6–8 for all microhematocrit tubes to make several buffy coat smears.

10) Allow the slides to dry for 5 minutes before staining.

References

1 Zini, G. (2014) Stability of complete blood count parameters with storage: toward defined specifications for different diagnostic applications. *Int. J. Lab. Hematol.*, **36** (2), 111–113.

2 Furlanello, T., Tasca, S., Caldin, M., *et al.* (2006) Artifactual changes in canine blood following storage, detected using the ADVIA 120 hematology analyzer. *Vet. Clin. Pathol.*, **35** (1), 42–46.

3 Basu, D., Veluru, H. (2019) A study of storage related changes and effect of refrigeration on hematological parameters and blood cell morphology in EDTA anticoagulated blood. *Ann. Pathol. Lab. Med.*, **6** (5), 289–296.

4 De Witte, F.G., Hebrard, A., Grimes, C.N., *et al.* (2020) Effects of different drying methods on smears of canine blood and effusion fluid. *Peer. J.*, **8**, e10092. doi: 10.7717/peerj.10092.

5 Houwen, B. (2002) Blood film preparation and staining procedures. *Clin. Lab. Med.*, **22** (1), 1–14.

6 Sun, P.L., Jeffery, U. (2021) Effect of dilution of canine blood samples on the specificity of saline agglutination tests for immune-mediated hemolysis. *J. Vet. Intern. Med.*, **34** (6), 2374–2383.

7 McManus, P.M. (1999) Frequency and severity of mastocytemia in dogs with and without mast cell tumors: 120 cases (1995–1997). *J. Am. Vet. Med. Assoc.*, **215** (3), 355–357.

8 Skeldon, N.C.A., Gerber, K.L., Wilson, R.J., *et al.* (2010) Mastocytemia in cats: prevalence, detection and quantification methods, haematological associations and potential implications in 30 cats with mast cell tumours. *J. Feline Med. Surg.*, **12** (12), 960–966.

9 Mylonakis, M.E., Koutinas, A.F., Billinis, C., *et al.* (2003) Evaluation of cytology in the diagnosis of acute canine monocytic ehrlichiosis (*Ehrlichia canis*): a comparison between five methods. *Vet. Microbiol.*, **91** (2–3), 197–204.

10 Schäfer, I., Müller, E., Nijhof, A.M., *et al.* (2022) First evidence of vertical Hepatozoon canis transmission in dogs in Europe. *Parasit. Vectors*, **15** (1), 296.

17

Erythrocytes

17.1 Approach to Evaluating Red Blood Cells

A thorough and accurate evaluation of erythrocytes can provide key insights for the diagnosis, treatment, and monitoring of disease in dogs and cats. Visual evaluation of red blood cells on a blood smear, combined with assessment of parameters from an automated CBC, provides the most comprehensive and powerful diagnostic information, and three major characteristics of erythrocytes (described in detail in this chapter) should be evaluated:

1) Distribution of red blood cells on the smear.
2) Morphology of red blood cells (including shape and color).
3) Inclusions.

Accurate assessment of red blood cells requires fresh samples that are appropriately prepared. A well-mixed, EDTA anticoagulated sample is preferred. The effect of storage on red blood morphology and CBC parameters is well documented and morphologic changes manifest within 3 hours when blood is stored at room temperature. Samples should be evaluated ideally within 2 hours or within 6–8 hours for refrigerated (4°C) samples [1–3]. It is best practice to make a blood smear within the first 2 hours of the blood draw, which should be fixed within the first hour of preparation to preserve red blood cell morphology. This slide can be evaluated at a later time and can be sent with the blood sample to the laboratory.

It is important to evaluate red blood cells on low- and high-power objectives. Red blood cell distribution including the length of the monolayer and initial evaluation of agglutination is best performed on low-power objectives (e.g., 10× or 20× objective), while morphology and inclusions are performed at higher objective magnification. Red blood cell morphology should be evaluated using a 100× objective in the monolayer of the smear, where half the cells are touching and half are individualized. If shape change (poikilocytosis) is noted, a minimum of 1000 cells would ideally be evaluated to provide a precise percentage of a particular poikilocyte [4, 5].

The following sections outline in detail the approach to evaluating and interpreting erythrocytes on a peripheral blood smear.

17.2 Red Blood Cell Distribution

The distribution of erythrocytes on a blood smear can give vital clues to underlying disease in a patient and is an important part of peripheral blood smear evaluation. Many of the parameters discussed in the following sections can be subjective, and should be correlated with other test results as available and may need to be complemented with other diagnostic procedures (e.g., saline agglutination test to help differentiate agglutination and rouleaux formation, or a PCV to evaluate red cell mass). Red blood cell distribution needs to be assessed on both low- and high-power objectives and involves evaluation of the monolayer and body of the smear. A high-quality blood smear is therefore imperative for accurate evaluation of red blood cell distribution; see Chapter 16, Section 16.2 for tips on blood smear preparation.

17.2.1 Anemia

17.2.1.1 Morphologic Appearance
Blood smears from anemic patients will have an elongated monolayer. A monolayer may be difficult to identify or nonexistent in severely anemic patients with very low red blood cell mass (Figure 17.1).

17.2.1.2 Clinical Considerations
- Anemia refers to a decrease in measures of erythrocyte mass (PCV, hematocrit, hemoglobin, and RBC concentration) below the reference intervals, ideally adjusted for age and breed.

Clinical Atlas of Small Animal Cytology and Hematology, Second Edition. Andrew G. Burton.
© 2024 John Wiley & Sons, Inc. Published 2024 by John Wiley & Sons, Inc.

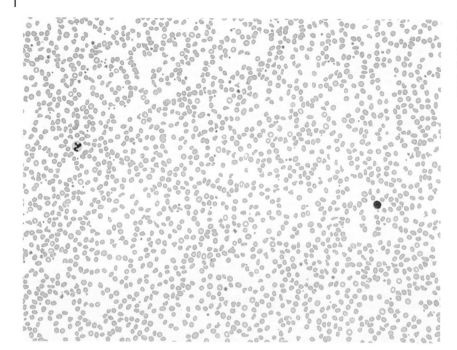

Figure 17.1 Blood smear, dog, 10× objective. Anemia (PCV = 16%). Note that the red blood cells are seldom touching, with no monolayer present even at low magnification. A neutrophil (left) and a lymphocyte (right) are also present.

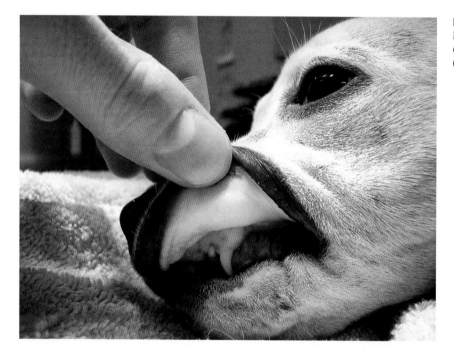

Figure 17.2 White mucous membranes in a puppy with severe anemia (PCV = 6%) secondary to *Ancylostoma caninum* (hookworm) infection.

- Clinical signs = patients often present with pale mucous membranes (Figure 17.2) and may also have an elevated heart rate or respiratory rate. Lethargy, obtunded mentation, or collapse may be seen in cases of severe or acute anemia.
- Anemia may be classified as regenerative or non-regenerative based on the bone marrow's ability to respond appropriately.

Regenerative Anemia
Destruction or loss of red blood cells will lead to a regenerative anemia if the bone marrow has sufficient time and substrates to upregulate erythropoiesis.

- Destruction: Often associated with immune-mediated anemia (see Section 17.3.7), infectious disease (see Section 17.5), or oxidative damage (see Sections 17.3.12 and 17.4.3).

- Loss: Hemorrhage may occur secondary to trauma, coagulopathy, bleeding ulcers or tumors, etc.

Note: It is also very important to evaluate the appropriateness of the regenerative response. A severe anemia (e.g., a PCV <15%) should be accompanied by a strong regenerative response (>300 000 reticulocytes μl^{-1} for dogs and >200 000 reticulocytes μl^{-1} for cats). If only a mild increase in the reticulocyte concentration is present, this regenerative response would be insufficient and may indicate an early or ineffective response. Serial monitoring of the erythrogram in these cases is imperative.

Non-regenerative Anemia The bone marrow may fail to produce an effective regenerative response seen in the periphery, and the major mechanisms responsible for this are as follows.

Pre-regenerative stage
- Upregulation of erythropoiesis and a regenerative response takes 3–5 days to produce a reticulocytosis. Acute hemolysis or hemorrhage may therefore initially be associated with a non-regenerative anemia.

Decreased production
- Anemia of inflammation: Anemia of inflammation is mediated by three major pathophysiologic mechanisms: [6]

    i) Hepcidin = an acute phase protein that causes retention of iron within macrophages and decreases iron absorption by degrading the iron transporter ferroportin.
    ii) Impaired erythropoiesis = inflammatory cytokines such as IL-1, TNF, and IL-6 can inhibit the formation of erythropoietin (EPO) and decrease the responsiveness of EPO receptors. IFN-γ may also induce apoptosis in erythroid precursors.
    iii) Decreased RBC survival.

Possibly associated with anemia of inflammation, anemia in geriatric patients has also been described in dogs [7].
- Iron deficiency: Can be associated with chronic hemorrhage, nutritional deficiency, or hepatic dysfunction.
- Chronic renal disease: Associated with decreased EPO production.
- Primary bone marrow disease: Including drug/toxin exposure, neoplasia (e.g., leukemia or metastatic disease), myelofibrosis, immune-mediated disease (including precursor-targeted immune-mediated anemia) [8], and infectious disease (e.g., retroviral disease in cats).

17.2.2 Erythrocytosis

17.2.2.1 Morphologic Appearance
Blood smears from patients with erythrocytosis have a very short or nonexistent monolayer (Figure 17.3).

Figure 17.3 Blood smear, dog (same dog as Figure 17.4), 20× objective. Erythrocytosis (PCV = 77%). Note that all red blood cells are touching, with no monolayer present even at low magnification.

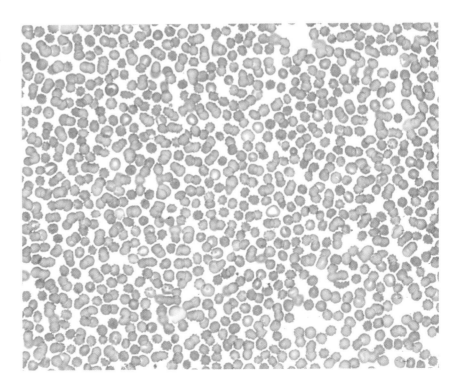

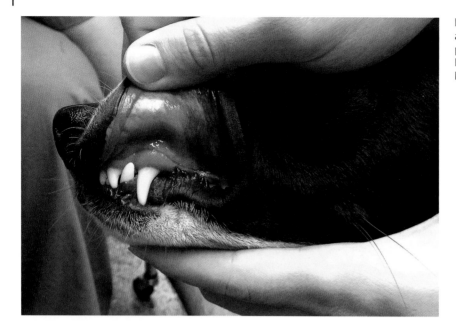

Figure 17.4 Red mucous membranes in a dog (same dog as Figure 17.3) with primary erythrocytosis and PCV of 77%. Note also the bright red color of the haired skin of the lower lip.

17.2.2.2 Clinical Considerations

- Erythrocytosis refers to an increase in measures of red blood cell mass (PCV, hematocrit, hemoglobin, and RBC concentration) above reference intervals, ideally adjusted for age and breed. For example, Greyhounds typically have higher measures of erythrocyte mass in health than most other dog breeds [9].
- Polycythemia is *not* an interchangeable term. Polycythemia vera is used in human medicine to describe a myeloproliferative neoplasm, and given species variation in manifestation of this disease, *primary erythrocytosis* is a more appropriate term in veterinary species.
- Clinical signs = patients often present with hyperemic mucous membranes (Figure 17.4). Clinical signs vary based on the underlying cause and may be absent or include signs of dehydration (in cases of relative erythrocytosis), bleeding tendencies, increased respiratory rate/effort, and neurologic signs (seizures and mentation changes) [10, 11].
- Erythrocytosis may be due to a relative process (altered ratio of erythrocytes to plasma), or an absolute process with increased production of erythrocytes by the bone marrow.

Relative Erythrocytosis

- Loss of isotonic fluid (dehydration).
- Redistribution of red blood cells (splenic contraction). Can be seen with epinephrine release, drug exposure such as acepromazine, exercise, or pain. Splenic HCT is approximately 80–90%, and contraction can increase peripheral HCT 1.5-fold in cats [12, 13].

Absolute Erythrocytosis
Primary

- Myeloproliferative disease (primary erythrocytosis) [10] (see Section 17.5.1 for more clinical details).

Secondary

- Appropriate: Chronic hypoxia, cardiac disease (such as right-to-left shunts) [14], chronic lung diseases [15].
- Inappropriate: EPO-secreting tumors [16].

17.2.3 Agglutination

17.2.3.1 Morphologic Appearance

On a peripheral blood smear, agglutination of red blood cells is characterized by aggregates of erythrocytes that appear as 'bunches of grapes' (Figures 17.5 and 17.6). These aggregates can be variably sized and variably dense. Evaluation for agglutination should ideally be performed in the monolayer to avoid overinterpretation that may occur in thick areas of the slide. Agglutination may also be seen macroscopically as red granules within a well-mixed blood tube or on a slide with a saline agglutination test (see Figures 16.11 and 16.12).

17.2.3.2 Clinical Considerations

- Agglutination indicates the presence of surface-bound anti-erythrocyte immunoglobulins binding multiple red blood cells. This is most frequently associated with IgM due to its pentameric structure with a greater number of, and greater distance between, binding sites [17].

Figure 17.5 Blood smear, dog, 50× objective. Agglutination secondary to immune-mediated hemolytic anemia. Note the numerous, dense, irregularly shaped aggregates of erythrocytes.

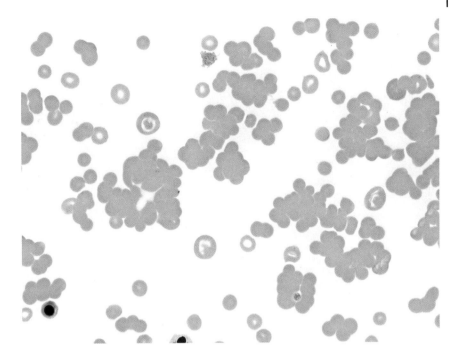

Figure 17.6 Blood smear, dog, 100× objective. Agglutination secondary to immune-mediated hemolytic anemia. Erythrocytes aggregate like 'bunches of grapes'.

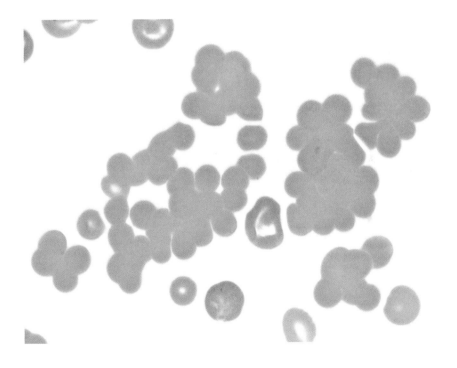

- Immune-mediated hemolytic anemia (IMHA) is the most common cause of agglutination [18].
- EDTA may rarely cause anticoagulant-induced agglutination reported in a cat, but not in dogs [19].
- Saline agglutination testing may be required to differentiate autoagglutination of red blood cells from marked rouleaux. A saline agglutination test may be performed by adding 1 drop of anticoagulated blood and 5–10 drops of physiologic saline to a test tube, mixing the sample well, and then placing a drop of this diluted blood on a glass slide with a coverslip and examining it as a wet mount. If rouleaux is present, the red blood cells will disperse, while agglutinated red blood cells will remain clumped. This procedure has high sensitivity, and specificity increases with increased dilution [20].

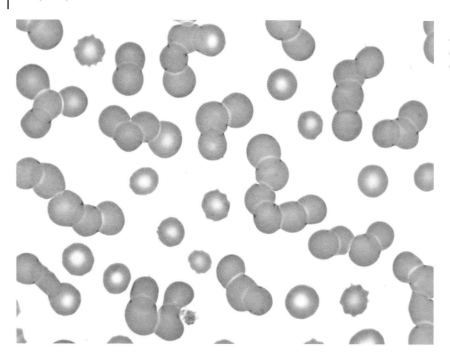

Figure 17.7 Blood smear, dog, 100× objective. Rouleaux formation. Note the organized, linear arrangement of the erythrocytes, like 'stacks of coins'.

17.2.4 Rouleaux Formation

17.2.4.1 Morphologic Appearance
Rouleaux is characterized by linear rows of erythrocytes that resemble 'stacks of coins' (Figure 17.7).

17.2.4.2 Clinical Considerations
- Rouleaux formation can be seen in blood smears from healthy cats due to less negatively charged cell membrane surfaces resulting in reduced electrostatic repulsive forces and is more common in the body of the smear than the monolayer.
- The finding of rouleaux formation in dogs and increased rouleaux in cats is an abnormal finding, most frequently associated with hyperglobulinemia.
- A saline agglutination test may be helpful to differentiate rouleaux formation from agglutination (see Section 17.2.3.2).

17.3 Red Blood Cell Morphology

17.3.1 Normal Erythrocytes

17.3.1.1 Morphologic Appearance
Dog   Mature canine erythrocytes are anucleated, discoid cells that are biconcave with an area of central pallor taking up approximately one-third of the cell (Figure 17.8). They are approximately 7 μm in diameter; however, breed variation may occur with some breeds having smaller (e.g., Akita, Shiba Inu, Shar Pei, and other Asian descent breeds), or larger (e.g., Poodles) erythrocytes normally

[21–23]. The life span of canine erythrocytes is approximately 110–120 days [24, 25].

Cat   Mature feline erythrocytes are anucleated, discoid cells that are biconcave but typically lack central pallor (Figure 17.9). They are smaller than canine erythrocytes, though their size is slightly more variable, approximately 5–6 μm in diameter. The life span of feline erythrocytes is approximately 65–80 days [25, 26].

17.3.2 Polychromatophils and Reticulocytes

17.3.2.1 Morphologic Appearance
Reticulocytes are immature, anucleate erythrocytes. Those that stain blue or blue-tinged on routine hematology stains are called polychromatophils. Polychromatophils are typically larger than normal erythrocytes and stain blue, blue-tinged, or purple with routine hematology stains due to increased proteins such as ribosomes in their cytoplasm (Figure 17.10). *Note*: Polychromatophils may be difficult to evaluate in overstained slides. Reticulocytes can be evaluated more accurately by using reticulocyte stains such as New Methylene Blue (NMB) which precipitates ribosomal RNA that is readily identified in reticulocytes as either chunky and coarse (aggregate reticulocytes) or fine (punctate reticulocytes) inclusions (Figure 17.11).

17.3.2.2 Clinical Considerations
- Low numbers of polychromatophils (less than 1.5% of erythrocytes) can be seen in healthy dogs. They are rare on blood smears from healthy cats.

Figure 17.8 Blood smear, dog, 100× objective. Normal erythrocyte morphology. The cells have central pallor taking up approximately one-third of the cell.

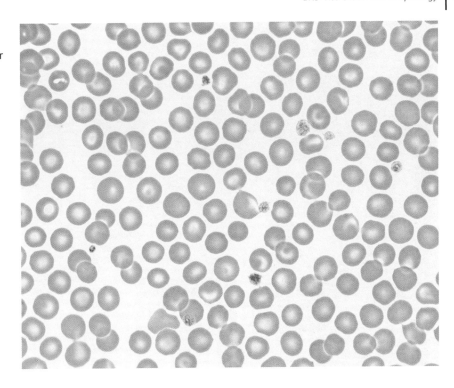

Figure 17.9 Blood smear, cat, 100× objective. Normal erythrocyte morphology. The erythrocytes lack central pallor and are mostly round with only rare, nonspecific shape changes.

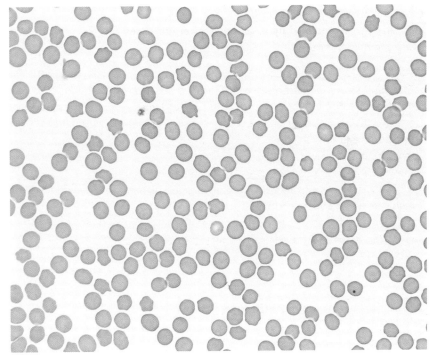

- Increased polychromatophils (and reticulocytes) in circulation typically indicate an appropriate regenerative response by the bone marrow toward anemia.
- In the absence of a reticulocyte concentration, polychromasia is a more accurate indicator of bone marrow regeneration to anemia than red blood cell indices such

as mean cell volume (MCV) and MCHC (e.g., macrocytic hypochromic) and red blood cell distribution width (RDW) (indicating anisocytosis) [27].
- A regenerative response by the bone marrow takes 3–5 days, and the absence of increased polychromatophils does not preclude an emerging regenerative response.

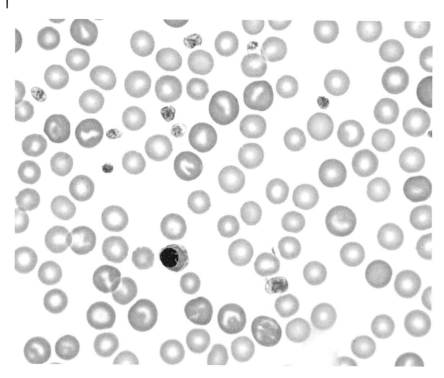

Figure 17.10 Blood smear, dog, 100× objective. Markedly increased polychromatophils (blue staining erythrocytes) in a dog with regenerative anemia due to hemorrhage secondary to rodenticide intoxication. Note the nucleated red blood cell (polychromatophilic rubricyte; lower left).

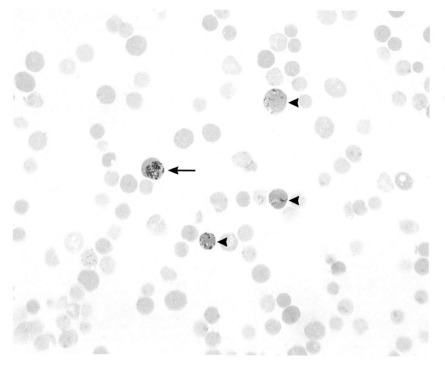

Figure 17.11 Blood smear, cat, 100× objective, New Methylene Blue stain. Reticulocytes stain blue and include punctate reticulocytes (arrowheads) with fine blue inclusions and an aggregate reticulocyte (arrow) with coarse aggregates of reticulin.

- Mild increases in the reticulocyte concentration with normal measures of erythrocyte mass may reflect normal variation, splenic contraction at the time of blood draw, a residual/ongoing regenerative response to previous or compensated anemia and may be seen with hypoxia secondary to cardiac disease and other disease states including inflammation and neoplasia [28–30].

- Punctate reticulocytes do not contain sufficient ribosomes to impart a blue tinge to the cells, and mild or early regenerative anemia in cats may not be associated with increased polychromatophils on routine stained blood smears.

17.3.3 Nucleated Red Blood Cells

17.3.3.1 Morphologic Appearance

The morphology of nucleated red blood cells (nRBCs) from most to least mature is described below:

- Metarubricytes: Metarubricytes are typically the size of a mature red blood cell and may have a polychromatophilic or pink cytoplasm. The nucleus is pyknotic, with a deep purple, homogeneous texture (Figure 17.12).
- Polychromatophilic rubricytes: These cells have lower N/C ratios than basophilic rubricytes, and the cytoplasm has a characteristic pink-blue appearance. Their nuclei have more condensed chromatin, but still have a coarse pattern with pale and dark areas (Figure 17.13).
- Basophilic rubricytes: Basophilic rubricytes are smaller than prorubricytes and have a greater volume of mid-blue cytoplasm. Their nuclei are round and have a coarse, marbled appearance with prominent light and dark areas (Figure 17.13).
- Prorubricytes: Prorubricytes appear similar to rubriblasts; however, they are slightly smaller, have more cytoplasm, lack nucleoli, and have more coarsely granular chromatin (Figure 17.14).
- Rubriblasts: Rubriblasts are large cells with round nuclei that have finely stippled, immature chromatin and typically a single, prominent nucleolus. They have high N/C ratios with a thin rim of deep-blue cytoplasm (Figure 17.15).

17.3.3.2 Clinical Consideration

The presence of increased nRBCs in circulation may be referred to as *rubricytosis* or *metarubricytosis*, though these terms are felt to be inadequate by the author due to the implication of a single stage of erythroid development in circulation, which is seldom the case.

Interpretation of nRBCs in circulation is often considered as either expected/appropriate or inappropriate.

Appropriate

- Normal variation: Low numbers of metarubricytes (<1–2 per 100 WBC) may be seen in healthy patients. Cats may have higher numbers in health than dogs due to the lack of a sinusoidal spleen.
- Splenectomy: Notably in dogs and most prominent in the perioperative stage.
- Splenic contraction: Epinephrine response, drug administration (e.g., acepromazine).
- Regenerative anemia: Low to moderately increased numbers of circulating nRBCs are considered an appropriate part of a regenerative response toward anemia by the bone marrow. *Note*: The presence of nucleated red blood cells alone does NOT indicate a regenerative response by the bone marrow, which requires an increase in reticulocytes/polychromatophils.

Inappropriate

- Drug/toxin exposure: Including lead poisoning and chemotherapeutic agents, which may also cause dysplastic changes [31, 32].

Figure 17.12 Blood smear, dog, 100× objective. Metarubricyte. Note the condensed chromatin pattern of the nucleus.

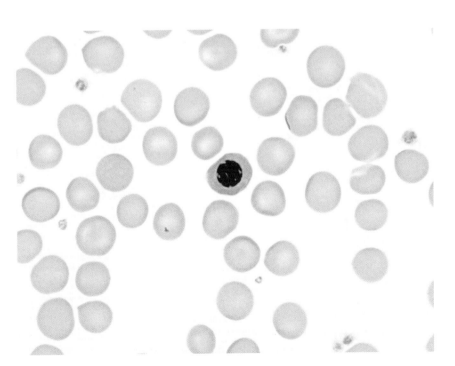

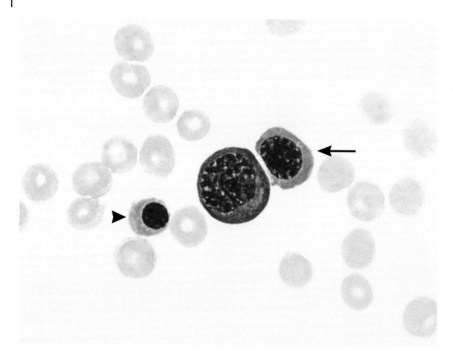

Figure 17.13 Blood smear, dog. Metarubricyte (arrowhead), polychromatophilic rubricyte (arrow), and basophilic rubricyte (center). Note the distinctive marbled chromatin pattern of the rubricytes and increasing blue intensity of the cytoplasm with younger precursors.

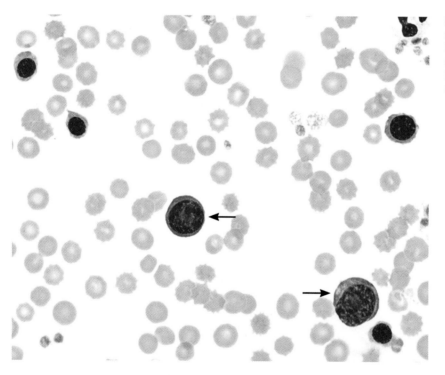

Figure 17.14 Blood smear, dog, 100× objective. Prorubricytes (arrows) that have finely stippled chromatin and a small volume of medium-blue cytoplasm. Polychromatophilic rubricytes and metarubricytes are also present.

- Bone marrow disease/damage: Including septicemia and heatstroke [33].
- Dyserythropoiesis [34].

17.3.3.3 Prognosis

Highly variable based on the underlying cause. In a case-controlled, retrospective study, dogs with an increased absolute nRBC count had a significantly higher mortality rate than controls, which increased with an increase in the absolute count [35]. Additionally, in cases of heatstroke, a marked increase in nRBCs at presentation was highly sensitive and specific for increased risk of death and was highly correlated with secondary complications such as DIC and acute kidney injury [33]. Increased nucleated red blood cells are also associated with increased mortality in acute trauma patients [36].

Figure 17.15 Blood smear, dog, 100× objective. A rubriblast is present with a large prominent nucleolus and a rim of deep blue cytoplasm. Two polychromatophilic rubricytes are also present.

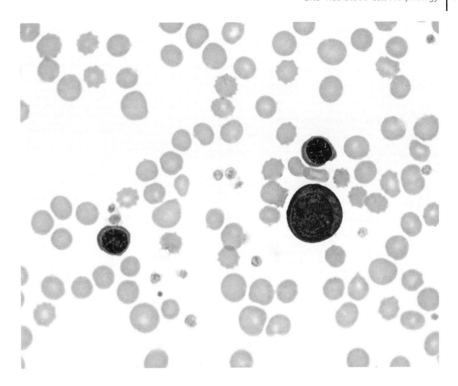

17.3.4 Hypochromatophils

17.3.4.1 Morphologic Appearance

Hypochromatophils are recognized by having increased central pallor in dogs, or the presence of any central pallor in cats, and less vibrant staining cytoplasm (Figure 17.16). Hypochromatophils should be distinguished from torocytes which represent an artifactual change and have sharp edges around the central pallor (compare to Figure 17.36).

17.3.4.2 Clinical Considerations

- Most frequently associated with iron-deficiency anemia.
- Iron-deficient erythrocytes are more fragile and may be associated with increased poikilocytosis (see Section 17.3.6).

Figure 17.16 Blood smear, dog, 100× objective. Hypochromatophils in a dog with portosystemic shunt. Note the increased central pallor exceeding one-third of the cells, and thin rim of pale staining red cytoplasm.

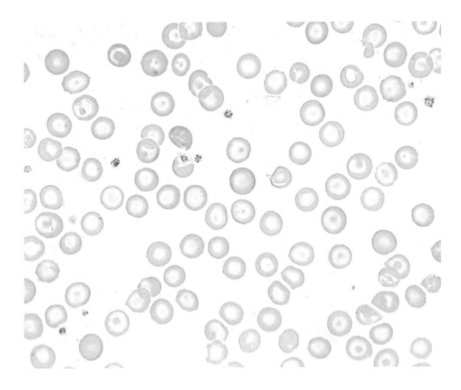

17.3.5 Anisocytosis

17.3.5.1 Morphologic Appearance
Anisocytosis refers to increased variation in the size of erythrocytes seen on a stained blood smear (Figure 17.17).

17.3.5.2 Clinical Considerations
- Anisocytosis is a subjective visual estimation of RDW.
- Variation in size may be due to increased numbers of small or large erythrocytes, or both.
- Potential causes for pathologic large and small erythrocytes may include:
  Large: Regenerative anemia (increased polychromatophils) and feline leukemia virus (FeLV) infection (cats) [37].
  Small: Iron-deficiency anemia, poikilocytosis, red blood cell fragmentation, and hyperthyroidism in cats [38].

17.3.6 Poikilocytes

Poikilocyte is an umbrella term for any red blood cell shape change. Red blood cells can take on innumerous different shapes; however, some have high clinical utility owing to being easily recognizable, reproducible, and associated with specific disease states, giving important clues into the underlying pathology (Figure 17.18). This concept is elegantly summarized by Bessis in his stunning book *Corpuscles: Atlas of red blood cell shapes*: 'The aim of classification could be defeated by the creation of special terms for each and every shape. A new shape deserves a new name only when it is of sufficient frequency and constancy, or its origin of sufficient interest' [39]. It is important to consider that although some poikilocytes lack specific names, this does not exclude the potential for clinical significance. Cats, for example, often have nonspecific poikilocytosis associated with underlying inflammation. It is also common that multiple different shape changes are present in a single blood smear.

When poikilocytes are noted, the number of such cells must be considered. In many cases, the degree of increase correlates to the severity of the underlying disease, and indeed rare instances of any shape change may not be clinically significant. The observation of poikilocytosis should always be interpreted in the context of all available diagnostic information. It is particularly critical for the evaluation of poikilocytes that only smears of high quality, made from fresh blood (EDTA anticoagulated blood less than 2 hours old), are used.

In the following sections, the most clinically important poikilocytes will be discussed, with an emphasis on their characteristic appearance and the underlying pathophysiology leading to their formation.

17.3.7 Spherocytes

17.3.7.1 Morphologic Appearance
Spherocytes are round/spherical, lack central pallor, and their coloration appears more dense than normal

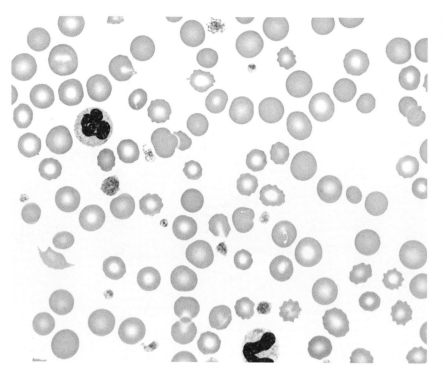

Figure 17.17 Blood smear, dog, 100× objective. Anisocytosis. Note the variation in size of red blood cells.

Figure 17.18 Blood smear, dog, 100× objective. Poikilocytosis. Note the many different shape changes including echinocytes (asterisks), blister cell (arrowhead), codocytes (open arrows), schistocyte (long arrow), acanthocyte (open arrowhead), and hemoglobin crystals (short arrow).

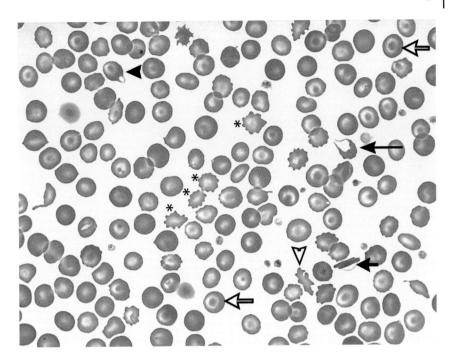

erythrocytes (Figure 17.19). They are formed through loss of cell membrane, resulting in sphering of the cells, and appear smaller than normal erythrocytes on a peripheral blood smear, though their volume remains similar to normal red blood cells, such that their presence does not usually affect MCV. Spherocytes can be evaluated on blood smears from dogs, but usually not cats, as feline erythrocytes routinely lack central pallor in health.

Note: It is critically important to evaluate spherocytes within the monolayer of the blood smear (see Chapter 16, Section 16.4.2). Erythrocytes close to the feathered edge may sphere due to the increased plasma volume in this area of the slide, losing central pallor, and they may be erroneously interpreted as spherocytes. It can be helpful to look for polychromatophils in the same area – if they also lack central pallor, then the red blood cell density is likely not optimal to evaluate morphology.

Figure 17.19 Blood smear, dog, 100× objective. Spherocytes in a case of immune-mediated hemolytic anemia. The spherocytes lack central pallor, are smaller and more densely colored than other erythrocytes. Note the increased number of polychromatophils supporting a regenerative response by the bone marrow, the metarubricyte (top right), and neutrophil (top center).

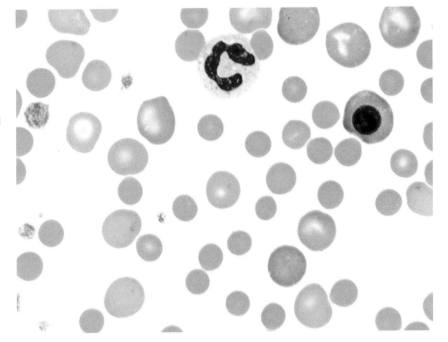

17.3.7.2 Clinical Considerations

Spherocytes may be seen in varying numbers in many different disease states:

- IMHA: IMHA is a common cause of spherocytosis, especially when large numbers of spherocytes are present [18]. In one study, >5 spherocytes per 100× objective field were associated with high specificity (95%) for the diagnosis of IMHA in dogs; however, sensitivity was 63% (i.e., low numbers of spherocytes can still be associated with IMHA) [40]. The absence of spherocytes also does not rule out IMHA, and correlation with clinical findings and other diagnostic testing may be required (e.g., evaluation for autoagglutination; see Section 17.2.3) [18].
- Drug/toxin exposure: Zinc toxicity [41], acetaminophen toxicity, envenomation including bee sting and snake envenomation [42, 43]. In cases of snake envenomation, spherocytes may also contain uniform small spikes known as spheroechinocytes (Figure 17.20) [44]. Spheroechinocytes can also be seen in low numbers in cases of pyruvate kinase deficiency [45].
- Fragmentation disease: Endocarditis [46] and microangiopathies (e.g., caused by hemangiosarcoma) [47].
- Bone marrow disease: Dyserythropoiesis [34].
- Post transfusion with stored blood [48].

17.3.8 Echinocytes

17.3.8.1 Morphologic Appearance

Echinocytes are spiculated erythrocytes (their name is derived from the Ancient Greek word *ekhînos* meaning hedgehog), with uniform, usually sharp spicules that are evenly spaced around the cells (Figure 17.21).

17.3.8.2 Clinical Considerations

Echinocytes frequently form as an *in vitro* artifact from excess EDTA (e.g., underfilling blood tubes), prolonged storage, or improper smear preparation (including slow drying of blood smears or delayed fixation). The term *crenation* may be used to describe echinocytes formed from artifacts. While artifact is a common cause of echinocytes, their presence may be an important indicator of underlying pathology, which may include:

- Renal disease: Notably glomerulonephritis and chronic kidney disease [49–51].
- Neoplasia: Most frequently with lymphoma but also reported in hemangiosarcoma and mast cell neoplasia [50].
- Drug/toxin exposure: Echinocytes have been associated with chemotherapeutic agents such as doxorubicin [52]. Echinocytes and (in severe cases) spheroechinocytes are reported in some cases of snake envenomation (Figure 17.20) [44, 53, 54].

17.3.9 Acanthocytes

17.3.9.1 Morphologic Appearance

Acanthocytes are characterized by irregularly spaced, variably sized, blunt-tipped projections (Figure 17.22). Their name is derived from the Ancient Greek word *ákantha* meaning thorn.

17.3.9.2 Clinical Considerations

Acanthocytes form when the erythrocyte membrane contains excess cholesterol relative to phospholipid. They can also occur secondary to fragmentation injury.

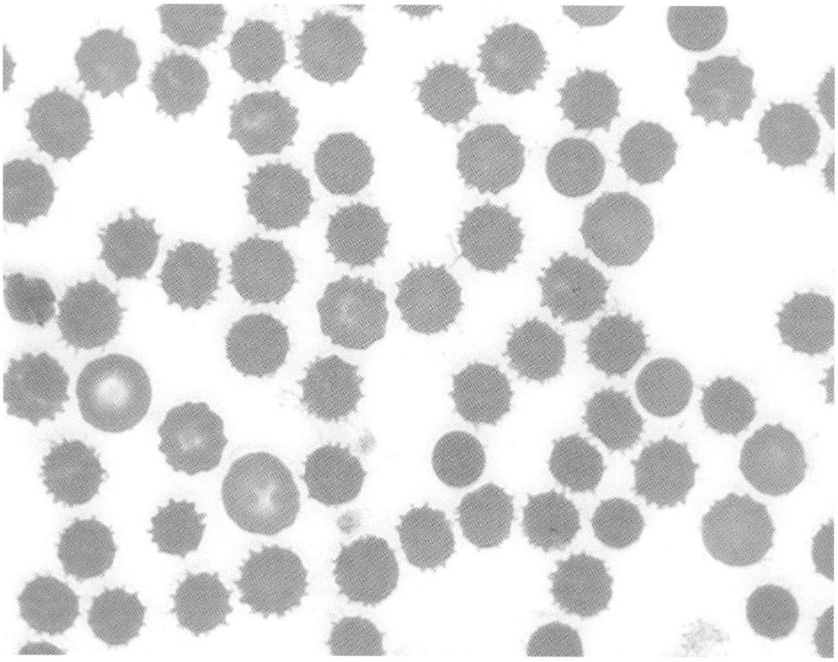

Figure 17.20 Blood smear, dog, 100× objective. Spheroechinocytes secondary to rattlesnake envenomation. Small, regularly spaced sharp spikes surround the spherocytes but not normal erythrocytes.

Figure 17.21 Blood smear, dog, 100× objective. Echinocytes from a dog with chronic renal disease. The erythrocytes have central pallor, with evenly spaced, regular, sharp spikes.

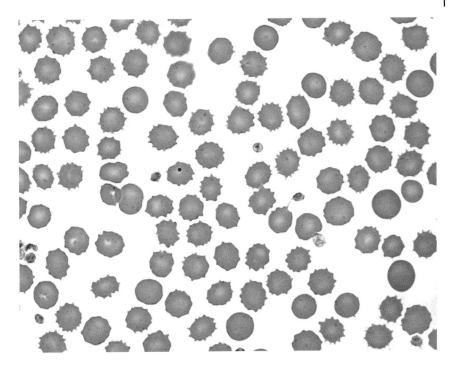

Figure 17.22 Blood smear, dog, 100× objective. Acanthocytes. The cells have irregular, variably spaced, and rounded projections.

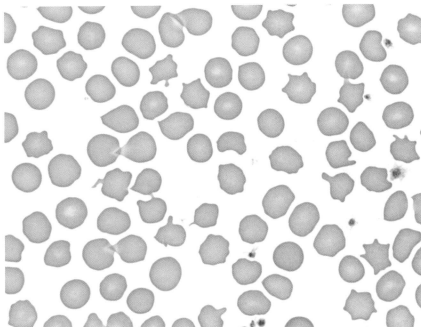

Alterations in lipid composition
- Liver disease [55, 56].
- High cholesterol diet [57].

Fragmentation disease
- Neoplasia: Including hemangiosarcoma, osteosarcoma, and lymphoma [58].
- Cardiac disease: Including ventricular outflow tract obstruction [59].
- Renal disease: Including chronic renal disease and glomerulonephritis [51, 58, 60].

- DIC [60].
- Dyserythropoiesis [34].

17.3.10 Schistocytes

17.3.10.1 Morphologic Appearance

Schistocytes (also referred to as schizocytes) are fragmented red blood cells that are smaller than normal erythrocytes. They are variably shaped (triangular, crescent-shaped, and elongated) and appear ragged, with

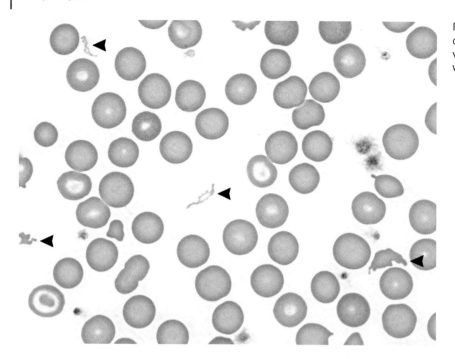

Figure 17.23 Blood smear, dog, 100× objective. Schistocytes (arrowheads) are variably shaped but mostly elongated with sharp, ragged points.

irregular, sharp/pointed projections (Figures 17.18, 17.23, and 17.24) [61]. Their name is derived from the Ancient Greek word skhízō meaning split.

17.3.10.2 Clinical Considerations

Schistocytes indicate fragmentation or mechanical injury to erythrocytes, which can be seen in many disease conditions:

- DIC: Formed via shearing of red blood cells when they pass through fibrin strands formed in small vessels (thrombotic microangiopathy) [62]. Common in dogs and variably present in cats [63–66]. Schistocytes and red blood cell fragments are a hallmark of DIC but are not specific for this condition.
- Iron deficiency: Erythrocytes are prone to mechanical injury due to increased fragility [67].
- Neoplasia: Especially hemangiosarcoma and lymphoma [47, 65].
- Cardiac disease: Including congestive heart failure and congenital ventricular outflow tract obstruction [59].
- Liver disease: Especially hepatic lipidosis in cats [55, 65].
- Myelofibrosis [68].

17.3.11 Keratocytes and Blister Cells

17.3.11.1 Morphologic Appearance

Erythrocytes that contain a hole or vesicle are called prekeratocytes or *blister cells*. The vesicles or blisters are eccentrically placed, with a fine rim of intact cell membrane (Figures 17.18 and 17.25). After the blister ruptures, it

creates a keratocyte with one or two variably long and thick hornlike projections on the same side of the cell (Figure 17.26), which is where the name is derived (the Ancient Greek word *kérato* meaning horn).

17.3.11.2 Clinical Considerations

Blister cells and keratocytes are mostly seen secondary to fragmentation disease and frequently accompany other poikilocytes including schistocytes and acanthocytes. They are also reported in other specific disease states.

Fragmentation disease

- Iron-deficiency anemia (associated with increased red blood cell fragility) [67].
- Cardiac disease [59].
- Neoplasia: Especially hemangiosarcoma [47].
- Drug/toxin exposure: Including doxorubicin therapy in cats [69].

Other disease states

Liver disease: Especially in cats with hepatic lipidosis [55].

17.3.12 Eccentrocytes

17.3.12.1 Morphologic Appearance

Eccentrocytes have an eccentrically placed region of increased pallor with a faint cell membrane border and hemoglobin localized to the remaining part of the cell (Figure 17.27). Their name is derived from the Ancient

Figure 17.24 Blood smear, dog, 100× objective. Schistocytes (arrowheads).

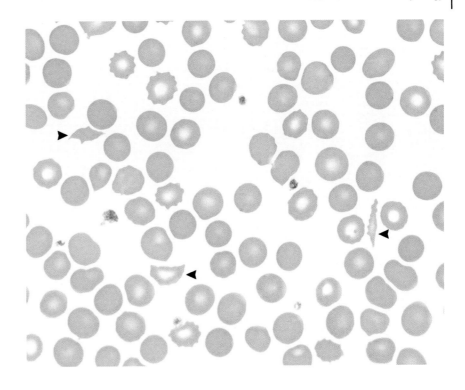

Figure 17.25 Blood smear, dog, 100× objective. A blister cell (arrow) and keratocyte (arrowhead) are present.

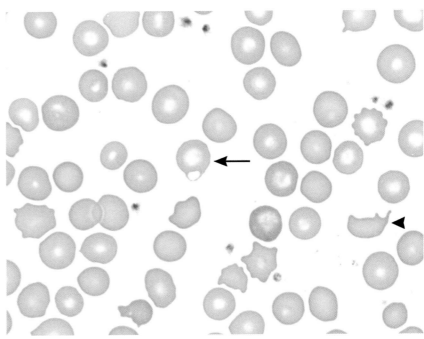

Greek word *ekkéntron* meaning 'out of center'. They have also been referred to as *hemighosts*.

17.3.12.2 Clinical Considerations

Eccentrocytes are associated with oxidative damage, which causes cross-linking of membrane proteins and adhesion of the opposing cell membranes, displacing hemoglobin to one side. They have been reported in the following diseases:

- Drug/toxin exposure: Allium toxicity (onion and garlic) [70–73], vitamin K1 and vitamin K antagonist intoxication [70], acetaminophen and nonsteroidal anti-inflammatory drugs [74], naphthalene [75], and prolonged propofol anesthesia [76].
- Neoplasia: Notably lymphoma [70, 77].
- Diabetic ketoacidosis [70].
- Infectious agents: Including *Babesia* spp. infection in dogs [78].

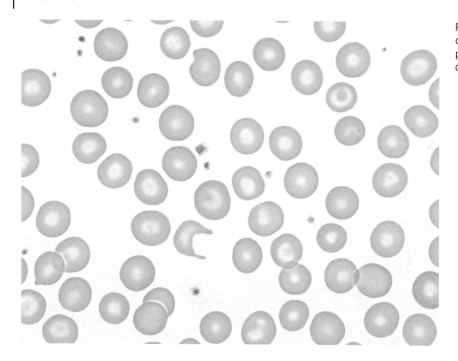

Figure 17.26 Blood smear, dog, 100× objective. Keratocyte. Note the projections giving the appearance of horns.

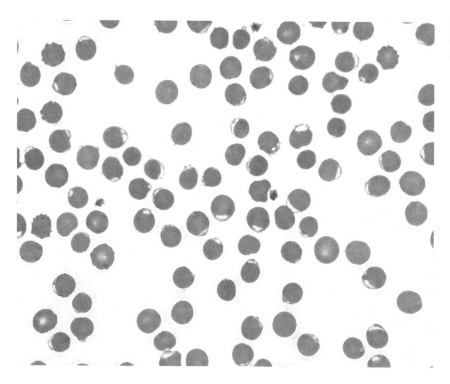

Figure 17.27 Blood smear, dog, 100× objective. Eccentrocytes in a dog secondary to acetaminophen toxicity.

17.3.13 Pyknocytes

17.3.13.1 Morphologic Appearance

Pyknocytes are small, dense, spherical erythrocytes that often have a focal tag or irregular area of ruffled cell membrane (Figure 17.28). The name is derived from the Ancient Greek word *puknós* meaning compact or condensed. They

can mimic spherocytes, but the latter have perfectly smooth membrane borders.

17.3.13.2 Clinical Considerations

Pyknocytes are associated with oxidative damage and often develop when the fused membrane of eccentrocytes ruptures or fragments off the cell (and therefore commonly

Figure 17.28 Blood smear, dog, 100× objective. Pyknocyte (arrow). Note the dense coloration of the cell and the delicate ruffled border of cell membrane around the eccentric pallor.

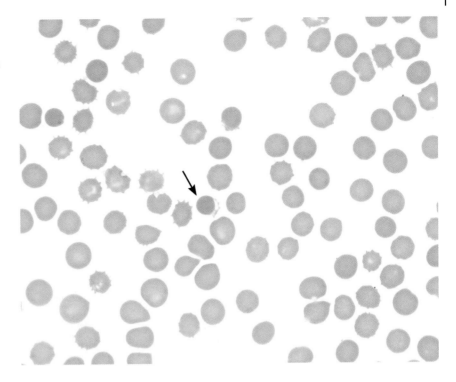

accompany eccentrocytes). They may also represent erythrocytes undergoing eryptosis (cell death). In addition to causes of oxidative damage causing eccentrocytes, they have also been reported in:

- Cardiac disease [59].
- Neoplasia: Notably hemangiosarcoma [47].

17.3.14 Elliptocytes (Ovalocytes)

17.3.14.1 Morphologic Appearance
Elliptocytes are variably elongated red blood cells whose length exceeds their width (Figure 17.29). They are also called *ovalocytes*. *Note*: Elliptocytes may form as an artifact of smear preparation from distortion of the cells in the direction of the smear. Relatively short elliptocytes all pointing in the same direction may be a clue for artifactual elliptocytosis, and elliptocytes with their line of axis pointing in different directions increase the confidence of formation *in vivo*.

17.3.14.2 Clinical Considerations
- Liver disease: Including hepatic lipidosis and portosystemic shunts in cats where elliptocytes may also be spiculated [55, 79].
- Neoplasia: Adrenocortical carcinoma in a cat [80].
- Bone marrow disease: Myelofibrosis [81, 82], and myelodysplasia in dogs [83].

- Drug/toxin exposure: Including doxorubicin chemotherapy in cats [69], and phenobarbital in dogs [84].
- Glomerulonephritis: Elliptocytes may be spiculated (Figure 17.30).
- Hereditary: Associated with membrane protein 4.1 deficiency and beta-spectrin abnormalities in dogs [85, 86].

17.3.15 Codocytes (Target Cells)

17.3.15.1 Morphologic Appearance
On a blood smear, codocytes appear like a 'bull's-eye' or target (hence their other name of *target cells*), with a central hemoglobinized region within the area of central pallor (Figure 17.31). On electron microscopy, the cells often appear bell-shaped; hence their name (derived from the Ancient Greek word *kódōn* meaning bell). This appearance occurs due to an increased cell membrane-to-volume ratio, resulting in the membranes touching in the middle of the cell and a central area of density.

17.3.15.2 Clinical Considerations
Codocytes are common in cases of regenerative anemia in dogs, as polychromatophils have an increased cell membrane-to-volume ratio. They can also be present in increased numbers in the following disease states:

- Hepatic disease.
- Iron-deficiency anemia.

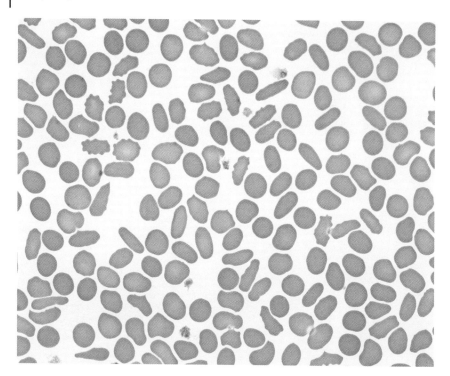

Figure 17.29 Blood smear, dog, 100× objective. Elliptocytes. Note the elongated shape and different orientation of the long-axis of the cells.

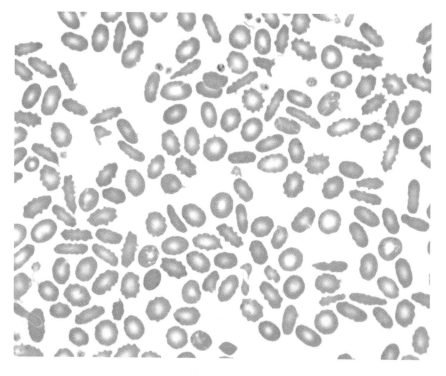

Figure 17.30 Blood smear, dog, 100× objective. Spiculated elliptocytes in a dog with Lyme nephritis.

- Neoplasia: Including hemangiosarcoma [47, 58].
- Dyserythropoiesis [34].

17.3.16 Dacryocytes

17.3.16.1 Morphologic Appearance
Dacryocytes are teardrop-shaped (their name is derived from the Ancient Greek word *dákruon* meaning teardrop),

with a rounded base tapering to a variably sharp, single, unipolar projection (Figure 17.32).

17.3.16.2 Clinical Considerations
This uncommon shape change is typically seen in low numbers and can be seen with:

- Bone marrow disease: Myelofibrosis [83], and congenital dyserythropoiesis [87].

Figure 17.31 Blood smear, dog, 100× objective. Codocytes (target cells).

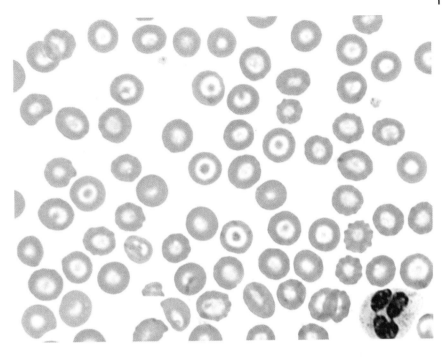

Figure 17.32 Blood smear, dog, 100× objective. Dacryocytes (arrowheads). Other dacrocytes are present, with their line of axis in different directions, supporting a pathologic etiology.

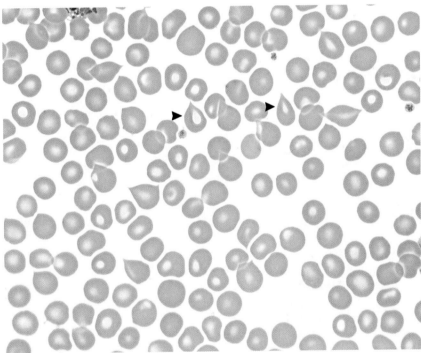

- Cardiac disease: Degenerative mitral valve disease [88].
- Glomerulonephritis.
- Hypersplenism [89].

17.3.17 Stomatocytes

17.3.17.1 Morphologic Appearance

Stomatocytes have an elongated or slitlike region of central pallor (Figure 17.33). Their name is derived from the Ancient Greek word *stoma* meaning mouth.

17.3.17.2 Clinical Considerations

Stomatocytes most frequently represent an artifactual change in blood smears from dogs and may be associated with thick smears, decreased blood pH, or the use of amphipathic drugs. Rare stomatocytes may also be present as an incidental finding in blood smears from dogs.

Pathologic stomatocytes form with an increased water content of erythrocytes and are present in variable numbers (10–50+% of red blood cells) in heritable syndromes in dogs, which may or may not be associated with clinical signs.

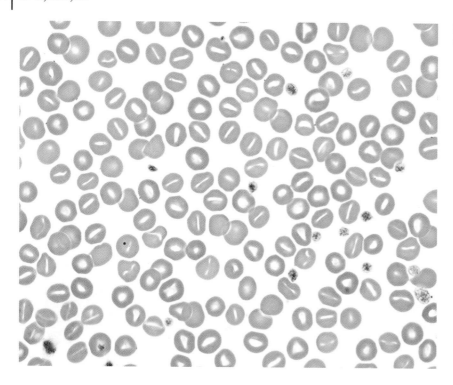

Figure 17.33 Blood smear, dog, 100× objective. Stomatocytes.

- Non-syndromic forms reported in Miniature Schnauzer, Standard Schnauzer, Beagle, and Australian Cattle Dogs [90–92].
- Syndromic forms reported in Alaskan Malamutes (associated with chondrodysplasia) and Drentsche Patrijshond dogs (associated with hypertrophic gastritis and polysystemic disease) [93, 94]. These dogs have shortened life spans associated with hemolytic anemia.

17.3.18 Ghost Cells

17.3.18.1 Morphologic Appearance

Lysed erythrocytes or 'ghost cells' have a distinct cell border but are very pale compared to intact erythrocytes and may be difficult to see on peripheral blood smears (Figure 17.34). Heinz bodies may be prominent in ghost cells caused by oxidative damage (Figure 17.35).

17.3.18.2 Clinical Considerations

- The presence of lysed or 'ghost' cells indicates hemolysis prior to blood smear preparation. This may occur *in vitro* (in the blood tube after collection) or *in vivo* associated with acute or active intravascular hemolysis (e.g., secondary to IMHA, oxidative damage, or hemotropic organisms).
- Markedly increased ghost cells likely indicate intravascular hemolysis.

17.3.19 Torocytes

17.3.19.1 Morphologic Appearance

Torocytes have central pallor with sharp edges, giving the center of red blood cells a 'punched out' appearance (Figure 17.36). This sharp-edged clear zone is also often surrounded by a concentric pale ring. Their name is derived from the Latin word *torus* for the rounded molding at the base of a column.

17.3.19.2 Clinical Considerations

Torocytes are considered to represent an artifactual change, with no clinical significance, and may occur due to prolonged storage of blood in EDTA. It is important to differentiate these cells from hypochromatophils (see Figure 17.16), in which the area of central pallor is less sharp and often more variable in size with mostly a thin rim of hemoglobin (the amount of central pallor of torocytes is typically more uniform, with a normal thick rim of surrounding hemoglobin).

17.3.20 Hemoglobin crystals

17.3.20.1 Morphologic Appearance

Hemoglobin crystals form within erythrocytes, resulting in variably deformed cells with angular, sharp, square/rectangular inclusions. They stain a similar color to normal red blood cells but often have a deeper color. They may be seen within red blood cells, surrounded by a thin rim of

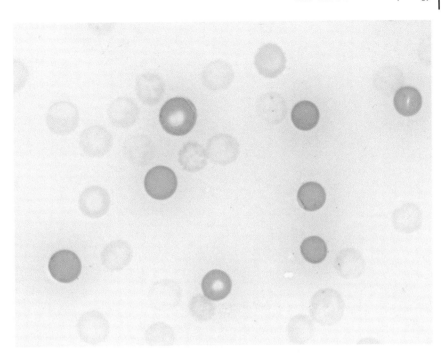

Figure 17.34 Blood smear, dog, 100×
objective. Ghost cells in a case of
immune-mediated hemolytic anemia.
Numerous ghost cells have faint pink
cytoplasm, accompanied by spherocytes
that are small with dense coloration.

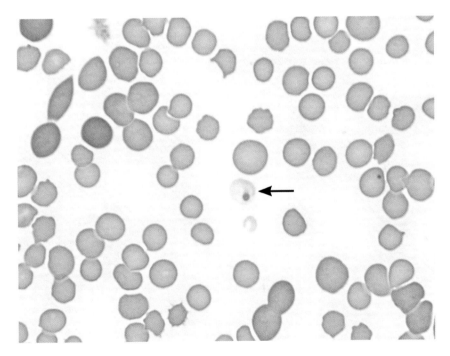

Figure 17.35 Blood smear, cat, 100×
objective. A Heinz body is seen within a
ghost cell (arrow).

membrane (Figures 17.18 and 17.37), or free (after rupture
of the cell) in the background of the slide (Figure 17.38).

17.3.20.2 Clinical Considerations

Hemoglobin crystals may be present in low numbers in
blood from healthy dogs and cats and often represent an
incidental finding. They may develop due to prolonged
storage of blood (for 12–24 hours after sampling) [95].

They have been reported with increased frequency in the
following disease states:

- Cardiac disease: Increased numbers of advanced heart
  failure when compared to control groups [88].
- Dyserythropoiesis [96].
- Infectious disease: Increased numbers of cats infected
  with *Mycoplasma haemofelis* [97].

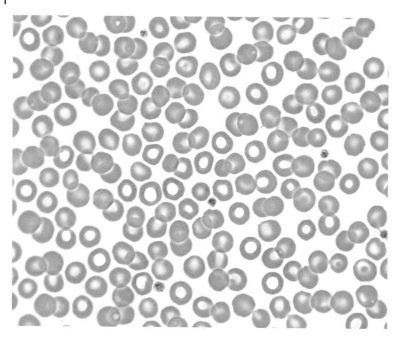

Figure 17.36 Blood smear, dog, 100× objective. Torocytes. Note the sharp border of the central pallor and the normal width and color of surrounding cell membrane.

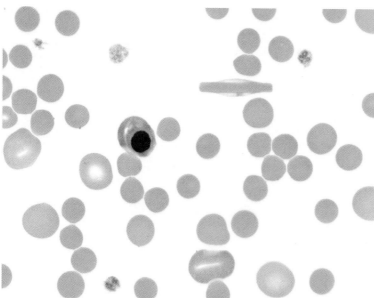

Figure 17.37 Blood smear, dog, 100× objective. Hemoglobin crystal in a dog with immune-mediated hemolytic anemia. Note the fine membrane of an intact red blood cell surrounding the crystal. Many spherocytes are present, as well as a metarubricyte.

17.4 Red Blood Cell Inclusions

17.4.1 Basophilic Stippling

17.4.1.1 Morphologic Appearance
Basophilic stippling is characterized by punctate blue/purple inclusions in the cytoplasm of erythrocytes stained with routine hematology stains. These inclusions are often noted diffusely and evenly throughout the cytoplasm and represent an aggregation of ribosomes and polyribosomes (Figure 17.39).

17.4.1.2 Clinical Considerations
Basophilic stippling may be seen in the following scenarios:

- Regenerative anemia: Usually only present in dogs and cats with a florid regenerative response.
- Lead poisoning: Considered to be a hallmark of lead toxicity (and often accompanied by increased nucleated red blood cells) due to inhibition of pyrimidine 5′-nucleotidase preventing degradation of ribosomal RNA which accumulates in the erythrocyte cytoplasm [98]. It is important to note that basophilic stippling is not consistently present in cases of lead toxicosis [99].
- Dyserythropoiesis: Basophilic stippling has been reported in a dog secondary to dyserythropoiesis and myelodysplasia associated with metastatic adenocarcinoma [100].

Figure 17.38 Blood smear, dog, 100× objective. Hemoglobin crystal.

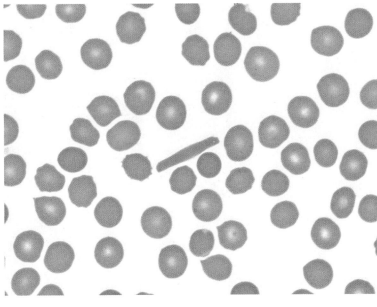

Figure 17.39 Blood smear, dog, 100× objective. Basophilic stippling associated with lead toxicity. Note the fine often diffuse distribution of the basophilic inclusions.

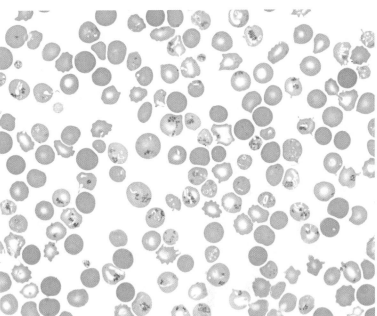

17.4.2 Siderotic Inclusions

17.4.2.1 Morphologic Appearance

Siderotic inclusions appear as variably chunky and variably shaped blue/basophilic inclusions and are often seen in focal aggregates toward the periphery of erythrocytes (compared to the diffuse, punctate inclusions of basophilic stippling) (Figure 17.40).

17.4.2.2 Clinical Considerations

- Anucleated erythrocytes containing siderotic inclusions are called *siderocytes*.
- Siderotic inclusions represent the accumulation of iron, either in the cytoplasm or in mitochondria. They stain blue with Prussian blue stain for iron, which can help differentiate them from basophilic stippling.
- Iron-laden mitochondria phagocytosed in autolysosomes are called *Pappenheimer bodies*.

Siderotic inclusions may be seen in the following conditions:

- Drug/toxin exposure: Including zinc/lead toxicity and chloramphenicol [101].
- Myelodysplasia and dyserythropoiesis [96, 102, 103].
- Inflammation (including hepatitis, pancreatitis, and glomerulonephritis) [102].

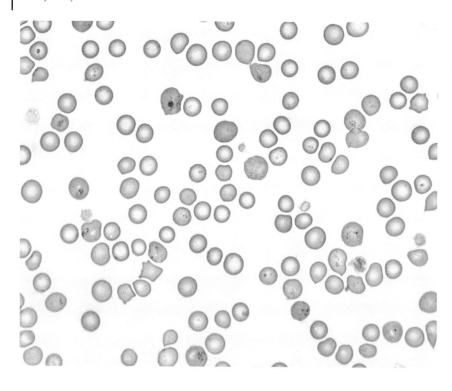

Figure 17.40 Blood smear, dog, 100× objective. Siderotic inclusions. The inclusions are often aggregated and suggest Pappenheimer bodies (upper left).

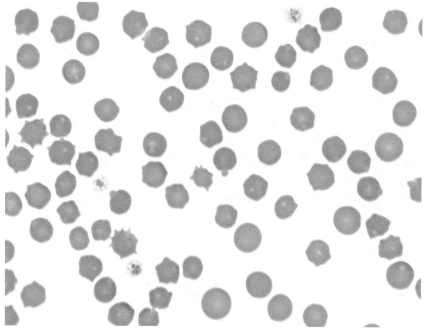

Figure 17.41 Blood smear, cat, 100× objective. Heinz bodies secondary to onion toxicity. Note that some Heinz bodies project from the side of erythrocytes, while others overlay the cell, giving the appearance of a small area of pallor.

17.4.3 Heinz Bodies

17.4.3.1 Morphologic Appearance

Heinz bodies are variably sized, round inclusions that stain a similar color to red blood cells on Romanowsky-stained blood smears. They may be seen protruding from the side of erythrocytes like a pimple but are also frequently seen over-lying red blood cells and often appear more pale than the

rest of the red blood cells (Figure 17.41). It is important to differentiate these from central pallor in dog erythrocytes. Heinz bodies stain dark blue with NMB stain (Figure 17.42).

17.4.3.2 Clinical Considerations

Heinz bodies represent oxidized hemoglobin that precipi-tates as intracellular aggregates attached to the internal

Figure 17.42 Blood smear, cat, 100× objective, new methylene blue stain (same case as Figure 17.41). The Heinz bodies stain intensely blue, allowing easy visualization and enumeration.

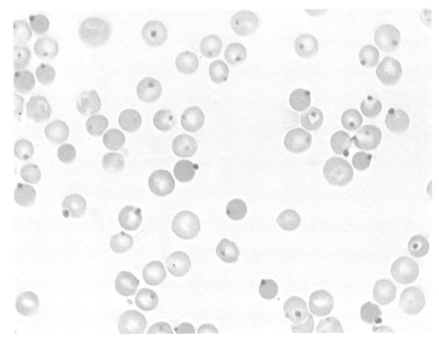

surface of red blood cell membranes. Small and large Heinz bodies are recognized:

Small Heinz bodies

- Seen primarily in cats.
- May be seen in low numbers (up to 5% of erythrocytes) in healthy cats.
- Increased numbers have been reported in cats secondary to diabetes mellitus (especially diabetic ketoacidosis), lymphoma, and hyperthyroidism [104, 105].
- May also form in cats secondary to ingestion of propylene glycol [106].

Large Heinz bodies

- Seen in cats and dogs.
- Drug exposure: Acetaminophen, vitamin K3 [107], repeat propofol anesthesia [108].
- Toxin exposure: Zinc [109], onion [110], skunk musk [111], and naphthalene [75].

17.4.4 Howell-Jolly Bodies

17.4.4.1 Morphologic Appearance

Howell-Jolly bodies (also known as micronuclei) appear as small, regular, round, densely basophilic red blood cell inclusions (Figure 17.43). They may be seen anywhere in the cell. Two or more Howell-Jolly bodies may be present in a single cell (Figure 17.44), though multiple inclusions within a single cell, atypical shapes, or large size are often associated with the underlying pathology (see below).

Note: Howell-Jolly bodies may mimic infectious agents such as *Mycoplasma* spp. or Distemper inclusions (see Figures 17.48 and 17.50). Careful examination and correlation with other findings are prudent.

17.4.4.2 Clinical Considerations

Howell-Jolly bodies represent nonfunctional nuclear fragments that may remain after the nucleus is extruded from immature cells. They are usually removed as red blood cells pass through the splenic sinuses.

Howell-Jolly bodies can be seen in low numbers in blood smears from healthy cats that have non-sinusoidal spleens. They are less common in blood from healthy dogs but may be seen in low numbers. Increased numbers of Howell-Jolly bodies may be seen in the following situations:

- Regenerative anemia (common).
- Drug/toxin exposure: Can be seen in increased numbers and atypical shapes secondary to chemotherapeutic agents [32]. They can also be seen secondary to glucocorticoid therapy.
- Splenectomy.
- Dyserythropoiesis: Including Poodle macrocytosis and metastatic neoplasia to the bone marrow [23, 100].
- FeLV infection: Increased Howell-Jolly bodies associated with erythroleukemia or myelodysplastic syndrome and may be large or multiple [112].
- Cobalamin deficiency: Reported in a cat [113].
- Chronic kidney disease: Increased Howell-Jolly bodies have been associated with disease progression of chronic kidney disease in dogs [51].

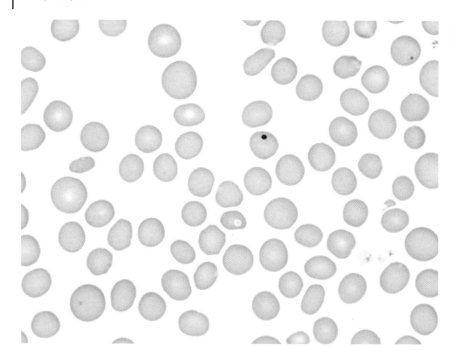

Figure 17.43 Blood smear, dog, 100× objective. Howell-Jolly body.

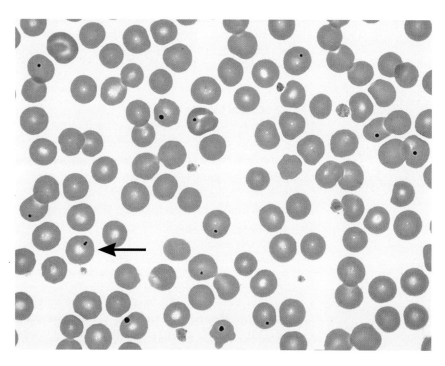

Figure 17.44 Blood smear, dog, 100× objective. Numerous Howell-Jolly bodies are seen within erythrocytes, including two within the same cell (arrow).

17.4.5 Red Blood Cell Artifacts

17.4.5.1 Morphologic Appearance

Common artifacts seen on red blood cells include refractile inclusions and stain precipitation. Refractile inclusions are often seen around the periphery of red blood cells and may give the cell border an irregular or moth-eaten appearance (Figure 16.7). They are variably sized and variable numbers may be present. These inclusions shine when the condenser of the microscope is moved up and down (compared to infectious agents or other pathologic inclusions).

Stain precipitation appears as stippled to aggregated, deep purple/basophilic material that may be diffuse or clumped on the surface of the cells (Figure 17.45). It is also often seen in the background of the smear, supporting this interpretation.

Figure 17.45 Blood smear, dog, 100× objective. Stain precipitation is seen both overlaying red blood cells and in the background of the slide (arrow). Compare to the perfectly round Howell-Jolly body (arrowhead).

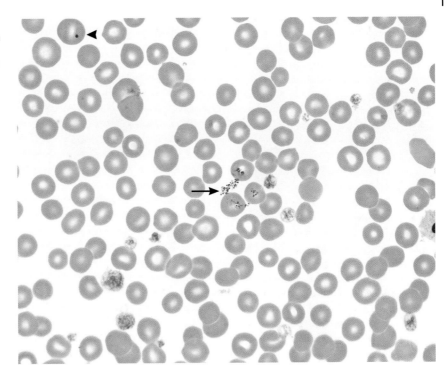

17.4.5.2 Clinical considerations

Refractile inclusions and stain precipitation are incidental findings; however, it is important to distinguish these from pathologic changes, including infectious organisms (see Section 17.5)

Refractile inclusions May result from slow drying of smears (particularly thick smears), staining of smears before they are fully dry, or contamination of the fixative with water.

Stain precipitation Usually results from the use of aged stains.

17.5 Red Blood Cell Neoplasia

17.5.1 Primary Erythrocytosis

17.5.1.1 Morphologic Appearance

Patients with primary erythrocytosis have increased red blood cell mass and a short, or nonexistent monolayer on the blood smear (Figure 17.3) with no other visual changes usually apparent.

17.5.1.2 Clinical Considerations

- Rare myeloproliferative disorder in dogs and cats.
- Clinical signs: Neurologic signs (seizures, paresis, and mentation changes) are common [10, 11].

- EPO concentrations are low or normal; however, low or normal EPO does not exclude causes of secondary erythrocytosis [114, 115].

17.5.1.3 Prognosis

Guarded to good. Prolonged survival times reported with appropriate medical management [10].

17.5.2 Erythroleukemia

17.5.2.1 Morphologic Appearance

Erythroleukemia is often associated with the presence of erythroblasts in circulation, typically with a concurrent non-regenerative anemia. These have nuclei approximately twofold to threefold the size of RBCs in diameter, with finely stippled chromatin and prominent nucleoli. The cells have a small to moderate rim of deep blue cytoplasm (Figure 17.46). Increased numbers of more mature nucleated RBCs are often noted, and dysplastic changes may be present in these cells, including binucleation or immature nuclei in fully hemoglobinized erythrocytes.

17.5.2.2 Clinical Considerations

- Cats > dogs.
- Subtype of acute myeloid leukemia (AML-M6/M6Er).
- Associated with FeLV infection in cats [116].

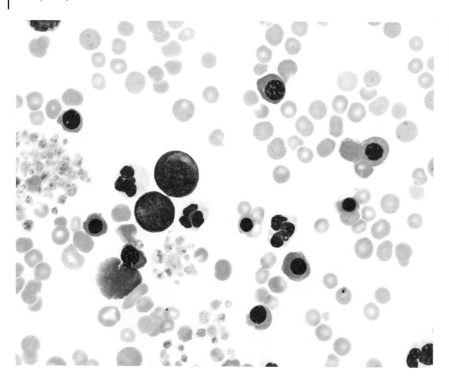

Figure 17.46 Blood smear, dog, 100× objective. Erythroleukemia. Note the two large erythroblasts, accompanied by many metarubricytes and rare rubricytes.

- Pancytopenia is common and erythroblasts may not be seen in circulation.
- Bone marrow evaluation is required for diagnosis (see Chapter 5, Section 5.4.4).

17.5.2.3 Prognosis

Grave prognosis in both dogs and cats, even with treatment [117, 118].

17.6 Red Blood Cell Infectious Agents

17.6.1 *Mycoplasma* spp.

17.6.1.1 Morphologic Appearance

Hemotropic *Mycoplasma* species are small (~0.3–1.0 μm diameter), basophilic, round to ring-shaped organisms, which may be seen in chains (Figures 17.47 and 17.48). They attach to the surface of erythrocytes and may be

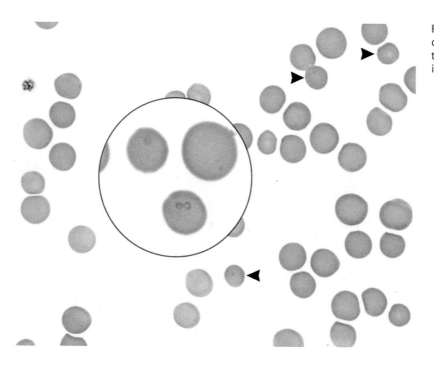

Figure 17.47 Blood smear, cat, 100× objective. *Mycoplasma haemofelis*. Note the ring-forms (magnified), also present in numerous other cells (arrowheads).

Figure 17.48 Blood smear, cat, 100× objective, Diff-Quik stain. *Mycoplasma haemofelis* organisms stain prominently with rapid Romanowsky-type stains and may be seen in chains (magnified and arrowheads).

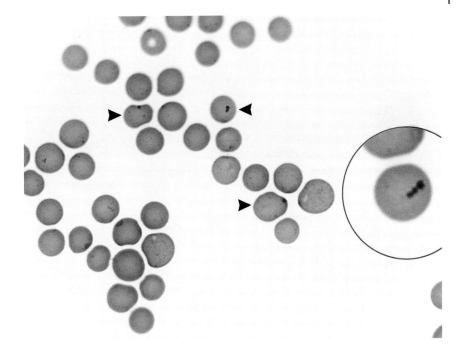

seen protruding from the side or overlying the cytoplasm of erythrocytes depending on cell orientation. It is important to not confuse *Mycoplasma* organisms with stain precipitation or basophilic stippling. Parasitemia is cyclic and organisms are not always present. *Note*: *Mycoplasma* organisms may detach from erythrocytes stored in EDTA and can be present in the background of the smears, often in aggregates or chains (Figure 17.49) [119].

17.6.1.2 Clinical Considerations
- Cats > Dogs.
- *Mycoplasma haemofelis* is the most pathogenic species in cats, causing severe hemolytic anemia. *Mycoplasma haemocanis* is most common in dogs but usually only causes disease in immunocompromised or splenectomized animals [120].
- Clinical Signs = lethargy, pallor, weakness, and intermittent fever.
- PCR testing is the most reliable test for diagnosis.

Figure 17.49 Blood smear, cat, 100× objective. Abundant *Mycoplasma haemofelis* organisms are seen in the background of the smear made from an EDTA sample >24 hours old. These are sometimes seen in linear chains, and intimately associated with the cell membranes, helping distinguish these from stain precipitation.

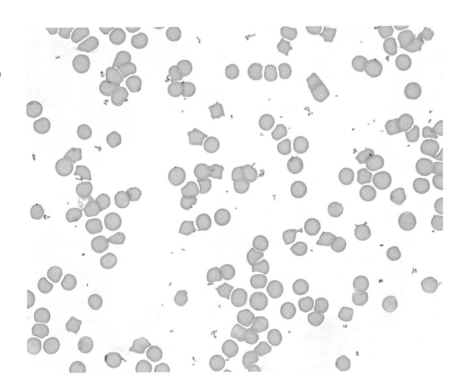

17.6.1.3 Prognosis

Generally good with prompt and appropriate therapy. Animals may remain subclinical carriers, and reactivation of disease is possible, though rare [121].

17.6.2 Distemper

17.6.2.1 Morphologic Appearance

Viral inclusions from canine Distemper virus are variably sized and shaped, ranging from 1 to 4 μm and varying from ovoid to polygonal, with some inclusions having straight edges. They stain more prominently with Diff Quik stains, where they appear deep red/basophilic (Figure 17.50) and are more commonly pale pink or blue with Wright Giemsa stains (Figures 17.51 and 17.52). Small Distemper inclusions can mimic Howell-Jolly bodies (compare to Figure 17.44); however, the variation in shape and red color of Distemper inclusions are useful morphologic features for differentiation on Diff Quik stained blood smears. Distemper inclusions may also be seen in conjunctival epithelial cells and leukocytes (see Chapter 18, Section 18.10.2).

17.6.2.2 Clinical Considerations

- Dogs affected; not seen in domesticated cats.
- Clinical signs = fever, cough, conjunctivitis, foot pad and nasal planum hyperkeratosis [122], and neurologic signs.
- Viral inclusions in erythrocytes are mostly seen early in the disease, and viremia is transient. The absence of inclusions does not preclude disease.

17.6.2.3 Prognosis

Variable. Dogs with mild signs often recover without therapy, while those with moderate gastrointestinal or respiratory signs often recover with supportive therapy. Prognosis is poor when CNS signs are present [123].

17.6.3 Cytauxzoon felis

17.6.3.1 Morphologic Appearance

Merozoites

Merozoites (piroplasms) are seen in erythrocytes. These are small (~0.5–1 μm in diameter), round to signet ring-shaped intracellular organisms (Figure 17.53). They are mostly seen singly but can also be seen in pairs or tetrads. *Cytauxzoon felis* piroplasms can be difficult to differentiate from other small organisms, including *Babesia felis* (compare to Figure 17.58) and *Mycoplasma haemofelis* (compare to Figure 17.47), and care should also be taken to not confuse these organisms with small artifacts (e.g., refractile drying artifacts).

Schizonts

Cytauxzoon felis schizonts may be seen in peripheral blood and are present in macrophages, which are often pushed to the feathered edge of blood smears due to their large size. The schizonts distend the cytoplasm of macrophages and contain numerous small, purple granular developing merozoites (Figure 17.54). The macrophages usually have a prominent, single basophilic nucleolus. In one study,

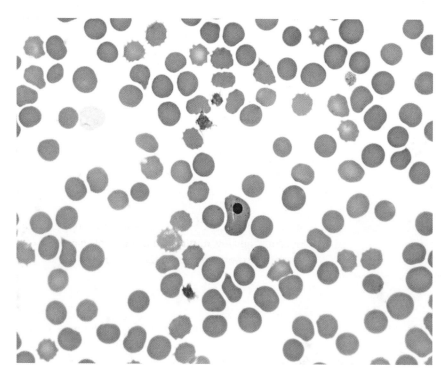

Figure 17.50 Blood smear, dog, 100× objective, Diff-Quik stain. Large Distemper inclusion staining deeply magenta with rapid Romanowsky-type stain.

Figure 17.51 Blood smear, dog, 100× objective. Distemper viral inclusion staining pale purple with Wright-Giemsa stain.

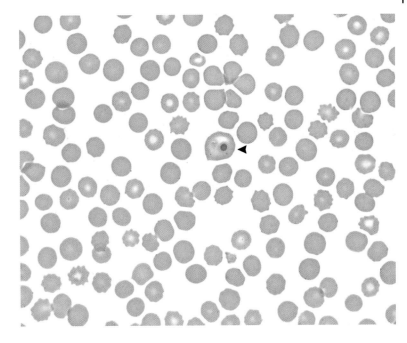

Figure 17.52 Blood smear, dog, 100× objective. Distemper viral inclusions (arrowheads) staining pale blue with Wright-Giemsa stain.

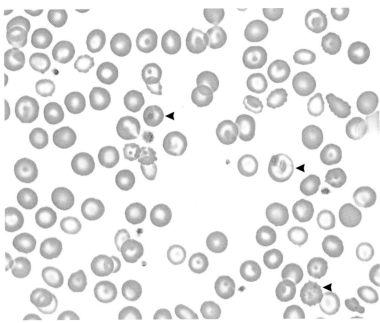

schizont-laden macrophages were seen in circulation in 33% of cases of acute cytauxzoonosis [124].

17.6.3.2 Clinical Considerations

- Cats only.
- Clinical signs = lethargy, fever, jaundice, variably regenerative anemia, thrombocytopenia, and neurologic signs (including seizures).
- Presence of piroplasms within erythrocytes in conjunction with clinical signs, or presence of schizonts in circulation, is considered diagnostic. PCR is a highly sensitive

method for diagnosis and may be positive days prior to clinical signs [125].
- Absence of organisms in circulation does not preclude infection, and low numbers of piroplasms may persist for years in recovered patients [126, 127].

17.6.3.3 Prognosis

Guarded to poor, with high morbidity and mortality rates, especially in untreated patients [126]. Subclinical infections may occur in some cats [127, 128].

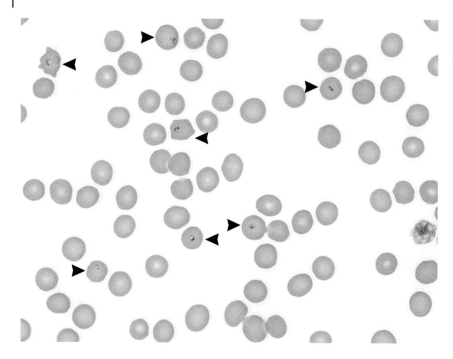

Figure 17.53 Blood smear, cat, 100× objective field. Numerous *Cytauxzoon felis* merozoites (piroplasms) are seen within erythrocytes (arrowheads). Note the signet ring shape of the organisms.

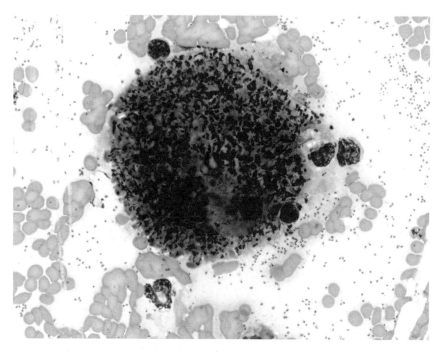

Figure 17.54 Blood smear, cat, 100× objective field. *Cytauxzoon felis* schizont. A macrophage contains numerous merozoites. Note the small merozoites free in the background and the macrophage nucleus with its prominent nucleolus. Courtesy of Dr. Maggie McCourt.

17.6.4 *Babesia* spp.

17.6.4.1 Morphologic Appearance

Babesial organisms can be broadly grouped into large and small via microscopic evaluation; however, further speciation is not possible visually. Large organisms such as *B. canis* and *B. vogeli* in dogs are approximately 3–6 μm in diameter/length and vary from round to often pear-shaped. They have a pale-blue cytoplasm with a prominent purple periphery and a dense purple, eccentrically placed nucleus.

They may be seen singly (Figure 17.55) as well as in pairs or tetrads (Figure 17.56).

Small organisms such as *B. gibsoni* or *B. conradae* in dogs and *B. felis* in cats are mostly round, approximately 1–2.5 μm in diameter, also with a clear to pale-blue cytoplasm and eccentrically placed, deep purple nuclei (Figures 17.57 and 17.58). Multiple merozoites within each red blood cell are also possible. Small *Babesia* spp. may be difficult to distinguish from *Mycoplasma* spp.

Figure 17.55 Blood smear, dog, 100× objective. Large *Babesia* organisms.

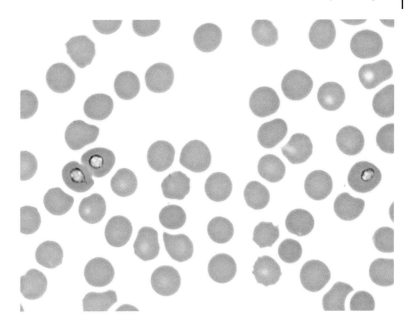

Figure 17.56 Blood smear, dog, 100× objective. Large *Babesia* organisms. Note the pairs of teardrop-shaped organisms within erythrocytes.

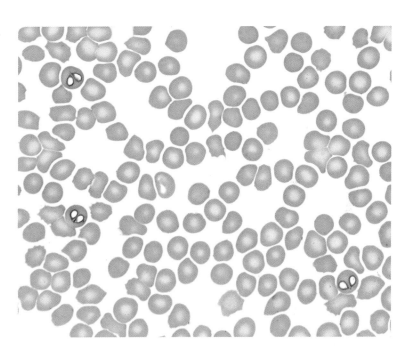

17.6.4.2 Clinical Considerations
- Dogs and cats.
- Greyhounds and American Pit Bull Terriers predisposed [129, 130].
- Clinical signs = lethargy, anorexia, pallor, lymphadenomegaly, and splenomegaly.
- Clinicopathologic findings = hemolytic anemia, thrombocytopenia, hyperglobulinemia, and proteinuria.
- Transmission may occur via ticks, bite wounds, transplacentally and via transfusion [131].

- Diagnosis via combination of evaluation of blood smear, PCR, and/or serology. Only PCR allows speciation [131].

17.6.4.3 Prognosis
Outcomes are variable and may be affected by disease severity, specific organisms, and various host factors [132]. Prognosis is generally good with appropriate therapy, but mortality can be high in untreated patients [133].

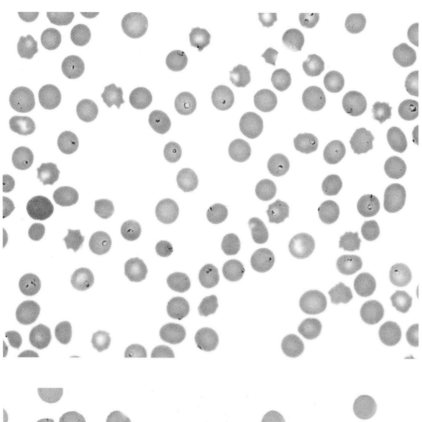

Figure 17.57 Blood smear, dog, 100× objective. *Babesia gibsoni.*

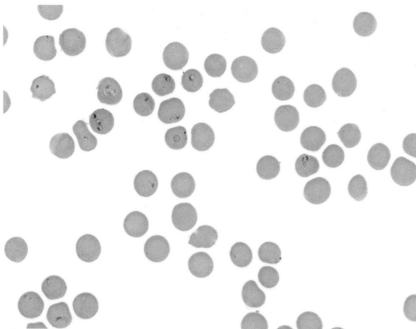

Figure 17.58 Blood smear, cat, 100× objective. *Babesia felis.* Multiple organisms are often present within the erythrocytes.

References

1 Zini, G. (2014) Stability of complete blood count parameters with storage: toward defined specifications for different diagnostic applications. *Int. J. Lab. Hematol.*, **36** (2), 111–113.

2 Furlanello, T., Tasca, S., Caldin, M., *et al.* (2006) Artifactual changes in canine blood following storage, detected using the ADVIA 120 hematology analyzer. *Vet. Clin. Pathol.*, **35** (1), 42–46.

3 Basu, D., Veluru, H. (2019) A study of storage related changes and effect of refrigeration on hematological parameters and blood cell morphology in EDTA anticoagulated blood. *Ann. Pathol. Lab. Med.*, **6** (5), 289–296.

4 Palmer, L., Briggs, C., McFadden, S., *et al.* (2015) ICSH recommendations for the standardization of nomenclature

and grading of peripheral blood cell morphological features. *Int. J. Lab. Hematol.*, **37** (3), 287–303.

5 Noutsos, T., Laidman, A.Y., Survela, L., *et al.* (2021) An evaluation of existing manual blood film schistocyte quantitation guidelines and a new proposed method. *Pathology*, **53** (6), 746–752.

6 Weiss, G., Ganz, T., Goodnough, L.T. (2019) Anemia of inflammation. *Blood*, **133** (1), 40–50.

7 Radakovich, L.B., Pannone, S.C., Truelove, M.P., *et al.* (2017) Hematology and biochemistry of aging – evidence of 'anemia of the elderly' in old dogs. *Vet. Clin. Pathol.*, **46** (1), 34–45.

8 Assenmacher, T.D., Jutkowitz, L.A., Koenigshof, A.M., *et al.* (2019) Clinical features of precursor-targeted immune-mediated anemia in dogs: 66 cases (2004-2013). *J. Am. Vet. Med. Assoc.*, **255** (3), 366–376.

9 Zaldívar-López, S. Marin, L.M., Lazbik, M.C., *et al.* (2011) Clinical pathology of Greyhounds and other sighthounds. *Vet. Clin. Pathol.*, **40** (4), 414–425.

10 Darcy, H., Simpson, K., Gajanayake, I., *et al.* (2018) Feline primary erythrocytosis: a multicentre case series of 18 cats. *J. Feline Med. Surg.*, **20** (12), 1192–1198.

11 Diogo, C.C., Fabretti, A.K., Camassa, J.A., *et al.* (2015) Diagnosis and treatment of primary erythrocytosis in a dog: a case report. *Top. Companion Anim. Med.*, **30** (2), 65–67.

12 Dane, D.M., Hsia, C.C., Wu, E.Y., *et al.* (2006) Splenectomy impairs diffuse oxygen transport in the lungs of dogs. *J. Appl. Physiol.*, **101** (1), 289–297.

13 Breznock, E.M., Strack D. (1982) Effects of the spleen, epinephrine and splenectomy on determination of blood volume in cats. *Am. J. Vet. Res.*, **43** (11), 2062–2066.

14 Greet, V., Bode, E.F., Dukes-McEwan, J., *et al.* (2021) Clinical features and outcome of dogs and cats with bidirectional and continuous right-to-left shunting patent ductus arteriosus. *J. Vet. Intern. Med.*, **35** (2), 780–788.

15 Holopainen, S., Laurila, H.P., Lappalainen, A.K., *et al.* (2022) Polycythemia in dogs with chronic hypoxic pulmonary disease. *J. Vet. Intern. Med.*, **36** (4), 1202–1210.

16 Hergt, F., Mortier, F., Werres, C., *et al.* (2019) Renal nephroblastoma in a 17-month-old Jack Russell Terrier. *J. Am. Anim. Hosp. Assoc.*, **55** (5), e55503.

17 Wardrop, K.J. (2005) The Coombs' test in veterinary medicine: past, present, future. *Vet. Clin. Pathol.*, **34** (4), 325–334.

18 Garden, O.A., Kidd, L., Mexas, A.M., *et al.* (2019) ACVIM consensus statement on the diagnosis of immune-mediated hemolytic anemia in dogs and cats. *J. Vet. Intern. Med.*, **33** (2), 313–334.

19 Schaefer, D.M.W., Priest, H., Stokol, T., *et al.* (2009) Anticoagulant-dependent in vitro hemagglutination in a cat. *Vet. Clin. Pathol.*, **38** (2), 194–200.

20 Sun, P.L., Jeffery, U. (2021) Effect of dilution of canine blood samples on the specificity of saline agglutination tests for immune-mediated hemolysis. *J. Vet. Intern. Med.*, **34** (6), 2374–2383.

21 Battison, A. (2007) Apparent pseudohyperkalemia in a Chinese Shar Pei dog. *Vet. Clin. Pathol.*, **36** (1), 89–93.

22 Conrado, F.O., Oliveira, S.T., Lacerda, L.A., *et al.* (2014) Clinicopathologic and electrocardiographic features of Akita dogs with high and low erythrocyte potassium phenotypes. *Vet. Clin. Pathol.*, **43** (1), 50–54.

23 Boyd, S.P., Best, M.P. (2018) Persistent reticulocytosis in a case of poodle macrocytosis. *Vet. Clin. Pathol.*, **47** (3), 400–406.

24 Rettig, M.P., Low, P.S., Gimm, J.A., *et al.* (1999) Evaluation of biochemical changes during in vivo erythrocyte senescence in the dog. *Blood*, **93** (1), 376–384.

25 Brown Jr, I.W., Eadie, G.S. (1953) An analytical study of in vivo survival of limited populations of animal red blood cells tagged with radio-iron. *J. Gen. Physiol.*, **36** (3), 327–343.

26 Kaneko, J.J., Green, R.A., Mia, A.S. (1966) Erythrocyte survival in the cat as determined by glycine-2-C14. *Proc. Soc. Exp. Biol. Med.*, **123** (3), 783–784.

27 Hodges, J., Christopher, M.M. (2011) Diagnostic accuracy of using erythrocyte indices and polychromasia to identify regenerative anemia in dogs. *J. Am. Vet. Med. Assoc.*, **238** (11), 1452–1458.

28 Choi, S., Yoon, W., Ahn, H., *et al.* (2022) Prevalence of reticulocytosis in the absence of anemia in dogs with cardiogenic pulmonary edema due to myxomatous mitral valve disease: a retrospective study. *Vet. Sci.*, **9** (6), 293.

29 Fuchs, J., Moritz, A., Grußendorf, E., *et al.* (2018) Reticulocytosis in non-anemic cats and dogs. *J. Small Anim. Pract.*, **59** (8), 480–489.

30 Pattullo, K.M., Kidney, B.A., Taylor, S.M., *et al.* (2015) Reticulocytosis in nonanemic dogs: increasing prevalence and potential etiologies. *Vet. Clin. Pathol.*, **44** (1), 26–36.

31 Moretti, P., Giordano, A., Stefanello, D., *et al.* (2017) Nucleated erythrocytes in blood smears of dogs undergoing chemotherapy. *Vet. Comp. Oncol.*, **15** (1), 215–225.

32 Collicutt, N.B., Garner, B. (2013) Erythrocyte dysplasia in peripheral blood smears from 5 thrombocytopenic dogs treated with vincristine sulfate. *Vet. Clin. Pathol.*, **42** (4), 458–464.

33 Aroch, I., Segev, G., Loeb, E., *et al.* (2009) Peripheral nucleated red blood cells as a prognostic indicator in heatstroke in dogs. *J. Vet. Intern. Med.*, **23** (3), 544–551.

34 Thomas-Hollands, A., Shelton, G.D., Guo, L.T., *et al.* (2021) Congenital dyserythropoiesis and polymyopathy without cardiac disease in male Labrador Retriever littermates. *J. Vet. Intern. Med.*, **35** (5), 2409–2414.

35 Dank, G., Segev, K., Elazari, M., *et al.* (2020) Diagnostic and prognostic significance of rubricytosis in dogs: a retrospective case-control study of 380 cases. *Isr. J. Vet. Med.*, **75** (4), 193–203.

36 Fish, E.J., Hansen, S.C., Spangler, E.A., *et al.* (2019) Retrospective evaluation of serum/plasma iron, red blood cell distribution width, and nucleated red blood cells in dogs with acute trauma (2009-2015): 129 cases. *J. Vet. Emerg. Crit. Care*, **29** (5), 521–527.

37 Weiser, M.G., Kociba, G.J. (1983) Erythrocyte macrocytosis in feline leukemia virus associated anemia. *Vet. Pathol.*, **20** (6), 687–697.

38 Gil-Morales, C., Costa, M., Tennant, K., *et al.* (2021) Incidence of microcytosis in hyperthyroid cats referred for radioiodine treatment. *J. Feline Med. Surg.*, **23** (10), 928–935.

39 Bessis, M. Corpuscles: atlas of red blood cell shapes. 1974, Springer-Verlag, Berlin Heidelberg.

40 Paes, G., Paepe, D., Meyer, E., *et al.* (2013) The use of the rapid osmotic fragility test as an additional test to diagnose canine immune-mediated haemolytic anaemia. *Acta Scanda*, **55** (1), 74–85.

41 Ambar, N., Tovar, T. (2022) Suspected hemolytic anemia secondary to acute zinc toxicity after ingestion of "max strength" (zinc oxide) diaper rash cream. *J. Vet. Emerg. Crit. Care*, **31** (1), 125–128.

42 Nair, R., Riddle, E.A., Thrall, M.A. (2019) Hemolytic anemia, spherocytosis, and thrombocytopenia associated with honey bee envenomation in a dog. *Vet. Clin. Pathol.*, **48** (4), 620–623.

43 Finney, E.R., Padula, A.M., Leister, E.M. (2020) Red-bellied black snake (*Pseudechis porphyriacus*) envenomation in 17 dogs: clinical signs, coagulation changes, haematological abnormalities, venom antigen levels and outcomes following treatment with a tiger-brown antivenom. *Aust. Vet. J.*, **98** (7), 319–325.

44 Walton, R.M., Brown, D.E., Hamar, D.W., *et al.* (1997) Mechanisms of echinocytosis induced by Crotalus atrox venom. *Vet. Pathol.*, **34** (5), 442–449.

45 Chandler Jr, F.W., Prasse, K.W., Callaway, C.S. (1975) Surface ultrastructure of pyruvate kinase-deficient erythrocytes in the Basenji dog. *Am. J. Vet. Res.*, **36** (10), 1477–1480.

46 Breitschwerdt, E.B., Kordick, D.L., Malarkey, D.E., *et al.* (1995) Endocarditis in a dog due to infection with a novel Bartonella subspecies. *J. Clin. Microbiol.*, **33** (1), 154–160.

47 Ng, C.Y., Mills, J.N. (1985) Clinical and haematological features of haemangiosarcoma in dogs. *Aust. Vet. J.*, **62** (1), 1–4.

48 Coll, A.C., Ross, M.K., Williams, M.L., *et al.* (2022) Effect of washing units of canine red blood cells on storage lesions. *J. Vet. Intern. Med.*, **36** (1), 66–77.

49 Christopher, M.M. (2008) Of human loss and erythrocyte survival: uremia and anemia in chronic renal disease. *Isr. J. Vet. Med.*, **63** (1), 4–11.

50 Weiss, D.J., Kristensen, A., Papenfuss, N., *et al.* (1990) Quantitative evaluation of echinocytes in the dog. *Vet. Clin. Pathol.*, **19** (4), 114–118.

51 Lippi, I., Perondi, F., Lubas, G., *et al.* (2021) Erythrogram patterns in dogs with chronic kidney disease. *Vet. Sci.*, 8 (7), 123.

52 Badylak, S.F., Van Vleet, J.F., Ferrans, V.J., *et al.* (1985) Poikilocytosis in dogs with chronic doxorubicin toxicosis. *Am. J. Vet. Res.*, **46** (2), 505–508.

53 Brown, D.E., Meyer, D.J., Wingfield, W.E., *et al.* (1994) Echinocytosis associated with rattlesnake envenomation in dogs. *Vet. Pathol.*, **31** (6), 654–657.

54 Masserdotti, C. (2009) Unusual "erythroid loops" in canine blood smears after viper-bite envenomation. *Vet. Clin. Pathol.*, **38** (3), 321–325.

55 Christopher, M.M., Lee, S.E. (1994) Red cell morphologic alterations in cats with hepatic disease. *Vet. Clin. Pathol.*, **23** (1), 7–12.

56 Shull, R.M., Bunch, S.E., Maribei, J., *et al.* (1978) Spur cell anemia in a dog. *J. Am. Vet. Med. Assoc.*, **173** (8), 978–982.

57 Cooper, R.A., Leslie, M.H., Knight, D., *et al.* (1980) Red cell cholesterol enrichment and spur cell anemia in dogs fed a cholesterol-enriched atherogenic diet. *J. Lipid Res.* **21** (8), 1082–1089.

58 Warry, E., Bohn, A., Emanuelli, M., *et al.* (2013) Disease distribution in canine patients with acanthocytosis. *Vet. Clin. Pathol.*, **42** (4), 465–470.

59 Passavin, P., Chetboul, V., Poissonnier, C., *et al.* (2021) Red blood cell abnormalities occur in dogs with congenital ventricular outflow tract obstruction. *Am. J. Vet. Res.*, **83** (3), 198–204.

60 Weiss, D.J., Kristensen, A., Papenfuss, N. (1993) Qualitative evaluation of irregularly spiculated red blood cells in the dog. *Vet. Clin. Pathol.*, **22** (4), 117–121.

61 Zini, G., d'Onofrio, G., Erber, W.N., *et al.* (2021) 2021 update of the 2012 ICSH recommendations for identification, diagnostic value, and quantification of schistocytes: Impact and revisions. *Int. J. Lab. Hematol.*, **43** (6), 1264–1271.

62 Bull, B.S., Kuhn, I.N. (1970) The production of schistocytes by fibrin strands (a scanning electron microscopy study). *Blood*, **35** (1), 104–111.

63 Feldman, B.F., Madewell, B.R., O'Neill, S. (1981) Disseminated intravascular coagulation: antithrombin, plasminogen, and coagulation abnormalities in 41 dogs. *J. Am. Vet. Med. Assoc.*, **179** (2), 151–154.

64 Stokol, T. (2012) Laboratory diagnosis of disseminated intravascular coagulation in dogs and cats: the past, the

present, and the future. *Vet. Clin. North Am. Small Anim. Pract.*, **42** (1), 189–202.

65 Peterson, J.L., Couto, C.G., Wellman, M.L. (1995) Hemostatic disorders in cats: a retrospective study and review of the literature. *J. Vet. Intern. Med.*, **9** (5), 298–303.

66 Tholen, I., Weingart, C., Kohn, B. (2009) Concentration of D-dimers in healthy cats and sick cats with and without disseminated intravascular coagulation (DIC). *J. Feline Med. Surg.*, **11** (10), 842–846.

67 Fulton, R., Weiser, M.G., Freshman, J.L., *et al.* (1988) Electronic and morphologic characterization of erythrocytes of an adult cat with iron deficiency anemia. *Vet. Pathol.*, **25** (6), 521–523.

68 Rebar, A.H., Lewis, H.B., DeNicola, D.B., *et al.* (1981) Red cell fragmentation in the dog: an editorial review. *Vet. Pathol.*, **18** (4), 415–426.

69 O'Keefe, D.A., Schaeffer, D.J. (1992) Hematologic toxicosis associated with doxorubicin administration in cats. *J. Vet. Intern. Med.*, **6** (5), 276–282

70 Caldin, M., Carli, E., Furlanello, T., *et al.* (2005) A retrospective study of 60 cases of eccentrocytosis in the dog. *Vet. Clin. Pathol.*, **34** (3), 224–231.

71 Harvey, J.W., Rackear, D. (1985) Experimental onion-induced hemolytic anemia in dogs. *Vet. Pathol.*, **22** (4), 387–392.

72 Yamato, O., Kasai, E., Katsura, T., *et al.* (2005) Heinz body hemolytic anemia with eccentrocytosis from ingestion of Chinese chive (*Allium tuberosum*) and garlic (*Allium sativum*) in a dog. *J. Am. Anim. Hosp. Assoc.*, **41** (1), 68–73.

73 Lee, K.W., Yamato, O., Tajima, M., *et al.* (2000) Hematologic changes associated with the appearance of eccentrocytes after intragastric administration of garlic extract to dogs. *Am. J. Vet. Res.*, **61** (11), 1446–1550.

74 Lieser, J., Schwedes, C., Walter, M., *et al.* (2021) Oxidative damage of canine erythrocytes after treatment with non-steroidal anti-inflammatory drugs. *Tierarztl. Prax. Ausg. K. Kleintiere. Heimtiere.*, **49** (6), 407–413.

75 Desnoyers, M., Hébert, P. (1995) Heinz body anemia in a dog following possible naphthalene ingestion. *Vet. Clin. Pathol.*, **24** (4), 124–125.

76 Romans, C.W., Day, T.K., Smith, J.J. (2020) Oxidative red blood cell damage associated with propofol and intravenous lipid emulsion therapy in a dog treated for 5-fluorouracil toxicosis. *J. Vet. Emerg. Crit. Care*, **30** (4), 481–486.

77 Parachini-Winter, C., Carioto, L.M., Gara-Boivin, C. (2019) Retrospective evaluation of anemia and erythrocyte morphological anomalies in dogs with lymphoma or inflammatory bowel disease. *J. Am. Vet. Med. Assoc.*, **254** (4), 487–495.

78 Carli, E., Tasca, S., Trotta, M., *et al.* (2009) Detection of erythrocyte binding IgM and IgG by low cytometry in sick dogs with Babesia canis or Babesia canis vogeli infection. *Vet. Parasitol.*, **162** (1–2), 51–57

79 Scavelli, T.D., Hornbuckle, W.E., Roth, L., *et al.* (1986) Portosystemic shunts in cats: seven cases (1976-1984). *J. Am. Vet. Med. Assoc.*, **189** (3), 317–325.

80 Attipa, C., Beck, S., Lipscomb, V., *et al.* (2018) Aldosterone-producing adrenocortical carcinoma with myxoid differentiation in a cat. *Vet. Clin. Pathol.*, **47** (4), 660–664.

81 Rautenbach, Y., Goddard, A., Clift, S.J. (2017) Idiopathic myelofibrosis accompanied by peritoneal extramedullary hematopoiesis presenting as refractory ascites in a dog. *Vet. Clin. Pathol.*, **46** (1), 46–53.

82 Bau-Gaudreault, L., Grimes, C. (2021) Pathology in practice. *J. Am. Vet. Med. Assoc.*, **258** (7), 721–724.

83 Weiss, D.J., Smith, S.A. (2002) A retrospective study of 19 cases of canine myelofibrosis. *J. Vet. Intern. Med.*, **16** (2), 174–178

84 Scott, T.N., Bailin, H.G., Jutkowitz, L.A., *et al.* (2021) Bone marrow, blood, and clinical findings in dogs treated with phenobarbital. *Vet. Clin. Pathol.*, **50** (1), 122–131.

85 Smith, J.E., Moore, K., Arens, M., *et al.* (1983) Hereditary elliptocytosis with protein band 4.1 deficiency in the dog. *Blood*, **61** (2), 373–377

86 Di Terlizzi, R., Gallagher P.G., Mohandas, N., *et al.* (2009) Canine elliptocytosis due to a mutant beta-spectrin. *Vet. Clin. Pathol.*, **38** (1), 52–58.

87 Holland, C.T., Canfield, P.J., Watson, A.D., *et al.* (1991) Dyserythropoiesis, polymyopathy, and cardiac disease in three related English springer spaniels. *J. Vet. Intern. Med.*, **5** (3), 151–159.

88 Kumiega, E., Michalek, M., Kasztura M., *et al.* (2020) Analysis of red blood cell parameters in dogs with various stages of degenerative mitral valve disease. *J. Vet. Res.*, **64** (2), 325–332.

89 Kuehn, N.F., Gaunt, S.D. (1986) Hypocellular marrow and extramedullary hematopoiesis in a dog: hematologic recovery after splenectomy. *J. Am. Vet. Med. Assoc.*, **188** (11), 1313–1315.

90 Bonfanti, U., Comazzi, S., Paltrinieri, S., *et al.* (2004) Stomatocytosis in 7 related Standard Schnauzers. *Vet. Clin. Pathol.*, **33** (4), 234–239.

91 Brown, D.E., Weiser, M.G., Thrall, M.A., *et al.* (1994) Erythrocyte indices and volume distribution in a dog with stomatocytosis. *Vet. Pathol.*, **31** (2), 247–250.

92 Castillo, D., Williams, T.L. (2021) Stomatocytosis in a Beagle and Australian Cattle Dog. *Vet. Clin. Pathol.*, **50** (4), 501–506.

93 Pinkerton, P.H., Fletch, S.M., Brueckner, P.J., *et al.* (1974) Hereditary stomatocytosis with hemolytic anemia in the dog. *Blood*, **44** (4), 557–567.

94 Slappendel, R.J., van der Gaag, I., van Nes, J.J., *et al.* (1991) Familial stomatocytosis-hypertrophic gastritis (FSHG), a newly recognised disease in the dog (Drentse Patrijshond). *Vet. Q.*, **13** (1), 30–40.

95 Beaudoin, S., Lanevschi, A., Dunn, M., *et al.* (2002) Peripheral blood smear from a dog. *Vet. Clin. Pathol.*, **31** (1), 33–35.

96 Canfield, P.J., Watson, A.D.J., Ratcliffe, R.C.C. (1987) Dyserythropoiesis, sideroblasts/siderocytes, and hemoglobin crystallization in dog. *Vet. Clin. Pathol.*, **16** (1), 21–28.

97 Simpson, C.F., Gaskin, J.M., Harvey, J.W. (1978) Ultrastructure of erythrocyte parasitized by *Haemobartonella felis. J. Parasitol.*, **64** (3), 504–511.

98 Huerter, L. (2000) Lead toxicosis in a puppy. *Can. Vet. J.*, **41** (7), 565–567.

99 King, J.B. (2016) Proximal tubular nephropathy in two dogs diagnosed with lead toxicity. *Aust. Vet. J.*, **94** (8), 280–284.

100 Lukaszewska, J., Lewandowski, K. (2008) Cabot rings as a result of severe dyserythropoiesis in a dog. *Vet. Clin. Pathol.*, **37** (2), 180–183.

101 Harvey, J.W., Wolfsheimer, K.J., Simpson, C.F., *et al.* (1985) Pathologic sideroblasts and siderocytes associated with chloramphenicol therapy in a dog. *Vet. Clin. Pathol.*, **14** (1), 36–42.

102 Weiss, D.J. (2005) Sideroblastic anemia in 7 dogs (1996-2002). *J. Vet. Intern. Med.*, **19** (3), 325–328.

103 Weiss, D.J., Lulich, J. (1999) Myelodysplastic syndrome with sideroblastic differentiation in a dog. *Vet. Clin. Pathol.*, **28** (2), 59–63.

104 Christopher, M.M., Broussard, J.D., Peterson, M.E. (1995) Heinz body formation associated with ketoacidosis in diabetic cats. *J. Vet. Intern. Med.*, **9** (1), 24–31.

105 Christopher, M.M. (1989) Relation of endogenous Heinz bodies to disease and anemia in cats: 120 cases (1978-1987). *J. Am. Vet. Med. Assoc.*, **194** (8), 1089–1095.

106 Fowles, J.R., Banton, M.I., Pottenger, L.H. (2013) A toxicological review of the propylene glycols. *Crit. Rev. Toxicol.*, **43** (4), 363–390.

107 Houston, D.M., Myers, S.L. (1993) A review of Heinz-body anemia in the dog induced by toxins. *Vet. Hum. Toxicol.* **35** (2), 158–161.

108 Bley, C.R., Roos, M., Price, J., *et al.* (2007) Clinical assessment of repeated propofol-associated anesthesia in cats. *J. Am. Vet. Med. Assoc.*, **231** (9), 1347–1353.

109 Bexfield, N., Archer, J., Herrtage, M. (2007) Heinz body haemolytic anaemia in a dog secondary to ingestion of a zinc toy: a case report. *Vet. J.*, **174** (2), 414–417.

110 Johnson, C.E., Seelig, D.M., Moore, F.M., *et al.* (2020) Spurious, marked leukocytosis in 2 cats with Heinz body hemolytic anemia. *Vet. Clin. Pathol.*, **49** (2), 232–239.

111 Fierro, B.R., Agnew, D.W., Duncan, A.E., *et al.* (2013) Skunk musk causes methemoglobin and Heinz body formation in vitro. *Vet. Clin. Pathol.*, **42** (3), 291–300.

112 Sykes, J.E., Hartmann, K. (2014) Feline leukemia virus infection. *Canine Feline Infect. Dis.* 224–238. doi: 10.1016/B978-1-4377-0795-3.00022-3. Epub 2013 Aug 26. Last accessed (June 8, 2023).

113 Stanley, E.L., Eatroff, A.E. (2017) Hypocobalaminaemia as a cause of bone marrow failure and pancytopenia in a cat. *Aust. Vet. J.*, **95** (5), 156–160.

114 Hasler, A.H., Giger, U. (1996) Serum erythropoietin values in polycythemic cats. *J. Am. Anim. Hosp. Assoc.*, **32** (4), 294–301.

115 Cook, S.M., Lothrop Jr, C.D. (1994) Serum erythropoietin concentrations measured by radioimmunoassay in normal, polycythemic and anemic dogs and cats. *J. Vet. Intern. Med.*, **8** (1), 18–25.

116 Rolph, K.E., Cavanaugh, R.P. (2022) Infectious causes of neoplasia in the domestic cat. *Vet. Sci.*, **9** (9), 467.

117 Park, D.S., Lee, J., Song, K.H., *et al.* (2022) Treatment of acute erythroleukemia with high dose cytarabine in a cat with feline leukemia virus infection. *Vet. Med. Sci.*, **8** (1), 9–13.

118 Tomiyasu, H., Fujino, Y., Takahashi, M., *et al.* (2011) Spontaneous acute erythroblastic leukaemia (AML-M6Er) in a dog. *J. Small Anim. Pract.*, **52** (8), 445–447.

119 Allison, R.W., Fielder, S.E., Meinkoth, J.H. (2010) What is your diagnosis? Blood film from an icteric cat. *Vet. Clin. Pathol.*, **39** (1), 125–126.

120 Pitorri, F., Dell'Orco, M., Carmichael, M., *et al.* (2012) Use of real-time quantitative PCR to document successful treatment of Mycoplasma haemocanis infection with doxycycline in a dog. *Vet. Clin. Pathol.*, **41** (4), 493–496.

121 Tasker, S. (2022) Hemotropic mycoplasma. *Vet. Clin. North Am. Small Anim. Pract.*, **52** (6), 1319–1340.

122 Areco, W.V.C., Aguiar, A., Barraza, V., *et al.* (2022) Macroscopic distribution, histopathology and viral antigen expression in dogs with canine distemper virus-induced hyperkeratosis in nasodigital and other regions. *J. Comp. Pathol.*, **193**, 9–19.

123 Gastellum-Leyva, F., Pena-Jasso, A., Alvarado-Vera, M., *et al.* (2022) Evaluation of the efficacy and safety of silver nanoparticles in the treatment of non-neurological and neurological distemper in dogs: a randomized clinical trial. *Viruses*, **14** (11), 2329.

124 Sleznikow, C.R., Granick, J.L., Cohn, A.L., *et al.* (2022) Evaluation of various sample sources for the cytologic diagnosis of Cytauxzoon felis. *J. Vet. Intern. Med.*, **36** (1), 126–132.

125 Kao, Y.F., Peake, B., Madden, R., *et al.* (2021) A probe-based droplet digital polymerase chain reaction assay for early detection of feline acute cytauxzoonosis. *Vet. Parasitol.*, **292**: 109413.

126 Sherrill, M.K., Cohn, A.L. (2015) Cytauxzoonosis: diagnosis and treatment of an emerging disease. *J. Feline Med. Surg.*, **17** (11), 940–948.

127 Brown, H.M., Lockhart, J.M., Latimer, K.S., *et al.* (2010) Identification and genetic characterization of *Cytauxzoon felis* in asymptomatic domestic cats and bobcats. *Vet. Parasitol.*, **172** (3–4), 311–316.

128 Wikander, Y.M., Anantatat, T., Kang, Q., *et al.* (2020) Prevalence of *Cytauxzoon felis* infection-carriers in Eastern Kansas domestic cats. *Pathogens*, **9** (10), 854.

129 Stayton, E., Lineberry, M., Thomas, J., *et al.* (2021) Emergence of Babesia conradae infection in coyote-hunting Greyhounds in Oklahoma USA. *Parasit. Vectors*, **14** (1), 402.

130 Barash, N.R., Thomas, B., Birkenheuer, A., *et al.* (2019) Prevalence of *Babesia* spp. and clinical characteristics of Babesia vulpes infection in North American dogs. *J. Vet. Intern. Med.*, **33** (5), 2075–2081.

131 Dear, J.D., Birkenheuer, A. (2022) Babesia in North America: an update. *Vet. Clin. North Am. Small Anim. Pract.*, **52** (6), 1193–1209.

132 Ayoob, A.L., Prittie, J., Hackner, S.G. (2010) Feline babesiosis. *J. Vet. Emerg. Crit. Care*, **20** (1), 90–97.

133 Condrad, P., Thomford, J., Yamane, I., *et al.* (1991) Hemolytic anemia caused by *Babesia gibsoni* infection in dogs. *J. Am. Vet. Med. Assoc.*, **199** (5), 601–605.

18

Leukocytes

18.1 Approach to Evaluating Leukocytes

Careful evaluation of leukocytes can provide critical information for the diagnosis, treatment, and monitoring of disease, especially inflammation, infectious organisms, and neoplasia. Visual inspection of leukocytes on a blood smear adds valuable information to that obtained from hematology analyzers, including information about left shifts and toxic changes in neutrophils, cell inclusions, infectious organisms, and neoplastic cells.

Evaluation of leukocytes should begin on low power (e.g., 10× objective) to gain an appreciation of cell distribution. Leukocytes may clump, sometimes in large aggregates at the feathered edge of the slide (e.g., leukergy) and large cells, including neoplastic cells, mast cells, and reactive monocytes, may also be pushed to the feathered edge. These findings may be missed if starting at a higher objective. Higher magnifications (using 40×, 50×, or 100× objectives) can then be used to evaluate morphology or perform a manual differential.

In the absence of a leukocyte concentration from an automated hematology analyzer, an estimated value may be achieved by the following methods:

1) A subjective estimate is categorized broadly as normal, elevated, or low. Such an estimate can be performed quickly and takes into account the uneven distribution of leukocytes across the blood smear, including the clumping of leukocytes at the feathered edge. The detection of severe alterations in leukocyte concentration (i.e., marked leukopenia or leukocytosis) is readily achieved with this method, providing strong clinical utility. Drawbacks include imprecision, high subjectivity, and required experience for comparing leukocyte concentrations to smears with known concentrations.
2) A more quantitative estimate may be obtained by counting the average number of leukocytes present in a field of view and multiplying it by the square of the objective. For example, if an average of 10 leukocytes is counted per field of view using a 40× objective lens, the estimated leukocyte concentration would be $10 \times (40)^2 = 16\,000$ cells μl^{-1}. This method provides freedom to count the leukocytes on the objective where the most accurate count can be performed (e.g., higher objectives in cases of leukocytosis, and lower objectives in cases of leukopenia). This method will underestimate the leukocyte concentration if cell clumping is present.

Visual inspection of leukocytes on a blood smear is recommended for all cases in which a CBC is performed, and is especially important when abnormalities are detected in the CBC, or in sick patients. A manual differential is often helpful, especially in cases with left shift, lymphocytosis, monocytosis, or circulating neoplastic cells. Manual differentials are inherently imprecise due to the low number of cells counted and uneven distribution of leukocytes across the smears; therefore, it is critical to scan the entire slide to gain an appreciation of the types of leukocytes present, and their distribution, including any clumping in the body or at the feathered edge of the smear [1]. Additionally, to increase the accuracy of the manual differential, a minimum of 200 cells should be counted [2], though this may not be possible in cases of severe leukopenia. It is beneficial to scan the monolayer of the smear prior to starting the differential to gain confidence in identifying the cell types present. If cells are encountered that are difficult to classify, compare the chromatin pattern, tinctorial properties of the cytoplasm, and the size of the cells with a known cell line to best classify their lineage. Comparison to the images in this chapter may also be helpful when evaluating leukocytes and leukocyte morphology.

Chapter 18 discusses in detail important morphologic and clinicopathologic changes in leukocytes in health and disease.

18.2 Neutrophils

18.2.1 Normal Neutrophils

18.2.1.1 Morphologic Appearance

Neutrophils in dogs and cats have segmented nuclei with multiple (typically 3–4) lobes joined by narrow regions or fine filaments, with condensed, regularly clumped chromatin. They have an abundant volume of clear to pale-pink cytoplasm (Figures 18.1 and 18.2). Neutrophil half-life in circulation is 5–10 hours.

Note: Low numbers of neutrophils from female dogs and cats may contain a small club-like or 'chicken drumstick' appendage attached to a terminal lobe of the nucleus by a fine chromatin strand known as a *Barr body* (Figure 18.3).

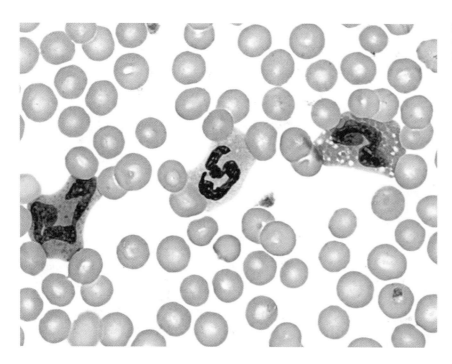

Figure 18.1 Blood smear, dog. Normal neutrophil (center), eosinophil (right), and basophil (left).

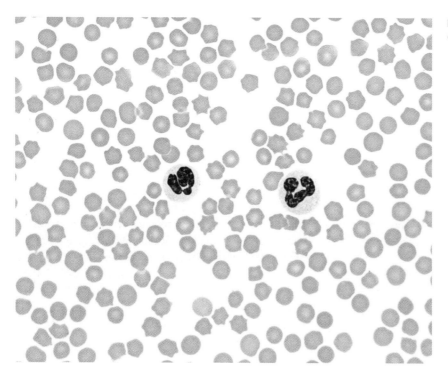

Figure 18.2 Blood smear, cat, 100× objective. Normal neutrophils.

Figure 18.3 Blood smear, dog, 100× objective. Normal neutrophil with a prominent Barr body extending from the 11 o'clock region of the nucleus.

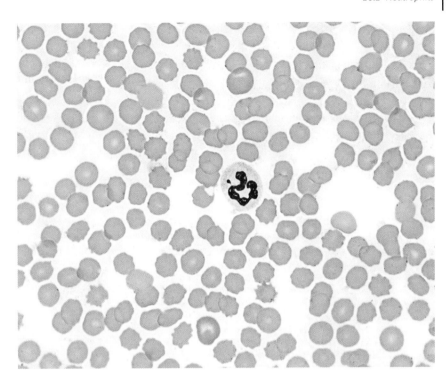

This appendage contains an inactivated X chromosome and is an incidental finding.

18.2.1.2 Clinical Considerations

Neutrophilia There are four major mechanisms for neutrophilia:

1) Increased production (appropriate)
   - Inflammation: May be due to infectious disease, sterile inflammation, immune-mediated disease, tissue necrosis, etc.
2) Increased production (inappropriate)
   - Primary neoplasia: Chronic granulocytic leukemia (see Section 18.9.5)
   - Paraneoplastic: Reported in lymphoma, renal carcinoma, hemangiosarcoma, mast cell tumors, thymoma, ovarian carcinoma, pulmonary adenocarcinoma, and pulmonary squamous cell carcinoma, among others [3–6].
3) Demargination
   - Epinephrine response: Also known as an *excitement response*. Mostly seen in cats and puppies. Typically resolves within 30 minutes. Often associated with lymphocytosis.
   - Corticosteroid response: Also known as a *stress response*. Associated with endogenous or exogenous corticosteroids. Typically causes a neutrophilia between 15 000 and 25 000µl^{-1}, but experimental studies have shown values up to 40 000µl^{-1} [7]. Maximal response occurs within 8 hours and will resolve within 24 hours if there is no further steroid release/exposure; though resolution takes longer with prolonged steroid exposure [7]. Lymphopenia is a hallmark of corticosteroid exposure and is helpful for differentiating it from epinephrine excitement responses.
4) Decreased transit into tissues
   - Corticosteroids
   - Leukocyte adhesion deficiency (LAD): Rare genetic disorder reported in Irish Setters, mixed breed dogs and cats [8–10]. Neutrophils lack surface receptor CD18, preventing binding to blood vessels and extravasation into tissues, resulting in marked neutrophilia (50 000–100 000+µl^{-1}). Affected animals are susceptible to infection and frequently die at a young age, though more prolonged life expectancy has been reported in cats [10].

Marked neutrophilia (>50 000 cells µl^{-1}) may be called a *leukemoid response* as it can mimic neoplasia, though this is seldom due to primary neoplasia of the granulocyte lineage. Commonly associated with a paraneoplastic response to non-hematogenous neoplasia (e.g., lymphoma, hemangiosarcoma, histiocytic sarcoma, and numerous carcinomas), inflammatory/infectious disease (abscess, pyometra, pancreatitis, septic peritonitis, and pneumonia), immune-mediated disease (e.g., IMHA, ITP, and IMPA), and tissue necrosis [3]. Often associated with high mortality rates, especially those with underlying neoplasia [3, 11, 12].

Neutropenia There are three major mechanisms for neutropenia:

1) Decreased production by the bone marrow
   - Infectious disease: Especially Parvovirus (dogs and cats) and FeLV/FIV (cats) [13–17].
   - Drug/toxin exposure: Including chemotherapeutic agents, estrogen exposure (exogenous or endogenous associated with Sertoli cell tumors), antimicrobial agents (chloramphenicol and trimethoprim sulfadiazine), anticonvulsants (phenobarbital and primidone), and miscellaneous (albendazole, methimazole, and griseofulvin) [13, 18, 19].
   - Bone marrow disease: Neoplasia, necrosis, myelofibrosis, and radiation therapy. Often associated with pancytopenia.
2) Utilization
   - Acute, fulminant inflammation: Marked inflammation, bacterial sepsis, and endotoxemia [13].
3) Destruction
   - Immune-mediated neutropenia is rare in dogs and cats.
   - Dogs with corticosteroid-responsive, idiopathic neutropenia are typically younger (<4 years) and have lower neutrophil concentrations (typically <200 cells μl^{-1}) than patients with known causes of neutropenia [20].

18.2.2 Hypersegmented Neutrophils

18.2.2.1 Morphologic Appearance

Neutrophils are considered hypersegmented when nuclei have five or more distinct lobes (Figure 18.4).

18.2.2.2 Clinical Considerations

Low numbers of hypersegmented neutrophils may be seen in aged blood samples. Hypersegmented neutrophils have been reported in the following pathologic conditions:

- Acute resolution of inflammation: In this scenario, neutrophil hypersegmentation and neutrophilia should be short lived. This scenario has been referred to as a 'right shift'.
- Drug/toxin exposure: Glucocorticoids and amphetamine toxicity [21].
- Leukocyte adhesion disorder (LAD): Decreased transit into tissues and aging of neutrophils in circulation results in hypersegmentation [9].
- Myelodysplastic syndrome [22, 23].
- Cobalamin/folate deficiency [24].

18.2.2.3 Prognosis

Highly variable based on the underlying cause. A good prognosis is seen with the resolution of inflammation and in cases where drug exposure is stopped. Myelodysplasia carries a guarded prognosis. Patients with LAD frequently die at a young age due to infection, though cats may have a more prolonged life expectancy [10].

18.2.3 Immature Neutrophils

18.2.3.1 Morphologic Appearance

The morphology of immature neutrophils from most to least mature is as follows:

- Band neutrophils: Band neutrophils (bands) classically have horseshoe-shaped nuclei forming parallel sides of

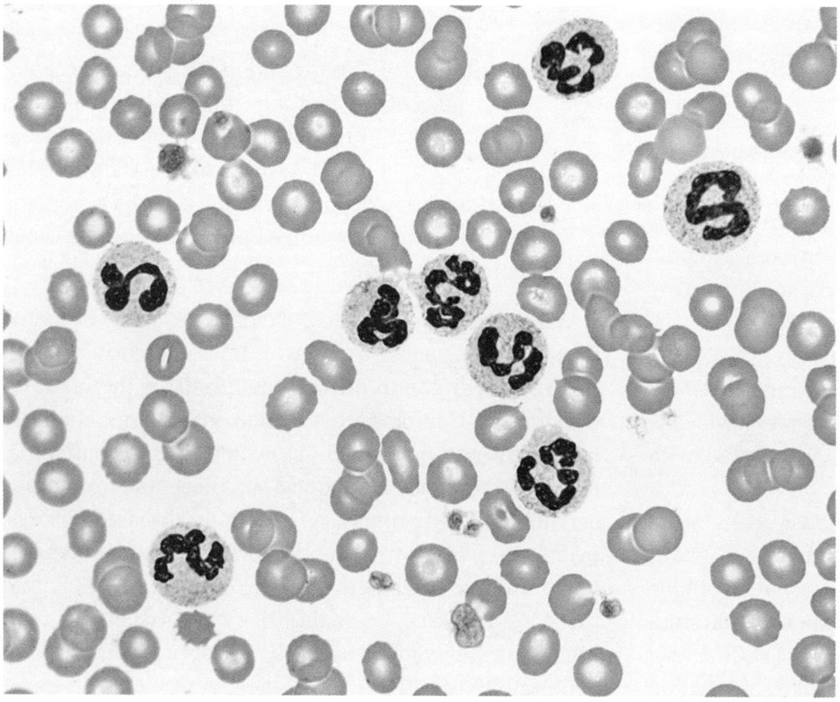

Figure 18.4 Blood smear, dog, 100× objective. Hypersegmented neutrophils in a dog, postoperative pyometra surgery. The hypersegmented neutrophils often have 5–9 distinct nuclear lobes.

equal width along the length of the nucleus (Figures 18.5 and 18.13). The nucleus may also twist to form an elongated or S-shape. The chromatin pattern is slightly more stippled compared to segmented neutrophils, and toxic changes may be present in the cytoplasm (see Section 18.2.5).

- Metamyelocytes: Metamyelocytes have reniform nuclei that have more finely stippled chromatin than bands and inapparent nucleoli (Figure 18.6). They have a moderate volume of pale-blue cytoplasm, often containing toxic changes when in peripheral blood.

Figure 18.5 Blood smear, dog, 100× objective. Band neutrophil (center) with two mature neutrophils. Note the parallel sides and equal width of the nucleus.

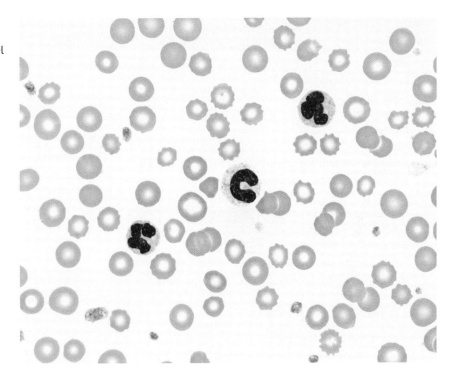

Figure 18.6 Blood smear, dog, 100× objective. Metamyelocyte. The nucleus has a kidney shape.

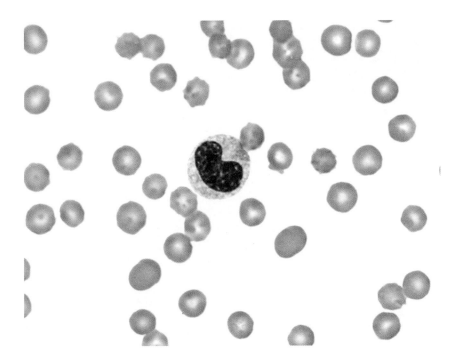

- Myelocytes: Myelocytes have round nuclei with no indentation, finely stippled chromatin, and inapparent nucleoli. They have a moderate volume of pale-blue cytoplasm (Figure 18.7).
- Promyelocytes: Promyelocytes are characterized by abundant pale- to mid-blue cytoplasm that contains diffuse pink granules (Figure 18.8). They have round nuclei with granular chromatin and inapparent nucleoli.
- Myeloblasts: Myeloblasts have round, centrally located nuclei with finely stippled chromatin and prominent single nucleoli. They have a moderate volume of encircling

medium-blue cytoplasm that may contain scant pink granules (Figure 18.9).

18.2.3.2 Clinical Considerations

- Inflammation: Immature neutrophils (usually bands) in circulation are a hallmark of inflammation, supporting upregulated granulopoiesis.
- May be associated with infection [25] and sterile inflammation (pancreatitis, necrosis, trauma, and immune-mediated disease) [26].

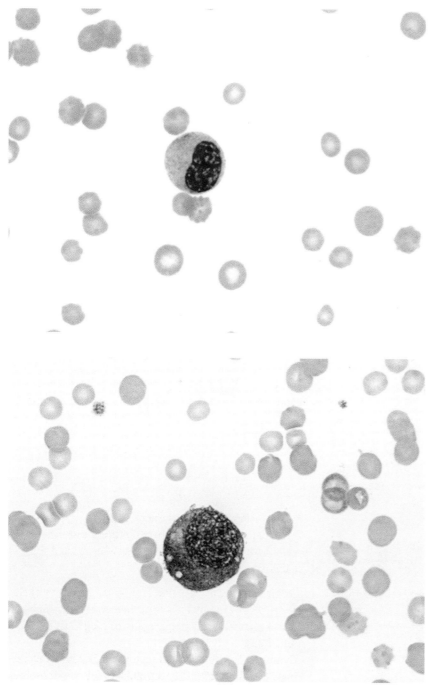

Figure 18.7 Blood smear, dog, 100× objective. Myelocyte. The nucleus is ovoid and the cytoplasm is pale to mid-blue.

Figure 18.8 Blood smear, dog, 100× objective. Promyelocyte. Note the prominent diffuse pink granulation of the cytoplasm.

Figure 18.9 Blood smear, dog, 100× objective. Myeloblast. Note the prominent nucleolus and faint pink cytoplasmic granulation.

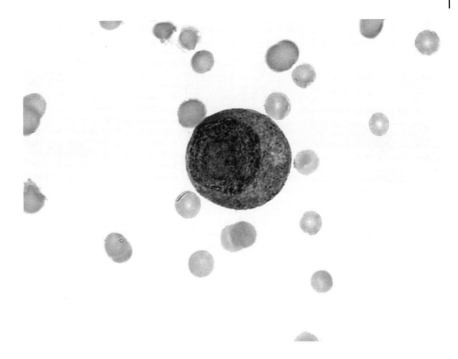

- Promyelocytes and myeloblasts may be seen in cases of severe (mostly septic) inflammation; however, their presence in circulation should raise concern for underlying leukemia.

18.2.3.3 Prognosis

Highly variable based on the underlying cause of the inflammation. A degenerative left shift (DLS) occurs when the number of immature neutrophils exceeds that of mature neutrophils in circulation and is associated with an increased risk of death or euthanasia in hospitalized dogs and cats, irrespective of total leukocyte concentration [27, 28].

18.2.4 Pelger-Huët Anomaly

18.2.4.1 Morphologic Appearance

Patients with Pelger-Huët anomaly have hyposegmented granulocytes with band, reniform, dumbbell, or round nuclei. They may mimic a left shift; however, many key features can be used to help differentiate Pelger-Huët anomaly from an inflammatory left shift:

- The nuclei have mature, clumped chromatin.
- Eosinophils are also frequently hyposegmented (Figure 18.10).
- Absence of toxic changes supports Pelger-Huët anomaly. Note, however, that patients with Pelger-Huët may have toxic changes with an inflammatory response.

18.2.4.2 Clinical Considerations

- Dogs > cats [29].

- Australian Shepherds overrepresented, but reported in many breeds including mixed breed dogs [30].
- Autosomal dominant hereditary disorder. Incomplete or decreased penetrance reported in Australian Shepherds [31].
- Pseudo-Pelger-Huët = acquired dysplastic change seen with infectious disease (FeLV), myeloid neoplasia [32], severe infections, and drug/toxin exposure [33].
- Affected leukocytes have normal function [34].

18.2.4.3 Prognosis

Homozygous inheritance is lethal, with death *in utero* or shortly after birth; often with skeletal deformities [35]. Heterozygous inheritance has little clinical consequence and is an incidental finding to the individual, though may factor into breeding considerations. Pseudo-Pelger-Huët changes resolve with the treatment of underlying disease.

18.2.5 Toxic Neutrophils

18.2.5.1 Morphologic Appearance

Toxic changes within neutrophils are most frequently noted in the cytoplasm (Figures 18.11–18.13) and include the following:

- Döhle bodies: Small, round to angular, blue/gray inclusions, often seen toward the periphery of the cytoplasm. Döhle bodies represent aggregates of rough endoplasmic reticulum.
- Cytoplasmic basophilia: The cytoplasm becomes increasingly deep blue with the accumulation of polyribosomes

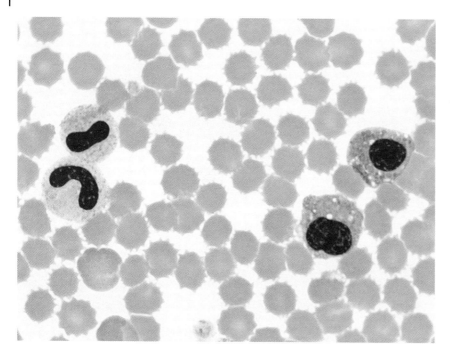

Figure 18.10 Blood smear, dog, Pelger-Huët anomaly. All granulocytes are hyposegmented, with mature, clumped chromatin. One neutrophil (upper left) has a classic 'dumbbell' shape, and no toxic changes are seen in the neutrophils.

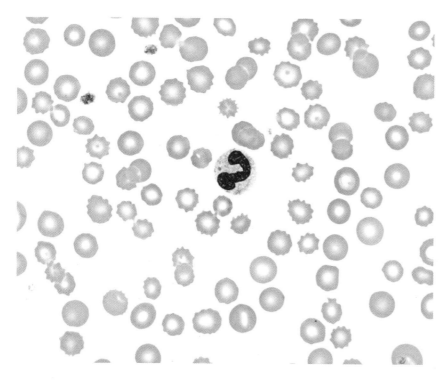

Figure 18.11 Blood smear, dog, 100× objective. Neutrophil with slight toxic changes including a small pale-blue Döhle body (left cytoplasm).

and rough endoplasmic reticulum associated with increased protein production.
- Vacuolation: Mild vacuolation appears lacy and irregular, with moderate to marked vacuolation associated with punctate clear vacuoles.

Nuclear changes may also be observed, including giant neutrophils and ring formation of the nucleus (Figure 18.14).

18.2.5.2 Clinical Considerations
- Small Döhle bodies may be present in some neutrophils from healthy cats, and their presence alone should not be overinterpreted as toxic change for this species [36].
- Toxic changes represent dysplastic changes that develop in the bone marrow secondary to accelerated or abnormal granulopoiesis, most frequently in response to inflammation or infection.

Figure 18.12 Blood smear, dog, 100×
objective. Neutrophils with moderate
toxic changes including numerous
prominent Döhle bodies and increased
cytoplasmic basophilia.

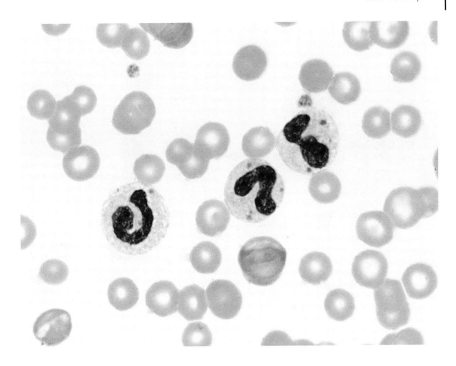

Figure 18.13 Blood smear, cat, 100×
objective. Neutrophils with marked toxic
changes including deep cytoplasmic
basophilia and vacuolation with small
Döhle bodies. Note the band neutrophil
(arrow) with parallel nuclear sides.

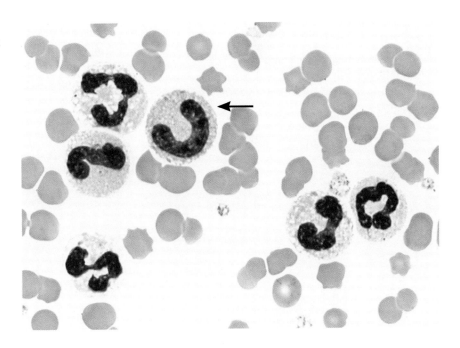

- Toxic changes can be semi-quantitatively graded as mild (Döhle bodies only) (Figure 18.11), moderate (moderate basophilia with variable vacuolation and Döhle bodies) (Figure 18.12), and marked (deep basophilia, prominent vacuoles, +/− Döhle bodies) (Figure 18.13).
- Slight toxic changes can form in aged or stored samples (pseudo-toxic changes). They can form as soon as 4 hours in blood stored at room temperature, and within 24

hours for refrigerated samples (4°C), and blood smears should be made as soon as possible after collection to evaluate toxic changes [37].

18.2.5.3 Prognosis
Toxic changes are associated with increased hospitalization time in both dogs and cats, and increased risk of mortality in hospitalized dogs with increased degree of toxicity [38, 39].

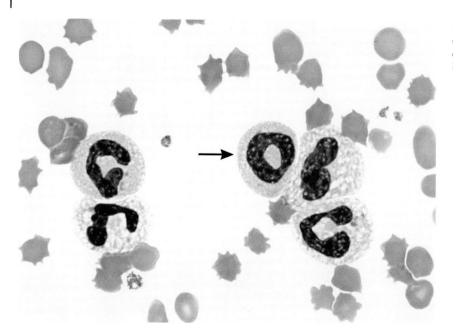

Figure 18.14 Blood smear, cat, 100× objective. Neutrophils with marked toxic changes and dysplastic changes, including a ring-form nucleus (arrow).

18.3 Neutrophil Inclusions

18.3.1 Lysosomal Storage Disease

18.3.1.1 Morphologic Appearance

Neutrophils contain mostly abundant, pink to magenta, fine, regularly sized granules diffusely throughout the cytoplasm (Figures 18.15 and 18.16). Granules frequently stain positively with toluidine blue.

18.3.1.2 Clinical Considerations

- Dogs and cats, though rare disease in both species [40, 41].
- Caused by enzyme or cofactor deficiencies causing abnormal accumulation of material within lysosomes of cells.
- >50 different lysosomal storage diseases organized into subgroups based on the metabolic pathway affected. Common subgroups include mucopolysaccharidoses (MPS), oligosaccharidosis, glycoproteinoses, sphingolipidoses, and proteinoses [41].

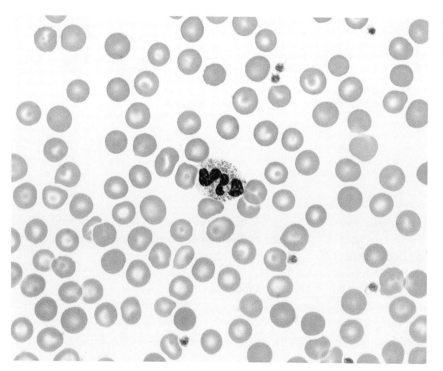

Figure 18.15 Blood smear, dog, 100× objective. Lysosomal storage disease, mucopolysaccharidosis (MPS) type VII.

Figure 18.16 Blood smear, dog, 100× objective. Lysosomal storage disease, mucopolysaccharidosis (MPS) type VI.

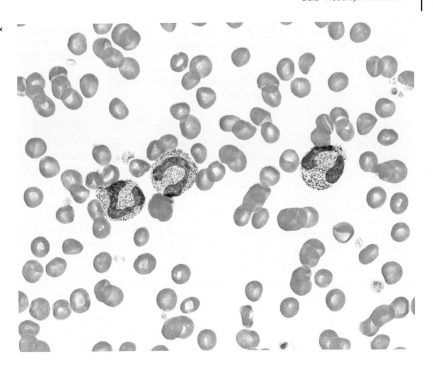

- Mostly diagnosed in juvenile patients, though some adult-onset forms exist [42].
- Clinical signs = neurologic signs (behavioral changes, ataxia, blindness, and seizures), heart failure, skeletal abnormalities, and ocular changes (corneal opacity and cataract formation).

18.3.1.3 Prognosis

Poor. Most cases are diagnosed shortly after birth and rapidly progress, with death usually within the first 12 months of life. Rarely animals with some disorders may survive years beyond the onset of clinical signs.

18.3.2 Neutrophil Granules in Cats

18.3.2.1 Morphologic Appearance

In some cat breeds, a variable number of fine, regularly sized, pink to red granules may be distributed diffusely throughout the cytoplasm (Figure 18.17).

Figure 18.17 Blood smear, cat, 100× objective. Clinically healthy adult Siamese cat with no signs of lysosomal storage disease.

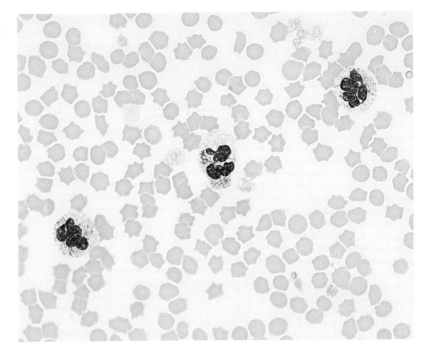

18.3.2.2 Clinical Considerations

- Reported in Birmans, as an autosomal recessive hereditary anomaly [43].
- Granules similar to those studied in Birman cats have also been reported in Siamese cats [44].

18.3.2.3 Prognosis

Excellent. This granulation is an incidental finding but must be distinguished from lysosomal storage disorders and toxic changes.

18.3.3 Mast Cell Granules

18.3.3.1 Morphologic Appearance

Mast cell granules phagocytosed by neutrophils are round, variably sized, and deep purple (Figure 18.18). They are diffusely scattered throughout the cytoplasm when multiple granules are present. The granules are usually more coarse than those seen in cases of inherited enzyme deficiencies and granulation of cats, and different color (deep purple) from the blue/green inclusions noted with sideroleukocytes.

18.3.3.2 Clinical Consideration

- Reported in both dogs and cats with mastocytemia, both with underlying mast cell neoplasia [45, 46].

18.3.3.3 Prognosis

Guarded given that reported cases (and those evaluated by the author) have been associated with underlying mast cell neoplasia.

18.3.4 Sideroleukocytes

18.3.4.1 Morphologic Appearance

Hemosiderin appears as variably sized and chunky inclusions with highly variable coloration ranging from light to dark brown as well as blue/green/aquamarine and may be present in the cytoplasm of neutrophils and monocytes/macrophages in circulation (sideroleukocytes) (Figure 18.19). Small inclusions may be difficult to differentiate from Döhle bodies (Section 18.2.5) and green-blue neutrophil inclusions (Section 18.3.5).

18.3.4.2 Morphologic Appearance

- Reported in dogs with hemolytic anemia treated with blood transfusions [47, 48].
- Stain positive (blue) with Prussian Blue stain for iron.

18.3.4.3 Prognosis

Variable, but often good with the treatment of underlying disease [47, 48].

18.3.5 Green-blue Neutrophil Inclusions

18.3.5.1 Morphologic Appearance

Green/blue, variably sized, irregular to globular material may be seen within the cytoplasm of neutrophils and monocytes (Figure 18.20). These inclusions can mimic hemosiderin in sideroleukocytes (see Section 18.3.4).

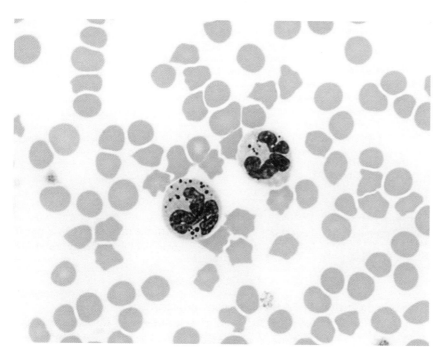

Figure 18.18 Blood smear, cat, 100× objective. Two neutrophils with mast cell granules seen within the cytoplasm in a cat with visceral mast cell neoplasia. The granules have uniform shape but vary in size and are deep purple.

Figure 18.19 Blood smear, cat, 100× objective. A neutrophil (center) contains green/blue inclusions that stained positively for Prussian Blue stain confirming iron and sideroleukocytes.

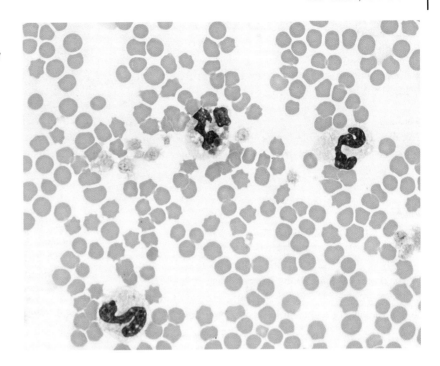

Figure 18.20 Blood smear, dog, 100× objective. A neutrophil contains green-blue cytoplasmic inclusions. The dog had acute liver failure and the inclusions were negative for Prussian Blue stain, with rule outs including bile or lipofuscin.

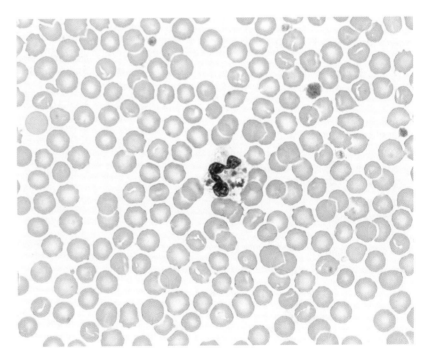

18.3.5.2 Clinical Considerations
- Rule outs include lipopigments (lipofuscin, ceroid), bile, or hemosiderin. These cannot be reliably distinguished with visual inspection of routine stained blood smears.
- Often associated with severe hepatic disease including acute liver failure, hepatic ischemia, and necrosis [49, 50].

18.3.5.3 Prognosis
Poor prognosis in humans with the moniker 'critical green inclusions' due to association with high mortality rates [49].

18.3.6 May-Hegglin Anomaly

18.3.6.1 Morphologic Appearance
Neutrophils contain inclusions that are variably sized (2–4 μm), elongated or fusiform, and mid-blue/gray

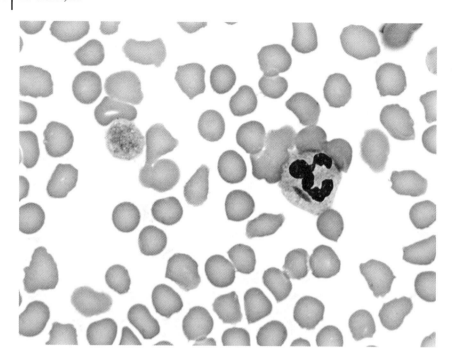

Figure 18.21 Blood smear, dog. May-Hegglin anomaly. Note the fusiform cytoplasmic inclusion in the neutrophil and the giant platelet. Slide courtesy of Dr. Bente Flatland.

(Figure 18.21). Single or multiple inclusions may be present within a single neutrophil. Macroplatelets are also present. The fusiform shape is helpful to distinguish from Döhle bodies and infectious agents such as Rickettsial morulae.

18.3.6.2 Clinical Considerations
- Single case reported in a Pug dog.
- Caused by a mutation in MYH9 gene that encodes non-muscle myosin heavy chain IIA [51].
- Neutrophil inclusions likely represent abnormal aggregates of myosin [52, 53].
- Normal neutrophil function.

18.3.6.3 Prognosis
Appears good based on limited veterinary data.

18.4 Eosinophils

18.4.1 Normal Eosinophils

18.4.1.1 Morphologic Appearance
Dogs: Eosinophils from dogs have segmented nuclei with an abundant volume of clear cytoplasm distended with numerous round, bright-pink granules (Figure 18.1).

Cats: Eosinophils from cats have segmented nuclei with an abundant volume of clear cytoplasm distended with numerous rod-shaped, bright-pink granules (Figure 18.22).

Eosinophil granules (especially in dogs) may coalesce to form larger or amorphous granules, and some cells may lose

granules with punctate, clear vacuoles noted in the cytoplasm (Figure 18.23). These are considered incidental findings. Mild vacuolation is a common, incidental finding, but must be distinguished from gray eosinophils (see Section 18.4.2).

18.4.1.2 Clinical Considerations
Eosinophilia
- Allergic/hypersensitivity disease [54].
- Parasitic disease [55–57].
- Primary eosinophilic inflammatory diseases: Including respiratory [58, 59], gastrointestinal [60, 61], neurologic [62], dermatologic [63, 64], and oral disease [65].
- Idiopathic hypereosinophilic syndrome [66].
- Hypoadrenocorticism [67, 68].
- Paraneoplastic response: Most frequently associated with mast cell neoplasia [69] and T-cell lymphoma [70]. Common cause of marked eosinophilia (>5000 cells μl^{-1}) [71].

Eosinopenia Typically not considered to be of clinical significance.

- Glucocorticoid exposure (endogenous or exogenous) the most common cause [72].

18.4.2 Gray Eosinophils

18.4.2.1 Morphologic Appearance
Gray eosinophils have a pale-blue/gray cytoplasm that appears highly vacuolated with numerous nonstaining granules and granules that appear pale-blue/gray or muddy pink (Figure 18.24).

Figure 18.22 Blood smear, cat, 100×
objective. Normal eosinophils. Note the
bright-pink, rod-shaped granules.

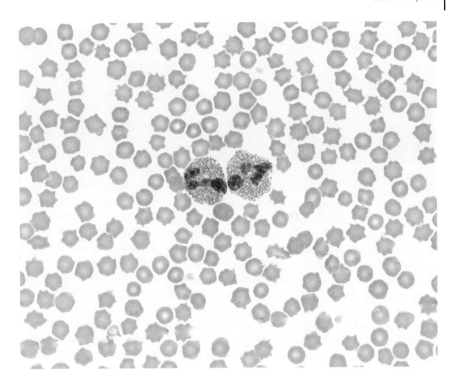

Figure 18.23 Blood smear, dog, 100×
objective. Normal eosinophils with some
coalesced granules and vacuoles.

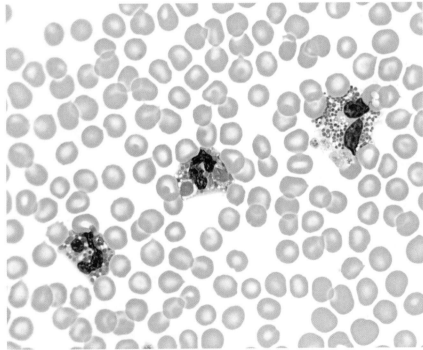

18.4.2.2 Clinical Considerations
- Dogs > Cats [73].
- Most common in Greyhounds and other Sighthounds [74].
  Reported less frequently in other dog breeds and cats [73, 75].
- Important to distinguish these cells from toxic neutrophils.

18.4.2.3 Prognosis
Excellent. Morphologic changes do not affect cell function.

18.5 Basophils

18.5.1 Normal Basophils

18.5.1.1 Morphologic Appearance
Dogs: Canine basophils have segmented nuclei that have a
distinct ribbon-like appearance with geometric or straight
edges (Figure 18.1). They have an abundant volume of pale

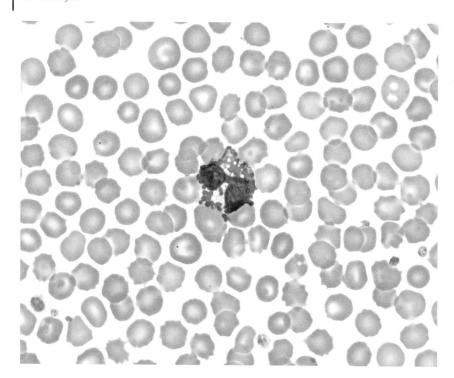

Figure 18.24 Blood smear, dog, 100× objective. Gray eosinophil in peripheral blood from a Greyhound. Note the blue gray to pale pink granules and prominent vacuolation. Slide courtesy of Dr. Maria Vandis.

purple cytoplasm that typically contains low numbers of pin-point to small purple granules that seldom fill the cytoplasm.

Cats: Feline basophils have segmented nuclei and an abundant volume of cytoplasm, usually heavily granulated with round, pale-lavender granules that do not obscure the nucleus, but may overlay it, giving a moth-eaten appearance to the edge of the nucleus (Figure 18.25).

18.5.1.2 Clinical Considerations

Basophilia Often accompanies eosinophilia. Seen most frequently in the following scenarios:

- Parasitic disease [76, 77].
- Allergic/hypersensitivity disease.
- Eosinophilic inflammatory disease [78].

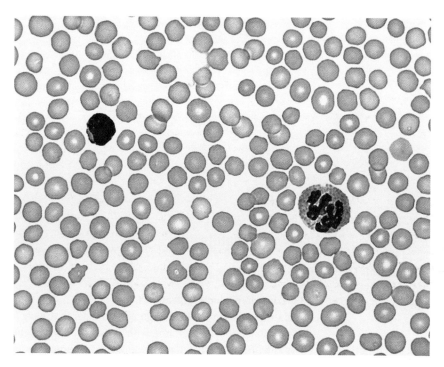

Figure 18.25 Blood smear, cat, 100× objective. Normal basophil (right) and small lymphocyte (left).

- Primary neoplasia: Basophilic leukemia and chronic myelogenous leukemia [79, 80].
- Paraneoplastic: Reported with mast cell neoplasia [81], lymphoma [82], thymoma [83], and essential thrombocythemia [84].

Basopenia Not of clinical significance

18.6 Mast Cells

18.6.1 Mast Cells

18.6.1.1 Morphologic Appearance

Mast cells have an abundant volume of clear to pale-pink cytoplasm that contains a variable number of metachromatic granules (Figures 18.26 and 18.27). They have round

Figure 18.26 Blood smear, dog, 100× objective. Mastocytemia.

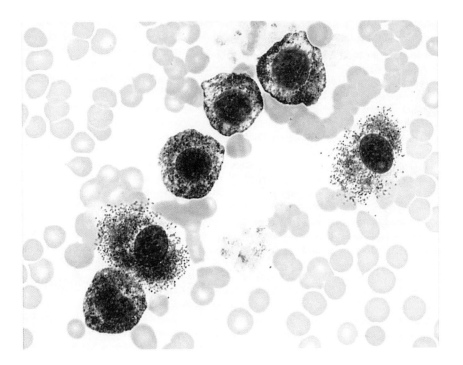

Figure 18.27 Blood smear, cat, 100× objective. Mastocytemia.

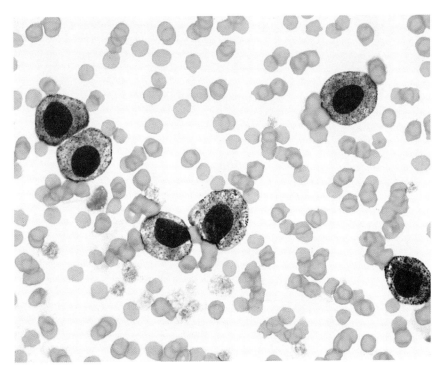

centrally located nuclei, distinguishing them from basophils that have segmented nuclei. They are most easily seen on lower objectives (10× or 20×) and are often pushed to the feathered edge of the slide. Evaluation of a buffy coat preparation may increase the chances of finding low numbers of mast cells in circulation.

18.6.1.2 Clinical Considerations
Dogs
- Most frequently seen with diseases other than mast cell neoplasia. Noted in cases of inflammation, neoplasia other than mast cell tumor, trauma/tissue injury, gastrointestinal disease (including parvoviral enteritis), and markedly regenerative anemia [85, 86].
- Mast cell neoplasia is an uncommon cause of mastocytemia in dogs [85].
- Although less common, mast cell neoplasia may still be associated with mastocytemia in dogs, especially when large numbers are present in circulation [45, 87].

Cats
- Most frequently associated with mast cell neoplasia [88, 89].
- Less common with non-mast cell neoplasia (lymphoid neoplasia and hemangiosarcoma) and possibly chronic renal failure, and mostly associated with low numbers of circulating mast cells (1–2 mast cells per smear) [88].

18.6.1.3 Prognosis
Variable based on species and underlying cause.

18.7 Monocytes

18.7.1 Normal Monocytes

18.7.1.1 Morphologic Appearance
Monocytes in cats and dogs are visually the largest leukocytes in circulation. They have an abundant volume of pale-blue/gray cytoplasm that may contain low numbers of punctate clear vacuoles. The nuclear shape is highly variable, even in the normal state, and may appear band-shaped, reniform, lobulated, or ameboid (Figures 18.28–18.30). The chromatin is lacy to reticulated with some clumping and condensation.

18.7.1.2 Clinical Considerations
Monocytosis
- Inflammation: Often associated with chronic inflammation, but also acute. Often associated with infectious disease, including fungal and protozoal agents [90, 91].
- Necrosis or tissue injury.
- Corticosteroid exposure: Endogenous (stress and hyperadrenocorticism) or exogenous. A three- to fourfold increase is seen within hours of exposure (maximal response by hour 8), and will return to normal within 24 hours with a single dose [7]. This is reliably present in dogs, and less consistent in cats.
- Neoplasia: May be primary (e.g., acute or chronic monocytic leukemia; see Section 18.9) or seen as a paraneoplastic process [4].

Monocytopenia   Not of clinical significance.

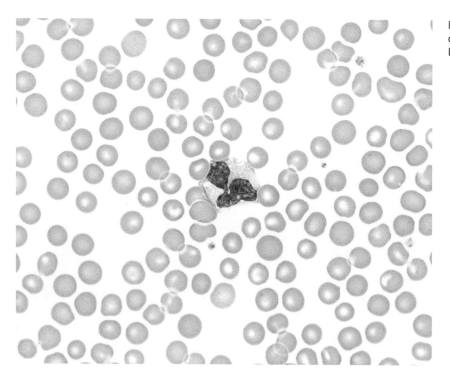

Figure 18.28 Blood smear, dog, 100× objective. Normal monocyte. Note the lobulated nucleus.

Figure 18.29 Blood smear, dog, 100× objective. Normal monocyte. Note the cleaved nucleus and rare punctate vacuoles.

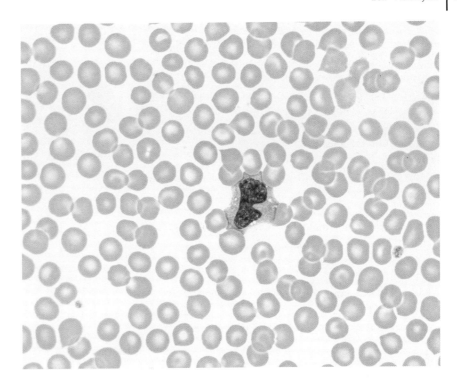

Figure 18.30 Blood smear, cat, 100× objective. Normal monocyte (left) with a reniform nucleus and clumped chromatin. Note the rare punctate vacuoles. A normal eosinophil (right) is also present.

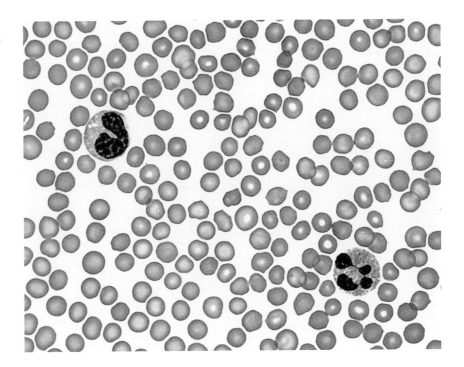

18.7.2 Reactive Monocytes

18.7.2.1 Morphologic Appearance

Reactive changes in monocytes are seen mostly in the cytoplasm, which becomes medium to deep blue and frequently more vacuolated (Figures 18.31 and 18.32). Nuclei may be less lobulated or indented. Monocytes with band or ovoid nuclei can be difficult to differentiate from toxic neutrophil precursors (Figure 18.33), though the ends of the nucleus of monocytes often form rounded knobs, and the chromatin pattern is less condensed than neutrophils, helping to differentiate these cells.

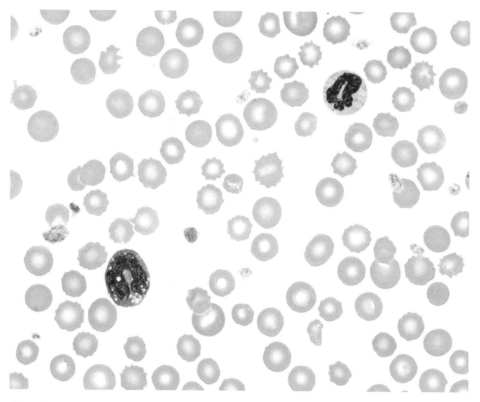

Figure 18.31 Blood smear, dog, 100× objective. Reactive monocyte (left) with medium-blue cytoplasm and increased vacuolation.

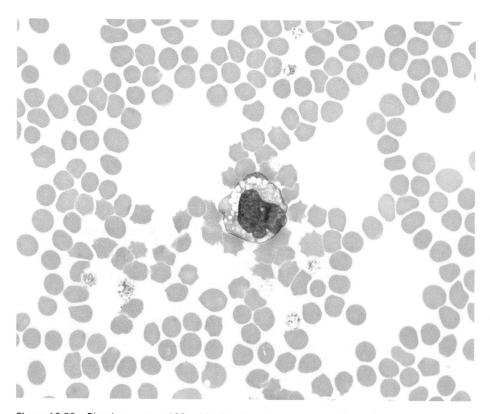

Figure 18.32 Blood smear, cat, 100× objective. Reactive monocyte with medium-blue cytoplasm and prominent vacuolation. Note the finely stippled nuclear chromatin.

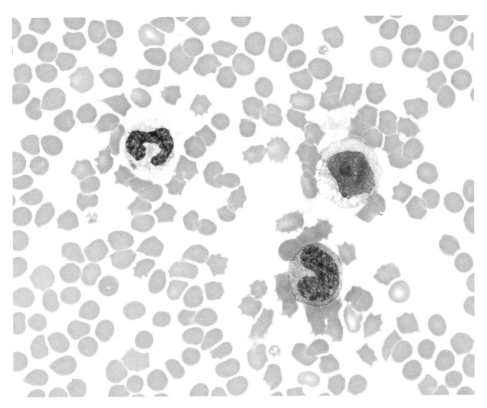

Figure 18.33 Blood smear, cat, 100× objective. A reactive monocyte (upper right) has an ovoid nucleus with finely stippled chromatin and prominent nucleolus. The cytoplasm is medium blue with prominent vacuolation. Compare the chromatin pattern to that of the metamyelocyte with moderate toxic changes (lower right). A neutrophil with marked toxic changes is also present (left).

18.7.2.2 Clinical Considerations
- Support active inflammation.

18.8 Lymphocytes

18.8.1 Normal Lymphocytes

18.8.1.1 Morphologic Appearance
Lymphocytes in both cats and dogs have nuclei approximately the size of a RBC in diameter with mature, regularly clumped chromatin and inapparent nucleoli. They have a scant rim of pale-blue cytoplasm, often forming a unipolar cap or wrapping halfway around the nucleus (Figures 18.34 and 18.35).

18.8.1.2 Clinical Considerations
Lymphocytosis
- Epinephrine excitement response (most common in cats and puppies).
- Physiologic: Young animals (<6 months), associated with antigenic stimulation.
- Antigenic stimulation: Especially in cases of chronic inflammation/infection [92].

- Hypoadrenocorticism [67].
- Neoplasia: Thymoma-associated lymphocytosis [83]. See Section 18.9 for primary neoplastic conditions of lymphocytes.
- Miscellaneous: Lymphocytosis of English Bulldogs [93].

Lymphopenia
- Corticosteroid response: Most common cause of lymphopenia [7].
- Acute inflammation/infection: Especially bacterial [94, 95] and viral infections [96, 97].
- Neoplasia: Including leukemia and lymphoma [98, 99].
- Radiation therapy [100].
- Lymphocyte depletion: Lymphangitis, protein-losing enteropathy [101], and chylous effusion [102].

18.8.2 Reactive Lymphocytes

18.8.2.1 Morphologic Appearance
Reactive lymphocytes are typically larger and have an increased volume of medium- to deep-blue cytoplasm (Figure 18.36). The cytoplasm of reactive lymphocytes may contain granules (Figure 18.37) or pink/blue globules (Russell bodies) (Figures 18.38); however, these inclusions

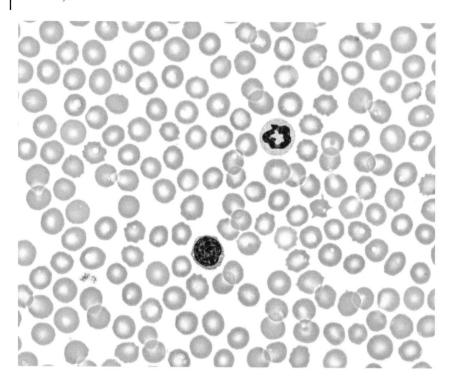

Figure 18.34 Blood smear, dog, 100× objective. Normal lymphocyte with mature, clumped chromatin and a scant volume of pale-blue cytoplasm. A normal neutrophil is also present.

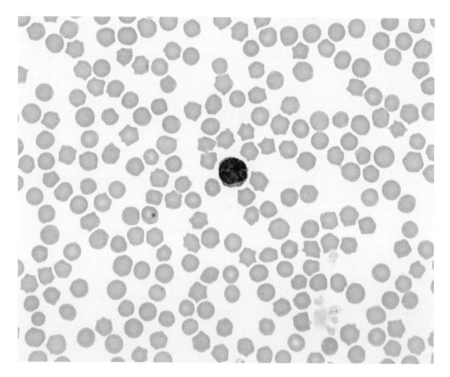

Figure 18.35 Blood smear, cat, 100× objective. Normal lymphocyte with mature, clumped chromatin and a scant rim of pale-blue cytoplasm.

can also be seen in neoplastic lymphocytes (see Section 18.9.1). Nuclei may become indented or convoluted. Nuclear chromatin mostly remains condensed but may become more open and stippled.

18.8.2.2 Clinical Considerations
- Response to antigenic stimulation.

- Chronic inflammatory conditions: Immune-mediated disease (including IMHA), allergic disease [103], pancreatitis, urinary disease, and inflammatory bowel disease [104].
- Infectious disease: Viral [105], fungal, and bacterial.
- Hyperthyroidism: Reported in cats [106].
- Neoplasia: Thymoma [83].

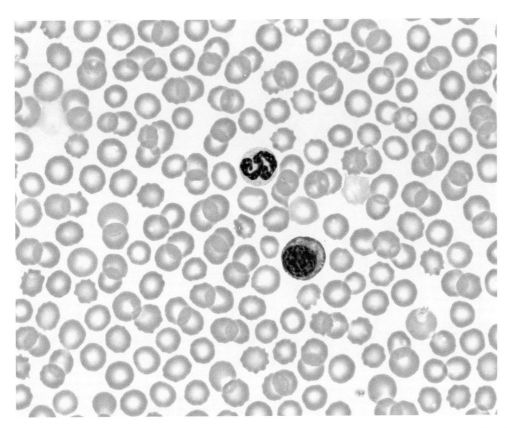

Figure 18.36 Blood smear, dog, 100× objective. Reactive lymphocyte. Note the increased volume of medium-blue cytoplasm.

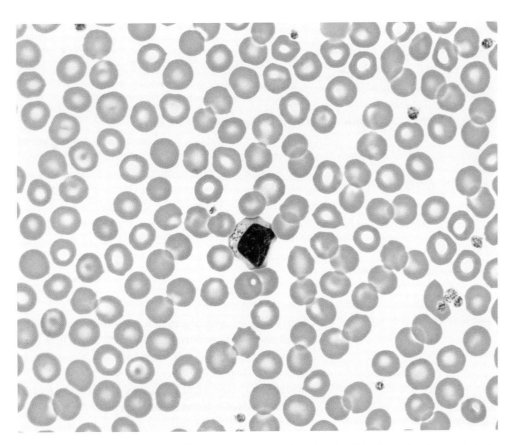

Figure 18.37 Blood smear, dog, 100× objective. Granular lymphocyte. Note the perinuclear packet of azurophilic granules.

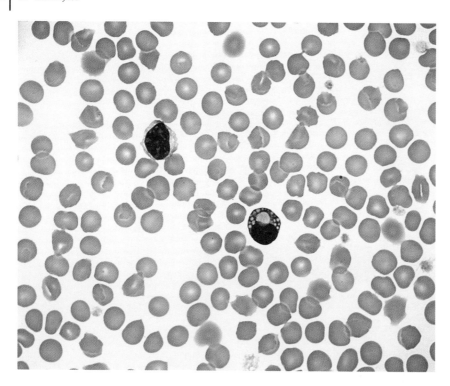

Figure 18.38 Blood smear, dog, 100× objective. Reactive lymphocytes with an increased volume of medium-blue cytoplasm and light blue Russell bodies (lower cell).

18.8.2.3 Prognosis

Typically good if the underlying cause of antigenic stimulation can be successfully treated or controlled.

18.8.3 Granular Lymphocytes

18.8.3.1 Morphologic Appearance

Lymphocyte granules may be seen in the cytoplasm of both small and large lymphocytes and are typically located in a localized perinuclear packet. They vary from fine to coarse/chunky and range from faint pink to deeply azurophilic (Figure 18.37).

18.8.3.2 Clinical Considerations

- Granules suggest either NK cell or CD8+ T-cell phenotype [107].
- Small, mature lymphocytes with granules may be seen in low numbers in healthy patients.
- May be present in increased numbers in inflammatory/infectious conditions [108] or neoplasia (see Sections 18.9.1 and 18.9.3).
- It is important to interpret granular lymphocytes in the context of the overall lymphoid population (heterogeneous or monomorphic morphology) to help differentiate inflammatory versus neoplastic disease.

18.8.3.3 Prognosis

Highly variable based on the underlying cause. Granular lymphocytes associated with inflammatory/infectious disease typically have a good prognosis with the treatment of underlying disease. Granular lymphocytes are often associated with indolent neoplastic disease in dogs (e.g., chronic lymphocytic leukemia [CLL]) but frequently portend a more aggressive disease in cats, irrespective of lymphocyte size.

18.9 Leukocyte Neoplasia

18.9.1 Chronic Lymphocytic Leukemia

18.9.1.1 Morphologic Appearance

CLL is characterized by a monomorphic population of small lymphocytes with nuclei approximately the size of a RBC in diameter, with mature, clumped chromatin and variably prominent nucleoli. The cells have a variable volume of cytoplasm, ranging from a scant rim wrapping halfway around the cell to abundant clear/pale-blue cytoplasm, which may contain a perinuclear packet of azurophilic granules (Figures 18.39 and 18.40).

18.9.1.2 Clinical Considerations

- Dogs > cats [109, 110].
- Most common in older patients.
- T-cell phenotype more common than B-cell in both dogs and cats. Granular T-cell most common phenotype in dogs [109, 111].
- Lymphocyte concentrations highly variable (15 000–1 600 000 cells μl^{-1} in one study [112], and the author has seen concentrations exceed 8 000 000 cells μl^{-1}).

Figure 18.39 Blood smear, dog, 100× objective. Chronic lymphocytic leukemia. There is a monomorphic expansion of small lymphocytes with mature clumped chromatin and a notable lack of any reactive changes. Note the indented and festooning nuclear membrane borders.

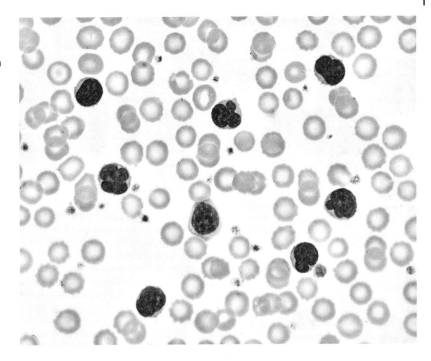

Figure 18.40 Blood smear, dog, 100× objective. Chronic lymphocytic leukemia. Note the perinuclear packet of azurophilic granules and mature clumped chromatin of the nuclei.

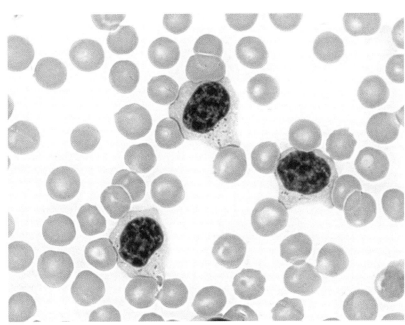

- Important to rule out inflammatory/reactive disorders for cases with lower lymphocyte concentrations (typically <30 000 cells μl^{-1}) including infectious/ inflammatory disease, thymoma-associated lymphocytosis [83], and hyperthyroidism. This may include testing for underlying disease, serial CBC evaluation of lymphocyte concentration and morphology, and/or immunophenotyping and PCR clonality testing on lymphocytes.

18.9.1.3 Prognosis

Typically good. CLL is mostly a slow progressive disease and is often detected as an incidental finding in middle-aged to older patients. Reported poor prognostic indicators include B-cell phenotype, young age (B-cell phenotype only), concurrent anemia (T-cell phenotype only), high Ki67 expression, clinical signs of disease at the time of diagnosis, and high lymphocyte concentrations (>60 000 cells μl^{-1}) [113, 114]. CLL can (rarely) transform to high-grade disease, including transformation to large cell lymphoma (Richter's syndrome) [115, 116].

18.9.2 Acute Lymphoblastic Leukemia

18.9.2.1 Morphologic Appearance

Acute lymphoblastic leukemia (ALL) is characterized by large cells with nuclei approximately twofold to threefold the size of RBCs in diameter with finely stippled immature chromatin and variably prominent nucleoli. Nuclei are often round but may be variably indented or irregular (Figure 18.41). The cells have a small to moderate rim of pale- to medium-blue cytoplasm, with moderate to high N/C ratios, and some cells may contain fine clear vacuoles (Figure 18.42). It is important to note that differentiating ALL cells from acute myeloid leukemia (AML) can be difficult or impossible, and further testing (including flow cytometry or immunocytochemistry) is frequently required.

18.9.2.2 Clinical Considerations

- Leukocytosis (due to neoplastic cells) common; however, normal white blood cell counts or leukopenia can be seen [117, 118].

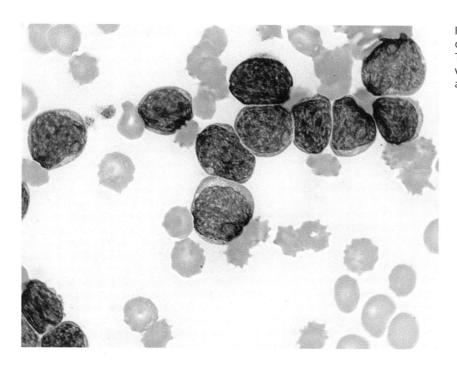

Figure 18.41 Blood smear, dog, 100× objective. Acute lymphoid leukemia (ALL), T-cell phenotype. Note the large nuclei with finely stippled, immature chromatin, and small rim of pale-blue cytoplasm.

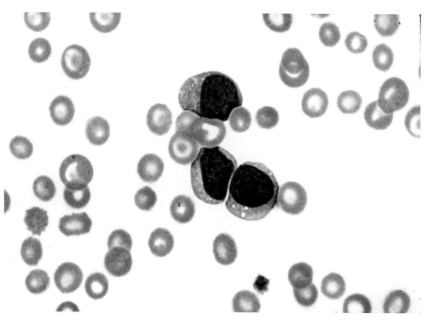

Figure 18.42 Blood smear, dog, 100× objective. Acute lymphoid leukemia (ALL), B-cell phenotype. The cells have finely stippled, immature chromatin, with an increased volume of pale-blue cytoplasm relative to those cells in Figure 18.41, which occasionally contains clear vacuoles. Photo courtesy of Dr. Bill Vernau.

- B-cell phenotype more common in dogs and cats [111, 118].
- Anemia, neutropenia, and thrombocytopenia common hematologic findings.
- Systemic infiltration may be present, including CNS [119], internal organs, and mediastinal lymph nodes [120].

18.9.2.3 Prognosis
Poor to grave [117, 118].

18.9.3 Large Cell Lymphomas

18.9.3.1 Morphologic Appearance
The leukemic phase of large cell lymphoma is characterized by variable numbers of cells with nuclei twofold to fourfold the size of RBCs in diameter, with finely stippled immature chromatin and variably prominent nucleoli (Figure 18.43). The nuclei may have indented or lobulated nuclear borders. The cells have a moderate volume of pale- to medium-blue cytoplasm, which may contain a perinuclear packet of azurophilic granules in the case of large granular lymphoma (LGL) (Figure 18.44).

Figure 18.43 Blood smear, dog, 100× objective. Leukemic phase of large cell lymphoma. The cells have large nuclei with finely stippled immature chromatin and prominent nucleoli.

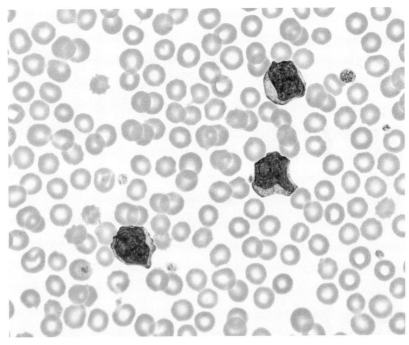

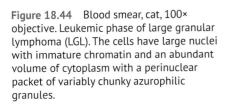

Figure 18.44 Blood smear, cat, 100× objective. Leukemic phase of large granular lymphoma (LGL). The cells have large nuclei with immature chromatin and an abundant volume of cytoplasm with a perinuclear packet of variably chunky azurophilic granules.

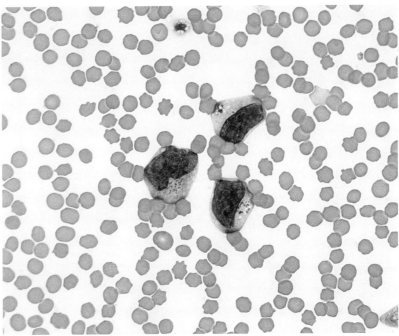

18.9.3.2 Clinical Considerations

- Morphologically similar to acute leukemias, warranting further diagnostic testing including investigation for enlarged lymph nodes or lymphoid organs, flow cytometry, and evaluation of bone marrow.
- Low numbers of large, immature lymphocytes may represent a reactive process or incipient neoplasia, further necessitating additional testing and correlation with clinical findings.
- Typically <100000 cells μl^{-1}. Acute leukemia becomes much more likely beyond this concentration.
- Thrombocytopenia often seen, and more prevalent and severe with a T-cell phenotype [111].

18.9.3.3 Prognosis

Guarded to poor. The leukemic phase of lymphoma supports stage V disease, though this may not affect remission or survival times [121]. LGL in cats carries a grave prognosis, especially with circulating neoplastic cells [122].

18.9.4 Acute Myeloid Leukemias

18.9.4.1 Morphologic Appearance

AML typically manifests with large, immature blast cells in circulation. They have large nuclei, often twofold to fourfold the size of RBCs in diameter, with finely stippled immature chromatin, and variably prominent nucleoli. Some cells may have indented or lobulated nuclei such as some monocytic leukemias (Figure 18.45). The cells have a variable volume of cytoplasm, which may contain diffuse, pink granules (which may be observed in granulocytic leukemia) (Figure 18.46) or clear vacuoles (which can be seen in monocytic leukemia) (Figure 18.45) or megakaryoblastic leukemia (see Chapter 19, Figures 19.14 and 19.15).

18.9.4.2 Clinical Considerations

- AML recognized in dogs and cats include AML-M1 (myeloblastic leukemia without differentiation), AML-M2 (myeloblastic leukemia with differentiation), AML-M4 (myelomonocytic leukemia; eosinophilic and basophilic variants reported), AML-M5a and M5b (monocytic leukemia without and with some monocyte differentiation, respectively), AML-M6 and M6Er (erythroleukemia and erythroleukemia with erythroblasts predominating), and AML-M7 (megakaryoblastic leukemia).
- >30% blasts in circulation support acute leukemia; though rare cases may lack neoplastic cells in circulation [123].
- Concentration of blasts ranged from 300 to 276500 cells μl^{-1} in dogs with AML in one study [124].
- Often associated with mediastinal mass lesions [120].
- Neoplastic cells often stain positively for CD34, which can help to differentiate them from the leukemic phase of large cell lymphoma (Figure 18.47) [111, 112].

18.9.4.3 Prognosis

Grave. Short survival times are reported, even with therapy [124, 125].

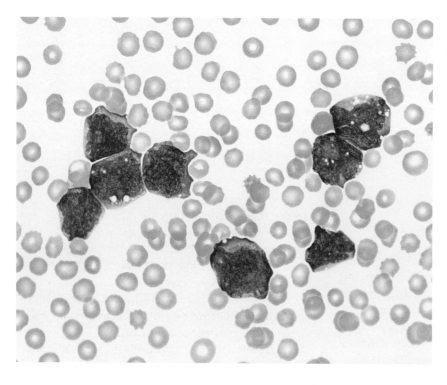

Figure 18.45 Blood smear, dog, 100× objective. Acute myeloid leukemia, AML-M5 monocytic leukemia. The cells have large indented nuclei with finely stippled immature chromatin and cytoplasmic vacuoles.

Figure 18.46 Blood smear, dog, 100× objective. Acute myeloid leukemia, AML-M1, myeloblastic leukemia. Note the fine pink diffuse granulation of the cytoplasm.

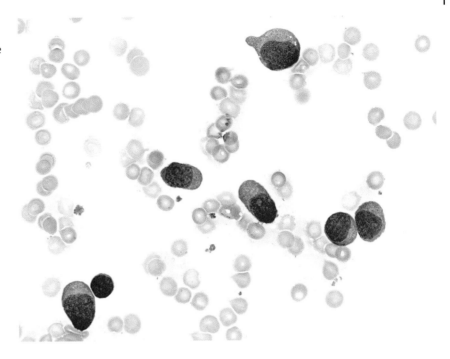

Figure 18.47 Blood smear, dog, 100× objective, CD34 stain, same case as Figure 18.46. Note the strong positive cytoplasmic staining, supporting acute leukemia.

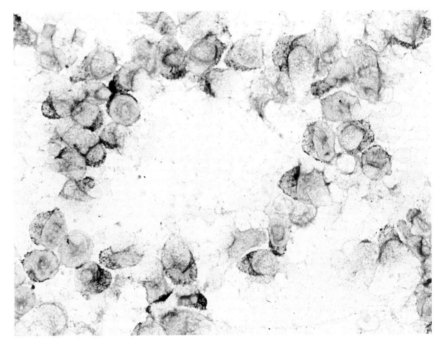

18.9.5 Chronic Myeloid Leukemias

18.9.5.1 Morphologic Appearance

Chronic myeloid leukemia (CML) is typically characterized by large numbers of relatively well-differentiated leukocytes that reflect the tumor lineage origin (Figure 18.48). Neutrophilic CML, for example, often presents with a 5–10-fold increase in differentiated neutrophils with modest increases in precursor cells and no to slight toxic changes, which may help differentiate from a florid inflammatory process (Figure 18.49) [126].

18.9.5.2 Clinical Considerations

- Rare disease in both dogs and cats.
- Neutrophilic, eosinophilic (reported in cats; often associated with FeLV infection) [127], basophilic [79, 128], and monocytic [129] lineages reported.
- Leukocyte concentrations typically >100 000 cells µl^{-1}.
- Important to differentiate from inflammatory (leukemoid) responses (see Section 18.2.1.2).
- May transform into acute leukemia (blast crisis) [130].

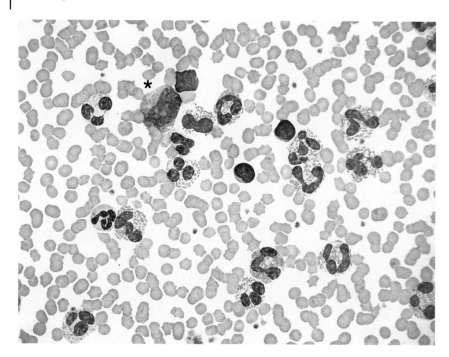

Figure 18.48 Blood smear, cat, 100× objective. Chronic myeloid leukemia, eosinophilic. Note the marked increase in eosinophils and the rare immature eosinophil precursors (asterisk). Photo courtesy of Dr. Andrea Siegel.

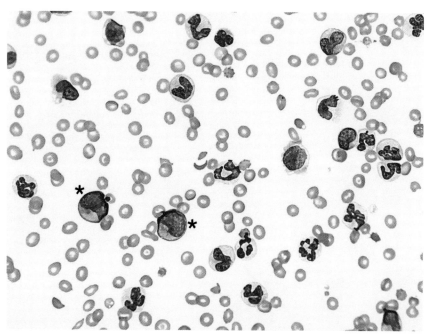

Figure 18.49 Blood smear, dog, 50× objective. Chronic myeloid leukemia. Note the markedly elevated leukocyte concentration dominated by neutrophils with dysplastic changes and rare immature precursors (asterisks). Slide courtesy of Dr. Maria Vandis.

18.9.5.3 Prognosis

Guarded, but prolonged survival possible with therapy [131]. Progression to blast crisis in circulation portends a grave prognosis.

18.10 Leukocyte Infectious Agents

18.10.1 Bacteria

18.10.1.1 Morphologic Appearance

Rickettsia: Rickettsial bacteria are small (0.5 μm) pleomorphic bacteria that replicate within phagolysosomes called morulae

(derived from the Latin *morum* meaning mulberry) in the cytoplasm of leukocytes (Figures 18.50 and 18.51). Differentiating species visually is not possible; however, morulae of *Ehrlichia canis* are typically seen in mononuclear cells (lymphocytes > monocytes), while those from *E. ewingii* and *Anaplasma phagocytophilum* infect granulocytes [132]. Reviewing large numbers of 100× objective fields (500–1000) on buffy coat smears increases the sensitivity of detection for *E. canis* infection where morulae are typically present in low numbers [133].

Rods/cocci: Rods and cocci are rarely seen intracellularly in leukocytes in peripheral blood smears. These are most frequently seen within phagolysosomes in

Figure 18.50 Blood smear, dog. 100× objective. A neutrophil contains a morula of *Anaplasma phagocytophilum*.

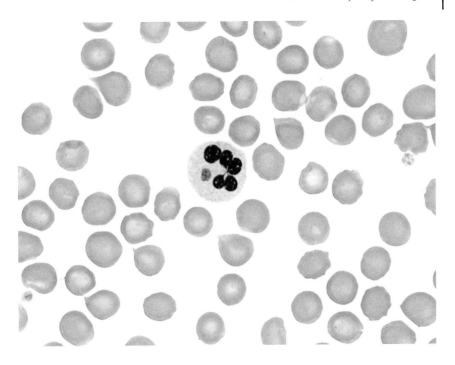

Figure 18.51 Blood smear, dog, 100× objective, Diff Quik stain. A neutrophil contains multiple morulae of *Ehrlichia ewingii*.

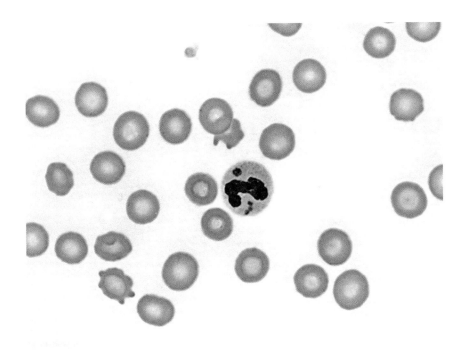

neutrophils and stain deeply basophilic (Figure 18.52). The neutrophils often appear toxic and degenerated. Mycobacteria may also be seen within circulating leukocytes with disseminated disease (Figure 18.53) [134]. *Note*: Neutrophils can phagocytose contaminating bacteria *in vitro*. In this instance, the neutrophils are

typically well preserved, are present in normal numbers, and lack toxic changes or left shifting.

18.10.1.2 Clinical Considerations
Rickettsial disease
- Dogs >> cats.

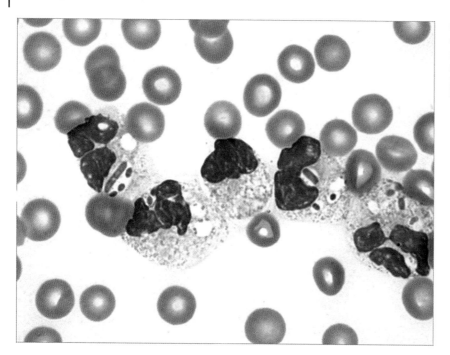

Figure 18.52 Blood smear, dog, 100× objective. Neutrophils contain phagocytosed bacteria of mixed morphology in prominent phagolysosomes. Photo courtesy of Dr. Bill Vernau.

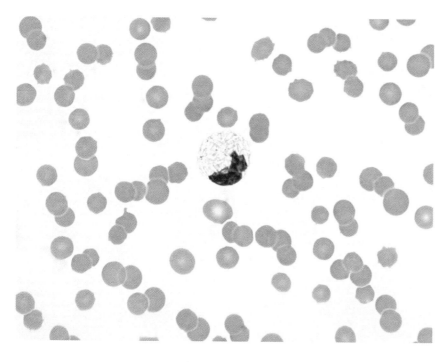

Figure 18.53 Blood smear, dog, 100× objective. A neutrophil contains abundant negatively staining rod-shaped bacteria (*Mycobacteria* spp.).

- Clinical signs = lethargy, fever, lymphadenopathy, neurologic signs, lameness/polyarthropathy, and bleeding diatheses (especially *E. canis*) [135].
- Hematologic changes = thrombocytopenia, neutrophilia (*A. phagocytophilum* and *E. ewingii*), neutropenia (*E. canis*), and anemia.
- A combination of PCR and serology testing provides the highest sensitivity for diagnosis [136].

Rods/Cocci
- Frequently associated with severe or disseminated disease.

18.10.1.3 Prognosis
Mostly good for Rickettsial infection with early detection and appropriate therapy. Severe, acute cases of *E. canis* carry a guarded prognosis [135]. Variable prognosis for bacterial sepsis based on underlying cause and therapy, but mostly poor.

18.10.2 Viral Inclusions

18.10.2.1 Morphologic Appearance

Distemper inclusions may be present within the cytoplasm of neutrophils. They vary from ovoid to polygonal and are most readily identified with Diff Quik stains as deep magenta inclusions. The inclusions stain pale-blue/gray with Wright Giemsa stains (compare Figures 18.54 and 18.55).

18.10.2.2 Clinical Considerations

- Dogs affected; not seen in domesticated cats.
- Clinical signs = fever, cough, conjunctivitis, foot pad and nasal planum hyperkeratosis [137], and neurologic signs.

18.10.2.3 Prognosis

Variable. Dogs with mild signs often recover without therapy, while those with moderate gastrointestinal or respiratory

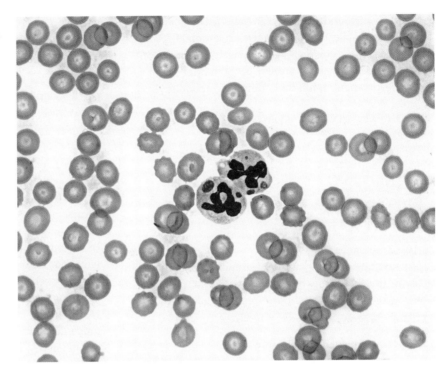

Figure 18.54 Blood smear, dog, 100× objective, Diff Quik stain. Two neutrophils contain multiple ovoid to polygonal, magenta Distemper viral inclusions.

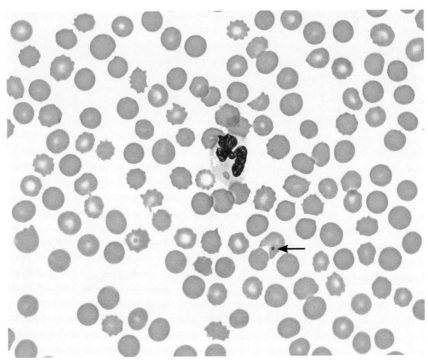

Figure 18.55 Blood smear, dog, 100× objective. A neutrophil contains a single pale-blue/gray Distemper viral inclusion (compare to the deep magenta staining with Diff Quik stain in Figure 18.53. Note also the small viral Distemper inclusion within an erythrocyte (arrow).

signs often recover with supportive therapy. Prognosis is poor when CNS signs are present [138].

18.10.3 Fungi

18.10.3.1 Morphologic Appearance

Fungal agents are rarely seen in circulation, with *Histoplasma capsulatum* most commonly reported. *H. capsulatum* organisms are small (~2–5 μm diameter), uniform, and round, surrounded by a clear halo (pseudo-capsule). They have pale-purple cytoplasm with a basophilic, eccentrically placed, and crescent-shaped nucleus (Figure 18.56). They are most frequently present in monocytes but may also be seen in neutrophils and rarely in eosinophils [139].

18.10.3.2 Clinical Considerations

- Dogs and cats.
- Associated with disseminated disease; noted in 29% of dogs in one retrospective study and 20–33% of feline cases [140–142].
- Evaluation of buffy coat smears increases the chances of finding organisms.

18.10.3.3 Prognosis

Associated with disseminated disease and a poor prognosis with high mortality rates reported [140, 142, 143].

18.10.4 Protozoa

18.10.4.1 Morphologic Appearance

Protozoal agents may be seen in leukocytes in circulation; most commonly *Hepatozoon* gamonts and *Cytauxzoon* schizonts, with *Leishmania* amastigotes reported rarely [144]. Cytauxzoon schizonts can be seen within macrophages and are discussed in Chapter 17; Section 17.6.3.

Hepatozoon gamonts may be seen within neutrophils and monocytes, often compressing the cell nucleus to the side. They are ovoid, ~8–11 μm long, ~4 μm wide, and stain pale-blue or may be negatively staining (Figure 18.57). Nuclei are variably visible. *H. canis* gamonts are slightly larger than those of *H. americanum* but cannot be reliably distinguished by cytology [145]. Evaluation of buffy coat smears increases the sensitivity of detection, especially for *H. americanum* where gamonts are usually present in low numbers [146].

18.10.4.2 Clinical Considerations

- Dogs > cats.
- *H. canis* and *H. americanum* (dogs); *H. felis*, *H. silvestris*, and *H. canis* (cats).
- Affected tissues include skeletal muscle and bone (*H. americanum*); spleen, bone marrow, lymph nodes, liver, kidney, lungs, +/− bone (*H. canis*); skeletal and cardiac muscles (*H. felis* and *H. silvestris*) [146].
- Clinical signs = subclinical infection common with *H. canis* in dogs and *H. felis* in cats [146, 147]. *H. canis* = lethargy, lymphadenomegaly, and splenomegaly. *H. americanum* = musculoskeletal signs (altered gait, weakness, muscle atrophy), pyrexia, and ocular discharge [146, 148].
- Hematologic changes = anemia, leukocytosis (often marked; especially with *H. americanum*), and thrombocytopenia (*H. canis*) [149].
- PCR up to 22 times more sensitive for the detection of *H. canis* than blood smear evaluation [150].

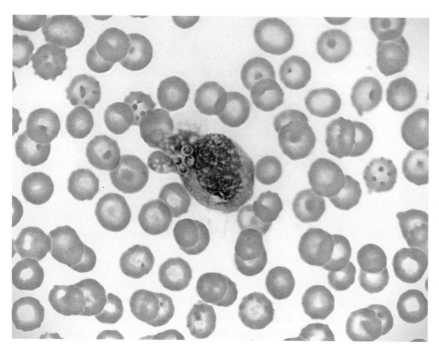

Figure 18.56 Blood smear, dog, 100× objective. A monocyte contains phagocytosed Histoplasma capsulatum organisms.

Figure 18.57 Blood smear, dog, 100×
objective. *Hepatozoon americanum*
gamonts within neutrophils.

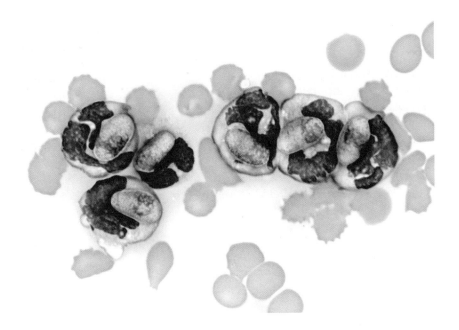

18.10.4.3 Prognosis

Short- and long-term control can be achieved with appropriate therapy [151]. Relapse may occur with *H. americanum*, and persistent infections may carry a more guarded prognosis due to complications from amyloidosis, glomerulopathy, and vasculitis [146, 152].

References

1 Kjelgaard-Hansen, M., Jensen, A.L. (2006) Is the inherent imprecision of manual leukocyte differential counts acceptable for quantitative purposes? *Vet. Clin. Pathol.*, **35** (3), 268–270.

2 Rock, W.A. Jr., Miale, J.B., Johnson, W.D. (1984) Detection of abnormal cells in white cell differentials: comparison of the HEMATRAK automated system with manual methods. *Am. J. Clin. Pathol.*, **81** (2), 233–236.

3 Ziccardi, C., Cohn, L.A., Janacek, B., *et al.* (2022) Etiology and outcome of extreme neutrophilic leukocytosis: a multi-institutional retrospective study of 269 dogs. *J. Vet. Intern. Med.*, **36** (2), 541–548.

4 Petterino, C., Luzio, E., Baracchini, L., *et al.* (2011) Paraneoplastic leukocytosis in a dog with a renal carcinoma. *Vet. Clin. Pathol.*, **40** (1), 89–94.

5 Weltan, S.M., Leisewitz, A.L., Goddard, A. (2008) A case-controlled retrospective study of the causes and implications of moderate to severe leukocytosis in dogs in South Africa. *Vet. Clin. Pathol.*, **37** (2), 164–172.

6 Dole, R.S., MacPhail, C.M., Lappin, M.R. (2004) Paraneoplastic leukocytosis with mature neutrophilia in a cat with pulmonary squamous cell carcinoma. *J. Feline Med. Surg.*, **6** (6), 391–395.

7 Jasper, D.E., Jain, N.C. (1965) The influence of adrenocorticotropic hormone and prednisolone upon marrow and circulating leukocytes in the dog. *Am. J. Vet. Res.*, **26** (113), 844–850.

8 Trowald-Wigh, G., Håkansson, L., Johannisson, A., *et al.* (1992) Leucocyte adhesion protein deficiency in Irish Setter dogs. *Vet. Immunol. Immunopathol.*, **32** (3–4), 261–280.

9 Zimmerman, K.L., McMillan, K., Monroe, W.E., *et al.* (2013) Leukocyte adhesion deficiency type I in a mixed-breed dog. *J. Vet. Diagn. Investig.*, **25** (2), 291–296.

10 Bauer, T.R. Jr., Pratt, S.M., Palena, C.M., *et al.* (2017) Feline leukocyte adhesion (CD18) deficiency caused by a deletion in the integrin β_2 (ITGB2) gene. *Vet. Clin. Pathol.*, **46** (3), 391–400.

11 Lucroy, M.D., Madewell, B.R. (1999) Clinical outcome and associated diseases in dogs with leukocytosis and neutrophilia: 118 cases (1996-1998). *J. Am. Vet. Med. Assoc.*, **214** (6), 805–807.

12 Lucroy, M.D., Madewell, B.R. (2001) Clinical outcome and diseases associated with extreme neutrophilic leukocytosis in cats: 104 cases (1991-1999). *J. Am. Vet. Med. Assoc.*, **218** (5), 736–739.

13 Brown, M.R., Rogers, K.S. (2001) Neutropenia in dogs and cats: a retrospective study of 261 cases. *J. Am. Anim. Hosp. Assoc.*, **37** (2), 131–139.

14 Castro, T.X., Cubel Garcia, R.C., Gonçalves, L.P., *et al.* (2013) Clinical, hematological, and biochemical findings in puppies with coronavirus and parvovirus enteritis. *Can. Vet. J.*, **54** (9), 885–888.

15 Turley, K., Bracker, K., Fernan, C., *et al.* (2023) A comparison on the Sepsis-2 and Sepsis-3 definitions for assessment of mortality risk in dogs with parvovirus. *J. Vet. Emerg. Crit. Care*, **33** (2), 208–216.

16 Kruse, B.D., Unterer, S., Horlacher, K., *et al.* (2010) Prognostic factors in cats with feline panleukopenia. *J. Vet. Intern. Med.*, 24 (6), 1271–1276

17 Stavroulaki, E.M., Mylonakis, M.E., Papanikolaou, E., *et al.* (2020) Steroid-responsive neutropenia in a cat with progressive feline leukemia virus infection. *Vet. Clin. Pathol.*, **49** (3), 389–393.

18 Withers, S.S., Lawson, C.M., Burton, A.G., *et al.* (2016) Management of an invasive and metastatic Sertoli cell tumor with associated myelotoxicosis in a dog. *Can. Vet. J.*, **57** (3), 299–304.

19 Schnelle, A.N., Barger, A.M. (2012) Neutropenia in dogs and cats: causes and consequences. *Vet. Clin. North Am. Small Anim. Pract.*, **42** (1), 111–122.

20 Brown, C.D., Parnell, N.K., Schulman, R.L., *et al.* (2006) Evaluation of clinicopathologic features, response to treatment, and risk factors associated with idiopathic neutropenia in dogs: 11 cases (1990-2002). *J. Am. Vet. Med. Assoc.*, **229** (1), 87–91.

21 Wilcox, A., Russell, K.E. (2008) Hematologic changes associated with Adderall toxicity in a dog. *Vet. Clin. Pathol.*, **37** (2), 184–189.

22 Weiss, D.J., Lulich, J. (1999) Myelodysplastic syndrome with sideroblastic differentiation in a dog. *Vet. Clin. Pathol.*, **28** (2), 59–63.

23 Shimoda, T., Shiranaga, N., Mashita, T., *et al.* (2000) A hematological study on thirteen cats with myelodysplastic syndrome. *J. Vet. Med. Sci.*, **62** (1), 59–64.

24 Gold, A.J., Scott, M.A., Fyfe, J.C. (2015) Failure to thrive and life-threatening complications due to inherited selective cobalamin malabsorption effectively managed in a juvenile Australian Shepherd dog. *Can. Vet. J.*, **56** (10), 1029–1034.

25 Kogan, D.A., Johnson, L.R., Jandrey, K.E., *et al.* (2008) Clinical, clinicopathologic, and radiographic findings in dogs with aspiration pneumonia: 88 cases (2004-2006). *J. Am. Vet. Med. Assoc.*, **233** (11), 1742–1747.

26 Gori, E., Pierini, A., Lippi, I., *et al.* (2021) Leukocytes ratio in feline systemic inflammatory response syndrome and sepsis: a retrospective analysis of 209 cases. *Animals*, **11** (6), 1644.

27 Burton, A.G., Harris, L.A., Owens, S.D., *et al.* (2013) The prognostic utility of degenerative left shifts in dogs. *J. Vet. Intern. Med.*, **27** (6), 1517–1522.

28 Burton, A.G., Harris, L.A., Owens, S.D., *et al.* (2014) Degenerative left shift as a prognostic tool in cats. *J. Vet. Intern. Med.*, **28** (3), 912–917.

29 Deshuillers, P., Raskin, R., Messick, J. (2014) Pelger-Huët anomaly in a cat. *Vet. Clin. Pathol.*, **43** (3), 337–341.

30 Vale, A.M., Tomaz, L.R., Sousa, R.S., *et al.* (2011) Pelger-Huët anomaly in two related mixed-breed dogs. *J. Vet. Diagn. Investig.*, **23** (4), 863–865.

31 Latimer, K.S., Campagnoli, R.P., Danilenko, D.M. (2000) Pelger-Huët anomaly in Australian Shepherds: 87 cases (1991-1997). *Comp. Hematol. Int.*, **10** (1), 9–13.

32 Toth, S.R., Onions, D.E., Jarrett, O. (1986) Histopathological and hematological findings in myeloid leukemia induced by a new feline leukemia virus isolate. *Vet. Pathol.*, **23** (4), 462–470.

33 Shull, R.M., Powell, D. (1979) Acquired hyposegmentation of granulocytes (pseudo-Pelger-Huët anomaly) in a dog. *Cornell. Vet.*, **69** (3), 241–247.

34 Latimer, K.S., Kircher, I.M., Lindl, P.A., *et al.* (1989) Leukocyte function in Pelger-Huët anomaly of dogs. *J. Leukoc. Biol.*, **45** (4), 301–310.

35 Latimer, K.S., Rowland, G.N., Mahaffey, M.B. (1988) Homozygous Pelger-Huët anomaly and chondrodysplasia in a stillborn kitten. *Vet. Pathol.*, **25** (4), 325–328.

36 Ward, J.M., Wright, J.F., Wharran, G.H. (1972) Ultrastructure of granulocytes in the peripheral blood of the cat. *J. Ultrastruct. Res.*, **39** (3), 389–396.

37 Bau-Gaudreault, L., Grimes, C.N. (2019) Effect of time and storage on toxic or pseudo-toxic change in canine neutrophils. *Vet. Clin. Pathol.*, **48** (3), 400–405.

38 Aroch, I., Klement, E., Segev, G. (2005) Clinical, biochemical, and hematological characteristics, disease prevalence, and prognosis of dogs present with neutrophil cytoplasmic toxicity. *J. Vet. Intern. Med.*, **19** (1), 64–73.

39 Segev, G., Klement, E., Aroch, I. (2006) Toxic neutrophils in cats: clinical and clinicopathologic features, and disease prevalence and outcome – a retrospective case control study. *J. Vet. Intern. Med.*, **20** (1), 20–31.

40 Bradbury, A.M., Gurda, B.L., Casal, M.L., *et al.* (2015) A review of gene therapy in canine and feline models of lysosomal storage disorders. *Hum. Gene. Ther. Clin. Dev.*, **26** (1), 27–37.

41 Skelly, B.J., Franklin, R.J.M. (2002) Recognition and diagnosis of lysosomal storage diseases in the cat and dog. *J. Vet. Intern. Med.*, **16** (2), 133–141.

42 Wilkerson, M.J., Lewis, D.C., Marks, S.L., *et al.* (1998) Clinical and morphologic features of mucopolysaccharide type II in a dog: naturally occurring model of Hunter syndrome. *Vet. Pathol.*, **35** (3), 230–233.

43 Hirsch, V.M., Cunningham, T.A. (1984) Hereditary anomaly of neutrophil granulation in Birman Cats. *Am. J. Vet. Res.*, **45** (10), 2170–2174.

44 Thompson, J.C. (2009) Unusual granulation of neutrophils from Siamese cats and possible link with granulation in Birman cats. *N. Z. Vet. J.*, **57** (1), 70.

45 Conrado, F.O., Raskin, R.E. (2017) What is your diagnosis? Purple granules within neutrophils of a dog. *Vet. Clin. Pathol.*, **46** (4), 639–640.

46 O'Neil, E., Burton, S. (2013) What is your diagnosis? Blood smear from a cat. *Vet. Clin. Pathol.*, **42** (3), 393–394

47 Gaunt, S.D., Baker, D.C. (1986) Hemosiderin in leukocytes of dogs with immune-mediated hemolytic anemia. *Vet. Clin. Pathol.*, **15** (3), 8–10.

48 Cluzel, C., Javard, R., Grimes, C. (2016) Pathology in practice. *J. Am. Vet. Med. Assoc.*, **249** (10), 1153–1155.

49 Hodgson, T.O., Ruskova, A., Shugg, C.J., *et al.* (2015) Green neutrophil and monocyte inclusions – time to acknowledge and report. *Br. J. Haematol.*, **170** (2), 229–235.

50 Yang, J., Gabali, A. (2018) Green neutrophilic inclusions: current understanding and review of the literature. *Curr. Opin. Hematol.*, **25** (1), 3–6.

51 Flatland, B., Fry, M.M., Baek, S.J., *et al.* (2011) May-Hegglin anomaly in a dog. *Vet. Clin. Pathol.*, **40** (2), 207–214.

52 Pecci, A., Noris, P., Invernizzi, R., *et al.* (2002) Immunocytochemistry for the heavy chain of the non-muscle myosin IIA as a diagnostic tool for MYH9-related disease. *Br. J. Haematol.*, **117** (1), 164–167.

53 Flatland, B., Kunishima, S. (2011) Successful immunostaining demonstrates abnormal intracytoplasmic MYH9 protein (NMMHC-IIA) in neutrophils of a dog with May-Hegglin anomaly. *Vet. Clin. Pathol.*, **40** (4), 409–410.

54 Walters, A.M., O'Brien, M.A., Selmic, L.E., *et al.* (2017) Comparison of clinical findings between dogs with suspected anaphylaxis and dogs with confirmed sepsis. *J. Am. Vet. Med. Assoc.*, **251** (6), 681–688.

55 Romano, A.E., Saunders, A.B., Gordon, S.G., *et al.* (2021) Intracardiac heartworms in dogs: clincial and echocardiographic characteristics in 72 cases (2010-2019). *J. Vet. Intern. Med.*, **35** (1), 88–97.

56 Sood, N.K., Mekkib, B., Singla, L.D., *et al.* (2012) Cytopathology of parasitic dermatitis in dogs. *J. Parasit. Dis.*, **36** (1), 73–77.

57 Dracz, R.M., Mozzer, L.R., Fujiwara, R.T., *et al.* (2014) Parasitological and hematological aspects of co-infection with Angiostrongylus vasorum and Ancylostoma caninum in dogs. *Vet. Parasitol.*, **200** (1–2), 111–116.

58 Johnson, L.R., Johnson, E.G., Hulsebosch, S.E., *et al.* (2019) Eosinophilic bronchitis, eosinophilic granuloma, and eosinophilic bronchopneumopathy in 75 dogs (2006-2016). *J. Vet. Intern. Med.*, **33** (5), 2217–2226.

59 Lee, E.A., Johnson, L.R., Johnson, E.G., *et al.* (2020) Clinical features and radiographic findings in cats with eosinophilic, neutrophilic, and mixed airway inflammation (2011-2018). *J. Vet. Intern. Med.*, **34** (3), 1291–1299.

60 Lyles, S.E., Panciera, D.L., Saunders, G.K., *et al.* (2009) Idiopathic eosinophilic masses of the gastrointestinal tract in dogs. *J. Vet. Intern. Med.*, **23** (4), 818–823.

61 Craig, L.E., Hardam, E.E., Hertzke, D.M., *et al.* (2009) Feline gastrointestinal eosinophilic sclerosing fibroplasia. *Vet. Pathol.*, **46** (1), 63–70.

62 Cardy, T.J.A., Cornelis, I. (2018) Clinical presentation and magnetic resonance imaging findings in 11 dogs with eosinophilic meningoencephalitis of unknown aetiology. *J. Small Anim. Pract.*, **59** (7), 422–431.

63 Bradley, C.W., Cain, C.L., Wong, T.S., *et al.* (2019) Discriminatory features of acute eosinophilic dermatitis with oedema (Wells-like syndrome) and sterile neutrophilic dermatosis (Sweet's-like syndrome) in dogs. *Vet. Dermatol.*, **30** (6), 517–e157

64 Santoro, D., Pucheu-Haston, C.M., Prost, C., *et al.* (2021) Clinical signs and diagnosis of feline atopic syndrome: detailed guidelines for a correct diagnosis. *Vet. Dermatol.*, **32** (1), 26-e6.

65 Mendelsohn, D., Lewis, J.R., Scott, K.I., *et al.* (2019) Clinicopathological features, risk factors and predispositions, and response to treatment of eosinophilic oral disease in 24 dogs (2000-2016). *J. Vet. Dent.*, **36** (1), 25–31.

66 Sykes, J.E., Weiss, D.J., Buoen, L.C., *et al.* (2001) Idiopathic hypereosinophilic syndrome in 3 Rottweilers. *J. Vet. Intern. Med.*, **15** (2), 162–166.

67 Reagan, K.L., McLarty, E., Marks, S.L., *et al.* (2022) Characterization of clinicopathologic and abdominal ultrasound findings in dogs with glucocorticoid deficient hypoadrenocorticism. *J. Vet. Intern. Med.*, **36** (6), 1947–1957.

68 Sieber-Ruckstuhl, N.S., Harburger, L., Hofer, N., *et al.* (2023) Clinical features and long-term management of cats with primary hypoadrenocorticism using desoxycorticosterone pivalate and prednisolone. *J. Vet. Intern. Med.*, **37** (2), 420–427.

69 Musser, M., Berger, E., Flaherty, H.A., *et al.* (2018) Marked paraneoplastic hypereosinophilia associated with a low-grade, metastatic canine mast cell tumour. *Vet. Rec. Case Rep.*, **6** (2), e000563.

70 Cave, T.A., Gault, E.A., Argyle, D.J. (2004) Feline epitheliotropic T-cell lymphoma with paraneoplastic eosinophilia – immunochemotherapy with vinblastine and human recombinant interferon alpha(2b). *Vet. Comp. Oncol.*, **2** (2), 91–97.

71 Guija-de-Arespacochaga, A., Kremer, L., Künzel, F., *et al.* (2022) Peripheral blood eosinophilia in dogs: prevalence and associated diseases. *Vet. Med. Sci.*, **8** (4), 1458–1465.

72 Lowe, A.D., Campbell, K.L., Barger, A., *et al.* (2008) Clinical, clinicopathological and histological changes observed in 14 cats treated with glucocorticoids. *Vet. Rec.*, **162** (24), 777–783.

73 Holmes, E., Raskin, R.E., McGill, P., *et al.* (2021) Morphologic, cytochemical, and ultrastructural features of gray eosinophils in nine cats. *Vet. Clin. Pathol.*, **50** (1), 52–56.

74 Giori, L., Gironi, S., Scarpa, P., *et al.* (2011) Grey eosinophils in sighthounds: frequency in 3 breeds and comparison of eosinophil counts determined manually and with 2 hematology analyzers. *Vet. Clin. Pathol.*, **40** (4), 475–483.

75 Irvine, K.L., Raskin, R.E., Smith, L.C., *et al.* (2019) Grey eosinophils in a Miniature Schnauzer with a poorly differentiated mast cell tumor. *Vet. Clin. Pathol.*, **48** (3), 406–412.

76 Schnyder, M., Di Cesare, A., Basso, W., *et al.* (2014) Clinical, laboratory and pathological findings in cats experimentally infected with Aelurostrongylus abstrusus. *Parasitol. Res.*, **113** (4), 1425–1433.

77 Karasuyama, H., Tabakawa, Y., Ohta, T., *et al.* (2018) Crucial role for basophils in acquired protective immunity to tick infestation. *Front. Physiol.*, **9**, 1769.

78 Almendros, A., Lai, S.Y., Giuliano, A. (2022) Eosinophilic pulmonary granulomatosis resembling a pulmonary carcinoma in a dog. *Open Vet. J.*, **12** (5), 612–617.

79 Azakami, D., Saito, A, Ochiai, K., *et al.* (2019) Chronic basophilic leukaemia in a dog. *J. Comp. Pathol.*, **166**, 5–8.

80 Mochizuki, H., Seki, T., Nakahara, Y., *et al.* (2014) Chronic myelogenous leukaemia with persistent neutrophilia, eosinophilia and basophilia in a cat. *J. Feline Med. Surg.*, **16** (6), 517–521.

81 Ramdass, K., Lunardon, T., Etzioni, A.L. (2021) An uncommon occurrence of bicavitary effusion due to mast cell neoplasia in a 12-year-old mixed breed dog. *Vet. Clin. Pathol.*, **50** (4), 593–596.

82 Balan, M., Hope, A., Cassidy, J., *et al.* (2017) Marked paraneoplastic basophilia accompanying eosinophilia in a cat with alimentary T-cell lymphoma. *JFMS Open. Rep.*, **3** (2), 2055116917730180.

83 Burton, A.G., Borjesson, D.L., Vernau, W. (2014) Thymoma-associated lymphocytosis in a dog. *Vet. Clin. Pathol.*, **43** (4), 584–588.

84 Mizukoshi, T., Fujino, Y., Yasukawa, K., *et al.* (2006) Essential thrombocythemia in a dog. *J. Vet. Med. Sci.*, **68** (11), 1203–1206.

85 McManus, P.M. (1999) Frequency and severity of mastocytemia in dogs with and without mast cell tumors: 120 cases (1995-1997). *J. Am. Vet. Med. Assoc.*, **215** (3), 355–357.

86 Stockham, S.L., Basel, D.L., Schmidt, D.A. (1986) Mastocytemia in dogs with acute inflammatory diseases. *Vet. Clin. Pathol.*, **15** (1), 16–21.

87 Palić, J., Heier, A., Acke, E., *et al.* (2023) Case of mastocytemia and systemic mastocytosis in a dog: ProCyte Dx and Sysmex XT-2000i scattergram findings, morphologic features, and c-kit somatic mutation analysis. *Vet. Clin. Pathol.*, **52** (2) 334–340.

88 Piviani, M., Walton, R.M., Patel, R.T. (2013) Significance of mastocytemia in cats. *Vet. Clin. Pathol.*, **42** (1), 4–10.

89 Lavabre, T., Betting, A., Bourgès-Abella, N., *et al.* (2019) Abnormal Sysmex XT-2000iV DIFF scattergram in a cat with a prominent mastocytemia. *Vet. Clin. Pathol.*, **48** (4), 624–629.

90 Arbona, N., Butkiewicz, C.D., Keyes, M., *et al.* (2020) Clinical features of cats diagnosed with coccidiomycosis in Arizona, 2004-2018. *J. Feline Med. Surg.*, **22** (2), 129–137.

91 Lilliehöök, I., Tvedten, H.W., Pettersson, H.K., *et al.* (2019) Hepatozoon canis infection causing a strong monocytosis with intra-monocytic gamonts and leading to erroneous leukocyte determinations. *Vet. Clin. Pathol.*, **48** (3), 435–440.

92 Avery, A.C., Avery, P.R. (2007) Determining the significance of persistent lymphocytosis. *Vet. Clin. North Am. Small Anim. Pract.*, **37** (2), 267–282.

93 Rout, E.D., Moore, A.R., Burnett, R.C., *et al.* (2020) Polyclonal B-cell lymphocytosis in English Bulldogs. *J. Vet. Intern. Med.*, **34** (6), 2622–2635.

94 Quilling, L.L., Outerbridge, C.A., White, S.D., *et al.* (2022) Retrospective case series: necrotizing fasciitis in 23 dogs. *Vet. Dermatol.*, **33** (6): 534–544.

95 Hodgson, N., Llewellyn, E.A., Schaeffer, D.J. (2018) Utility and prognostic significance of neutrophil-to-lymphocyte ratio in dogs with septic peritonitis. *J. Am. Anim. Hosp. Assoc.*, **54** (6), 351–359.

96 Carlton, C., Norris, J.M., Hall, E., *et al.* (2022) Clinicopathological and epidemiological findings in pet cats naturally infected with feline immunodeficiency virus (FIV) in Australia. *Viruses*, **14** (10), 2177.

97 Watanabe, R., Eckstrand, C., Liu, H., *et al.* (2018) Characterization of peritoneal cells from cats with experimentally-induced feline infectious peritonitis (FIP) using RNA-seq. *Vet. Res.*, **49** (1), 81.

98 Museux K., Turinelli, V., Rosenberg, D., *et al.* (2019) Chronic lymphopenia and neutropenia in a dog with large granular lymphocytic leukemia. *Vet. Clin. Pathol.*, **48** (4), 721–724.

99 Mutz, M., Boudreaux, B., Kearney, M., *et al.* (2015) Prognostic value of baseline absolute lymphocyte concentration and neutrophil/lymphocyte ratio in dogs with newly diagnosed multi-centric lymphoma. *Vet. Comp. Oncol.*, **13** (4), 337–347.

100 Kent, M.S., Emami, S., Rebhun, R., *et al.* (2020) The effects of local irradiation on circulating lymphocytes in dogs receiving fractionated radiotherapy. *Vet. Comp. Oncol.*, **18** (2), 191–198.

101 Craven, M.D., Washabau, R.J. (2019) Comparative pathophysiology and management of protein-losing enteropathy. *J. Vet. Intern. Med.*, **33** (2), 383–402.

102 Myers 3rd, N.C., Engler, S.J., Jakowski, R.M. (1996) Chylothorax and chylous ascites in a dog with mediastinal lymphangiosarcoma. *J. Am. Anim. Hosp. Assoc.*, **32** (3), 263–269.

103 Bowlt, K., Cattin, I., Stewart, J. (2014) Carbimazole-associated hypersensitivity vasculitis in a cat. *J. Small Anim. Pract.*, **55** (12), 643–647

104 Rout, E.D., Labadie, J.D., Curran, K.M., *et al.* (2020) Immunophenotypic characterization and clinical outcome in cats with lymphocytosis. *J. Vet. Intern. Med.*, **34** (1), 105–116.

105 Gleich, S., Hartmann, K. (2009) Hematology and serum biochemistry of feline immunodeficiency virus-infected and feline leukemia virus-infected cats. *J. Vet. Intern. Med.*, **23** (3), 552–558.

106 Thoday, K.L., Mooney, C.T. (1992) Historical, clinical and laboratory features of 126 hyperthyroid cats. *Vet. Rec.*, **131** (12), 257–264.

107 McDonough, S.P., Moore, P.F. (2000) Clinical hematologic, and immunophenotypic characterization of canine large granular lymphocytosis. *Vet. Pathol.*, **37** (6), 637–646.

108 Sprague, W.S., TerWee, J.A., VandeWoude, S. (2010) Temporal association of large granular lymphocytosis, neutropenia, proviral load, and FasL mRNA in cats with acute feline immunodeficiency virus infection. *Vet. Immunol. Immunopathol.*, **134** (1–2), 115–121.

109 Workman, H.C., Vernau, W. (2003) Chronic lymphocytic leukemia in dogs and cats: the veterinary perspective. *Vet. Clin. North Am. Small Anim. Pract.*, **33** (6), 1379–1399.

110 Campbell, M.W., Hess, P.R., Williams, L.E. (2013) Chronic lymphocytic leukaemia in the cat: 18 cases (2000-2010). *Vet. Comp. Oncol.*, **11** (4), 256–264.

111 Tasca, S., Carli, E., Caldin, M., *et al.* (2009) Hematologic abnormalities and flow cytometric immunophenotyping results in dogs with hematopoietic neoplasia: 210 cases (2002-2006). *Vet. Clin. Pathol.*, **38** (1), 2–12.

112 Vernau, W., Moore, P.F. (1999) An immunophenotypic study of canine leukemias and preliminary assessment of clonality by polymerase chain reaction. *Vet. Immunol. Immunopathol.*, **69** (2–4), 145–164.

113 Rout, E.D., Labadie, J.D., Yoshimoto, J.A., *et al.* (2021) Clinical outcome and prognostic factors in dogs with B-cell chronic lymphocytic leukemia: a retrospective study. *J. Vet. Intern. Med.*, **35** (4), 1918–1928.

114 Comazzi, S., Gelain, M.E., Martini, V., *et al.* (2011) Immunophenotype predicts survival time in dogs with chronic lymphocytic leukemia. *J. Vet. Intern. Med.*, **25** (1), 100–106.

115 Conway, E.A., Waugh, E.M., Knottenbelt, C. (2020) A case of T-cell lymphocytic leukemia progressing to Richter syndrome with central nervous system involvement in a dog. *Vet. Clin. Pathol.*, **49** (1), 147–152.

116 Comazzi, S., Martini, V., Riondato, F., *et al.* (2017) Chronic lymphocytic leukaemia transformation into high-grade lymphoma: a description of Richter's syndrome in eight dogs. *Vet. Comp. Oncol.*, **15** (2), 366–373.

117 Ferrari, A., Cozzi, M., Aresu, L., *et al.* (2021) Tumor staging in a Beagle dog with concomitant large B-cell lymphoma and T-cell acute lymphoblastic leukemia. *J. Vet. Diagn. Investig.*, **33** (4), 792–796.

118 Tomiyasu, H., Doi, A., Chambers, J.K., *et al.* (2018) Clinical and clinicopathological characteristics of acute lymphoblastic leukemia in six cats. *J. Small Anim. Pract.*, **59** (12), 742–746.

119 Vernau, K.M., Terio, K.A., LeCouteur, R.A., *et al.* (2000) Acute B-cell lymphoblastic leukemia with meningeal metastasis causing primary neurologic dysfunction in a dog. *J. Vet. Intern. Med.*, **14** (1), 110–115.

120 Epperly, E., Hume, K.R., Moirano, S., *et al.* (2018) Dogs with acute myeloid leukemia or lymphoid neoplasms (large cell lymphoma or acute lymphoblastic leukemia) may have indistinguishable mediastinal masses on radiographs. *Vet. Radiol. Ultrasound*, **59** (5), 507–515.

121 Flory, A.B., Rassnick, K.M., Stokol, T., *et al.* (2007) Stage migration in dogs with lymphoma. *J. Vet. Intern. Med.*, **21** (5), 1051–1047.

122 Finotello, R., Vasconi, M.E., Sabattini, S., *et al.* (2018) Feline large granular lymphocyte lymphoma: an Italian Society of Veterinary Oncology (SIONCOV) retrospective study. *Vet. Comp. Oncol.*, **16** (1), 159–166.

123 Jain, N.C., Blue, J.T., Grindem, C.B., *et al.* (1991) Proposed criteria for classification of acute myeloid leukemia in dogs and cats. *Vet. Clin. Pathol.*, **20** (3), 63–82.

124 Davis, L.L., Hume, K.R., Stokol, T. (2018) A retrospective review of acute myeloid leukaemia in 35 dogs diagnosed by a combination of morphologic findings, flow cytometric immunophenotyping and cytochemical staining results (2007-2015). *Vet. Comp. Oncol.*, **18** (2), 268–275.

125 Juopperi, T.A., Bienzle, D., Bernreuter, D.C., *et al.* (2011) Prognostic markers for myeloid neoplasms: a comparative review of the literature and goals for future investigation. *Vet. Pathol.*, **48** (1), 182–197.

126 Fine, D.M., Tvedten, H.W. (1999) Chronic granulocytic leukemia in a dog. *J. Am. Vet. Med. Assoc.*, **214** (12), 1809–1812.

127 Gelain, M.E., Antoniazzi, E., Bertazzolo, W., *et al.* (2006) Chronic eosinophilic leukemia in a cat: cytochemical and immunophenotypical features. *Vet. Clin. Pathol.*, **35** (4), 454–459.

128 Shimoda, T., Tanabe, M., Shoji, Y., *et al.* (2022) Monoblastic leukemia (M5a) with chronic basophilic leukemia in a cat. *J. Vet. Med. Sci.*, **84** (2), 251–256.

129 Cruz Cardona, J.A., Milner, R., Aleman, A.R., *et al.* (2011) BCR-ABL translocation in a dog with chronic monocytic leukemia. *Vet. Clin. Pathol.*, **40** (1), 40–47.

130 Comazzi, S., Aresu, L., Marconato, L. (2015) Transformation of canine lymphoma/leukemia to more aggressive diseases: anecdotes or reality? *Front. Vet. Sci.*, 2, 42

131 Anjos, D.S.D., Costa, P.B., Magalhães, L.F., *et al.* (2018) Hydroxyurea-induced onychomadesis in a dog with chronic myeloid leukemia: a case report. *Top. Companion Anim. Med.*, **33** (3), 73–76.

132 Allison, R.W., Little, S.E. (2013) Diagnosis of rickettsial diseases in dogs and cats. *Vet. Clin. Pathol.*, **42** (2), 127–144.

133 Mylonakis, M.E., Koutinas, A.F., Billinis, C., *et al.* (2003) Evaluation of cytology in the diagnosis of acute canine monocytic ehrlichiosis (*Ehrlichia canis*): a comparison between five methods. *Vet. Microbiol.*, **91** (2–3), 197–204.

134 Etienne, C.L., Granat, F., Trumel, C., *et al.* (2013) A mycobacterial coinfection in a dog suspected on blood smear. *Vet. Clin. Pathol.*, **42** (4), 516–521.

135 Diniz, P.P.V.P., Moura de Aguiar, D. (2022) Ehrlichiosis and Anaplasmosis: an update. *Vet. Clin. North Am. Small Anim. Pract.*, **52** (6), 1225–1266.

136 Kidd, L. (2019) Optimal vector-borne disease screening in dogs using both serology-based and polymerase chain reaction-based diagnostic panels. *Vet. Clin. North Am. Small Anim. Pract.*, **49** (4), 703–718.

137 Areco, W.V.C., Aguiar, A., Barraza, V., *et al.* (2022) Macroscopic distribution, histopathology and viral antigen expression in dogs with canine distemper virus-induced hyperkeratosis in nasodigital and other regions. *J. Comp. Pathol.*, **193**, 9–19.

138 Gastellum-Leyva, F., Pena-Jasso, A., Alvarado-Vera, M., *et al.* (2022) Evaluation of the efficacy and safety of silver nanoparticles in the treatment of non-neurological and neurological distemper in dogs: a randomized clinical trial. *Viruses*, **14** (11), 2329.

139 Clinkenbeard, K.D., Cowell, R.L., Tyler, R.D. (1988) Identification of Histoplasma organisms in circulating

eosinophils of a dog. *J. Am. Vet. Med. Assoc.*, **192** (2), 217–218.

140 Mitchell, M., Stark, D.R. (1980) Disseminated canine histoplasmosis: a clinical survey of 24 cases in Texas. *Can. Vet. J.*, **21** (3), 95–100.

141 Davies, C., Troy, G.C. (1996) Deep mycotic infections in cats. *J. Am. Anim. Hosp. Assoc.*, **32** (5), 380–391.

142 Clinkenbeard, K.D., Cowell, R.L., Tyler, R.D. (1987) Disseminated histoplasmosis in cats: 12 cases (1981-1986). *J. Am. Vet. Med. Assoc.*, **190** (11), 1445–1448.

143 VanSteenhouse, J.L., DeNovo, R.C. Jr (1986) Atypical Histoplasma capsulatum infection in a dog. *J. Am. Vet. Med. Assoc.*, **188** (5), 527–528.

144 Giudice, E., Passantino, A. (2011) Detection of Leishmania amastigotes in peripheral blood from four dogs – short communication. *Acta Vet. Hung.*, **59** (2), 205–213.

145 Vincent-Johnson, N.A., Macintire, D.K., Lindsay, D.S., *et al.* (1997) A new Hepatozoon species from dogs: description of the causative agent of canine hepatozoonosis in North America. *J. Parasitol.*, **83** (6), 1165–1172.

146 Baneth, G., Allen, K. (2022) Hepatozoonosis of dogs and cats. *Vet. Clin. North Am. Small Anim. Pract.*, **52** (6), 1341–1358.

147 Baneth, G., Aroch, I., Tal, N., *et al.* (1998) Hepatozoon species infection in domestic cats: a retrospective study. *Vet. Parasitol.*, **79** (2), 123–133.

148 Marchetti, V., Lubas, G., Baneth, G., *et al.* (2009) Hepatozoonoiss in a dog with skeletal involvement and meningoencephalomyelitis. *Vet. Clin. Pathol.*, **38** (1), 121–125.

149 Thongsahuan, S., Chethanond, U., Wasiksiri, S., *et al.* (2020) Hematological profile of blood parasitic infected dogs in Southern Thailand. *Vet. World*, **13** (11), 2388–2394.

150 Aktas, M., Özübek, S., Altay, K., *et al.* (2015) A molecular and parasitological survey of Hepatozoon canis in domestic dogs in Turkey. *Vet. Parasitol.*, **209** (3–4), 264–267.

151 Macintire, D.K., Vincent-Johnson, N.A., Kane, C.W., *et al.* (2001) Treatment of dogs infected with Hepatozoon americanum: 53 cases (1989-1998). *J. Am. Vet. Med. Assoc.*, **218** (1), 77–82.

152 Macintire, D.K., Vincent-Johnson, N.A., Dillon, A.R., *et al.* (1997) Hepatozoonosis in dogs: 22 cases (1989-1994). *J. Am. Vet. Med. Assoc.*, **210** (7), 916–922.

19

Platelets

19.1 Approach to Evaluating Platelets

Visual inspection of a blood smear is a critical component of accurate platelet evaluation. Platelets (especially those from cats) are prone to activation during venipuncture, resulting in clumping or even clot formation, which can result in an artifactually low platelet concentration (pseudothrombocytopenia). A blood smear should always be evaluated to confirm the platelet concentration and to assess platelet morphology, which may provide important clues to underlying disease or patient response to therapy.

Well-mixed, EDTA anticoagulated blood is the preferred sample for platelet evaluation.

To minimize platelet activation during venipuncture, collection of blood using the largest vein and needle appropriate for the patient is recommended; though needle gauges may not have a major effect on platelet clumping and concentration results when jugular venipuncture is performed in cats by experienced phlebotomists [1]. Atraumatic venipuncture without redirection of the needle is also recommended. The EDTA tube should be filled according to manufacturer guidelines and inverted gently 10 times immediately after filling to ensure adequate mixing of the sample. The tube should be inspected for any gross clots, and the wooden end of a cotton swab can be used to stir the sample to further evaluate for any clots.

A well-prepared, high-quality blood smear is essential for accurate evaluation of platelet concentration and morphology. These should be made from either fresh whole blood or well-mixed EDTA anticoagulated blood. For detailed instructions on blood smear preparation, please see Chapter 16, Section 16.2. Blood smears should be evaluated on both low- and high-power objectives. On low power, scan the feathered edge and the body of the smear for any large platelet aggregates, or fibrin clots. Counting platelets and evaluation of platelet morphology are performed at 1000× magnification.

An estimate of the platelet concentration can be performed on a well-prepared blood smear with no platelet aggregates or clots present. To perform an estimate, count the number of platelets present within the monolayer in a 100× objective field. Repeat this step 5–10 times, and divide the number of platelets counted by the number of fields reviewed to obtain an average of platelets per 100× objective field. A single platelet within the monolayer represents approximately 15 000 platelets μl^{-1} [2]. Therefore, multiply the average number of platelets per 100× objective field by 15 000 to obtain a platelet estimate.

Chapter 19 outlines these approaches in detail and discusses important features of platelet morphology and pathology.

19.2 Platelet Distribution

19.2.1 Platelet Clumping

19.2.1.1 Morphologic Appearance
Often seen at the feathered edge of the slide, but may also be seen in the body of the smear. Platelet clumps vary from small (3–5 platelets) to large aggregates comprising tens or even hundreds of platelets (Figure 19.1).

19.2.1.2 Clinical Considerations
- Common cause of pseudothrombocytopenia (up to 71% of feline samples) [3, 4].
- Blood tubes should be evaluated for clots using the wooden end of a cotton swab.
- EDTA is the anticoagulant of choice to evaluate platelets. Clumping more common with citrate than with EDTA in dogs. Clumping is also more likely to occur in refrigerated samples (4°C) as compared to samples stored at room temperature, irrespective of the anticoagulant [5, 6]. Rarely, EDTA-dependent pseudothrombocytopenia may occur in dogs [7].

Clinical Atlas of Small Animal Cytology and Hematology, Second Edition. Andrew G. Burton.
© 2024 John Wiley & Sons, Inc. Published 2024 by John Wiley & Sons, Inc.

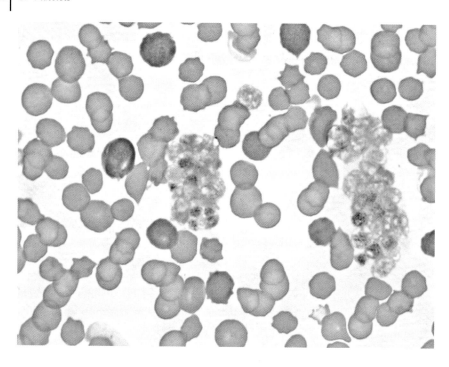

Figure 19.1 Blood smear, cat, 100× objective. Large platelet aggregates.

- Platelet clumps within blood tubes dissociate over time, and rerunning samples with platelet clumping after 24 hours may provide a more accurate concentration [8].

19.2.2 Thrombocytopenia

19.2.2.1 Morphologic Appearance
Thrombocytopenia is characterized by a decreased number of platelets within the monolayer (typically less than 10 platelets per 100× objective field in dogs and cats) (Figure 19.2) in the absence of any platelet aggregates/clumps and any clots within the blood tube. *Note*: It may be necessary to evaluate a slide made from fresh, whole blood collected via clean venipuncture to avoid platelet clumping affecting interpretation.

19.2.2.2 Clinical Considerations
Thrombocytopenia must be verified with evaluation of a blood smear to rule out platelet clumping. If verified, four

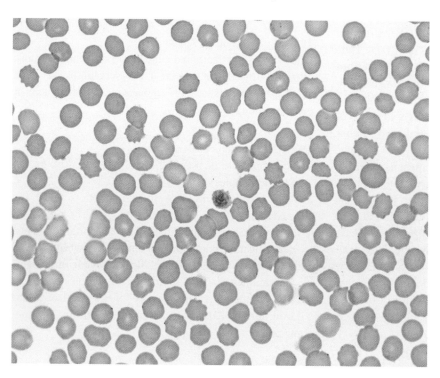

Figure 19.2 Blood smear, dog, 100× objective. Thrombocytopenia. Note the single platelet within the field of view.

major mechanisms may lead to pathologic thrombocytopenia. *Note*: Multiple of these mechanisms may contribute to the development of thrombocytopenia in a single patient:

- Destruction: Most commonly associated with immune thrombocytopenia (ITP) [9]. ITP is more likely to cause severe thrombocytopenia (<10000–30000 platelets μl^{-1}) than other mechanisms in both dogs and cats [10, 11].
- Decreased production by the bone marrow: Consider drug/toxin exposure, including chemotherapy [12] and estrogens (endogenous or exogenous) [13], among others; infectious disease (including Rickettsial disease in dogs and retroviral disease in cats) [11, 14, 15]; neoplasia [16]; and myelofibrosis.
- Consumption of platelets: DIC, [17] snake envenomation, [18] vasculitis, [19] neoplasia, [16, 20] and hemorrhage [21].
- Splenic sequestration: May be associated with drug/toxin exposure [22] as well as infiltrative disease and hypersplenism [23].

Thrombocytopenia often manifests with spontaneous bleeding, especially causing petechiae in the skin, and bleeding along mucous membranes (Figure 19.3). Spontaneous bleeding frequently occurs at a platelet concentration of ~40 000 platelets μl^{-1}; however, there is heterogeneity in bleeding tendency with thrombocytopenia, which may occur at higher concentrations, and some patients do not experience spontaneous bleeding with platelet concentrations less than 30000 platelets μl^{-1} [24, 25].

19.2.3 Thrombocytosis

19.2.3.1 Morphologic Appearance

Blood smears from patients with thrombocytosis have increased numbers of platelets within the monolayer, with often greater than 50 platelets per 100× objective field (Figure 19.4). The platelets usually have regular morphology, and platelet clumping may also be present (see Section 19.2.1). *Note*: Platelet clumping with a platelet concentration within the reference interval may mask a thrombocytosis – always correlate automated platelet concentrations with degree of clumping on blood smear evaluation.

19.2.3.2 Clinical Considerations

Thrombocytosis itself does not usually result in clinical signs or disease, though the underlying cause may. Thrombocytosis is categorized as primary or secondary, with secondary thrombocytosis significantly more common than primary thrombocytosis.

Primary thrombocytosis
- Myeloproliferative disorder with aberrant increased production of platelets by the bone marrow (see Section 19.5.1).

Secondary thrombocytosis
- Neoplasia: Often the most common reported cause of thrombocytosis in dogs [26, 27]. Carcinomas (especially transitional cell carcinoma) and round-cell neoplasia (especially lymphoma and mast cell neoplasia) are most

Figure 19.3 Mucosal bleeding and petechia formation in a dog with marked thrombocytopenia (platelet concentration <5000 platelets μl^{-1}) due to immune-mediated thrombocytopenia.

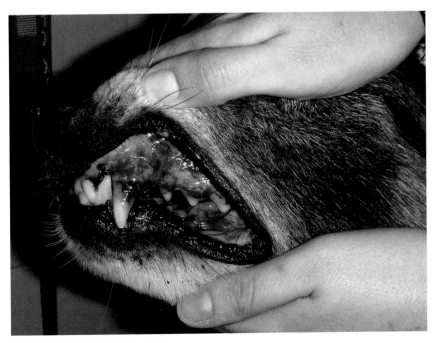

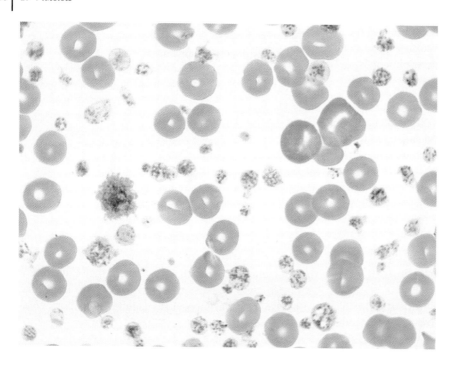

Figure 19.4 Blood smear, dog, 100× objective. Thrombocytosis.

common. Thrombocytosis may also be seen in cases of acute megakaryoblastic leukemia (see Section 19.4.2).

- Inflammation: Mostly IL-6 mediated [28]. Often associated with immune-mediated disease in dogs [27].
- Iron-deficiency anemia: Iron deficiency appears to increase thrombopoiesis through a thrombopoietin (TPO)-independent process [29].
- Splenic contraction or splenectomy: ~30% of circulating platelets are stored in the spleen. Splenic contraction (e.g., due to epinephrine excitement) can cause a transient thrombocytosis that resolves in minutes to hours. Splenectomy may also cause thrombocytosis that typically resolves 2–3 months postoperatively [30, 31]. Thrombocytosis secondary to splenectomy for splenic masses has been correlated with hypercoagulability in dogs [31].
- Drug exposure: Including vincristine, glucocorticoids, and epinephrine.

Thrombocytosis may also be associated with pseudohyperkalemia, characterized by an elevation in potassium concentration greater in serum than plasma due to release from platelets during clotting [32].

19.3 Platelet Morphology

19.3.1 Normal Platelets

19.3.1.1 Morphologic Appearance
Dogs Canine platelets are anucleated, and typically round to ovoid, though elongated shapes may be present. They have clear to pale blue cytoplasm with faint pink, diffusely

scattered granules (Figure 19.5). They are approximately 2–4 μm in diameter. Mean platelet lifespan in circulation is 5–7 days [33].

Cats Platelets from cats are round to ovoid, anucleated, and have clear to pale blue cytoplasm with prominent, diffuse, intensely staining pink to magenta granules (Figure 19.6). They are larger than other species (up to 6 μm, or larger, in diameter), and have more variation in size, which may be attributed to an altered M-loop region in β-1 tubulin, resulting in the production of larger platelets [34]. Mean platelet lifespan in circulation is 4–6 days. Feline platelets are especially prone to activation, forming platelet aggregates and may be degranulated (see Section 19.3.3 and 19.3.4).

19.3.2 Macroplatelets

19.3.2.1 Morphologic Appearance
Macroplatelets are those that are the same size or larger than the diameter of a mature erythrocyte (Figure 19.7).

19.3.2.2 Clinical Considerations
- Also called *giant platelets* or *shift platelets*.
- Low numbers frequently seen in healthy patients, especially in cats.
- Common with regenerative response to thrombocytopenia, though macroplatelets are not always immature or young platelets [35].
- Macrothrombocytopenia: Commonly seen in Cavalier King Charles Spaniels, and less commonly in other

Figure 19.5 Blood smear, dog, 100× objective. Normal platelets. The platelets are small, uniform, and have faint diffuse pink granulation.

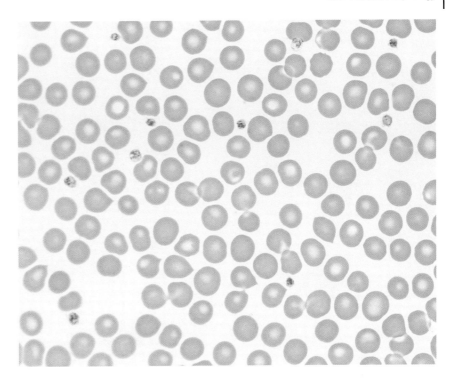

Figure 19.6 Blood smear, cat, 100× objective. Normal platelets. Note the variation in size and prominent diffuse magenta granules.

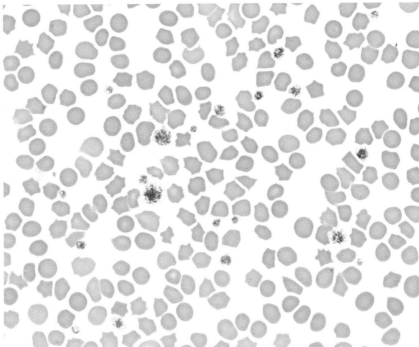

breeds [36–38]. Due to a heritable, autosomal, recessive trait causing mutation in the gene encoding β-1 tubulin resulting in macroplatelets and thrombocytopenia, with normal platelet function and normal platelet mass [36].

- May-Hegglin Anomaly: Rare heritable condition characterized by giant platelets and thrombocytopenia accompanied by pale blue, fusiform inclusions within neutrophils (Figure 19.8) [39].

19.3.3 Activated Platelets

19.3.3.1 Morphologic Appearance

Activated platelets lose their discoid shape, and often form thin cytoplasmic processes and tendrils (filopods). Their granules are often condensed centrally (Figure 19.9), and some activated platelets may be hypo- or agranular (see Section 19.3.4).

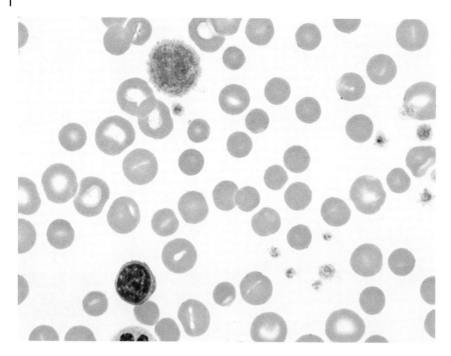

Figure 19.7 Blood smear, dog, 100× objective. A macroplatelet (top) is larger than red blood cells and even leukocytes (compare to the small lymphocyte present).

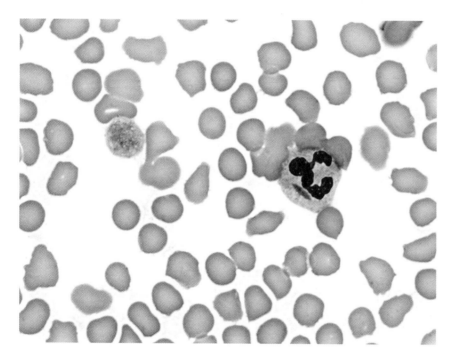

Figure 19.8 Blood smear, dog. May-Hegglin anomaly. Note the fusiform cytoplasmic inclusion in the neutrophil and the giant platelet. Slide courtesy of Dr. Bente Flatland.

19.3.3.2 Clinical Considerations

- Platelet activation often occurs *in vitro* as a consequence of blood collection.
- Activated platelets *in vivo* have been identified in cases of inflammation, immune-mediated disease, and neoplasia, and may be associated with thromboembolic disease [40–42].

19.3.4 Hypogranular Platelets

19.3.4.1 Morphologic Appearance

Hypogranular platelets appear as clear discs, devoid of granules, with a thin translucent border. They may be seen individually or in aggregates (Figure 19.10).

19.3.4.2 Clinical Considerations

- Most commonly result from activation of platelets with loss of granules.

Figure 19.9 Blood smear, cat, 100× objective. A large activated platelet is seen (center) with centrally condensed granules. Similar condensed granules and filopod formation are also seen (inset).

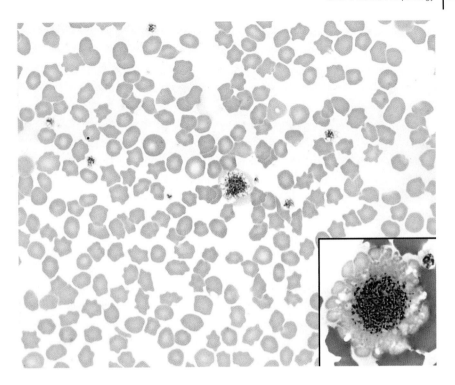

Figure 19.10 Blood smear, cat, 100× objective. Platelet aggregates with hypogranular platelets. Compare to the single well-granulated platelet (center).

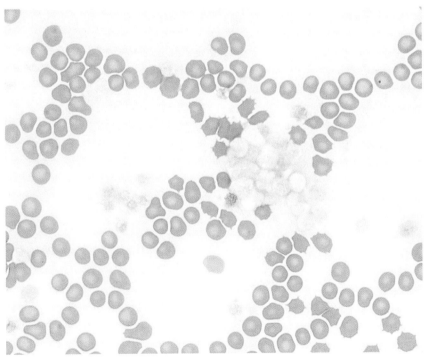

- Also rarely represent dysplastic changes associated with myeloid neoplasia [43].
- Can be difficult to see. Careful examination of the blood smear at 1000× magnification is important to avoid a false interpretation of thrombocytopenia.
- Must also not be confused with fragments of cytoplasm from other cells.

19.3.5 Vacuolated Platelets

19.3.5.1 Morphologic Appearance

Vacuolated platelets contain variably sized, punctate, clear vacuoles varying from 1 to 3 μm, often consuming most of the diameter of the platelet (Figure 19.11). A single, large vacuole may be present, giving the appearance of central pallor.

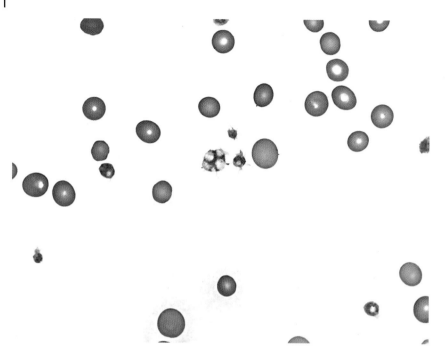

Figure 19.11 Blood smear, dog, 100× objective. Vacuolated platelets. Single and multiple vacuoles are noted in platelets in a dog with autophagic vacuoles of unknown cause. Photo courtesy of Dr. Emily Walters.

19.3.5.2 Clinical Considerations
- Reported rarely in dogs.
- May represent distension of the open canalicular system (OCS) or autophagy [44].
- Most often associated with neoplasia including acute megakaryoblastic leukemia and essential thrombocythemia [43, 45].

19.3.5.3 Prognosis
Guarded to poor. Often represent dysplastic changes associated with serious bone marrow disease; notably neoplasia in the megakaryoblast lineage.

19.4 Platelet Neoplasia

19.4.1 Primary Thrombocytosis

19.4.1.1 Morphologic Appearance
An increased number of platelets is noted, and platelets may be seen in clumps (Figure 19.12). Abnormal platelet morphology may be present, with giant platelets, variable granulation (including hypogranular platelets), and bizarre platelet shapes [46].

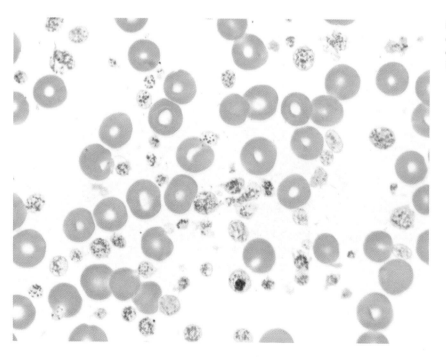

Figure 19.12 Blood smear, dog, 100× objective. Thrombocytosis (platelet concentration > 1 000 000 platelets μl^{-1}) in a dog with primary thrombocytosis.

19.4.1.2 Clinical Considerations

- Myeloproliferative disease, causing increased platelet production.
- Also called *essential thrombocythemia*.
- Often accompanied by paraneoplastic basophilia, which may be marked and resolved with therapy (Figure 19.13) [46, 47].

19.4.1.3 Prognosis

Variable, but can be good with appropriate therapy [47].

19.4.2 Acute Megakaryoblastic Leukemia

19.4.2.1 Morphologic Appearance

When present in circulation, neoplastic cells have nuclei approximately twofold to threefold the size of RBCs in diameter, with finely stippled chromatin and prominent nucleoli. They have a variable volume of mid-to-deep blue cytoplasm that may contain punctate clear vacuoles (Figures 19.14 and 19.15). Thrombocytopenia or thrombocytosis (often with 1 million+ platelets μl^{-1}) may be present. For bone marrow findings, see Chapter 5, Section 5.4.5).

Figure 19.13 Blood smear, dog, 100× objective. Primary thrombocytosis. Note the marked increase in platelets and the two basophils. Photo courtesy of Dr. Andrea Siegel.

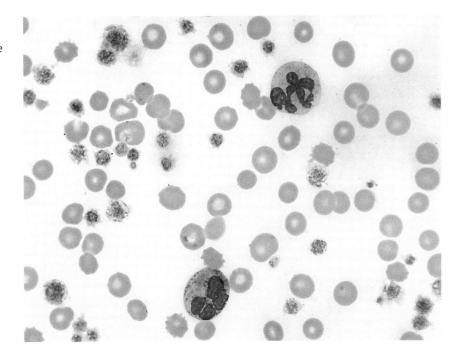

Figure 19.14 Blood smear, dog, 100× objective. Acute megakaryoblastic leukemia (AML-M7). The neoplastic cells have deep blue cytoplasm with punctate vacuoles. Note the concurrent thrombocytosis.

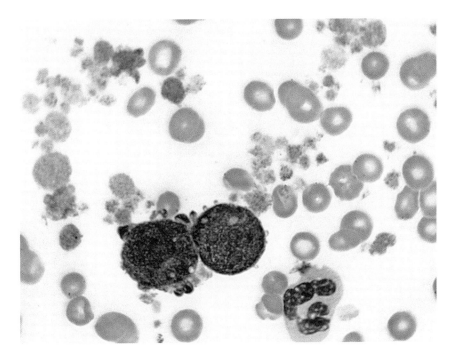

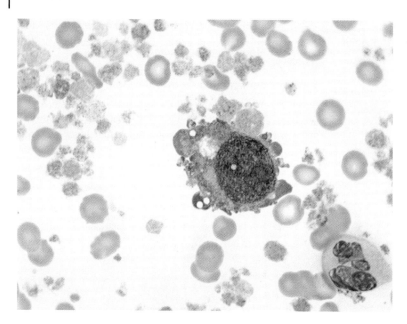

Figure 19.15 Blood smear, dog, 100× objective. Acute megakaryoblastic leukemia (AML-M7).

19.4.2.2 Clinical Considerations

- Rare subtype of acute myeloid leukemia (AML-M7 subtype).
- Dogs > cats.
- Thrombocytopenia common, but thrombocytosis reported [48, 49]. Platelet dysfunction also reported [43].
- Diagnosis based on CBC and blood morphologic changes, bone marrow evaluation ± flow cytometry with markers such as CD9 and CD61 if leukemic cells present in circulation [50].

19.4.2.3 Prognosis

Mostly grave with short survival times, though rare reports of prolonged survival with chemotherapy reported [51].

19.5 Platelet Infectious Agents

19.5.1 Anaplasma platys

19.5.1.1 Morphologic Appearance

Tightly packed, round clusters of red to basophilic bacterial organisms (morulae) may be seen within platelets (Figure 19.16). These can be difficult to differentiate from platelet granules.

Note: Evaluation of a buffy coat preparation that concentrates platelets may increase the chance of seeing morulae.

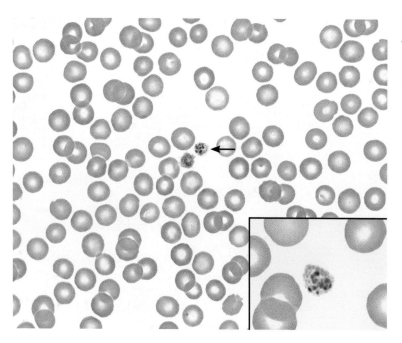

Figure 19.16 Blood smear, dog, 100× objective. *Anaplasma platys* organisms (arrow and inset) are seen within platelets. Compare these regular purple clustered organisms with the faint granulation of the normal platelet present.

19.5.1.2 Clinical Considerations

- Dogs >> cats [52].
- The only known obligate intracellular pathogen in platelets of dogs and cats [53].
- Acute infection associated with recurrent thrombocytopenia in 10–14 day cycles [14].
- Wide variation in disease severity from asymptomatic or mild, to severe.

- Clinical signs = fever, lethargy, lymphadenopathy, and signs of primary hemostatic disorder (petechiae, ecchymoses, and epistaxis).

19.5.1.3 Prognosis

Variable, but mostly good with appropriate therapy. Many dogs are asymptomatic or are subclinical carriers. May be life threatening in patients with severe diseases associated with coagulopathy.

References

1 Solbak, S., Epstein, S.E., Hopper, K. (2019) Influence of needle gauge used for venipuncture on measures of hemostasis in cats. *J. Feline Med. Surg.*, **21** (2), 143–147.

2 Weiss, D.J. (1984) Uniform evaluation and semiquantitative reporting of hematologic data in veterinary laboratories. *Vet. Clin. Pathol.* 13 (2), 27–31.

3 Norman, E.J., Barron, R.C.J., Nash, A.S., *et al.* (2001) Prevalence of low automated platelet counts in cats: comparison with prevalence of thrombocytopenia based on blood smear estimation. *Vet. Clin. Pathol.*, **30** (3), 137–140.

4 Engelmann, A.M., Veleda, P.A., Mello, C.B.E., *et al.* (2022) Amikacin prevents platelet aggregation in feline venous blood samples. *Vet. Clin. Pathol.*, **51** (1), 51–56.

5 Stokol, T., Erb, H.N. (2007) A comparison of platelet parameters in EDTA- and citrate-anticoagulated blood in dogs. *Vet. Clin. Pathol.*, **36** (2), 148–154.

6 Mylonakis, M.E., Leontides, L., Farmaki, R., *et al.* (2008) Effect of anticoagulant and storage conditions on platelet size and clumping in healthy dogs. *J. Vet. Diagn. Investig.* **20** (6), 774–779.

7 Wills, T.B., Wardrop, K.J. (2008) Pseudothrombocytopenia secondary to the effects of EDTA in a dog. *J. Am. Anim. Hosp. Assoc.*, **44** (2), 95–97.

8 Riond, B., Waßmuth, A.K., Hartnack, S., *et al.* (2015) Study on the kinetics and influence of feline platelet aggregation and deaggregation. *BMC Vet. Res.*, **11** (276), doi: 10.1186/s12917-015-0590-7. Last accessed May 8, 2023.

9 LeVine, D.N., Brooks, M.B. (2019) Immune thrombocytopenia (ITP): pathophysiology update and diagnostic dilemmas. *Vet. Clin. Pathol.*, **48**, 17–28.

10 Botsch, V., Küchenhoff, H., Hartmann, K., *et al.* (2009) Retrospective study of 871 dogs with thrombocytopenia. *Vet. Rec.*, **164** (21), 647–651.

11 Ellis, J., Bell, R., Barnes, D.C., *et al.* (2018) Prevalence and disease associations in feline thrombocytopenia: a retrospective study of 194 cases. *J. Small Anim. Pract.*, **59** (9), 531–538.

12 Musser, M. L., Curran, K.M., Flesner, B.K., *et al.* (2021) A retrospective evaluation of chemotherapy overdoses in dogs and cats. *Front. Vet. Sci.*, **8**, 718967.

13 Salyer, S.A., Lapsley, J.M., Palm, C.A., *et al.* (2022) Outcome of dogs with bone marrow suppression secondary to Sertoli cell tumor. *Vet. Comp. Oncol.*, **20** (2), 484–490.

14 Diniz, P.P.V.P., Moura de Aguiar, D. (2022) Ehrlichiosis and Anaplasmosis: an update. *Vet. Clin. North Am. Small Anim. Pract.*, **52** (6), 1225–1266.

15 Pare, A., Ellis, A., Juette, T. (2022) Clinicopathological findings of FeLV-positive cat at a secondary referral center in Florida, USA (2008-2019). *PLoS One*, **17** (4), e:0266621.

16 Grindem, C.B., Breitschwerdt, E.B., Corbett, W.T., *et al.* (1994) Thrombocytopenia associated with neoplasia in dogs. *J. Vet. Intern. Med.*, **8** (6), 400–405.

17 Goggs, R., Mastrocco, A., Brooks, M.B. (2018) Retrospective evaluation of 4 methods for outcome prediction in overt disseminated intravascular coagulation in dogs (2009-2014): 804 cases. *J. Vet. Emerg. Crit. Care*, **28** (6), 541–550.

18 Kopke, M.A., Botha, W.J. (2020) Thromboelastographic evaluation of 2 dogs with boomslang (Dispholidus typus) envenomation. *J. Vet. Emerg. Crit. Care*, **30** (6), 712–717.

19 Innerå, M. (2013) Cutaneous vasculitis in small animals. *Vet. Clin. North Am. Small Anim. Pract.*, **43** (1), 113–134.

20 Masyr, A.R., Rendahl, A.K., Winter, A.L., *et al.* (2022) Retrospective evaluation of thrombocytopenia and tumor stage as prognostic indicators in dogs with splenic hemangiosarcoma. *J. Am. Vet. Med. Assoc.*, **258** (6), 630–637.

21 Lewis, D.C., Bruyette, D.S., Kellerman, D.L., *et al.* (1997) Thrombocytopenia in dogs with anticoagulant rodenticide-induced hemorrhage: eight cases (1990-1995). *J. Am. Anim. Hosp. Assoc.*, **33** (5), 417–422.

22 Noguchi, K., Matsuzaki, T., Ojiri, Y., *et al.* (2006) Prostacyclin causes splenic dilation and haematologic changes in dogs. *Clin. Exp. Pharmacol. Physiol.*, **33** (1–2), 81–88.

23 Spangler, W.L., Kass, P.H. (1999) Splenic myeloid metaplasia, histiocytosis, and hypersplenism in the dog (65 cases). *Vet. Pathol.*, **36** (6), 583–593.

24 Makielski, K.M., Brooks, M.B., Wang, C., *et al.* (2018) Development and implementation of a novel immune

thrombocytopenia bleeding score for dogs. *J. Vet. Intern. Med.*, **32** (3), 1041–1050.

25 O'Marra, S.K., Delaforcade A.M., Shaw, S.P. (2011) Treatment and predictors of outcome in dogs with immune-mediated thrombocytopenia. *J. Am. Vet. Med. Assoc.*, **238** (3), 346–352.

26 Neel, J.A., Snyder, L., Grindem, C.B. (2012) Thrombocytosis: a retrospective study of 165 dogs. *Vet. Clin. Pathol.*, **41** (2), 216–222.

27 Woolcock, A.D., Keenan, A., Cheung, C., *et al.* (2017) Thrombocytosis in 715 dogs (2011-2015). *J. Vet. Intern. Med.*, **31** (6), 1691–1699.

28 Kaser, A., Brandacher, G., Steurer, W., *et al.* (2001) Interleukin-6 stimulates thrombopoiesis through thrombopoietin: role in inflammatory thrombopoiesis. *Blood*, **98** (9), 2720–2725.

29 Evstatiev, R., Bukaty, A., Jimenez, K., *et al.* (2014) Iron deficiency alters megakaryopoiesis and platelet phenotype independent of thrombopoietin. *Am. J. Hematol.* **89** (5), 524–529.

30 Jain, N.C., ed. (1986) Platelet disorders. *Schalm's Veterinary Hematology*, 4th ed. Philadelphia: Lea and Febiger, 469–470.

31 Phipps, W.E., de Laforcade, A.M., Barton, B.A., *et al.* (2020) Postoperative thrombocytosis and thromboelastographic evidence of hypercoagulability in dogs undergoing splenectomy for splenic masses. *J. Am. Vet. Med. Assoc.*, **256** (1), 85–92.

32 Reimann, K.A., Knowlen, G.G., Tvedten, H.W. (1989) Factitious hyperkalemia in dogs with thrombocytosis. The effect of platelets on serum potassium concentration. *J. Vet. Intern. Med.*, **3** (1), 47–52.

33 Tanaka, R., Murota, A., Nagashima, Y., *et al.* (2002) Changes in platelet lifespan in dogs with mitral valve regurgitation. *J. Vet. Intern. Med.*, **16** (4), 446–451.

34 Boudreaux, M.K., Osborne, C.D., Herre, A.C., *et al.* (2010) Unique structure of the M loop region of β-1 tubulin may contribute to size variability of platelets in the family Felidae. *Vet. Clin. Pathol.*, **39** (4), 417–423.

35 Handtke, S., Thiele, T. (2020) Large and small platelets – (when) do they differ? *J. Thromb. Haemost.* **18** (6), 1256–1267.

36 Davis, B., Toivio-Kinnucan, M., Schuller, S., *et al.* (2008) Mutation in beta 1-tubulin correlates with macrothrombocytopenia in Cavalier King Charles Spaniels. *J. Vet. Intern. Med.*, **22** (3), 540–545.

37 Gelain, M.E., Tutino, G.F., Pogliani, E., *et al.* (2010) Macrothrombocytopenia in a group of related Norfolk Terriers. *Vet. Rec.*, **167** (13), 493–494.

38 Hawakawa, S., Spangler, E.A., Christopherson, P.W., *et al.* (2016) A novel form of macrothrombocytopenia in Akita dogs. *Vet. Clin. Pathol.*, **45** (1), 103–105.

39 Flatland, B., Fry, M.M., Baek, S.J., *et al.* (2011) May-Hegglin anomaly in a dog. *Vet. Clin. Pathol.*, **40** (2), 207–214.

40 Weiss, D.J., Brazzell, J.L. (2006) Detection of activated platelets in dogs with primary immune-mediated hemolytic anemia. *J. Vet. Intern. Med.*, **20** (3), 682–686.

41 Moritz, A., Walcheck, B.K., Weiss, D.J. (2005) Evaluation of flow cytometric and automated methods for detection of activated platelets in dogs with inflammatory disease. *Am. J. Vet. Res.*, **66** (2), 325–329.

42 Phillips, C., Naskou, M.C., Spangler, E. (2022) Investigation of platelet measurands in dogs with hematologic neoplasia. *Vet. Clin. Pathol.*, **51** (2), 216–224.

43 Cain, G.R., Feldman, B.F., Kawakami, T.G., *et al.* (1986) Platelet dysplasia associated with megakaryoblastic leukemia in a dog. *J. Am. Vet. Med. Assoc.*, **188** (5), 529–530.

44 Pieczarka, E.M., Yamaguchi, M., Wellman, M.L., *et al.* (2014) Platelet vacuoles in a dog with severe nonregenerative anemia: evidence of platelet autophagy. *Vet. Clin. Pathol.*, **43** (3), 326–329.

45 Tablin, F., Jain, N.C., Mandell, C.P., *et al.* (1989) Ultrastructural analysis of platelets and megakaryocytes from a dog with probable essential thrombocythemia. *Vet. Pathol.*, **26** (4), 289–293.

46 Hopper, P.E., Mandell, C.P., Turrell, J.M., *et al.* (1989) Probable essential thrombocythemia in a dog. *J. Vet. Intern. Med.* **3** (2), 79–85.

47 Mizukoshi, T., Fujino, Y., Yasukawa, K., *et al.* (2006) Essential thrombocythemia in a dog. *J. Vet. Med. Sci.*, **68** (11), 1203–1206.

48 Comazzi, S., Gelain, M.E., Bonfanti, U., *et al.* (2010) Acute megakaryoblastic leukemia in dogs: a report of three cases and review of the literature. *J. Am. Anim. Assoc.*, **46** (5), 327–335.

49 Rochel, D., Abadie, J., Robveille, C., *et al.* (2018) Thrombocytosis and central nervous system involvement in a case of canine acute megakaryoblastic leukemia. *Vet. Clin. Pathol.*, **47** (3), 363–367.

50 Valentini, F., Tasca, S., Gavazza, A., *et al.* (2012) Use of CD9 and CD61 for the characterization of AML-M7 by flow cytometry in a dog. *Vet. Comp. Oncol.*, **10** (4), 312–318.

51 Willmann, M., Müllauer, L., Schwendenwein, I., *et al.* (2009) Chemotherapy in canine acute megakaryoblastic leukemia: a case report and review of the literature. *In Vivo*, **23** (6), 911–918.

52 Lima, M., Soares, P., Ramos, C., *et al.* (2010) Molecular detection of *Anaplasma platys* in a naturally-infected cat in Brazil. *Braz. J. Microbiol.*, **41** (2), 381–385.

53 Llanes, A., Rajeev, S. (2020) First whole genome sequence of *Anaplasma platys*, an obligate intracellular Rickettsial pathogen of dogs. *Pathogens*, **9** (4), 277.

20

Background Features and Miscellaneous Cells

20.1 Approach to Blood Smear Background Features

An important component of blood smear evaluation includes an assessment of the background of the slide. Important pathologic changes or clues for disease may be missed if only the cellular components of the slide are evaluated.

A thorough examination of background features requires active evaluation at low- and high-power objectives. Large objects (including some infectious agents, neoplastic cells, or megakaryocytes) may be missed if the slide is not reviewed at low-power objective, especially the feathered edge where they may be pushed during slide preparation. Small extracellular elements (including some infectious agents or stain precipitation) may also be missed or mis-characterized if not carefully evaluated on higher objectives.

The following sections will describe some of the more common important extracellular features and miscellaneous cells/cellular elements to be recognized on peripheral blood smears. Some of these are critical for disease diagnosis, while others may represent an incidental or clinically insignificant finding, though it is important that these are not mistaken or overlooked for pathologic changes.

20.2 Acellular Elements

20.2.1 Stain Precipitation

20.2.1.1 Morphologic Appearance
The appearance of stain precipitation varies and may present as fine, purple, granular material seen diffusely across the slide, to variably sized aggregates/clumps (Figure 20.1). It is often seen in the background of the smear, but may also overlay both erythrocytes and leukocytes and mimic inclusions or infectious agents (Figure 20.2).

20.2.1.2 Clinical Considerations
- May be present in increased amounts with old stains.
- Important to differentiate from infectious organisms or pathologic inclusions if overlying erythrocytes or leukocytes.

20.2.2 Cryoglobulin

20.2.2.1 Morphologic Appearance
Cryoglobulin appears as variably large, amorphous pools of smooth, pale blue-grey material (Figure 20.3). It is often pushed to the feathered edge of the slide.

20.2.2.2 Clinical Considerations
- Most frequently associated with neoplasia (including multiple myeloma and lymphoma) and rarely infectious disease including Leishmaniasis [1–3].
- Defined by abnormal proteins in blood that precipitate below 37°C. Ischemic lesions may therefore be present in affected patients in areas associated with cooler peripheral temperatures such as pinnae or distal extremities where proteins precipitate in the microvasculature [4].
- A white precipitate may be visible in cooled serum, which disappears with warming, as precipitation of these proteins is reversible [1].
- Cryoglobulin may be present in the absence of hyperglobulinemia (due to precipitation of proteins), highlighting the importance of noticing this finding on examination of a blood smear.

20.2.2.3 Prognosis
Guarded. Prognosis often poor, given that most cases are associated with neoplasia.

Clinical Atlas of Small Animal Cytology and Hematology, Second Edition. Andrew G. Burton.
© 2024 John Wiley & Sons, Inc. Published 2024 by John Wiley & Sons, Inc.

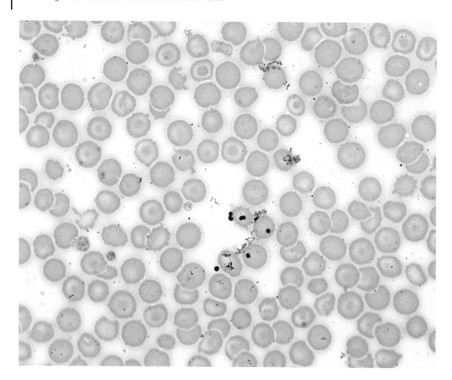

Figure 20.1 Stain precipitation, varying from fine pink to deep purple and chunky material seen in the background and on top of erythrocytes. Care is required to distinguish this from infectious agents.

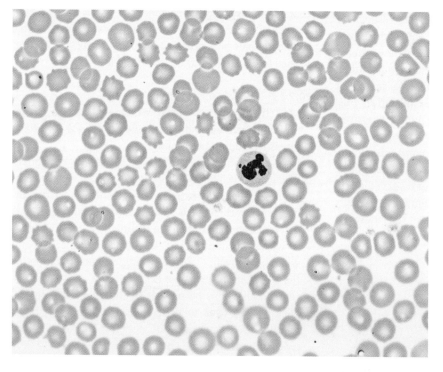

Figure 20.2 Stain precipitation. Note the amorphous green/black stain precipitation overlying the cytoplasm of the neutrophil, which could mimic inclusions including hemosiderin (sideroleukocytes; see Figure 18.19).

20.3 Miscellaneous Cells

20.3.1 Megakaryocytes

20.3.1.1 Morphologic Appearance

Megakaryocytes are large cells (ranging from 50 to more than 100 μm in diameter) with an abundant volume of pink, granular purple cytoplasm. Their nuclei are variably lobulated depending on the stage of maturation, with mature cells having numerous lobes (Figure 20.4). Megakaryocytes are most likely to be seen at the feathered edge of blood smears due to their large size.

20.3.1.2 Clinical Considerations

- Single, well-differentiated megakaryocytes are seen rarely and typically represent an incidental finding [5].

Figure 20.3 Blood smear, dog, 10× objective. Cryoglobulin. Note the large pools of smooth, pale-blue material, seen mostly at the feathered edge of the smear.

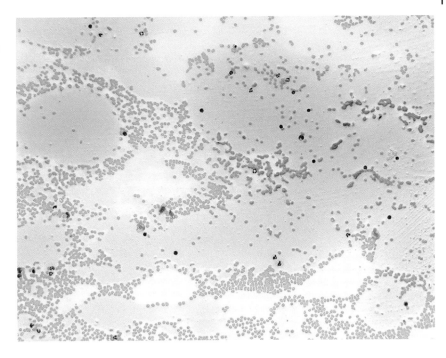

Figure 20.4 Blood smear, cat, 50× objective. A mature megakaryocyte is seen at the feathered edge of the smear. Note the large size relative to leukocytes.

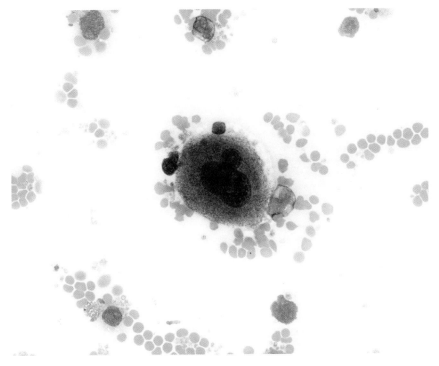

- Increased numbers of variably well-differentiated cells may indicate underlying bone marrow disease or mega-karyoblastic leukemia (see Chapter 19, Section 19.4.2).

20.3.1.3 Prognosis

Good prognosis when rare cells noted as an incidental finding. Guarded to poor prognosis if associated with bone marrow disease including leukemia.

20.3.2 Macrophages

20.3.2.1 Morphologic Appearance

Macrophages may contain phagocytosed material such as hemosiderin pigment (Figure 20.5), or infectious agents, including *Cytauxzoon felis* schizonts (see Chapter 17, Section 17.6.3).

20.3.2.2 Clinical Considerations

- Rare finding in circulation

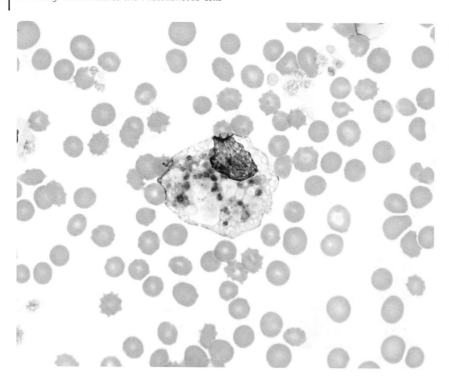

Figure 20.5 Blood smear, dog, 100× objective. Macrophage with abundant cytoplasm containing blue/brown globular hemosiderin pigment.

- May be seen in inflammatory disease states (including IMHA) and infectious diseases.
- Sampling of tissue macrophages during venipuncture can also be seen, including macrophages with hemosiderin, if resampling through a hematoma of a previous venipuncture site.

20.3.2.3 Prognosis
Variable based on underlying etiology.

20.3.3 Plasma Cells

20.3.3.1 Morphologic Appearance
Plasma cells have a moderate volume of pale- to mid-blue cytoplasm that frequently has a prominent perinuclear clearing (Golgi zone) and may have a pink coloration at the periphery of the cell (Figures 20.6 and 20.7). They have round nuclei that are often eccentrically placed and have regularly condensed chromatin with multiple, small, basophilic nucleoli.

Figure 20.6 Blood smear, dog. A plasma cell is seen at the feathered edge of the slide. Note the prominent perinuclear clearing (Golgi zone).

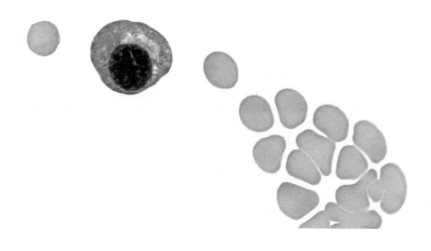

Figure 20.7 Blood smear, dog, 100× objective. Plasma cell. Note the pink coloration of the periphery of the cytoplasm (flame cell) and the eccentric nucleus.

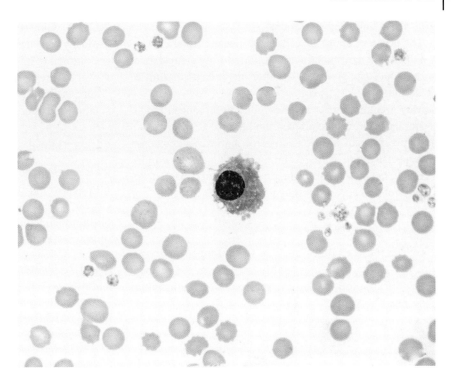

20.3.3.2 Clinical Considerations
- Rarely seen in circulation.
- Reported in patients with underlying plasma cell neoplasia [6].
- May also be present in cases of inflammatory disease.

20.3.3.3 Prognosis
Variable, based on the underlying disease process.

20.3.4 Apoptotic Cells

20.3.4.1 Morphologic Appearance
The nuclei of cells undergoing apoptosis (programmed cell death) become pyknotic and appear smaller and densely basophilic. These then undergo karyorrhexis with breakdown of the nucleus into variably sized, often perfectly round nuclear fragments (Figure 20.8).

Figure 20.8 Blood smear, dog, 100× objective. An apoptotic cell (right) undergoing karyorrhexis with dense nuclear fragments. A normal neutrophil is seen on the left.

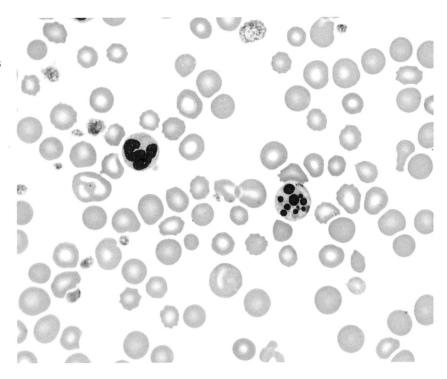

20.3.4.2 Clinical Considerations

- The origin of apoptotic cells cannot be accurately determined, but can sometimes be inferred from cytoplasmic material (e.g., granules) or other intact cells present in circulation.
- Most frequently occurs *in vitro* due to prolonged blood storage prior to slide preparation [7].
- May also occur *in vivo* in cases of marked leukocytosis (especially with acute resolution of inflammatory conditions), neoplasia (e.g., acute or chronic leukemias), or in cases of leukocyte adhesion disorder (LAD).

20.3.4.3 Prognosis

Good, if these changes are due to prolonged or inappropriate blood storage. Highly variable based on the origin of apoptotic cells, if associated with underlying disease.

20.3.5 Ruptured Cells

20.3.5.1 Morphologic Appearance

The nuclei of ruptured cells often have a characteristic appearance and are large and round, with a lacy or netted web of fine nuclear strands (Figure 20.9). These are also referred to as "basket cells."

20.3.5.2 Clinical Considerations

- Mostly considered an incidental finding.
- Common in low numbers on blood smears.
- May be present in increased numbers if excessive pressure used during slide preparation, or if fragile cell populations are present such as some neoplastic cells.

20.3.6 Mitotic Cells

20.3.6.1 Morphologic Appearance

Mitotic figures in cells in peripheral blood smears are similar to those seen in cytology samples (see Chapter 2, Section 2.5.1) and mostly reflect one of the normal stages of mitosis (Figure 20.10).

20.3.6.2 Clinical Considerations

- Rarely seen in cells in circulation and are suggestive of increased cell production/proliferation.
- May be seen with neoplastic conditions, including acute leukemias.
- May be present in non-neoplastic populations including nucleated red blood cell precursors with strong regenerative responses.

20.3.6.3 Prognosis

Variable based on the biologic behavior of the underlying cell population.

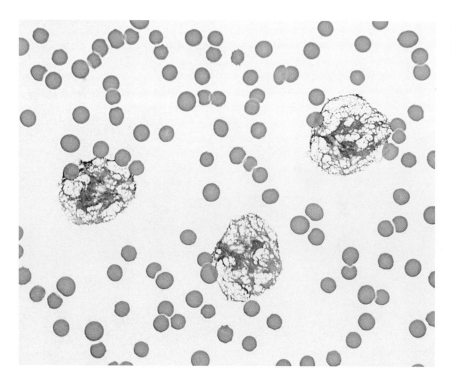

Figure 20.9 Blood smear, cat, 100× objective. Nuclei from three ruptured cells (basket cells) form round webs of lacy nuclear chromatin strands.

Figure 20.10 Blood smear, dog, 100× objective. A mitotic figure is seen (arrow) in a case of erythroleukemia in a dog.

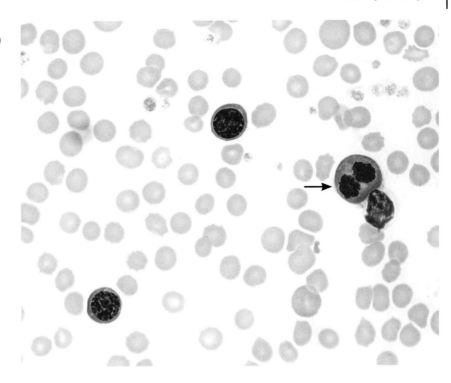

20.4 Infectious Agents

20.4.1 Microfilariae

20.4.1.1 Morphologic Appearance
Microfilariae (nematoid larvae) in the peripheral blood of dogs and cats are large, serpiginous organisms, typically ranging from 200 to 350 μm in length, and 4 to 10 μm in width. They are usually pale blue with basophilic internal organs (Figure 20.11). They are most easily seen on low-power objectives, and are frequently pushed to the feathered edge of the slide.

20.4.1.2 Clinical Considerations
- Dogs > cats.
- Most common species include *Dirofilaria immitis*, *Dirofilaria repens*, and *Acanthocheilonema reconditum*.

Figure 20.11 Blood smear, dog, 50× objective. Microfilaria (*Dirofilaria immitis*) in a dog with heartworm disease.

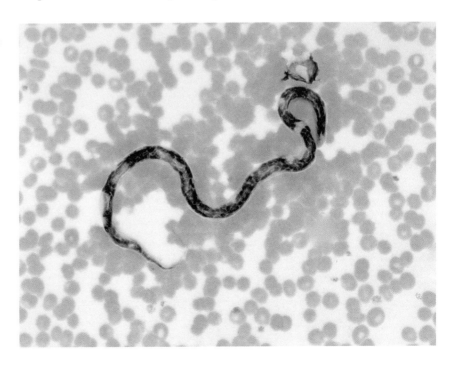

• These are difficult to distinguish morphologically on peripheral blood smears alone and are most readily distinguished based on size (length and width), head and tail shape, and movement in a Knott or modified Knott test.

20.4.1.3 Prognosis

Animals with asymptomatic or mild clinical disease associated with *D. immitis* typically have a good prognosis with appropriate therapy. Those with severe heartworm disease have a more guarded prognosis even with treatment [8, 9]. *D. repens* and *A. reconditum* are less pathogenic, mostly associated with localized skin disease [10, 11].

20.4.2 Bacteria

20.4.2.1 Morphologic Appearance

Rods and cocci: Rod and cocci bacteria may be seen in the background of blood smears, either as single or mixed populations and can have variable morphology. It is important to differentiate possible extracellular bacteria from stain precipitation (Figure 20.12).

Spirochetes: Spirochete bacteria are approximately 10–20 μm in length and have a characteristic tightly coiled and spiraled appearance (Figure 20.13). They may be seen individually or in tight mats.

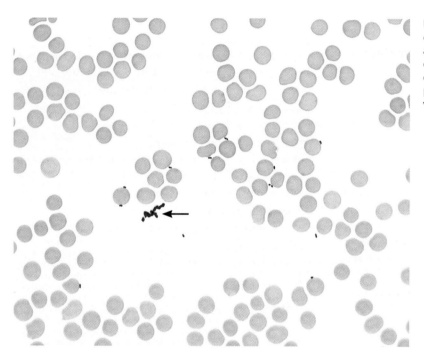

Figure 20.12 Blood smear, dog, 100× objective. Bacteremia. Small bacterial cocci are seen in the background of the smear; often attached to the surface of red blood cells. Note the small aggregate of stain precipitation (arrow), which could be confused with bacteria.

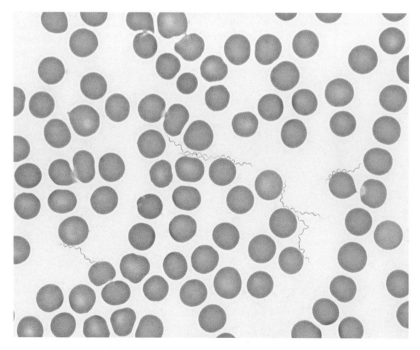

Figure 20.13 Blood smear, dog, 100× objective. Spirochete bacteria in a dog with tick-borne relapsing fever (TBRF).

20.4.2.2 Clinical Considerations
Rods and cocci

- May represent contamination of the sample (e.g., from skin during venipuncture or from contaminated stains).
- Extracellular bacteria may also represent bacteremia, especially if a monomorphic population is present. Bacteremia is frequently associated with neutrophilia, left shift and toxic changes, and clinical signs such as fever, tachycardia, bradycardia (cats), and other signs of sepsis [12].
- Bacteremia is more common in immunocompromised patients [13].
- Intracellular bacteria (especially those associated with degenerated cells) are usually indicative of true infection (see Chapter 18; Section 18.10.1).
- Mortality rates in patients with bacteremia are high [12].

Spirochetes

- Associated with tick-borne relapsing fever (TBRF).
- Dogs > cats.
- Caused by *Borrelia* spp. including *Borrelia turicatae, Borrelia hermsii,* and *Borrelia persica* [14, 15]. *Note*: *Borrelia burgdorferi* (the causative agent of lyme borreliosis) has not been observed in peripheral blood smears.
- Clinical signs = Fever, lethargy, inappetence, musculoskeletal signs (stiffness, lameness, and joint effusion), ocular disease (uveitis), and neurologic disease (ataxia and vision loss) [14, 16].
- Clinicopathologic findings = Thrombocytopenia invariably present.

20.4.2.3 Prognosis

Rods and cocci: Contamination is an incidental finding with no clinical significance, while bacteremia is associated with a guarded prognosis with high risk of sepsis and death.

Spirochetes: Most reported cases of TBRF have a good prognosis, with many making a full recovery with appropriate therapy, though rare cases succumb to their disease [16, 17].

20.4.3 Protozoa

20.4.3.1 Morphologic Appearance

Trypomastigotes of *Trypanosoma cruzi* are elongated, fusiform, and flagellated organisms approximately 10–20 μm long and 2–3 μm wide. They have clear-to pale pink cytoplasm with a delicate undulating border on one side. There is a prominent, basophilic nucleus that is mostly centrally located, and a subterminal basophilic kinetoplast posterior to the nucleus (Figure 20.14).

20.4.3.2 Clinical Considerations

- Dogs >> cats. Cats can become infected, but clinical disease is rare.
- Also known as Chagas's disease.
- *T. cruzi* the most common species.
- Trypomastigotes may be seen in peripheral blood in acute stages of disease only.
- Clinical signs = Subclinical infection common [18, 19]. Lethargy, fever, lymphadenopathy, cardiac disease (arrhythmias, myocarditis, and heart failure) [20], and neurologic disease (pelvic limb ataxia) [21].

Figure 20.14 Blood smear, dog, 100× objective. *Trypanosoma cruzi* trypomastigotes.

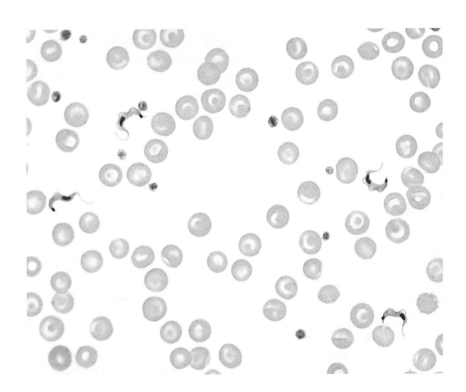

20.4.3.3 Prognosis

Many dogs have subclinical disease. Those that develop clinical signs have a guarded to poor prognosis, especially those with right heart enlargement and complex ventricular arrhythmias [22, 23]. Dogs infected at a young age appear more susceptible to severe disease and have short survival times [24].

References

1 Hickford, F.H., Stokol, T., van Gessel, Y.A., *et al.* (2000) Monoclonal immunoglobulin G cryoglobulinemia and multiple myeloma in a domestic shorthair cat. *J. Am. Vet. Med. Assoc.*, **217** (7), 1029–1033.

2 Hurvitz, A.I., MacEwen, E.G., Middaugh, C.R., *et al.* (1977) Monoclonal cryoglobulinemia with macroglobulinemia in a dog. *J. Am. Vet. Med. Assoc.*, **170** (5), 511–513.

3 Stein, L., Wertheimer, E. (1942) A new fraction of a cold-susceptible protein in blood of dogs with kala-azar. *Ann. Trop. Med. Parasitol.*, **36** (1), 17–27.

4 Nagata, M., Nanko, H., Hashimoto, K., *et al.* (1998) Cryoglobulinaemia and cryofibrinogenaemia: a comparison of canine and human cases. *Vet. Dermatol.*, **9** (4), 277–281.

5 Roszel, J., Prier, J.E., Koprowska, I. (1965) The occurrence of megakaryocytes in the peripheral blood of dogs. *J. Am. Vet. Med. Assoc.*, **147** (2), 133–137.

6 Patel, R.T., Caceres, A., French, A.F., *et al.* (2005) Multiple myeloma in 16 cats: a retrospective study. *Vet. Clin. Pathol.*, **34** (4), 341–352.

7 Houwen, B. (2002) Blood film preparation and staining procedures. *Clin. Lab. Med.*, **22** (1), 1–14.

8 Ames, M.K., Atkins, C.E. (2020) Treatment of dogs with severe heartworm disease. *Vet. Parasitol.*, **283**, 109131.

9 Maxwell, E., Ryan, K., Reynolds, C., *et al.* (2014) Outcome of a heartworm treatment protocol in dogs presenting to Louisiana State University from 2008 to 2011: 50 cases. *Vet. Parasitol.*, **206** (1–2), 71–77.

10 Albanese, F., Abramo, F., Braglia, C., *et al.* (2013) Nodular lesions due to infestation by Dirofilaria repens in dogs from Italy. *Vet. Dermatol.*, **24** (2), 255–256.

11 Brianti, E., Gaglio, G., Napoli, E., *et al.* (2012) New insights into the ecology and biology of Acanthocheilonema reconditum (Grassi, 1889) causing canine subcutaneous filariosis. *Parasitology*, **139** (4), 530–536.

12 Greiner, M., Wolf, G., Hartmann, K. (2008) A retrospective study of the clinical presentation of 140 dogs and 39 cats with bacteremia. *J. Small Anim. Pract.*, **49** (8), 378–383.

13 Saarenkari, H.K., Sharp, C.R., Smart, L. (2022) Retrospective evaluation of the utility of blood cultures in dogs (2009-2018): 45 cases. *J. Vet. Emerg. Crit. Care*, 32 (1), 141–145.

14 Piccione, J., Levine, G.J., Duff, C.A., *et al.* (2016) Tick-borne relapsing fever in dogs. *J. Vet. Intern. Med.*, **30** (4), 1222–1228.

15 Baneth, G., Dvorkin, A., Ben-Shitrit, B., *et al.* (2022) Infection and seroprevalence of *Borrelia persica* in domestic cats and dogs in Israel. *Parasit. Vectors*, **15** (1), 102.

16 Baker, K., Piccione, J. (2021) What is your diagnosis? Peripheral blood smear from a dog. *Vet. Clin. Pathol.*, **50** (2), 287–289.

17 Whitney, M.S., Schwan, T.G., Sultemeier, K.B., *et al.* (2007) Spirochetemia caused by *Borrelia turicatae* infection in 3 dogs in Texas. *Vet. Clin. Pathol.*, **36** (2), 212–216.

18 Allen, K.E., Lineberry, M.W. (2022) *Trypanosoma cruzi* and other vector-borne infections in shelter dogs in two counties of Oklahoma, United States. *Vector. Borne. Zoonotic. Dis.*, **22** (5), 273–280.

19 Elmayan, A., Weihong, T., Duhon, B., *et al.* (2019) High prevalence of Trypanosoma cruzi infection in shelter dogs from southern Louisiana, USA. *Parasit. Vectors*, **12** (1), 322.

20 Hamer, S.A., Saunders, A.B. (2022) American Chagas disease (American Trypanosomiasis) in the United States. *Vet. Clin. Small. Anim. Pract.*, **52** (6), 1267–1281.

21 Berger, S.L., Palmer, R.H., Hodges, C.C., *et al.* (1991) Neurologic manifestations of Trypanosomiasis in a dog. *J. Am. Vet. Med. Assoc.*, **198** (1), 132–134.

22 Matthews, D.J., Saunders, A.B., Meyers, A.C., *et al.* (2021) Cardiac diagnostic test results and outcomes in 44 dogs naturally infected with Trypanosoma cruzi. *J. Vet. Intern. Med.*, **35** (4), 1800–1809.

23 Malcolm, E.L., Saunders, A.B., Vitt, J.P., *et al.* (2022) Antiparasitic treatment with itraconazole and amiodarone in 2 dogs with severe, symptomatic Chagas cardiomyopathy. *J. Vet. Intern. Med.*, **36** (3), 1100–1105.

24 Meurs, K.M., Anthony, M.A., Slater, M., *et al.* (1998) Chronic Trypanosoma cruzi infection in dogs: 11 cases (1987-1996). *J. Am. Vet. Med. Assoc.*, **213** (4), 497–500.

Index

a

Abdominal fluid *see* Body
 cavity fluids
Abscess
 cutaneous 127, 128f
 leukemoid response and 477
 mammary gland 366
 pancreatic 278, 279f
 tooth root 218
Acanthocheilonema reconditum see
 Microfilariae
Acanthocytes 445f, 446, 447f
Acantholytic cells, pemphigus
 foliaceus
 132–133, 132f
Acid fast
 Cryptosporidium spp. 64, 64f
 Mycobacterium spp. 69, 70f
 Nocardia spp. 69
Acral lick granuloma 126
Actinomyces spp. 69, 71f, 126
Acute leukemia
 bone marrow 176–179, 176f–179f
 lymph node infiltration 150, 151f
 non-regenerative
  anemia and 435
 peripheral blood 461, 462f,
  500–502, 500f–503f
 spleen 160, 160f–161f
Acute lymphoid leukemia (ALL)
 bone marrow 178, 179f
 peripheral blood 500–502, 500f
Acute myeloid leukemia (AML)
 bone marrow 176–178, 176f–178f
 erythroid 160, 161f, 176, 178f,
  459, 461, 462f, 502

granulocytic/monocytic 160f,
 176, 176f–177f, 481, 492
lymph node infiltration 150, 151f
megakaryoblastic 177, 178f, 502,
 523, 523f–524f, 529
peripheral blood 461, 462f,
 500–502, 500f–503f
spleen 160, 160f–161f
Adenocarcinoma
 adrenocortical 339, 340f
 anal sac apocrine gland
  111, 112f
 ceruminous gland 412, 413f–414f
 clitoral 374, 374f
 colon 264f
 intestinal 262, 263f
 lung 317, 318f–319f
 mammary 361, 365f
 nasal 312, 314f
 neutrophilia 477
 ovarian 359, 360f
 pancreatic 274, 274f–275f
 parathyroid 335, 336f
 perianal gland 111, 111f
 prostatic 355, 355f
 renal 285, 288f
 salivary 255, 257f
 sweat gland 105, 106f
 thyroid 332, 332f–334f
Adenoma
 adrenocortical 338, 338f–339f
 bile duct 250, 251f
 ceruminous gland 412, 413f
 intestinal 262, 263f
 mammary 34f, 361, 362f–363f
 ovarian 359, 360f

pancreatic 272, 273f
parathyroid 335, 335f
perianal gland 110, 110f
salivary 255, 256f
sebaceous 105, 107f
sweat gland 105, 106f
thyroid 331, 331f
Adipocytes *see also* Lipoma
 incidental 15, 22f
Adrenal gland 338–340
 adenocarcinoma 339, 340f
 adenoma 338, 338f–339f
 extramedullary hematopoiesis
  339, 339f
 pheochromocytoma 340, 341f
Aelurostrongylus abstrusus
 65, 67f, 322
Algae 56–58
Alimentary tract *see* Intestines
Allergic disease
 basophilia 490
 cutaneous 131, 131f
 eosinophilia 488
 respiratory 324, 325f
Amastigotes, in *Leishmania* 60,
 60f, 184f
Amelanotic melanoma *see*
 Melanoma
Ammonium urate crystals *see* Urine,
 crystals
Amyloid
 liver 249, 249f
 spleen 165, 166f
Anal sac apocrine gland
  adenocarcinoma 111, 112f
Anaphase 33–34, 41f

Clinical Atlas of Small Animal Cytology and Hematology, Second Edition. Andrew G. Burton.
© 2024 John Wiley & Sons, Inc. Published 2024 by John Wiley & Sons, Inc.

Anaplasma platys   524, 524f
Anaplasma spp.   72, 72f, 221, 221f, 504, 505f, 524, 524f
Anaplastic mammary carcinoma   362, 365f
Anaplastic sarcoma with giant cells   37f, 120, 121f
Ancylostoma spp.   269, 270f
Anemia   433–435
   Immune-mediated hemolytic anemia (IMHA)   430f–431f, 437, 437f, 445f, 455f, 456f
   of inflammatory disease   435
   Iron deficiency   435, 443, 448, 451, 518
   Non-regenerative   435
   Regenerative   434–435, 439, 440f
Anestrus, vaginal cytology   367, 370f
Anisocytosis
   tissue cells   31, 34f
   red blood cells   444, 444f
Anisokaryosis   32, 36f
Anisonucleosis   32
Antinuclear antibodies (ANA)   221
Aortic body tumor   337
Apocrine gland adenocarcinoma, anal sac   111, 112f
Apoptotic cells
   peripheral blood   531–532, 531f
   tissue   14, 19f, 24, 29f
Arthritis
   immune-mediated   221, 222f
   osteoarthritis   219
   septic   219, 220f
Arthrospores, *Dermatophyte* spp.   46, 48f
Artifacts
   cell lysis   14, 18f–19f, 428f
   crystal formation   13, 16f
   formalin   14, 20f
   gel   13, 16f
   glove powder/starch crystals   13, 15f
   hemoglobin crystals   13, 17f, 427, 428f
   nuclear material   14, 18f

pollen grains   14, 20f
   stain precipitation   8, 13, 15f, 427, 427f, 460, 461f, 527, 528f
Ascites *see* Body cavity fluids
Aspergillus spp.   53, 54f, 218, 406, 415
Astrocytoma   379, 382f

b

Babesia spp.   449, 466, 467f–468f
Bacteremia   534–535, 534f
Bacteria
   abscess   127, 128f, 279f
   acid fast   69, 70f
   arthritis   219, 220f
   Borrelia spp.   534–535, 534f
   bile   252, 252f
   branching   69, 71f
   cerebrospinal fluid   391f, 395–396
   fecal flora   267, 267f–268f
   fluids   194–195, 195f, 200f
   identification of   69–75, 69f–75f
   osteomyelitis   217
   otitis externa   413, 414f–415f
   peripheral blood   534–535, 534f
   pneumonia   321–323, 323f
   prostatitis   357, 357f
   rickettsial   72, 72f, 220–221, 221f, 504, 505f, 524, 524f
   spiral   73, 74f, 267
   spirochetes   534, 534f
   spore forming   73, 73f
   vaginitis   373, 374f
Bactibilia   252, 252f
Band neutrophils   173f, 478, 479f, 483f
Bare nuclei, artifact   14, 19f
Barium, pneumonia   326, 327f
Barr body   476, 477f
Basal cell carcinoma   104, 105f
Basal cells, vaginal cytology   366, 368f
Basal cell tumor *see* Cutaneous basilar epithelial neoplasia
Basket cells   532, 532f

Basophilic stippling   456, 457f
Basophils   476f, 489–490, 490f
Bence-Jones urine protein   162, 185, 216
Benign mammary tumors   34f, 361, 362f–363f,
Benign neoplasia   30, 33f–34f
Benign prostatic hyperplasia (BPH) *see* Prostate hyperplasia
Beta islet cell tumors *see* Insulinoma
Bile duct adenoma   250, 251f
Bile duct carcinoma   250, 251f
Bile duct cystadenoma   250, 251f
Bile peritonitis
   classic   197, 197f
   white bile   197, 198f
Biliary epithelium   250, 250f
Biliary hyperplasia   250, 250f
Biliary tract   250–252
Bilirubin
   concentration in body fluids   197
   crystals *see* Urine crystals
   pigment, hepatocytes   246, 247f
Bladder   291–294
   hyperplasia   291, 292f
   papilloma/polyp   292, 293f
   transitional cell carcinoma   293, 293f
Blastocystis   63, 63f
Blastomyces dermatitidis   48, 49f
Blister cells   445f, 448, 449f
Blood
   background features   527–528
   components   430, 431f
   erythrocytes   433–468
   leukocytes   475–509
   platelets   515–525
Blood smear
   approach to evaluation   427–430
   artifacts
      of preparation   424f, 425t
      of staining   425–426, 426f
   background features   527–528
   monolayer   429, 429f
   preparation   421–423, 422f–423f
   stain precipitation   427, 427f, 527, 528f
   staining procedure   425–426

Body cavity fluids   193–208
  bile peritonitis   197–198,
      197f–198f
  blood-to-fluid glucose
      difference   195
  cell concentration in   193
  cestodiasis   65, 66f, 194
  cholesterol-to-triglyceride
      ratio   199
  chylous effusion   198–199, 198f
  classification of   193
  exudate, eosinophilic
      195–196, 196f
  exudate, high
      protein   196–197, 196f
  exudate, neutrophilic   195, 195f
  exudate, septic   194–195, 194f
  exudate, sterile   195, 195f
  feline infectious peritonitis   197
  fluid-to-serum creatinine
      ratio   200
  fluid-to-serum potassium
      ratio   200
  hemorrhagic   200, 201f
  histiocytic sarcoma   206f, 207
  lymphocyte-rich
      effusion   199, 199f
  lymphoma   205, 206f
  mast cell neoplasia   207,
      207f–208f
  mesothelial hyperplasia   200–201,
      201f–202f
  mesothelioma   202–203, 203f
  modified transudate   193
  neoplastic   202–207, 203f–208f
  pericardial   195, 196, 200, 206f,
      207, 338
  protein concentration in   193
  transudate
      low protein   193, 194f
      high protein   193
  triglyceride concentration in   199
  uroabdomen   193, 199–200, 200f
Bone
  chondrosarcoma   212–213, 214f
  fibrosarcoma   215, 216f
  hemangiosarcoma   214, 215f
  histiocytic sarcoma   216, 217f

  metastatic neoplasia
      216–217, 218f
  multilobular osteochondrosarcoma
      (MLO)   214, 215f
  multiple myeloma   216, 217f
  osteoma   211, 212f
  osteomyelitis   217–218, 218f
  osteosarcoma   211–212, 212f–213f
Bone marrow   170–187
  acute leukemia   176–179,
      176f–179f
  aplasia   185
  chronic lymphocytic leukemia
      183, 184f
  erythroid hyperplasia   180, 181f
  granulocytic/erythroid ratio
      (G/E ratio)   176
  granulocytic hyperplasia
      180, 180f
  hemophagocytic histiocytic
      sarcoma   182, 182f
  hemophagocytosis
      180–181, 181f
  histiocytic sarcoma   182, 183f
  hypoplasia   185, 187f
  inflammation/infection
      182, 183f–184f
  lymphoma   179, 179f
  metastatic disease   185, 186f
  multiple myeloma   185, 185f
  normal   170, 176, 170f–175f
Bordetella bronchiseptica   70, 71f,
      322, 324f
Borrelia spp.   534f, 535
Bowel *see* Intestines
Brain   379–386
  astrocytoma   379, 382f
  choroid plexus carcinoma
      385, 386f
  choroid plexus papilloma
      384, 385f
  encephalitis   386, 387f
  ependymoma   386, 387f
  histiocytic sarcoma   383, 385f
  lymphoma   380–381, 384f
  meningioma   379, 380f–381f
  neuroblastoma   382, 384f
  oligodendroglioma   379, 383f

  primitive neuroectodermal tumors
      (PNET)   381–382, 384f
  psammoma body, meningioma
      379, 381f
Branchial cyst   169, 169f
Bronchoalveolar lavage (BAL)
      320–327
  allergic disease   324
  bacteria   320, 322, 322f–324f
  Curschmann's spirals
      320–321, 323f
  eosinophilic
      inflammation   323–324, 325f
  foreign material   326, 327f
  goblet cells   320, 322f
  hemorrhage   326, 327f
  hyperplastic epithelium   320, 322f
  hypersensitivity   324
  infectious agents   322–323,
      323f–324f
  lymphocytic
      inflammation   326, 326f
  macrophages   325, 325f
  mononuclear inflammation
      325, 325f
  mucus   320–321, 322f–323f
  neoplasia   327, 328f
  neutrophilic
      inflammation   321, 323f
  normal epithelium   320, 321f
  oropharyngeal contamination
      320, 322f
Brucella canis   349
Brush
  sampling procedure   7
Buffy coat   430, 431f
  infectious agents   64, 504, 508
  mast cells   492

C

C cell carcinoma, thyroid
      334–335, 334f
Calcareous corpuscles   65, 66f
Calcinosis circumscripta
      129, 129f–130f
Calcinosis cutis   129, 130f
Calcium oxalate crystals *see* Urine
      crystals

Campylobacter spp.   73, 74f, 267

Candida spp.   50, 51f, 297f, 406, 415

Canine
   cutaneous mast cell neoplasia
      85–87, 85f–88f
   histiocytoma   90–91, 91f–92f
   lymphoma   143–144, 144f–146f
   sterile nodular panniculitis
      124–125, 125f

Cannibalism, cells in neoplasia
   31, 35f, 202, 203f

Capillaria plica   298, 298f

Capillaries   15, 21f, 115, 116f, 121,
   122f, 239, 240f, 285, 338f, 347,
   349f, 379, 383f

Carcinoid
   gall bladder   240
   intestine   263, 264f
   liver   239, 241f

Carcinoma *see also* Adenocarcinoma
   adrenocortical   339, 340f
   BAL/TTW   327, 328f
   basal cell   104, 105f
   bile duct   250–251, 251f
   body cavity fluids   204, 204f–205f
   choroid plexus   385, 386f,
      398, 399f
   clear cell adnexal   112, 113f
   hepatocellular   21f, 32f, 238–239,
      240f–241f
   lung   317, 318f–319f
   mammary   36f, 361–362,
      363f–365f
   Merkel cell   93–94, 95f
   metastatic
      bone   216–217, 218f
      bone marrow   185, 186f
      cutaneous   108, 109f
      liver   241, 242f
      lymph node   151, 151f
      spleen   164, 164f
      synovial fluid   222, 224f
   parathyroid   335, 336f
   perianal gland   35f, 111
   pituitary   340, 341f
   prostatic   12f, 30f, 355, 355f
   pulmonary   317, 318f–319f
   renal   285, 287f–288f

   sebaceous   107, 108f
   squamous cell   109, 110f, 315,
      315f, 317, 319f, 405, 407f
   thymic   167, 168f
   thyroid   332–333, 332f–334f
   thyroid C cell carcinoma   334, 334f
   transitional cell   36f, 289f, 293,
      293f, 296f, 355, 356f

Carcinoma *in situ*   262

Carcinomatosis   263

Carcinosarcoma, mammary
   gland   365

Carotid body tumor   336, 336f–338f

Casts, urinary *see* Urine casts

Cell count
   body cavity fluids   193
   cerebrospinal fluid   386
   synovial fluid   219

Cells, categorization   15, 24, 29–30

Cellulitis *see* Panniculitis

Central nervous system   379–401

Cerebrospinal fluid (CSF)   386–400
   blood contamination of   394
   cell concentration   386
   choroid plexus carcinoma
      398, 399f
   choroid plexus cells, incidental
      389, 389f
   eosinophilic inflammation
      391, 391f
   ependymal cells   39, 399f
   feline infectious peritonitis
      395, 396f
   granulomatous meningoencephalitis
      395, 395f
   hemorrhage   394, 394f
   histiocytic sarcoma   397, 398f
   infectious agents   391f,
      395–396, 396f
   intervertebral disc
      material   387, 388f
   lymphocytic
      inflammation   392, 392f
   lymphoma   397, 397f
   mast cell neoplasia   399, 400f
   meningitis-arteritis   390
   mononuclear inflammation
      392, 393f

   mononuclear reactivity   392, 393f
   myelin-like material   388, 389f
   neoplasia   397–400
   neutrophilic inflammation   390,
      390f–391f
   normal   386, 388f
   protein concentration   386
   septic meningitis   391f,
      395–396, 396f
   surface epithelial cells   389,
      389f–390f
   xanthochromia   394

Ceruminous gland adenocarcinoma
   412, 413f–414f

Ceruminous gland
   adenoma   412, 413f

Cestodiasis *see* Body cavity fluids

Chagas' disease *see*
   Trypanosoma cruzi

Chemodectoma   336–338
   aortic body tumor   337
   carotid body tumor   336f–338f

Chemoreceptor tumors *see*
   Chemodectoma

Chlamydia spp,
   conjunctival   409, 410f

Cholangiocarcinoma   250, 251f

Cholangiohepatitis   245, 250, 252

Cholangitis   246, 250

Cholecystitis   252, 252f

Cholestasis   246, 247f, 248

Cholesterol crystals   11, 11f, 101,
   224, 225f, 278, 279f, 290, 292

Cholesterol-to-triglyceride ratio *see*
   Body cavity fluids

Chondroid   212, 214f, 315, 367f

Chondrosarcoma
   bone   212–213, 214f
   mammary gland   362
   nasal   315, 316f

Choroid plexus carcinoma
   brain   385, 386f
   cerebrospinal fluid   398, 399f

Choroid plexus cells   389, 389f

Choroid plexus papilloma   384, 385f

Chronic lymphocytic leukemia (CLL)
   bone marrow   183–184, 184f
   liver   243

peripheral blood   498–499, 499f
    spleen   161, 161f
Chylous effusion   198–199, 198f
Ciliated epithelium
    branchial cyst   169, 169f
    respiratory   320, 321f
Clear cell adnexal carcinoma
        112, 113f
Clitoral adenocarcinoma   374, 374f
Clostridium spp.   73, 73f
Coccidioides spp.   63, 63f–64f
Coccidiosis *see Cystoisospora* spp.
Codocytes   445f, 451, 453f
Colitis   267
Collagen
    extracellular matrix   12, 13f,
    in feline gastrointestinal
        eosinophilic sclerosing
        fibroplasia   266
    in keloidal fibromas   115, 115f
    mast cell tumors   85, 85f, 86
Colloid, thyroid   331–332,
        331f–332f
Colon *see* Intestines
Conjunctiva   409–412
    Chlamydia felis   409, 410f
    inflammation   409, 410f–411f
    lymphoma   411, 412f
    mast cells   410, 411f
    Mycoplasma felis   409, 411f
    neoplasia   411–412
Copper pigment, in hepatocytes
        247–248, 248f–249f
Cornea   405–409
    bacterial keratitis   405, 407f
    chronic superficial keratitis
        408, 409f
    eosinophilic keratitis   407, 408f
    fungal keratitis   406, 408f
    hyperplasia   405, 406f
    inflammation   406f
    normal epithelium   405, 406f
    pigmentary keratitis   409, 410f
    squamous cell carcinoma
        405, 407f
Corticosteroid
    hepatopathy   235
    stress response   477

Cranial mediastinal mass
    chemodectoma   336–337
    lymphoma   168, 169f
    thymoma   167, 167f–168f
Creatinine, in body fluids   200
Crenation   422, 423f, 446
Criteria of malignancy
        31–32, 34f–39f
Crown cells   115, 117f
Cryoglobulin   527, 529f
Cryptococcus spp.   45, 46f–47f, 218,
        322, 396f
Cryptosporidium spp.   64, 64f
Crystals
    ammonium urate   300, 301f
    background artifact   13, 16f
    barium   326, 327f
    bilirubin   303, 303f
    calcium oxalate
        dihydrate   298, 299f
    calcium oxalate monohydrate
        299, 300f
    cholesterol   11, 11f, 101, 224,
        225f, 278, 279f, 290, 292
    cystine   302, 302f
    glove power   13, 15f
    hematoidin   12f, 200, 201f, 202,
        203f, 255, 257f
    hemoglobin   13, 17f, 445f,
        454–455, 456f–457
    struvite   298, 299f
    uric acid   301, 301f–302f
    urinary   298–303
CSF *see* Cerebrospinal fluid (CSF)
Curschmann's spirals   320–321, 323f
Cutaneous basilar epithelial
        neoplasia   102–103, 103f
    granular   104f
    pigmented   104f
Cutaneous lymphoma   93, 94f
Cutaneous metastatic carcinoma
        108, 109f
Cuterebra spp.   75, 76f
Cyniclomyces guttulatus
        53, 53f, 267
Cyst
    background   11, 11f
    Giardia lamblia   61, 62f

infundibular/epidermal
        101, 101f–103f
    kidney   290, 292f
    pancreas   278, 279f
    Pneumocystis spp.   50, 51f–52f
    prostate   356, 357f
    synovial   224, 225f
    thymic branchial   169, 169f
Cystadenoma, of bile duct   250, 251f
Cystine *see* Urine crystals
Cystitis *see* Urine, infection/
        inflammation
Cystoisospora spp.   272, 272f
Cytauxzoon felis
    merozoites   60, 61f, 464, 466f
    schizonts   60, 61f, 464, 466f, 508
Cytologic analysis of cells   11–43
Cytologic artifacts   13–15, 14f–20f
Cytology samples
    collection of   1–7, 2f–3f, 6f
    fine-needle aspiration   2, 3f
    needle collection   2–3, 2f–3f
    selection of cases   1
    slide preparation   3–4, 4f–5f
    staining   7–8, 7f
Cytoplasmic fragments   12, 14f

d
Dacryocytes   452, 453f
Degenerative joint disease   219, 224
Degenerative left shift   481
Degenerative neutrophils   24, 28f
Demodex spp.   75, 77f, 415, 417f
Dermatophyte spp.   46, 48f
Diatoms   57, 57f
Diestrus, vaginal cytology   373, 373f
Diff-Quik stain   7–8, 7f, 85, 88f, 90f,
        146f, 350, 425, 463f–464f,
        505f, 507, 507f
Dipylidium caninum   271, 271f
Dirofilaria spp. *see* Microfilariae
Disseminated intravascular
        coagulation (DIC)   442, 447,
        448, 517
Distemper
    conjunctiva   409
    erythrocytes   464, 464f–465f
    leukocytes   507, 507f

Döhle bodies   24, 28f, 481–483, 482f–483f

Dracunculus   67, 68f

Dry-mount fecal cytology   267–268

Dysgerminoma   358, 358f

Dystrophic mineralization   129

e

Ear mites *see Otodectes cynotis*

Ears   412–417

  ceruminous gland adenocarcinoma 412–413, 413f

  ceruminous gland adenoma   412, 413f

  otitis externa   413–415, 414f–417f

Eccentrocytes   448, 450f

Echinocytes   445f, 446, 447f

Ectoparasites   75–78

Effusions *see* Body cavity fluids

Ehrlichia spp.   72, 221, 504, 505f

Elliptocytes   451, 452f

Encephalitis   386, 387f

Endocrine tumors   331–341

Endospores

  Clostridium spp.   73, 73f

  Coccidioides spp.   49, 50f

  Prototheca spp.   56, 57f

  Rhinosporidium seeberi   58, 58f

Enteritis   267, 268f

Eosinopenia   488

Eosinophilia   488

Eosinophilic effusion   195–196, 196f

Eosinophilic granuloma   131, 131f

Eosinophilic inflammation

  body cavity fluids   195–196, 196f

  bronchoalveolar lavage   323, 325f

  cerebrospinal fluid   391, 391f

  cornea   407, 408f

  cutaneous lesions   130–131, 130f–131f

  feline gastrointestinal eosinophilic sclerosing fibroplasia   266, 266f

  lymphadenitis   142, 143f

  mast cell tumor   85, 85f

Eosinophilic keratitis   407, 408f

Eosinophilic meningoencephalomyelitis   391, 391f

Eosinophils

  gray   488, 490f

  peripheral blood   476f, 488, 489f

  tissue   24, 25f

Ependymal cells   389, 389f

Ependymoma   386, 387f

Epidermal inclusion cyst *see* Infundibular/epidermal cyst

Epithelial cells

  cerebrospinal fluid   389, 389f–390f

  identification of   29, 30f

Epithelioid macrophages   126

Epithelioma, sebaceous   107, 107f

Epitheliotropic lymphoma   93

Erythrocytes *see also* Red blood cells (RBCs)

  body cavity fluids   200, 201f

  cerebrospinal fluid   394, 394f

  hemorrhage   11, 12f

  peripheral blood *see* Red blood cells (RBCs)

  synovial fluid   223, 224f

Erythrocytosis   435–436, 435f–436f

  paraneoplastic   285, 289, 316

  primary   436f, 461

Erythroid precursors

  adrenal gland   339f

  bone marrow   170f–171f, 180, 181f

  peripheral blood   441, 441f–443f

  spleen   155, 155f

Erythroleukemia

  bone marrow   176–177, 178f

  peripheral blood   461, 462f

  spleen   160, 161f

Erythrophagocytosis

  hemophagocytic syndrome   166, 166f

  hemorrhage   11, 12f, 200, 202, 326, 327f

  histiocytic sarcoma   162, 182, 182f

Escherichia coli   252, 285, 358, 365, 373

Estrogen

  bone marrow hypoplasia   185, 478, 517

  granulosa cell tumor   359

  sertoli cell tumor   346

  serum concentration   370, 373

  in squamous metaplasia, prostate   356

Estrous cycle   366–373

  cytologic staging of   366, 370f–373f

Estrus, vaginal cytology   370, 372f

Ethylene glycol toxicity   299–300, 300f

Excitement response   477, 495, 518

Extracellular matrix

  background   12, 13f

  chondroid   212, 214f, 315, 316f, 367f

  collagen   12, 13f, 85, 85f, 86, 115, 115f

  colloid   331–332, 331f–332f

  mesenchymal cells   29–30

  osteoid   211, 212f–213f

Extramedullary hematopoiesis (EMH)

  adrenal gland   339, 339f

  spleen   155, 155f

Extramedullary plasmacytoma

  cutaneous   95, 96f–98f

  gastrointestinal   261, 261f

  nasal   311, 313f

Exudate *see* Body cavity fluids

Eyes   405–412

  conjunctiva   409–412

  cornea   405–409

f

Fatty cast, urinary   305, 307f

Fatty liver *see* Hepatic lipidosis

Fecal cytology   267–272

  bacteria   267, 267f

  bacterial overgrowth   267, 269f

  Campylobacter spp.   73, 74f, 267

  Clostridium spp.   73, 73f, 267

  Coccidia   272, 272f

  Cryptosporidium spp.   64, 64f, 267

Cyniclomyces guttulatus 53, 53f, 267
Cystoisospora spp. 272, 272f
Giardia spp. 61, 62f, 267
hookworm 269, 270f, 434f
inflammation 267, 268f
normal 267, 267f–268f
parasite ova 268–272
roundworm 268, 269f
tapeworm 271, 271f
trichomonads 62, 63f
whipworm 270–271, 270f
Feline
eosinophilic keratitis 407, 408f
gastrointestinal eosinophilic
sclerosing fibroplasia
266, 266f
hepatic lipidosis 235, 237f–238f
visceral mast cell neoplasia 89,
163–164, 164f, 207, 486f
Feline herpesvirus,
conjunctival 408–409
Feline immunodeficiency
virus (FIV)
lymphoma 144
neutropenia 478
Toxoplasma gondii 59
Feline infectious peritonitis (FIP)
cerebrospinal fluid 395, 396f
exudate 196–197, 196f, 199
Feline leukemia virus (FeLV)
acute erythroid leukemia 461
acute lymphoid leukemia 179
bone marrow hypoplasia 185
chronic myeloid leukemia
(CML) 503
Cryptosporidium spp. 64
erythroleukemia 461
Howell-Jolly bodies 459
lymphoma 144
macrocytosis 444
mediastinal lymphoma 169
nasal lymphoma 314
neutropenia 478
pseudo-Pelger-Huët 481
Feline mast cell neoplasia
cutaneous 87–89, 89f–90f
visceral 163, 164f, 486f

FeLV *see* Feline leukemia
virus (FeLV)
Fibrocartilagenous emboli
(FCE) 390
Fibroma
cutaneous 13f, 33f, 113, 114f
keloidal 115, 115f
Fibroplasia
reactive 112, 113f
reactive, in mast cell
tumors 85, 86f
Fibrosarcoma
bone 215, 216f
cutaneous 114–115, 114f
keloidal 115
mammary 362
metastatic 153f, 165f, 243f
nasal 315, 316f
Filaroides hirthi 65, 67f, 322
Fine-needle aspiration 2–3, 2f–3f
FIP *see* Feline infectious
peritonitis (FIP)
FIV *see* Feline immunodeficiency
virus (FIV)
Flame cell
blood smear 531f
identification 24, 27f
multiple myeloma 216, 217f
plasmacytoma 96, 97f, 311, 313f
reactive lymphoid
hyperplasia 139
Fluid-to-serum creatinine ratio 200
Fluid-to-serum potassium ratio 200
Fluids *see* Body cavity fluids;
Cerebrospinal fluid (CSF);
Synovial fluid
Follicular cyst *see* Infundibular/
epidermal cyst
Foreign body
cutaneous reaction 126
nasal 311
otitis externa 414–415
respiratory 325
septic peritonitis 195
sialocele and 256
Formalin artifact 8, 14, 20f
Fungal agents 45–56
Furunculosis 126

g
Gallbladder
carcinoid 240, 252, 252f
white bile and 198, 198f
Gamonts, *Hepatozoon* spp. 64, 65f,
508, 509f
Gastrinoma 276f, 277
Gastritis *see* Intestines
Gastrointestinal stromal tumor
(GIST) 265, 265f
Gastrointestinal tract *see* Intestines
Gel, artifact 13, 16f
Ghost cells 454, 455f
Giant cells
anaplastic sarcoma with giant
cells 37f, 120, 121f
macrophages, multinucleated
125f, 127f
osteoclasts 213f, 218f
osteosarcoma 211
Giant cell tumor of soft tissue *see*
Anaplastic sarcoma with
giant cells
Giardia spp. 61, 62f
Gliomas 379
Glomerular tuft 285, 286f
Glove powder crystals, artifact
13, 15f
Glucose, in body cavity fluids 195
Goblet cells 320, 322f
Gram stain
Actinomyces spp. 69
Clostridium spp. 73
Helicobacter spp. 74
Mycobacterium spp. 69
Nocardia spp. 69
Simonsiella spp. 75
Granular casts, urinary 303, 304f
Granular lymphoma
blood 501, 501f
intestinal 259, 261f
pancreas, metastatic 277f
Granulocytic/Erythroid ratio (G/E
ratio) 176
Granulocytic leukemia
acute 176, 502, 503f
bone marrow 176f–177f
chronic 477, 503, 504f

Granulocytic leukemia (*cont'd*)
  lymph node   151
  spleen   160, 160f
Granulocytic precursors
  bone marrow   170, 172f–174f, 180, 180f
  spleen   155, 155f–156f
Granuloma
  acral lick   126
  eosinophilic   131, 131f
Granulomatous inflammation
  cutaneous   126, 127f
  lymph node   143, 144f
  osteomyelitis   218, 218f
Granulomatous meningoencephalitis (GME)   395, 395f
Granulosa cell tumor   18f, 359, 359f

h

Hair follicular tumors *see* Cutaneous basilar epithelial neoplasia
Hair shaft fragments   101, 102f
Heartworm   533–534, 533f
Heinz bodies   455f, 458–459, 458f–459f
  New methylene blue   426, 459f
Helicobacter spp.   73, 74f
Helminths   65–69
Hemangioma   116–117, 118f
Hemangiopericytoma   115
Hemangiosarcoma
  bone   214, 215f
  cutaneous   118, 118f–119f
  hemorrhagic effusion with   200
  kidney   290, 291f
  mammary   362
  neutrophilia and   477
  poikilocytosis and   446–448, 451–452
  spleen   157, 157f
Hemarthrosis   223, 224f
Hematoidin crystals   11, 12f, 200, 201f, 203f, 257f
Hematopoiesis *see* Extramedullary hematopoiesis (EMH)
Hemoabdomen   158–159, 200, 201f

Hemoglobin crystals
  artifact   13, 17f, 427, 428f
  peripheral blood   445f, 454–455, 456f–457f
Hemophagocytic histiocytic sarcoma
  bone marrow   182, 182f
  spleen   162, 163f
Hemophagocytic syndrome   166, 166f
Hemorrhage
  background   11, 12f
  body cavity fluids   200, 201f
  bronchoalveolar lavage   326, 327f
  cerebrospinal fluid   394, 394f
  iatrogenic   200, 223, 394
  regenerative anemia   435, 440f
  synovial fluid   223, 224f
Hemorrhagic effusion   200, 201f
Hemosiderin
  chronic hemorrhage   11, 12f, 118f, 143f, 200, 201f, 327f, 530f
  liver   246–247, 248f
Hepatic disease *see* Liver
Hepatic lipidosis   235, 237f–238f, 245f
  poikilocytosis and   447–448, 451
Hepatitis *see* Liver, inflammation
Hepatocellular carcinoma
  high-grade   32f, 164f, 239, 241f
  well-differentiated   21f, 238–239, 240f
Hepatocytes *see* Liver
Hepatoid gland tumor *see* Perianal gland adenoma
Hepatoma   236–237, 239f
Hepatosplenic lymphoma   159, 160f
Hepatozoon spp.   64, 65f, 429, 431, 508, 509f
Herpesvirus, conjunctival   409
Histiocytic sarcoma *see also* Hemophagocytic histiocytic sarcoma
  body fluids   206f, 207
  bone   216, 217f
  bone marrow   182, 183f
  brain   383, 385f
  cerebrospinal fluid   397, 398f

criteria of malignancy   37f–39f, 42f
  cutaneous   92, 92f–93f
  lungs   318, 320f
  neutrophilia and   477
  periarticular   225, 226f
  spleen   162, 163f
  synovial fluid   222, 223f
Histiocytoma   32f, 90, 91f–92f
Histoplasma capsulatum
  feces   267
  osteomyelitis   218
  peripheral blood   508, 508f
  tissue   45, 47f
Hodgkin's-like lymphoma   149, 150f
Hookworm   269, 270f, 434f
Howell-Jolly bodies   459, 460f–461f
Hyaline cast, urine   303, 304f
Hygroma   128
Hypercalcemia
  anal sac apocrine gland adenocarcinoma   112
  clitoral adenocarcinoma   375
  leiomyoma   227
  lymphoma, large cell   144
  lymphoma, lymphoblastic   148
  lymphoma, mediastinal   168–169
  multiple myeloma   162, 185, 216
  parathyroid adenocarcinoma   335
  parathyroid adenoma   335
  renal carcinoma   285
  thymoma   167
Hyperchromasia, nuclear   32, 38f
Hyperplasia
  biliary   250, 250f
  corneal   405, 406f
  erythroid, bone marrow   180, 181f
  granulocytic, bone marrow   180, 180f
  liver, nodular   235, 238f
  lung   317, 317f
  lymph node   139, 140f–141f
  mesothelial   200, 201f–202f
  pancreas, nodular   272, 273f
  prostatic   350, 354f
  respiratory epithelial   312, 313f, 320, 322f
  spleen, nodular   154, 154f–155f

synovial 219
thyroid, adenomatous 331
transitional cell 292f,
    293–294, 295f
Hypersensitivity reaction
    basophilia, blood 490
    bronchoalveolar lavage 324
    conjunctivitis 410
    cutaneous 130, 131f
    eosinophilia, blood 488
    eosinophils in 24
Hyphae, fungal
    Aspergillus spp. 53, 54f
    Candida spp. 50, 51f
    Conidiobolus spp. 324f
    keratitis 406, 408f
    osteomyelitis 218f
    Penicillium spp. 53, 54f
    Phaeohyphomycosis 54, 55f
    Pythium insidiosum 56, 56f
Hypocellular, bone marrow
    185, 187f

i

Iatrogenic hemorrhage
    cerebrospinal fluid 394
    hemorrhagic effusion 200
    synovial fluid 223
Idiopathic
    calcinosis cutis 129
    chylous effusion 199
    eosinophilic airway disease 324
    eosinophilic granuloma 132
    eosinophilic meningoencephalitis
        391, 391f
    hypereosinophilic syndrome 488
    neutropenia 478
    pericardial effusion,
        hemorrhagic 200
    sialadenosis 255
    sialocele 256
    xanthoma 124
Immune mediated polyarthritis
    (IMPA) 125, 221, 222f
Immunoglobulins
    flame cells 24, 27f
    mott cells 24, 27f
    ragocytes 221, 222f

Immunophenotype, lymphoma *see*
    Phenotype, lymphoma
In vitro artifacts
    background crystal formation
        13, 16f
    cell lysis 14, 19f
    formalin 8, 14, 20f
    hemoglobin crystal formation
        cytology 13–14, 17f
        blood 427, 428f
    urine crystal formation 298
Infectious agents 45–78
Infiltrative lipoma *see* Lipoma
Inflammation
    bile 252
    body cavity fluids 193–196
    bone 217, 218f
    bone marrow 182–183, 183f–184f
    brain 386, 387f
    bronchoalveolar lavage 321–326,
        323f–326f
    cerebrospinal fluid 390–393,
        390f–394f
    characterization, cells 24, 25f–28f
    conjunctiva 409–410, 410f–411f
    cornea 405–409, 406f–409f
    cutaneous disorders 124–132,
        125f–132f
    ears 413–415, 414f–417f
    feces 267, 268f
    granulomatous 126, 127f
    intestine 258, 259f
    joint 219–222, 220f–222f
    kidney 285, 287f
    liver 244–246, 245f–246f
    lung 320, 321f
    lymph node 140–143, 142f–144f
    mammary gland 365, 367f
    nasal cavity 311, 312f
    pancreas 277–278, 278f–279f
    prostate 357, 357f
    pyogranulomatous 126, 127f
    salivary gland 257, 258f
    testicle 348, 350f
    urine 296, 297f
    vagina 373, 374f
Inflammatory bowel disease (IBD)
    258, 496

Inflammatory cells, identification
    24, 25f–28f
Infundibular/epidermal cyst 101,
    101f–103f
Injection site reaction 126
Insulinoma 275, 276f
Intermediate cells, vaginal
    cytology 366, 369f
Interstitial cell tumor 347, 349f
Intervertebral disc material
    387, 388f
Intestines 258–267
    adenocarcinoma 262, 263f
    adenoma 262
    carcinoid 263, 264f
    feline gastrointestinal eosinophilic
        sclerosing fibroplasia
        266, 266f
    gastrointestinal stromal tumor
        (GIST) 265, 265f
    inflammation 258, 259f
    leiomyosarcoma 265f, 266
    lymphoma, large cell 259–260,
        260f–261f
    lymphoma, small cell 258,
        259f–260f
    mast cell neoplasia 262, 262f
    plasmacytoma 261, 261f
    polyp 262, 263f
Intracellular bacteria 13, 72f, 127,
    128f, 144f, 194, 194f, 200f,
    220f–221f, 279f, 297f, 312f,
    323f, 357f, 367f, 373f–374f,
    391f, 407f, 411f, 505f–506f, 524f
Ischemia 305, 393, 487
Ischemic myelopathy *see*
    Fibrocartilagenous
    emboli (FCE)
Islet cell tumors 275
Isospora see Cystoisospora spp.

j

Joint fluid *see* Synovial fluid
Joints 219–226
    degenerative disease 219, 224
    hemarthrosis 223, 224f
    immune mediated disease
        221, 222f

Joints (*cont'd*)
  infection   219–221, 220f–221f
  inflammation   219–222,
    220f–223f
  neoplasia
    metastatic   222, 223f–224f
    primary   225, 226f
  synovial cyst   224, 225f
  systemic lupus erythematosus
    221, 223f
Juvenile cellulitis   141, 142f

k
Karyolysis   24, 28f
Karyorrhexis   24, 28f, 531, 531f
Keloidal fibroma/fibrosarcoma
  115, 115f
Keratin debris
  incidental   15, 23f
  infundibular/epidermal cysts
    101, 102f
Keratinization   109, 110f, 319f, 355,
  356f, 405, 407f
Keratinocytes   132, 132f
Keratitis   405–409
  bacterial   405, 407f
  chronic superficial   408, 409f
  eosinophilic   407, 408f
  fungal   406, 408f
  pigmentary   409, 410f
Keratocytes   448, 449f–450f
Keratohyaline granules, squamous
  papilloma   108, 109f
Kerion   47, 48f
Kidney   285–291
  carcinoma   285, 287f–288f
  cyst   290, 292f
  inflammation   285, 287f
  glomerulus   285, 286f
  lymphoma   288, 290f
  nephroblastoma   286, 289f–290f
  normal   285, 286f
  pyelonephritis   285, 287f
  sarcoma   289, 291f
  transitional cell carcinoma
    285, 289f
Kinetoplasts, in *Leishmania* spp.
  60, 60f

l
Large granular lymphoma (LGL)
  intestines   259, 261f
  pancreas   277f
  peripheral blood   501, 501f
Large intestine *see* Intestines
Larynx
  rhabdomyoma   227f
Lead toxicity   456–457, 457f
Left shift   478–481
  degenerative   481
Leiomyoma   227, 229f, 265, 294, 373
Leiomyosarcoma   30f, 228, 230f,
    265, 265f, 266, 373
Leishmania spp.   60
  amastigotes   60, 60f
  bone marrow   184f
  orchitis   349
  peripheral blood   508
Leukemia
  acute erythroid   160, 161f, 176,
    178f, 459, 461, 462f, 502
  acute granulocytic/
    monocytic   160f, 176,
    176f–177f, 481, 492, 502f
  acute lymphoid   178, 179f,
    500–502, 500f
  acute megakaryoblastic   177,
    178f, 502, 523, 523f–524f, 529
  acute myeloid   176–179,
    461–462, 500–503
  chronic lymphocytic   161,
    161f, 183, 184f, 243,
    498–499, 499f
  lymph node infiltration   150, 151f
  spleen   160, 160f–161f
Leukemoid response   477
Leukergy   475
Leukocyte adhesion deficiency
  (LAD)   477–478, 532
Leukocytes *see also* White blood
  cells (WBC)
  peripheral blood   475–509
  tissue   24, 25f–28f
Leukogram
  excitement   477, 495, 518
  inflammatory   477–481
  stress   477, 492

Leydig cells   345, 346f
Leydig cell tumor   347, 349f
Lipid, background   15, 22f
Lipid droplets, fatty cast   305, 307f
Lipidosis
  hepatic   235, 237f–238f, 245f
  poikilocytosis and   448, 451
Lipofuscin   235, 246, 247f, 487, 487f
Lipoma
  infiltrative   122
  myelolipoma   156, 156f
  subcutaneous   121, 121f–122f
Liposarcoma   115, 122, 122f–123f
Liver   235–250
  amyloid   249, 249f
  bile pigment   246, 247f
  carcinoid   239, 241f
  carcinoma   238
    high-grade   239, 241f
    well-differentiated   238, 240f
  cholangiohepatitis   245, 250, 252
  cholestasis   246, 247f
  copper pigment   247, 248f–249f
  cytoplasmic changes
    235, 237f–238f
  hemosiderin pigment   246, 248f
  hepatic lipidosis   235, 237f–238f
  hepatoma   236, 239f
  inflammation   244–246,
    245f–246f
  lipofuscin pigment   246, 247f
  lymphoma
    large cell   242, 243f–244f
    small cell   243, 244f
  metastatic disease   241, 242f–243f
  nodular hyperplasia   235, 238f
  normal   235, 236f
  nuclear inclusion   235, 236f
  steroid hepatopathy   235
  vacuolar hepatopathy   235,
    237f–238f
Lubricant gel, artifact   13, 16f
Lung   317–320
  bronchoalveolar lavage of
    320–328
  carcinoma   317, 318f–319f
  histiocytic sarcoma   318, 320f
  hyperplasia   317, 317f

infection   320, 321f

inflammation   320, 321f

parasites   65–66, 67f

squamous cell carcinoma   317, 319f

Lungworm

   Aelurostrongylus abstrusus
     65, 67f

   Filaroides hirthi   65, 67f

   Oslerus osleri   65

Lupus erythematosus (LE) cells,
   synovial fluid   221, 223f

Luteinizing hormone (LH)   370, 373

Lymph node   139–153

   eosinophilic lymphadenitis
     142, 143f

   hyperplasia   139, 140f–141f

   infectious organisms   142f,
     143, 144f

   leukemia infiltration   150, 151f

   lymphoma

     Hodgkin's-like   149, 150f

     large cell   143, 144f–146f

     lymphoblastic   148, 148f

     mott cell differentiation
      149, 149f

     small cell   145–147, 146f–147f

   metastatic disease   151, 151f–153f

   neutrophilic lymphadenitis
     140, 142f

   normal   139, 139f–140f

   reactive hyperplasia
     139, 140f–141f

   salmon poisoning disease
     143, 144f

Lymphadenitis

   eosinophilic   142, 143f

   neutrophilic   140, 142f

   septic   142f

Lymphocytes

   granular   259, 261f, 277f, 497f,
     498–499, 499f, 501, 501f

   in bone marrow   176

   in bronchoalveolar lavage   326f

   in cerebrospinal fluid   388f, 392,
     392f, 394f

   in histiocytoma   92f

   identification of   24, 26f

   lymph nodes   139

peripheral blood   495–498,
     496f–498f

reactive   495, 497f

in seminoma   348f

in synovial fluid   219

Lymphocytic inflammation

   bronchoalveolar lavage   326, 326f

   cerebrospinal fluid   388f, 392,
     392f, 394f

   intestines   258

   liver   244, 245f

   nasal cavity   311, 312f

Lymphoglandular bodies *see*
     Cytoplasmic fragments

Lymphoid leukemia *see* Leukemia

Lymphoma

   B-cell   144, 147, 149, 159, 179, 412

   bladder   294, 294f

   body cavity fluids   205, 206f

   bone marrow   179, 179f

   brain   380, 384f

   cerebrospinal fluid   397, 397f

   conjunctiva   411, 412f

   cutaneous   93, 94f–95f

   cytoplasmic fragments and   14f

   epitheliotropic   93

   hepatosplenic   159, 160f

   Hodgkin's-like   149, 150f

   intestinal   258–259, 259f–261f

   large cell   143, 144f–146f

   large granular   259, 261f, 277f,
     501, 501f

   leukemic phase   501, 501f

   liver   242–243, 243f–244f

   lymphoblastic   148, 148f

   marginal zone   159, 159f

   mediastinal   148, 168, 169f

   mott cell differentiation   149, 149f

   nasal   314, 314f

   nodal   143–149

   pancreas   277, 277f

   peripheral blood   501, 501f

   renal   288, 290f

   small cell   145–147, 146f–147f

   spleen   158–159, 158f–160f, 161

   T-cell   24, 93, 142, 144–148, 159,
     168–169, 259, 412, 488, 502

   thymic   168, 169f

Lymphoplasmacytic inflammation

   brain   386, 387f

   intestines   258, 259f

   liver   244, 245f

   nasal cavity   311, 312f

Lysis, of cells   14, 18f–19f

Lysosomal storage disease   484,
     484f–485f

m

Macrophages

   alveolar   325, 325f

   body cavity fluids   193

   cerebrospinal fluid   386, 388f

   epithelioid   126

   granulomatous inflammation
     126, 127f

   hemorrhage   201f

   identification of   24, 26f

   multinucleated   126, 127f

   peripheral blood   529, 530f

   synovial fluid   219, 219f,
     224f, 225f

   xanthoma   124, 124f

Magnesium ammonium phosphate
     crystals *see* Urine crystals,
     struvite

Malassezia spp.

   identification   51, 52f

   otitis externa   415, 416f

Malignancy, criteria of
     30–33, 34f–39f

Malignant fibrous histiocytoma *see*
     Anaplastic sarcoma with
     giant cells.

Malignant mammary tumors   36f,
     361–362, 363f–365f

Malignant melanoma   33f, 99,
     100f–101f, 153f

Mammary gland   361–366

   adenocarcinoma   361, 365f

   adenoma   361, 362f

   benign tumors   361, 362f–363f

   carcinoma   36f, 361–362,
     363f–365f

   carcinosarcoma   365

   complex tumor   364, 366f

   hyperplasia   361

Mammary gland (*cont'd*)
    inflammation 365, 367f
    mastitis 365, 367f
    metastatic 218f, 242f
    mixed tumor 364, 367f
    sarcoma 362, 366f
Marginal zone lymphoma 159, 159f
Mast cell neoplasia
    body fluid 207, 207f–208f
    bone marrow 185, 187f
    canine 31f, 85, 85f–88f
    cerebrospinal fluid 399, 400f
    collagen in 85, 85f
    cutaneous 85–90, 85f–90f
    Diff-Quik 8, 88f
    eosinophilic inflammation in
        85, 86f, 88f
    feline 87–88, 89f–90f
    fibroplasia in 85, 86f
    grading 85
    high-grade 85, 86f–88f
    intestine 262, 262f
    low-grade 85, 85f–86f
    metastatic 152, 152f, 164, 165f,
        187f, 242f
    spleen 163–164, 164f–165f
    subcutaneous 85
    visceral 163, 164f
Mast cell granules
    in leukocytes 486, 486f
Mast cells
    allergic disease 130, 131f
    in bone marrow 185
    buffy coat and 431
    conjunctivitis 410, 411f
    in eosinophilic keratitis 407
    in feline gastrointestinal
        eosinophilic sclerosing
        fibroplasia 266–267
    in hemangioma 117, 118f
    lymph nodes 152
    paraneoplastic 117, 118f,
        167, 168f
    peripheral blood 491, 491f
    staining 8, 88f
    in thymoma 167, 168f
Mastitis 365, 367f
Mastocytemia 491, 491f

Matrix *see* Extracellular matrix
May Hegglin anomaly
    487–488, 488f
Mediastinal lesions
    branchial cyst 169, 169f
    chemodectoma 336
    lymphoma 148, 168, 169f
    thymic carcinoma 167, 168f
    thymoma 167, 167f–168f
Medulloblastoma 382
Megakaryoblastic leukemia 177,
    178f, 502, 523, 523f–524f, 529
Megakaryocytes
    bone marrow 170, 176, 174f–175f
    extramedullary hematopoiesis
        156f
    identification of 174f–175f
    myelolipoma 156f
    peripheral blood 528, 529f
Melamed-Wolinska bodies 293,
    293f, 355, 356f
Melanocytoma 99, 100f
Melanoma
    amelanotic 101f
    benign 99, 100f
    malignant 33f, 99, 100f–101f
    metastatic 153f
    poorly melanotic 101f
Meningeal cells 389, 390f
Meningioma 379, 380f–381f
Meningitis
    eosinophilic 391, 391f
    mononuclear 392
    septic 390, 391f, 395, 396f
    steroid responsive meningitis-
        arteritis 390, 390f, 392–393
Meningoencephalitis
    granulomatous
        meningoencephalitis
        392, 395, 395f
    necrotizing meningoencephalitis
        392, 395
    of unknown etiology 392, 393
Merkel cell carcinoma 93, 95f
Merozoites, *Babesia* spp.
    466, 467f–468f
Merozoites, *Cytauxzoon felis*
    60, 61f, 464, 466f

Mesenchymal tissue cells
    identification of 29, 30f–31f
    origin of 29
Mesocestoides 65, 66f
Mesomycetozoea 58
Mesothelioma 34f–35f, 202,
    203f–204f
Mesothelium
    body cavity fluids 200, 201f–202f
    hyperplasia 200, 201f–202f
    identification of 15, 200–201
    neoplasia *see* Mesothelioma
    normal 15, 24f
    reactive 200, 201f–202f
Metamyelocytes
    bone marrow 173f, 180, 180f
    peripheral blood 479, 479f, 495f
Metaphase 33, 40f–41f, 43f
Metaplasia, squamous, prostate
    355, 356f
Metarubricytes
    bone marrow 171f
    peripheral blood 441, 441f–442f,
        445f, 456f, 462f
Metastatic disease
    bone 216, 218f
    bone marrow 179f, 185,
        186f–187f
    cutaneous 108, 109f
    joints 222, 223f–224f
    kidney 285
    liver 241, 242f–243f
    lungs 317
    lymph nodes 151–152, 151f–153f
    pancreas 277f
    spleen 164, 164f–165f
Metritis 373
Microfilariae 533, 533f
Microsporum spp. 47
Mineralization
    calcinosis circumscripta 129, 129f
    dystrophic 129
    identification of 12–13, 14f
    infundibular/epidermal cysts
        101, 102f
    prostatic carcinoma 355
    prostatic cyst 356, 357f
    psammoma body 379, 381f

Mites
  Demodex spp.   75, 77f, 415, 417f
  Otodectes cynotis   78, 78f,
      415, 416f
  Sarcoptes scabiei   77, 77f
Mitotic figures
  atypical/bizarre   34–35, 42f–43f
  in blood   532, 533f
  criteria of malignancy
      32–33, 40f–43f
  normal   33, 40f–42f
Modified transudate *see* Body
      cavity fluids
Monocytes   492, 492f–495f
Monocytic leukemia   150, 151f, 176,
      177f, 492, 502, 502f
Mononuclear inflammation
  bronchoalveolar lavage   325,
      325f–326f
  cerebrospinal fluid   392, 393f
  synovial fluid   219, 220f
Mononulcear reactivity
  cerebrospinal fluid   392, 393f
  synovial fluid   219, 220f
Mott cell
  identification of   24, 27f
  lymph nodes   139,
  lymphoma, differentiation in
      149, 149f
  rhinitis   312f
  Russell bodies   149f, 313f, 495, 498f
Mucin
  biliary cystadenoma   250, 251f
  bronchoalveolar lavage   321, 323f
  cholecystitis   252, 252f
  myxoma   119f
  myxosarcoma   120f
  nasal cavity   312f
  respiratory epithelium   321f–322f
  salivary gland   255,
  sialocele   255, 257f
  synovial cyst   224, 225f
  synovial fluid   219, 219f
  white bile   198f
Mucocele, salivary   255, 257f
Mucus   320–321, 323f
Multilobular osteochondrosarcoma
      (MLO)   214, 215f

Multinucleation
  criterion of malignancy   32, 37f
  crown cells   115, 117f
  giant cells   121f
  macrophages   126, 127f
  osteoclasts   213f
Multiple myeloma
  bone   216, 217f
  bone marrow   185, 185f
  spleen   162, 162f
Muscle
  skeletal muscle, normal   15, 23f
  tumors of   226–229, 227f–230f
Mycobacterium spp.
  airway   322, 325
  mastitis   365
  peripheral blood   505, 506f
  pyelonephritis   285
  pyogranulomatous
      inflammation   69f–70f, 126
  tissues   69, 69f–70f
Mycoplasma spp.
  airway   324
  conjunctiva   409, 411f
  peripheral blood   462, 462f–463f
Myelin, in cerebrospinal
      fluid   388, 389f
Myeloblasts   172f, 180, 180f,
      480, 481f
Myelocytes   173f, 480, 480f
Myelofibrosis   185
Myeloid leukemia *see* Leukemia
Myeloid/erythroid (M/E) ratio *see*
      Granulocytic/Erythroid
      (G/E) ratio
Myelolipoma   156, 156f
Myelomonocytic leukemia
  bone marrow   176, 177f
  lymph node infiltration   150, 151f
  peripheral blood   502
Myiasis   75, 76f
Myxoma   119, 119f
Myxosarcoma   120, 120f

n

Nasal cavity   311–317
  adenocarcinoma   312, 314f
  chondrosarcoma   315, 316f

epithelial hyperplasia   312, 313f
extramedullary plasmacytoma
      311, 313f
fibrosarcoma   315, 316f
infection   311, 312f
inflammation   311, 312f
lymphoma   314, 314f
squamous cell carcinoma
      315, 315f
N/C ratios   31, 36f
Necrosis   11, 12f
Necrotizing cholecystitis   197
Necrotizing meningoencephalitis
      (NME)   392, 395
Nematodes   65–67
Neoplasia *see also* specific
      tumor types
  benign   30, 34f
  criteria of malignancy   30–32
  malignant   30, 35f–39f
  mitoses in   33–34, 40f–43f
Neorickettsia helminthoeca   72, 72f,
      143, 144f
Neospora caninum   58, 59f
Nephroblastoma
  renal   286, 289f–290f
  spinal   400, 401f
Nerve sheath tumor   400, 401f
Neuroblastoma   382, 384f
Neuroendocrine tumor
  chemodectomas   336, 336f–338f
  hepatic carcinoid   239, 241f
  gastrinoma   276f, 277
  insulinoma   275, 276f
  intestinal carcinoid   263, 264f
  pancreas   275–277, 276f
  parathyroid tumors   335–336,
      335f–336f
  thyroid tumors   331–334,
      331f–334f
Neutropenia   478
Neutrophilia   477
Neutrophilic inflammation
  abscess   127, 128f
  body cavity fluids   194f, 195, 195f
  bronchoalveolar lavage   321, 323f
  cerebrospinal fluid   390, 390f–391f
  conjunctiva   409, 410f–411f

Neutrophilic inflammation (*cont'd*)
  cornea   405, 406f–407f
  feces   267, 268f
  kidney   285, 287f
  liver   245, 246f
  lymphadenitis   140, 142f
  pancreas   277–278, 278f–279f
  salivary gland   257, 258f
  semen   354f
  synovial fluid   219–221,
      220f–223f
  urine   296, 297f
Neutrophils
  bands   478, 173f, 478, 479f, 483f
  degenerative   24, 28f
  Döhle bodies   24, 28f, 481–483,
      482f–483f
  hypersegmented   478, 478f
  identification of   24, 25f
  inclusions   484–488
  karyolysis   24, 28f
  karyorrhexis   24, 28f, 531, 531f
  left shift   478–481, 479f–481f
  lysosomal storage disease   484,
      484f–485f
  normal   24, 25f, 476, 476f
  Pelger-Huët anomaly
      481, 482f
  peripheral blood   476–478, 476f
  pyknosis/pyknotic   24, 29f
  right shift   478
  toxic changes   24, 28f, 481–483,
      482f–484f, 495f
New methylene blue (NMB)
  Heinz bodies   459f
  procedure   426
  reticulocytes   438, 440f
Nocardia spp.   69
Nodular hyperplasia
  liver   235, 238f
  pancreas   272, 273f
  spleen   154, 154f–155f
Nodular panniculitis, canine
      sterile   124–125, 125f
Nose *see* Nasal cavity
Nuclear fragmentation   32, 38f
Nuclear streaming   14, 18f

Nuclear to cytoplasmic ratios (N/C
      ratios)   31, 36f
Nucleated red blood cells (nRBC)
  bone marrow   170f–171f
  peripheral blood   441, 441f–443f
Nucleoli, criteria of
      malignancy   32, 39f

o

Oligodendroglioma   379, 383f
Oncocytoma   226
Oocysts
  Cryptosporidium spp.   64, 64f
  Cystoisospora spp.   272, 272f
  Toxoplasma gondii   59
Oomycetes   56, 56f
Orchitis   348, 350f
Oropharyngeal contamination   75,
      320, 322f
Oslerus osleri   65
Osteoarthritis   219–220
Osteoblast   211, 212f, 218f
Osteoclast   213f, 218f
Osteoid   212f–213f
Osteoma   211, 212f
Osteomyelitis   217, 218f
Osteosarcoma   31f, 38f, 39f, 211,
      212f–213f, 362, 366f
Otitis externa
  bacterial   413, 414f–415f
  fungal   415, 416f
  parasitic   415, 416f–417f
Otodectes cynotis   78, 78f,
      415, 416f
Ovalocytes   451, 452f
  Ovary   358–361
  adenocarcinoma   359, 360
  adenoma   359, 360
  dysgerminoma   358, 358f
  granulosa cell tumor   18f,
      359, 359f
  teratoma   360, 361f

p

Pancreas   272–279
  abscess   278, 279f
  adenocarcinoma

poorly-differentiated
      274, 275f
  well-differentiated
      274, 274f
  adenoma   272, 273f
  beta islet cell tumor   275, 276f
  cyst   278, 279f
  gastrinoma   276f, 277
  inflammation   277–278, 278f
  insulinoma   275, 276f
  lymphoma   277, 277f
  metastatic neoplasia   277, 277f
  nodular hyperplasia   272, 273f
Pancreatitis   277–278, 278f
  exudate   195, 195f
Panniculitis   124, 125f, 126
Pannus   409, 409f
Papilloma
  bladder   292
  choroid plexus   384, 385f
  squamous   108, 109f
Pappenheimer bodies   457, 458f
Parabasal cells, vaginal
      cytology   366–367, 368f,
      370–371, 370f, 373
Paragonimus kellicotti   68, 68f
Parasites
  ectoparasites   75–78, 76f–78f,
      415, 416f
  effusions   65, 66f
  gastrointestinal   61–64, 62f–64f
  ova   268–272, 269f–272f
  respiratory   65–66, 67f
Parathyroid
      adenocarcinoma   335, 336f
Parathyroid adenoma   276, 277f
*Pearsonema plica see Capillaria
      plica*
Pelger-Huët anomaly   481, 482f
Pemphigus foliaceus   132, 132f
Penicillium spp.   53, 54f
Penis   358
Pentatrichomonas hominis   62
Perianal gland adenocarcinoma
      111, 111f
Perianal gland adenoma
      110, 110f

Pericardial effusion
  hemorrhagic   200, 201f
  idiopathic   200
  neoplastic   203–205, 206f
  reactive mesothelial
      hyperplasia   200–201, 202f
  septic   195
Perinuclear vacuolation   109, 110f,
      202f, 315, 318
Peripheral nerve sheath tumor   115
Peritonitis
  bile   197, 197f–198f
  feline infectious peritonitis
      196–197, 196f, 199
  parasitic   65, 66f
  septic   194–195, 194f
  sterile   195, 195f
Perivascular wall tumors
      115, 116f–117f
Phaeohyphomycosis   54, 55f
Phenotype, lymphoma
  B-cell   144, 147, 149, 159, 179, 412
  T-cell   24, 93, 142, 144–148, 159,
      168–169, 259, 412, 488, 502
Pheochromocytoma   340, 341f
Pigmentary keratitis   409, 410f
Pigments, hepatic   246–248,
      247f–249f
Pilomatricoma   103
Piroplasms, *Cytauxzoon felis*   60,
      61f, 464–465, 466f
Pituitary carcinoma   340, 341f
Plaque, eosinophilic   132
Plasma cells *see also* Plasmacytoma
      and Multiple myeloma
  bone marrow   176, 182, 183f
  brain   386, 387f
  flame cells   24, 27f
  identification of   24, 26f
  intestines   258, 259f
  liver   244, 245f
  lymph node   139, 140f
  mott cells   24, 27f
  nasal cavity   311, 312f
  peripheral blood   530,
      530f, 531f
  spleen   154, 155f

Plasmacytoma
  colon   261, 261f
  cutaneous   95, 96f–98f
  nasal   311, 313f
Platelets   515–525
  activated   519, 521f
  aggregates   515, 516f
  Anaplasma platys   524, 524f
  approach to evaluation   515
  clumping   515, 516f
  estimating concentration   515
  giant platelets / macroplatelets
      518, 520f
  hypogranular   520, 521f
  macrothrombocytopenia
      518–519
  neoplasia   522–524, 522f–524f
  normal   518, 519f
  pseudothrombocytopenia   515
  thrombocytopenia
      516, 516f–517f
  thrombocytosis   517, 518f
  vacuolated   521, 522f
Pleural effusion *see* Body cavity fluids
Pneumocystis spp.   50, 51f–52f
Pneumonia   320–321, 323,
      323f–324f
Poikilocytes *see* Red blood cells
      (RBCs), poikilocytes
Pollen grains   14, 20f
Polyarthritis   221, 222f–223f
Polychromatophils   171f, 426,
      438–439, 440f, 445f
Polycythemia *see* Erythrocytosis
Polyp
  bladder   292, 293f
  gastrointestinal   262, 263f
  nasal, *Rhinosporidium seeberi*   58
Polypoid cystitis   293
Potassium, in body cavity fluids   200
Primary erythrocytosis   436f, 461
Primary thrombocytosis   517,
      522–523, 522f–523f
Primitive neuroectodermal tumors
      (PNET)   381–382, 384f
Proestrus, vaginal cytology
      370, 371f

Progesterone, concentration
  estrous cycle staging
      370, 373
  granulosa cell tumor   359
Promegakaryocytes   175f
Promyelocytes
  bone marrow   172f, 180, 180f
  peripheral blood   480–481, 480f
Prophase   33, 40f
Prorubricytes
  bone marrow   170f, 180
  peripheral blood   441, 442f
Prostate   350, 354–358
  carcinoma   355, 355f
  cyst   356, 357f
  hyperplasia   350, 354, 354f
  septic prostatitis   357, 357f
  squamous metaplasia
      355–356, 356f
  transitional/urothelial cell
      carcinoma   355, 356f
Protein concentration
  body cavity fluids   193–194
  cerebrospinal fluid   386
Prototheca spp.   56, 57f
Protozoa   58–65
Psammoma bodies, meningioma
      379, 381f
Pseudohyperkalemia   518
Pseudohyphae, *Candida* spp.
      50, 51f
Pseudothrombocytopenia   515
Pulmonary *see* Lung
Pulmonary carcinoma   317,
      318f–319f
  cutaneous metastases
      108, 109f
Pyelonephritis   285, 287f
Pyknocytes   450, 451f
Pyknosis/pyknotic cells   24, 29f
Pyogranulomatous inflammation
      126, 127f
Pyometra   359, 373, 477, 478f
Pyothorax   194–195
Pythium insidiosum   56, 56f
Pyuria *see* Urine, infection/
      inflammation

r

Rabies, vaccine reaction 127f

Ragocytes 221, 222f

Ranula 256

Reactive fibrohistiocytic nodule
 124, 125f

Reactive fibroplasia 112, 113f

Reactive lymphoid hyperplasia
 139, 140f–141f

Rectal

 adenoma 262

 carcinoid, prognosis in 264

 plasmacytoma 261, 261f

 prolapse 262

 scrape 267

Rectum *see* Intestines

Red blood cells (RBCs) *see also*
  Erythrocytes

 agglutination 436, 437f

 anemia 433–435, 434f

 anisocytosis 444, 444f

 approach to evaluation 433

 artifacts 426f, 454, 456f, 460, 461f

 Babesia spp. 466, 467f–468f

 basophilic stippling 456, 457f

 Cytauxzoon felis 60, 61f,
  464–465, 466f

 Distemper 464, 464f–465f, 507f

 distribution 433–438

 erythrocytosis 435–436,
  435f–436f

 ghost cells 454, 455f

 Heinz bodies 455f, 458,
  458f–459f

  New methylene blue 426, 459f

 hemoglobin crystals 445f, 454,
  456f–457f

 Howell-Jolly bodies 459,
  460f, 461f

 hypochromatophils 443, 443f

 inclusions 456–461, 457f–461f

 infectious agents 462–467,
  462f–468f

 monolayer 422–423, 429,
  429f, 433

 morphology 438–455

 Mycoplasma spp. 462, 462f–463f

neoplasia of 461–462, 462f

normal 438, 439f

nucleated 440f, 441–442,
 441f–443f

Pappenheimer bodies
 457, 458f

poikilocytes 444–455

 acanthocytes 445f, 446, 447f

 blister cells 445f, 448, 449f

 codocytes 445f, 451, 453f

 dacryocytes 452, 453f

 eccentrocytes 448–449, 450f

 echinocytes 445f, 446, 447f

 elliptocytes 451, 452f

 ghost cells 454, 455f

 keratocytes 448, 449f–450f

 ovalocytes 451, 452f

 pyknocytes 450, 451f

 schistocytes 445f, 447,
  448f–449f

 spherocytes 444–446, 445f,
  455f–456f

 spheroechinocytes 446, 446f

 stomatocytes 453, 454f

 target cells 445f, 451, 453f

 torocytes 454, 455f

polychromatophils 171f, 426,
 438–439, 440f, 445f

reticulocytes 426, 435, 438, 440f

rouleaux 438, 438f

saline agglutination test 430,
 430f–431f

siderocytes 457, 458f

siderotic inclusions 457, 458f

Reed-Sternberg cells 149, 150f

Renal 285–291

 carcinoma 285, 287f–288f

 cyst 290, 292f

 inflammation 285, 287f

 glomerulus 285, 286f

 lymphoma 288, 290f

 nephroblastoma 286, 289f–290f

 normal 285, 286f

 pyelonephritis 285, 287f

 sarcoma 289, 291f

 transitional cell carcinoma
  285, 289f

Reproductive system

 female 358–375

 male 345–358

Respiratory tract 311–328

Reticulocytes 426, 435, 438, 440f

Reticulum 426, 440f

Rhabdomyoma 226, 227f

Rhabdomyosarcoma 227, 228f–229f

Rhinitis 311, 312f

Rhinosporidium seeberi 58, 58f

Rickettsia spp.

 identification 72, 72f

 joints 220, 221f

 lymph nodes 143, 144f

 peripheral blood 72f, 504, 505f,
  524, 524f

Ringworm *see Dermatophyte* spp.

Romanowsky stains 7–8, 7f, 425

Round cell tumors,
  classification of 29

Roundworm 268, 269f

Rubriblasts

 bone marrow 170f, 178f, 180

 peripheral blood 441, 443f, 462f

Rubricytes

 bone marrow 170f–171f,
  180, 181f

 peripheral blood 440f, 441,
  442f–443f, 462f

Russell bodies, mott cells 149f,
 313f, 495, 498f

s

Saline agglutination test 430,
 430f–431f, 436–438

Salivary gland 255–258

 adenocarcinoma 255, 257f

 adenoma 255, 256f

 inflammation 257, 258f

 mucocele 255, 257f

 normal 255, 256f

 sialocele 255, 257f

Salmon poisoning disease 72, 72f,
 143, 144f

Sample collection 1–7

 brush 7

 cytology 1–7

fine-needle aspiration 2–3, 2f–3f
impression smear 6
needle collection 2–3, 2f–3f
procedure 2–7
scrape 5–6
swab 5, 6f
techniques 2–7
Sample preparation
 blood 421–425, 422f–424f
 cytology 3–4, 4f–5f
Sample staining
 blood 425
 cytology 7–8, 7f
Sarcoma
 anaplastic sarcoma with giant
  cells 37f, 120, 121f
 chondrosarcoma 212–213, 214f,
  315, 316f, 362
 fibrosarcoma 114–115, 114f, 115,
  153f, 165f, 215, 216f, 315,
  316f, 362
 hemangiosarcoma 118,
  118f–119f, 157, 157f, 200, 214,
  215f, 290, 291f, 362, 477
 hemophagocytic histiocytic
  sarcoma 162, 163f, 182, 182f
 histiocytic sarcoma *see*
  Histiocytic sarcoma
 keloidal fibrosarcoma 115
 leiomyosarcoma 30f, 228, 230f,
  265, 265f, 266, 373
 liposarcoma 115, 122, 122f–123f
 metastatic
  liver 241, 242f–244f
  lymph node 151, 151f–153f
  spleen 164, 164f–165f
  synovial fluid 222, 223f–224f
 myxosarcoma 120, 120f
 osteosarcoma 31f, 38f, 39f, 211,
  212f–213f, 362, 366f
 renal sarcoma 289, 291f
 rhabdomyosarcoma 227,
  228f–229f
 soft tissue sarcoma 43f, 115,
  116f–117f
 synovial cell sarcoma 13f,
  225, 226f

Sarcoptes scabiei 77, 77f
Satellite nuclei 32, 37f
Schistocytes 445f, 447, 448f–449f
Schizont, *Cytauxzoon felis* 60, 61f,
 464, 466f, 508
Scrapes
 corneal 406
 deep skin 76
 rectal 267
 sampling procedure 5–6
Sebaceous adenoma 105–106, 107f
Sebaceous carcinoma 107, 108f
Sebaceous epithelioma 107, 107f
Semen analysis 350, 351f–354f
Seminoma 345, 348f
Septic
 abscess 127, 128f, 218, 278, 279f,
  366, 477
 arthritis 219, 220f
 body cavity fluids 194, 194f, 200f
 lymphadenitis 142f
 mastitis 365, 367f
 meningitis 390, 391f, 395, 396f
 pancreatic abscess 278, 279f
 prostatitis 357, 357f
 rhinitis 311, 312f
 urine 296, 297f
 vaginitis 373, 374f
Seroma 128, 128f
Sertoli cell 345, 346f
Sertoli cell tumor 345, 348f
Sialadenitis 257, 258f
Sialadenosis 255
Sialocele 255, 257f
Siderocytes 457, 458f
Siderotic inclusions 457, 458f
Simonsiella-like spp.
 identification 75, 75f
 oropharyngeal contamination
  320, 322f
Skeletal muscle, normal 15, 23f
Skin 85–133
Skin surface debris 15, 23f
Small cell lymphoma *see* Lymphoma
Small intestines *see* Intestines
Soft tissue sarcoma 43f, 115,
 116f–117f

Spermatozoa morphology 350,
 351f–354f
Spherocytes 444–446, 445f,
 455f–456f
Spheroechinocytes 446, 446f
Spherules, *Coccidioides* spp. 49, 49f
Spinal cord 400–401
 ependymoma 401
 meningioma 401
 nephroblastoma 400, 401f
 nerve sheath tumor 400, 401f
Spindle cells, identification of
 29, 30f
Spirochetes 534, 534f
Spleen 153–167
 amyloid 165, 166f
 chronic lymphocytic leukemia
  161, 161f
 extramedullary hematopoiesis
  155, 155f
 hemangiosarcoma 157, 157f
 hemophagocytic histiocytic
  sarcoma 162, 163f
 hemophagocytic syndrome
  166, 166f
 histiocytic sarcoma 162, 163f
 hyperplasia, nodular 154, 154f
 leukemia 160, 160f–161f
 lymphoma
  hepatosplenic 159, 160f
  large cell 158, 158f
  marginal zone 159, 159f
  small cell 161
 mast cell neoplasia 163, 164f
 metastatic disease 164,
  164f–165f
 multiple myeloma 162, 162f
 myelolipoma 156, 156f
 nodular hyperplasia 154, 154f
 normal 153, 154f
Sporothrix schenckii 45, 48f
Squamous cell carcinoma
 cornea 405, 407f
 cutaneous 109, 110f
 lung 317, 319f
 lymph node, metastatic 151f
 nasal 315, 315f

Squamous metaplasia, prostate 355, 356f
Squamous papilloma 108, 109f
Stain
Acid fast 64, 64f, 69, 70f
Alkaline Phosphatase (ALP) 211
artifacts 425, 426f
Diff-Quik 7–8, 7f, 425
Grocott methenamine silver (GMS) 55, 55f
handling and storage 7–8
New methylene blue (NMB) 426
precipitation 8, 15f, 427, 427f, 461, 461f, 527, 528f, 534f
procedure 7–8, 425
Prussian blue 457
Romanowsky-type 7–8, 7f
Wright Giemsa 7, 425
Starch crystals, artifact 13, 15f
Steatitis 126, 126f
Sterile nodular panniculitis 124, 125f, 126
Steroid hepatopathy 235
Steroid responsive meningitis-arteritis 390, 392–393
Stomach *see* Intestines
Stomatocytes 453, 454f
Strap cells 227
Stress leukogram 477
Struvite crystals *see* Urine crystals
Superficial cells, vaginal cytology 366–367, 369f, 370, 371f, 373
Suppurative inflammation *see* Neutrophilic inflammation
Surface epithelial cells, in cerebrospinal fluid 389, 389f–390f
Swab
sampling procedure 5, 6f
Sweat gland
adenocarcinoma 105, 106f
Sweat gland adenoma 105, 106f
Synovial cell sarcoma 13f, 225, 226f
Synovial cyst 224, 225f
Synovial fluid
cell concentration 219
degenerative joint disease 219, 224

hemarthrosis 223, 224f
immune mediated polyarthritis (IMPA) 221, 222f
inflammation 219–222, 220f–223f
metastatic neoplasia 222, 223f–224f
mononuclear inflammation 219, 220f
mononuclear reactivity 219, 220f
normal 219, 219f
ragocytes 221, 222f
rickettsial disease 220–221, 221f
septic 219–221, 220f–221f
systemic lupus erythematosus 221, 223f
Systemic lupus erythematosus (SLE) 221, 223f

t

Tachyzoites
Neospora caninum 58, 59f
Toxoplasma gondii 59, 59f, 321f
Tamm-Horsfall proteins 303
Tapeworm 271, 271f
Telophase 33–34, 42f
Teratoma 360, 361f
Testes 345–349
inflammation 348, 350f
interstitial (Leydig) cell tumor 347, 349f
normal 345, 346f–347f
orchitis 348, 350f
seminoma 345, 348f
sertoli cell tumor 345, 348f
Thoracic fluid *see* Body cavity fluids
Thrombocytopenia 516, 516f–517f
pseudothrombocytopenia 515
Thrombocytosis 517, 518f
Thymic branchial cyst 169, 169f
Thymic carcinoma 167, 168f
Thymic lymphoma 168, 169f
Thymoma 167, 167f–168f
Thyroid adenoma 331, 331f
Thyroid C cell carcinoma 334, 334f

Thyroid carcinoma 332–334, 332f–334f
Thyroid medullary carcinoma *see* Thyroid C cell carcinoma
Tick-borne relapsing fever (TBRF) 534f, 535
Tissue cells, types 24, 29
Torocytes 454, 456f
Total nucleated cell count
body cavity fluids 193
cerebrospinal fluid 386
synovial fluid 219
Total protein concentration
body cavity fluids 193
cerebrospinal fluid 386
Toxascaris leonina 268
Toxic neutrophils 24, 28f, 481–483, 482f–484f, 495f
Toxocara spp. 268, 269f
Toxoplasma gondii 59, 59f, 321f
Transitional cell carcinoma 36f
bladder 293, 293f
kidney 285, 289f
prostate 355, 356f
in urine 295, 296f
Transitional cell papilloma/polyp 292, 293f
Transitional epithelium
hyperplasia 294–295, 295f
normal 294–295, 295f
Transmissible venereal tumor (TVT) 98, 98f–99f, 152, 152f
Transtracheal wash *see* Bronchoalveolar lavage
Transudate *see* Body cavity fluids
Traumatic catheterization, urethra 296
Trichoblastoma 103, 103f
Trichoepithelioma 103, 104f
Trichomoniasis 62, 63f
Trichophyton spp. 47
Trichuris vulpis 270f, 271
Triglycerides, in chylous effusion 199
Tritrichomonas foetus 62, 63f

Trophozoites
  Giardia spp. 61, 62f
  Pneumocystis spp. 50
Trypanosoma cruzi 535, 535f
Tumors *see also* specific tumor types
  epithelial 29, 30f, 34f
  mesenchymal 29, 30f–31f, 33f
  round cell 29, 31f–32f
TVT *see* Transmissible
    venereal tumor

u

Ultrasound gel, artifact 13, 16f
Uncinaria spp. 269
Urine 294–307
  Capillaria plica 298, 298f
  hyperplastic cells 294, 295f
  infection/inflammation
      296–297, 297f
  neoplastic cells 295, 296f
  normal cells 294, 295f
Urine casts 303–307
  cellular 305, 306f
  granular 303, 304f
  hyaline 303, 304f
  fatty 305, 307f
  waxy 303, 305f
Urine crystals 298–303
  ammonium urate 300, 301f
  bilirubin 303, 303f
  calcium oxalate dihydrate
      298, 299f
  calcium oxalate
      monohydrate 299, 300f
  cystine 302, 302f
  struvite 298, 299f
  uric acid 301, 301f–302f
Uric acid crystals, urine
    301, 301f–302f
Uroabdomen 199, 200f

v

Vaccination reaction 126, 127f
Vacuolar hepatopathy 235, 237f–238f
Vagina
  inflammation 373, 374f
  neoplasia 373–374, 374f

Vaginal cytology 366–373
  anestrus 367, 370f
  cell types 366, 368f–369f
  diestrus 373, 373f
  estrous cycle staging 366–373
  estrus 370, 372f
  proestrus 370, 371f
Vaginitis 373, 374f
Venereal tumor, transmissible *see*
    Transmissible venereal
    tumor (TVT)
Virus
  canine distemper virus
      409, 464, 464f–465f, 507, 507f
  feline herpesvirus 408–409
  feline immunodeficiency virus
      (FIV) 59, 144, 478
  feline infectious peritonitis
      (FIP) 196–197, 196f, 199,
      395, 396f
  feline leukemia virus *see* Feline
      leukemia virus (FeLV) 179,
      185, 461, 503
  papilloma virus 108
  parvovirus 185, 478, 492

w

Wart *see* Squamous papilloma
Waxy casts, urinary 303, 305f
Whipworm 270, 270f
White bile peritonitis 197, 198f
White blood cells (WBCs) *see also*
    Leukocytes
  approach to evaluation 475
  bacteria 504, 506f
  bands 478, 173f, 478,
      479f, 483f
  basophils 476f, 489–490, 490f
  degenerative left shift 481
  Distemper 507, 507f
  Döhle bodies 24, 28f, 481–483,
      482f–483f
  eosinophils 488–489
    eosinopenia 488
    eosinophilia 488
    gray 488, 490f
    normal 476f, 488, 489f

  infectious agents 504–509,
      505f–509f
  left shift 478–481
  leukemoid response 477
  leukergy 475
  lymphocytes 495–498
    granular 498, 499f
    lymphocytosis 495
    lymphopenia 495
    normal 495, 496f
    reactive 495–496, 497f
  mastocytemia 491–492, 491f
  monocytes 492–495
    monocytosis 492
    normal 492, 492f–493f
    reactive 493, 494f–495f
  neoplasia 498–504
    acute lymphoid leukemia
        (ALL) 500, 500f
    acute myeloid leukemia
        (AML) 502, 502f–503f
    chronic lymphocytic leukemia
        (CLL) 498, 499f
    chronic myeloid leukemia
        (CML) 503, 504f
    leukemic phase of
        lymphoma 501, 501f
  neutrophils
    granules in cats 485, 485f
    immature 478–481,
        479f–481f
    inclusions 484–488
    lysosomal storage disease 484,
        484f–485f
    May Hegglin
        anomaly 487–488, 488f
    neutropenia 478
    neutrophilia 477
    normal 24, 25f, 476, 476f
    toxic 24, 28f, 481–483,
        482f–484f, 495f
  Pelger-Huët anomaly
      481, 482f
  Rickettsial spp. 504, 505f
  sideroleukocytes 486, 487f
  toxic changes 24, 28f, 481–483,
      482f–484f, 495f

Windrowing
    salivary gland   255
    synovial fluid   220f, 222f, 225, 226f

x
Xanthochromia, of cerebrospinal
       fluid   394
Xanthoma   124, 124f

y
Yeast

candida   50, 51f
enteric   267, 268f
malassezia   51, 52f, 415, 416f

z
Zoonoses
    Blastocystis   64
    Bordetella bronchiseptica   71
    Brucella canis   349
    Campylobacter spp.   73

Cryptosporidium spp.   64
Dermatophytes spp.   47
giardia   61
hookworms   270
Leishmania spp.   60
Mycobacterium spp.   69
roundworms   268
Sporothrix schenckii   45
tapeworms   272
Toxoplasma gondii   59